IRAN UNDER ALLIED OCCUPATION IN WORLD WAR II

The Bridge to Victory & A Land of Famine

Mohammad Gholi Majd

University Press of America,® Inc.
Lanham · Boulder · New York · Toronto · Plymouth, UK

4501 Forbes Boulevard
Suite 200
Lanham, Maryland 20706
UPA Acquisitions Department (301) 459-3366

Unit A, Whitacre Mews, 26-34 Stannary Street,
London SE11 4AB, United Kingdom

Printed in the United States of America
British Library Cataloging in Publication Information Available

Library of Congress Control Number: 2016930753
ISBN: 978-0-7618-6738-8 (clothbound : alk. paper)
eISBN: 978-0-7618-6739-5

™ The paper used in this publication meets the minimum requirements of American National Standard for Information Sciences—Permanence of Paper for Printed Library Materials, ANSI Z39.48-1992

Dedicated to the Memory of Asghar Mahlouji (1920-2014)

Contents

Chapter 1

Introduction

Having experienced occupation and famine in World War I, Iran endured a similar fate in World War II. The two World Wars thus inflicted vast suffering on the people of Iran: as shown in a previous study[1] at least 8-10 million died of starvation and disease in World War I, and, as shown in this study, another 4 million Iranians suffered the same fate in World War II. In all, 12-14 million Iranians perished in the two world wars, victims of starvation and disease. Iran's population in 1944 (12 million) was the same as 1900, an indication that nearly half a century of population growth had been wiped out due to war and famine, a catastrophe of Malthusian proportions.

Given the importance of Iran as the only year-round and the most secure supply route to Russia, and as the principal source of fuel to the Allied armies, it is difficult to see how Iran could have escaped invasion and occupation.[2] The critical importance of Iranian oil was further enhanced by the loss of the Indonesian and Burmese oil fields to Japan and the rapid German advance towards the Baku fields. Because of its oil and its function as supply route to Russia, Iran was dubbed the "Bridge to Victory."[3] Of the 17½ million tons of lend-lease supplies sent to Russia, nearly 5 million tons went via Iran, making the "Persian Corridor" the second most important in terms of tonnage. However, the Persian Corridor was strategically the most important route because of its proximity to the titanic battles being waged in southern Russia. The decisive victory at Stalingrad in 1942-43 and the subsequent ones were made possible by American aid delivered via Iran.[4]

After the occupation of the country, Great Britain and Russia commandeered nearly all of Iran's trucks and buses as well its railways, seized all the food they could lay their hands on, and brought in tens of thousands of Polish refugees from Russia, thereby creating a severe food, transport as well as a public health crisis. Prevention by Russia of grain shipment from the northern regions, especially Azerbaijan, to Tehran had created a serious bread shortage in the capital. Given the limitations of Iran's port and inland transport system, importing supplies for Iran could only be accomplished at the expense of aid to Russia. In response to Iranian pleas for help, the Allied powers had committed themselves in formal treaty and solemn declarations, including one by the three Allied heads of state, that "the minimum needs" of the Iranian people would be met. As the 1942-43 famine and typhus epidemic indicate, the Allies failed to deliver. In September 1944, moreover, citing the imperative to assist the newly liberated countries of Europe, and seizing on some flimsy excuse, the Allied powers had wiggled out of their obligation to ship wheat to Iran, the solemn Tehran Declaration by Roosevelt, Stalin and Churchill on December 1, 1943, notwithstanding. Fortunately, the approaching end of the war and the improved domestic transportation situation had rendered wheat shipments to Iran unnecessary.

Painfully aware of what had happened to them in World War I, and terrified at the specter of a similar calamity in World War II, the Iranian people had fought to avoid a repetition. The violent bread riots in Tehran and in other towns, the spreading chaos and the tribal uprisings during 1942-44 were manifestations of this struggle. Fearing a collapse of the Iranian government, and concerned for the safety of the main supply route to Russia and source of fuel for their forces, the Allied powers in the fall of 1943 had taken steps to assist Iran and had thus prevented an extension of the famine into the third year, as it had happened in World War I. Although 4 million died in the famine of 1942-43, by their resistance the Iranian people had prevented a calamity similar to that of World War I. In their struggle for survival, they had found sympathetic and helpful friends in the persons of the American Minister to Iran, Louis G. Dreyfus, Jr (1889-1973), and his wife, Grace Dreyfus.

World War II Famine in Iran

Having shed light on the Great Famine of 1917-1919 in a previous book, this study aims to complete the story by examining the causes and consequences of the Iranian famine of 1942-1943. The famine is described in the context of the political and diplomatic history of Iran during this period. The study is rooted in the belief expressed by the late economic historian, Charles Philip Issawi (1916-2000), that the best way to study the political, social and economic history of the Middle East is to examine primary documents. This study is based on US State Department archives, the records of the US Military Intelligence Division pertaining to Iran (MID-Iran), reports of the Office of Strategic Services (OSS), and the reports of several British intelligence agencies that were active in the Middle East in World War II, of which the Combined Intelligence Centre Iraq (CICI) was possibly the most prolific. The wealth of documentation in these sources has enabled me to tell the untold story of the World War II famine in Iran. The book begins with the onset of occupation in September 1941 and takes us through November 1944 when signs of improved economic conditions were visible, the famine had ended, and the typhus epidemic was receding. As the documents attest, despite the valiant efforts of the Administrator General of Finances, Arthur C. Millspaugh and his team of American assistants, real improvements had only come with the approaching end of the war. With Allied victory in sight, and having shaken off famine, Iran had immediately faced a crisis with its northern neighbor over Russian demand for an oil concession and the Azerbaijan crisis of 1945-46. These are beyond the scope of the present study and merit a separate treatment.

Other countries including India, China, and Indo-China also suffered famine in World War II. The 1942-43 Bengal famine in which 3-5 million Indians died is perhaps the best known, and certainly the most discussed in the literature. A 2010 study blames the British and Winston Churchill in particular.[5] In contrast, there is no mention in the literature of the Iranian famine which, after all, had coincided with the Bengal famine, and in which as many Iranians—4 million—had died. For instance, a highly praised 2012 book on the strategic role of food in World War II devotes much space to the Bengal and Tonkin (Indo-China) famines but does not mention Iran.[6] In the appendant index at the end of the book, there is not even an entry for "Iran" or "Persia". It contains much information on the amount of lend-lease food shipped to Russia, but no mention of the routes by which this aid was delivered. Given that the author is acquainted with the British diplomatic archives, and given the large amount of correspondence between the Foreign Office and the State Department over the food situation in Iran, most of which is given in this study, it is difficult to believe that she remained unaware of the famine in Iran. Moreover, her description of the Middle East Supply Center (MESC) in Cairo as an altruistic aid agency meeting the essential needs of the Middle East countries is vastly different from its portrayal in State Department records as an outfit ruthlessly restricting imports of food and medicine and other essential goods and working feverishly to expand the post-war British share of the Middle East trade. It is hoped that the present study will rectify some of these ommissions and commissions, and pave the way for additional research into this crucial phase of modern Iranian history.

Notes

1. Majd, Mohammad Gholi. *The Great Famine & Genocide in Iran: 1917-1919.* Lanham: University Press of America, 2013 (2nd Edition). 71-80.

2. Majd, Mohammad Gholi. *August 1941: The Anglo-Russian Occupation of Iran and Change of Shahs.* Lanham, MD: University Press of America, 2012.

3. Axelrod, Alan. *Encyclopedia of World War II, Volume 1.* New York: Facts on File, Inc., 2007. 456.

4. Motter, T.H. Vail. *United States Army in World War II: The Middle East Theater: The Persian Corridor and Aid to Russia.* Washington D.C.: Office of the Chief of Military History, Department of the Army, 1952. The following from Motter (pages 4-6) illustrates the point: "In committing munitions and equipment to the titanic defense of Stalingrad, the USSR knew that material losses could be mitigated by ever mounting quantities by future lend-lease receipts . . . How important for the Russians Anglo-American reinforcement through the Persian Corridor might prove was accurately anticipated as early as the spring of 1942 by a German study prepared for Hitler. It reads, in part, as follows: '. . . All British or American war material which reaches Russia by way of the Near East and the Caucasus is extremely disadvantageous to our land offensive. Every ton of supplies which the enemy manages to get through to the Near East means a continuous reinforcement of the enemy war potential, makes our own operations in the Caucasus more difficult, and strengthens the British position in the Near East and Egypt.' Written before El Alamein and Stalingrad extinguished the German drive for the Middle East, the document stands as eloquent tribute to the effectiveness of the political partnership of Great Britain and the United States in the Persian Corridor." As documented in this study, however, the Anglo-American "political partnership" in Iran was far from harmonious.

5. Mukerjee, Madhusree. *Churchill's Secret War: The British Empire and the Ravaging of India during World War II.* New York: Basic Books, 2010.

Another book, also published in 2010, quotes Churchill as having said on numerous occasions that famine was an excellent way to "cull the surplus population of the coloured and inferior races." The two world wars had provided Churchill an excellent opportunity to "cull the surplus population" of the Near East. Toye, Richard. *Churchill's Empire: The World that Made Him & the World He Made*. New York: Henry Holt & Company, 2010. For an excellent review of the book, where the quotation in the text is obtained, see Johann Hari, "Not His Finest Hour: The Dark Side of Winston Churchill." *The Independent*, October 28, 2010.

6. Collingham, Lizzie. *The Taste of War: World War II and the Battle for Food*. New York: The Penguin Press, 2012.

Chapter 2

Fear of Soviet Mischief in Northern Iran and the Tripartite Treaty of Alliance

The immediate task of Mohammad Ali Foroughi's post-Reza Shah Cabinet, which was presented to Majlis (Parliament) on September 21, 1941, was to get the ex-Shah safely out of the country and keep his son, Mohammad Reza, on the throne. It soon became apparent that Foroughi also had to negotiate a "treaty of alliance" with Great Britain and Russia. In a report of September 29, 1941, Dreyfus discusses the new cabinet (Dispatch 119, 891.00/1841): "Although this is an appeasement cabinet, it is not fair to brand it solely as such for several appointments are based on merit and none appears to have been made for appeasement alone."

Dreyfus next discusses the cabinet's program which resembled a "New Deal" for the Iranians:

> This program was discussed by the Majlis and approved in principle on September 23rd, after which a vote of confidence was given the cabinet. The Majlis, in discussing these reforms, is indulging in a great deal of loose talk, deputies reveling in their new found freedom of speech. This will result beyond doubt in a great amount of delay, confusion and incompetence in putting the Government's program into effect.

Anxiety about the food situation was already on the rise. Dreyfus on October 1, 1941 (Dispatch 130, 891.5017/15):

> I have the honor to inform the Department that, as one of the reforms aimed directly at aiding the peasants, the Government on September 26 increased its price for the purchase of wheat by almost one hundred percent, that is, from 650 rials a ton to 1,200 rials. In addition to the above increases, a premium of 300 rials a ton will be given for wheat sold in the current month of Mehr and 150 rials a ton for that sold in the coming month of Aban. To pay at least part of the additional costs, it was announced that the price of bread is increased by about 0.30 rials a kilogram. In explaining this increase, it was said that greater attention will be paid in the future to the quality of bread, which in the past months has been admittedly low. The Minister of Finance, to reassure the people on the important question of wheat shortage, announced by radio on September 26 that 100,000 tons of wheat have been purchased in India, of which 3,000 tons have already arrived. He urged the farmers to return to their work with the assurance that their wheat would be bought at a high price and the consumers in Tehran to have patience since their needs of 1,000 kharvars of wheat a day were being adequately supplied. It was further announced on September 27, by way of improvement in the food situation, that each purchaser will now be permitted to purchase up to six kilograms of rice instead of the former maximum of two.

Of course, the claim concerning the purchase of 100,000 tons of Indian wheat was false. Dreyfus on October 17, 1941 (Telegram 193, 891.602/112): "The Council of Ministers on October 15 abolished the monopolies on tea, sugar, cloth, automobiles and spare parts and tires and tubes." These items were extremely scarce during the war years.

Dreyfus on November 4, 1941 (Dispatch 147 and enclosure, 891.0177/3):

> I have the honor, in continuation of the Legation's despatches on reforms being put into effect in Iran, to enclose the full text of a law voted by the Majlis on October 28, 1941, by which government salaries are considerably increased as of October 23, 1941 (first of the present month of Aban) . . . There was urgent need for this legislation, for the burden on common people of low wages, high taxes and increased living costs was reaching the breaking point. The result of this combination of adverse factors was an increase in graft and bribery to

the point where many employees depended upon such outside revenue to meet their living expenses. This fact was recognized by the Government and the present law is intended to correct the evil system. The Prime Minister in a speech to the Majlis on October 23 stated that the cost of living in Iran had increased fourfold in recent years, a figure which most observers and officials believe to be too conservative.

Growing Fear of Soviet Intentions

In addition to worsening economic conditions, Iranians grew increasingly fearful of the Russians. US Ambassador Steinhardt from Moscow on September 8, 1941 (Telegram 1641, 740.0011 EW 1939/14783):

> The following Tass denial is published in today's newspapers. "German newspapers and German radio are disseminating reports that Soviet troops are allegedly organizing local Soviets in the regions of Iran which they have occupied. Tass has been authorized to deny these reports as being not in accord with the facts."

Soon after, the British had expressed anxiety. On September 23, 1941, Foreign Secretary Anthony Eden had cabled Sir Stafford Cripps, the British Ambassador in Moscow:

> When the Soviet Ambassador came to see me this afternoon I spoke to His Excellency about the position of Iranian Azerbaijan. I understood that there had been movement, especially among the Armenian minority, in favor of the separation of that province from Iran and its eventual federation with the Soviet Union. Considerable apprehension appeared to exist lest these separatist tendencies should be encouraged by the Soviet military authorities in Tabriz. It appeared that, on their first arrival, Soviet forces had armed many Armenian irregulars to keep order in Azerbaijan, but that these Armenians have since been disarmed. About first September an open air meeting had been held at Tabriz which was chiefly attended by Armenians, who demanded independence for Azerbaijan and its federation with the Soviet Union; but that the Soviet military authorities had wisely prevented a second meeting being held with the same object in view. A petition, however, had been circulated in the same sense. It seemed to me most important that no encouragement should be given to the movement for autonomy in Azerbaijan by the Soviet Government. The effect of any such action on Turkey and on the Moslem population in the other parts of Iran would be deplorable. The Ambassador replied that he felt sure that the

> Soviet authorities had no such intention. Indeed, I myself had told him that the Soviet military authorities had prevented the second meeting. I replied that though this was so, I attached so much importance to the matter that I hoped that the Ambassador would telegraph to his government reporting what I had said. M. Maisky undertook to do so.

Where Eden left off, Sir Reader Bullard, the British Minister in Tehran, took up. Dreyfus on September 26, 1941 (Telegram 167, 891.00/ 1784):

> The British Minister is much perturbed about the difficult position in which Iran has been placed by Russian occupation of the north. In telegrams to London and Moscow he has described Iran's present economic situation as very bad, cut off as it is from revenue and food and other necessary products formerly supplied by the rich northern provinces. He told me frankly that he does not see how present unsatisfactory conditions can continue much longer. In addition to remarking on the harm being done to Iran, he stated "furthermore I do not see how the British can utilize the railways and transportation facilities efficiently until conditions in Iran are restored to normal." In support of this statement he mentioned interference in connection with a recent shipment of jute by the British to Russia, in which the Soviet soldiers in the north of Iran confiscated the gasoline the trucks were carrying. Factories, he said, are closing for want of raw materials, food is short and many businesses are at a standstill. Although Russian forces entered Iran a month ago, no effort seems to have been made by them to reopen communications or establish commerce. The Minister said for example that although there are four telegraph lines to Tabriz and Russian military are using only two no one can explain why communications have not been reestablished on the other two.
>
> There appears to be no coordination between Russian civilian and military and dealings with either are a complete enigma. The British Consul at Tabriz in a series of reports shown me by the British Minister paints a very sorry picture of conditions in that area, including opening of jails, requisitioning of houses and crops, political intrigue, looting by rabble and sympathy on the part of the Russians to separatist movements. I must point out, however, that Dr. Cochrane, an American missionary doctor who was in Tabriz until a few days ago gives a much more moderate report. While admitting there was looting by Armenian and Turkish rabble at the beginning, mainly of premises of Germans and fleeing Iranians, he reports that public security on the

> whole is good and the troops well disciplined. He confirms, however, what other observers report—namely intrigue and open sympathy on the part of the Russians to aspirations of Armenians and others in separatist movements. In this regard as reported in my No. 158 the Russian Ambassador has recommended to the Iranians that elections be held and that a greater amount of local autonomy be granted.
>
> My own impressions based on investigations which are still continuing are that Russian forces are well disciplined and that public security is being adequately maintained. Iranian sources report numerous cases of looting and violence on the part of Russians at Kazvin but I have been unable to confirm them. From the political and economic angles, however, there is much to cause worry. By their political intrigue and failure to reestablish communications, and commerce, the Russians are not only doing great harm to Iran but are failing to live up to their pledge to respect the territorial integrity and independence of the country. The Iranians are willing to accept the pledged word of Great Britain referred to in the Department's No. 95 but they have serious reason to doubt the parallel promise of Russia. How little confidence the British have in the promises or intentions of their ally may be judged from the above views of the British Minister. The Department may wish to urge Russia at the Moscow Conference to cease interfering in the political life of this unfortunate country and to cooperate in or, at least, to refrain from obstructing a return to normal communications and commerce.

Next, Cripps had joined in. Steinhardt on September 27, 1941 (Telegram 1716, 891.00/1785):

> The British Ambassador in response to my inquiry told me this afternoon that he had reason to believe that the Soviet forces occupying Iran are carrying on propaganda but he was unable to give me details. He also stated that the Soviet forces now number seven divisions of which two or three are mechanized. He stated that he had suggested to London that the Soviet and British armed forces in Iran be reduced to one division each but that the suggestion had not (repeat not) been favorably received by the British military authorities.

Dreyfus on September 28, 1941 (Telegram 171, 891.00/1787):

> Foreign Minister yesterday expressed to me his great preoccupation at the present unsatisfactory political and economic position of the coun-

try. Iran, he says has willingly met every demand only to be presented with new ones. Deputies and others are asking when will the allies stop making demands and do something concrete to help Iran out of its difficulties. Since this conversation the British Minister has informed me his Government is presenting to the Iranians a draft of a treaty of alliance which will make definite guarantees and give substantial assistance. In addition Wavell is here discussing among other things the withdrawal of troops from Tehran. Telegraph service has been reestablished with almost all points in the north including Tabriz. While British indicate their desire to assist Iran and live up to their formal assurances Russian propaganda continues. A Russian newspaper printed in Persian called "thoughts of the people" is disseminating Russian propaganda. In a recent number it refers to high prices in Iran and asks when will the people stop living an impoverished life and begin to live like human beings. It prints a caricature of the former Shah, it criticizes the Foroughi Government. . . . While public security is being adequately maintained by occupying forces in the cities it is degenerating in the rural areas. There are widespread and apparently true reports of restlessness and disorder among the tribes particularly the Kurds and Lurs who have obtained arms abandoned by Iranian forces.

The deteriorating political situation is described by Dreyfus in a report of October 6, 1941 (Dispatch 136, 891.00/1843):

Although there has been no breakdown in governmental machinery and probably will not be as long as the British are standing watch, there is much confusion, inefficiency, loose talk and personal ambition. The spirits of the people have become so depressed by the Russian occupation that it is difficult for them to rally to the concerted and sustained effort necessary to solve their problems. Stories of robbery, bodily harm, extortion and requisition by Russian forces, some true, some exaggerated, and others false, form the principle topic of conversation. The most discussed case of this kind is the robbery, allegedly by Russians, of the Minister of Roads and his wife on the Shemiran road several days ago. Whether or not these stories are true is unimportant in considering this question since they are fully believed by the Iranians. The result of this has been a growing conviction that little can be accomplished in healing the nation's wounds until the Russians withdraw. The British, who were during the first days of occupation looked upon as saviors of the Iranian people from the Russian menace, are also coming in for their share of criticism, since it is generally believed they are unwilling or unable to control their Russian ally or require his withdrawal. Too, the Iranians feel impotent to solve their own problems without consulting the British oracle. As one high official expressed it, the Iranians before taking any action wait for inspiration from heaven, meaning the B.B.C. daily Persian broadcast from London.

Dreyfus on October 7, 1941, just two weeks after the formation of a new cabinet (Telegram 178, 740.0011 EW 1939/15695):

> Increasingly unfavorable public reaction to Russian occupation is causing Iranian political situation to deteriorate. This will, in my opinion, result soon in cabinet changes particularly in the dismissal of the Minister of Roads. There are persistent rumors this forenoon that Shah will either abdicate or be forced out and that a republic will be instituted. A sense of futility and impotency pervade official quarters. . . . British Minister informs me that his relations with Russian authorities continue to be difficult and enigmatic and that Iranian political and economic situation cause him worry. He has received a stiff note from Iran Government asking for withdrawal of troops from Tehran to which he will reply today verbally to effect that harsh notes of this kind serve no useful purpose particularly at this time when British relations with Russians in Iran are so difficult. A political party called Azadi or freedom now being formed offers some hope for unity and strong leadership. It includes as members several cabinet members, Hossein Ala and other influential conservative persons and in addition seems to have British blessing. Foreign Minister told me this forenoon that he takes an unfavorable view of the treaty which it seems to him to demand much and gives little. He added that the British Minister furnished him only a rough draft with paragraph 7 on economic assistance to Iran entirely missing. He is of the opinion that Iran should not sign the treaty unless troops are withdrawn from Tehran.

Eden's telegram of September 23, 1941 to Cripps, given above, was forwarded to Washington by Ambassador John Winant on October 4, 1941 (Telegram 4724, 891.00/1792):

> Secret and personal for the Secretary and Under Secretary. I communicated with Mr. Eden at once. I have followed the situation in all its details and know for a fact that Mr. Eden has considered Russian interference in Iran internal affairs or efforts towards separatist movements by them as harmful and unwarranted. He told me some time ago that he had taken up this situation with the Soviet Ambassador and has

pressed the matter since. He has also pointed out to the Russian Ambassador that political activity on the part of his country in Iran will inevitably have harmful effects in Turkey. It is his intention to continue "his endeavors to implement the assurances that His Majesty's Government and the Soviet Government have given to respect the political independence and territorial integrity of Iran." He asked me to tell you that he is deeply grateful for your interest in the matter. Mr. Eden suggests that you might instruct me to take up with Mr. Maisky the interest of our Government in supporting the political independence and territorial integrity of Iran. This might enable us to coordinate our efforts with greater precision.

Cable to Winant on October 8, 1941 (Telegram 4298, 891.00/1792):

Your 4724, October 4, 8 p.m. In accordance with Mr. Eden's suggestion, you may discuss with the Soviet Ambassador the interest of this Government in the preservation of the political independence and territorial integrity of Iran, explaining the attitude of this Government as set forth in the Department's 4218, October 3, 11 p.m. You should thank Mr. Eden for his helpfulness, state that you are complying with his suggestion that you discuss the matter with the Soviet Ambassador, and inform him that our Embassy at Moscow has been instructed to take the matter up directly with the Soviet authorities. For your information there is repeated the following telegram which has been sent to Moscow by the Department.

The telegram repeated to Moscow is dated October 8, 1941, and reads:

Triple priority. Subsequent to the Department's 1078, September 25, 7 p.m., the Legation at Tehran has submitted to the Department further telegraphic reports, substantiated by information supplied by the British Minister to Iran, that the Russians in the occupied zones are engaging in political intrigue, dissemination of Soviet propaganda, and displaying open sympathy toward Armenian and other separatist movements. Russian Government support of this activity has been indicated by the recent suggestion by the Russian Ambassador in Tehran to the Iranian Government that special elections should be held and a greater degree of autonomy granted to certain areas in Iran. Mr. Eden has taken up this matter with Mr. Maisky in London, pointing out that Soviet political activities in Iran will inevitably have harmful effects in Turkey, and he has informed Ambassador Cripps by cable of this conversation. You should seek the earliest opportunity to inform the

Foreign Office that this Government views with concern reports which have been received concerning Russian political activities in Iran and is extremely apprehensive of the effect upon Turkey of any display of Russian sympathy toward an Armenian separatist movement in Iran. In this connection you should refer to the assurances that the territorial integrity and political independence of Iran will be respected, contained in the Soviet note of August 25 to the Iranian Ambassador, and you should refer also to Dekanosov's reaffirmation of these assurances reported in section four of your 1632, September 6, 2 p.m. Referring to the President's message of reassurance to the Shah (Department's 1026, September 4, 2 p.m.) you should state that this Government is confident that the Soviet Government will make sure that effective measures are being taken to implement the assurances which it has given to respect the territorial integrity and political independence of Iran.

Steinhardt on October 9, 1941 (Telegram 1778, 740.0011 EW 1939/15719):

The Moscow papers yesterday carried a Tass denial in the following terms: "The Berlin and Rome radio are disseminating a report that the Soviet Union has demanded the annexation of northwest Iran to Soviet Armenia and that General Wavell has approved this demand. Tass has been authorized to deny this report as being false and provocative."

Steinhardt on October 11, 1941 (Telegram 1788, 891.00/1794):

Department's 1124, October 8, 1 p.m. I called on Vyshinski this afternoon and conveyed to him the substance of the Department's telegram under reference. He stated that reports that the Soviets in the occupied zone of Iran were engaged in political activities or propaganda or were displaying open sympathy toward Armenians or other separatist movements must be of German origin. And were not in accordance with the facts. He added that the Soviet Government had no knowledge of any such activities by agents of the Soviet Government and that all that the Soviet authorities in the occupied zone of Iran are interested is in "the maintenance of law and order." I stressed the harmful effect upon Turkey of any display of Soviet sympathy toward an Armenian separatist movement in Iran to which Vyshinski replied that he "quite understood" this viewpoint.

The State Department, however, needed first-hand information on conditions in Azerbaijan. Instruction to Dreyfus on October 11, 1941 (Telegram 109, 740.0011 EW 1939/15972A):

> The Department desires that Moose visit Tabriz and such portions of the Tabriz area as you and he may deem desirable and possible for him to visit for the following purposes: One. To ascertain discreetly the nature of the Soviet occupation with particular reference to separatist movements and the treatment of local population. Two. To ascertain the present state of construction and condition of the railway line between Kazvin and Tabriz as well as plans for completing and improving it, with particular reference to the future transport thereon of lend-lease supplies. Three. To discuss with American citizens in Tabriz their problems and prospects. Four. To make preliminary and discreet investigation of the availability of consular office and living quarters in Tabriz. For the strictly confidential information of the Legation and Consulate, the Department is considering the reestablishment of a consulate at Tabriz and sending of an additional officer to Iran for that purpose. The Department deems it highly desirable that the visit be made without delay, and that you should take every appropriate step to facilitate it. Upon Moose's return, reports on the above matters are desired by telegraph.

Dreyfus on October 13, 1941 (Telegram 187, 891.00/1975):

> With reference to the Department's 104, there has been an improvement in the situation in the north of Iran. The Soviet authorities have prevented further meetings of Armenian separatists; relative free road communication between important cities has been reestablished; the British Minister reports better cooperation on the part of Soviet authorities in transportation matters; the British Consul at Tabriz reports an improvement in the general conduct of the Russians; and the Foreign Minister informs me that the Iranian police are being rearmed. In addition, the British Minister advises me confidentially that the forces occupying Tehran will be withdrawn, a fact which when made known will have a favorable effect.

Dreyfus on October 29, 1941 (Telegram 201, 740.0011 EW 1939/16232):

> Reference Department's 109, October 11, 6 p.m. Moose returned here Sunday evening after having visited Tabriz, Rezaieh and Resht and is

now preparing a report on his trip which includes the following: all evidence obtained tends to show that Soviet discipline has been uniformly good and that minor disturbances which have occurred were caused by local people. Open separatist movements were early discouraged by the Soviet military authorities though Communist propaganda continues to be spread by word of mouth, motion pictures and in Tabriz by the theater and the registration of Soviet sympathizers.

The Shah's position remained precarious. Dreyfus on October 25, 1941 (Telegram 207, 891.00/1803):

> The political situation in Iran remains quiet. Unfortunate factors which have created a state of nervous confusion are the political uncertainty, lack of strong leadership, growth of personal opportunism, abuse of newly found freedom of speech, economic stagnation, and decline in public morale due to Soviet occupation. One of the most potentially and permanent dangerous factors in the present situation is the deterioration in security in rural areas where tribes have obtained arms abandoned by Iranian forces. . . . The Shah has strengthened his precarious position by acts of charity, evidence of willingness to govern constitutionally and by showing a democratic and cooperative spirit. Hossein Ala told me yesterday and he speaks for an important and influential group that believes the Shah has taken hold well and deserves a chance. His ultimate destiny however will depend not only on Iranian political developments but also on the future attitude of the Allies. The Egyptian Ambassador confidentially informs me he has been instructed to indicate to the Shah that Egypt would welcome him and the Queen should they have to leave Iran.

Dreyfus adds:

> The British do not view with favor the present unlimited freedom of speech or the advance of self-seeking elements and are taking steps to assert control. As indicated in my 200 the treaty as amended would require the institution of censorship. A step in the direction of firmer control was taken two days ago when the military governor of Tehran announced that newspapers publishing statements against the Government will be suppressed and the meetings and gatherings will not be permitted.

Despite the reassuring report by Consul James S. Moose, Jr, the situation in Azerbaijan remained chaotic. Dreyfus in a report of January

29, 1942, the day the Tripartite Treaty of Alliance was signed, and entitled, "Situation in Northern Iran; Soviet-Iranian Relations; Soviet Government is Opening Twelve Consulates in Iran." (Dispatch 191 and enclosure, 740.0011 EW 1939/19521):

> I have the honor to enclose a translation of a confidential communication addressed to me by the Minister of Foreign Affairs touching on the situation in Azerbaijan and to offer the following comments on the general situation in northern Iran and on Soviet-Iranian relations. As suggested in my telegram No. 19 of January 27, 2 p.m., the situation in northern Iran has shown little sign of improvement. It is difficult to get a clear picture of conditions there because of the evasions, exaggerations and distortions of fact in which both the Iranian and Soviet officials indulge. Rumors, often entirely without foundation, fly about like snow in a blizzard only to disappear to make way for others equally questionable. Out of the welter of conflicting reports and prejudiced statements, however, two facts emerge with some clarity—the situation is serious and the Russians have considerable responsibility therefor. Just how far the Russians have gone, that is, whether they have openly connived, officially inspired or merely passively permitted, is not fully clear. The Foreign Minister told me that he has been assured by the Soviet Ambassador that instructions had been given Soviet officials in the occupied area to refrain from interfering in internal Iranian affairs but that in his opinion these instructions are being disregarded. As the Department is aware, the Soviets have also given formal assurances to the Turkish Government in this sense but such assurances are apparently given as little weight by the Turkish as by the Iranian and British governments. . . . The investigations of the British intelligence officers, the Turkish Government, the Iranian authorities, and this Legation all point to the same conclusion—that while the Russians have refrained from open acts of interference in Iranian internal affairs they have accomplished this indirectly by encouraging minorities, particularly Kurds, to resist Iranian authority. They have made this resistance on the part of the minorities easier by refusing to permit Iranian armed forces to operate in Soviet occupied areas and by permitting insufficient numbers of Iranian police officers. While, as stated above, they may have committed few acts of direct interference, they have shown their sympathy towards the Kurds and other minorities in small ways. A group of Kurds was recently given a propaganda and pleasure jaunt to Baku and on their return, according to an American missionary source, were given gifts of sugar, a scarce and highly desired commodity. Kurds are encouraged to enter the towns in native costume,

sometimes armed. Murders and acts of violence go unpunished and in some cases the Kurdish perpetrators are protected from the Iranian police. Although the situation in several places in northern Iran is of a disturbing nature, that in the Rezaiyeh area is most aggravated. There is no doubt whatsoever that there have been many murders and acts of violence, some for political motives but most of a personal nature. An American missionary reports that . . . hundreds of Iranians have fled Rezaiyeh for Tabriz and this report is fully substantiated from other sources. . . . The situation at Rezaiyeh has been brought into the limelight by the case of the expulsion of the Iranian Governor, a matter referred to in my despatch No. 11 of January 15. The Governor has returned to Tehran and gives the following version of this affair: A Kurdish chief attacked the tax collection agency on the outskirts of the town, was arrested by Iranian police and put in jail but was ordered released by the Soviet officials. After attacking the agency again, the Kurd proceeded to the hotel around which the Iranian police threw a cordon. The Soviet commander then required the Iranian police to withdraw and informed the Governor, when he protested, that he might come and talk the matter over with him. The Governor thereupon left Rezaiyeh for Tehran.

The Soviet answer to the above and similar cases is that Iranian authorities have consistently, since the beginning of the invasion, fled in terror leaving their work to be done by the Soviets who are not prepared to assume civilian duties. They accuse the Iranians of lack of cooperation and deny hotly that they are interfering in the internal affairs of the country or permitting others to resist authority. There is little doubt, as I have reported since the country was invaded on August 26, that the Iranians have improved on "he who fights and runs away" by not fighting and still running away. Their attitude of defeatism and impotency has been harmful to their own cause. Much good could be done in the present situation were both the Russians and Iranians to make an honest endeavor to understand the viewpoint of the other and offer some degree of cooperation. In certain areas of the north, there is tribal unrest which warrants mention. The Khalkhalis, near Ardebil, have gained possession of arms and are committing depredations; in southern Mazenderan, between Semnan and Firuzkuh, the tribesmen are said to be robbing and raiding; the Karadaghis near Julfa are said to be agitating for union with Russia; and disturbances of a rather serious nature have broken out in Khorrasan where there have been cases of highway robbery and violence. A Colonel, who was a relative of the Legation interpreter, was killed by bandits near Zabol.

The case of Khorrasan reveals the difficulty of relations with the Russians. The Iranians have been trying for some time to send Ali Mansour, former Prime Minister, to Meshed as Governor. They obtained Soviet consent, which was later withdrawn because Mansour was allegedly anti-Russian, but it is now understood that consent has again been given. . . .

The Soviets have demanded to open 22 Soviet Consulates in Iran and, after some negotiation, have been granted permission to open twelve at the following places: Pahlevi, Resht, Tabriz, Bandar Shapur, Meshed, Kermanshah, Gorgan, Bandar Shah, Rezaiyeh, Nowshahr, Maku and Bajgiran. The agreement was reached on the basis of reciprocity, the concession to the Iranians being that they might open one consulate at Ashkabad but only after the war. The Iranians, it should be mentioned, had in former times consulates in southern Russia at Rostov, Tashkent, Tiflis, Batum, Baku, and Bajgiran, while the Russians had several consulates in Iran. Shah Reza wished to limit Russian influence in Iran and reduced Russian consular representation to one consulate at Pahlevi while the Iranians retained only the consulate at Baku. The significance of the opening of these consulates, which is proceeding apace, seems to have been missed by some observers. The Iranians, however, realize the danger to their country but they have at present neither the means nor the energy to resist. It may well be that the Soviets have limited the historic ambition of their Czarist forbears to press ever southward toward the Persian Gulf. To the Iranians, who have long feared Russian penetration, the future is far from bright.

I have wished to develop the background picture given above before announcing a new development which may alter the situation materially. The Soviet authorities have at long last given permission for Iranian troops to proceed to certain areas of Russian occupied Iran to put down disturbances. Troops have already left for Meshed to quell disorders in Khorrasan and others have departed for the Ardebil area to reestablish order among the Khalkhalis. Agreement is about to be reached, although there may still be a slip, for the sending of Iranian troops to Tabriz and Rezaiyeh. Although this may be an indication of a new attitude on the part of the Soviet authorities which will permit the Iranians to reestablish their control, it would be unwise to make any predictions. Unless these forces are given full support by the Soviet authorities, particularly in the Rezaiyeh area, the situation might well deteriorate rather than improve. The Kurds are clearly getting out of hand, the British authorities reporting that the Iranian forces in south-

> ern Kurdistan are afraid to proceed too far north of Senna for fear the Soviets will incite the Kurds against them. We should for the moment consider this Soviet permission to send troops northward as a hopeful indication rather than as a sure sign of coming improvement. . . . In conclusion, there would seem little hope for immediate improvement in the situation. There is, however, a ray of hope in the dispatch of Iranian troops to the north, particularly if permission be granted for operations against the Kurds near Rezaiyeh. If the Russians were honestly to cooperate, troops operating southward from Rezaiyeh in liaison with those now working in southern Kurdistan could possibly accomplish something of value.

Foreign Minister Ali Soheily's letter to Dreyfus, marked "confidential and direct," is dated January 18, 1942:

> I have the honor to bring to Your Excellency's attention the latest reports received from Rezaiyeh: 1. Three days ago an automobile came to the door of the Grand Hotel and took the Kurdish chiefs staying there to a place where a bigger crowd and a number of Assyrians had gathered. Speeches were delivered for them that they should obtain their independence and unite themselves with the Assyrians. They encouraged them to ask for their independence. There were several Russian officers with two ladies in that gathering. 2. In Jame Mosque at Rezaiyeh a group of people have come together, taken votes for Governor General and Governor. They want to appoint Omar Aqa, the Kurd, as Governor General and the son of Seyid Taha as Governor. The Kurds have gathered in the city of Rezaiyeh and intend to do away with the road guards and put their own men in their place. 3. The threatening of Government officials is intensifying, and several of them have found themselves forced to leave that place and go to Tabriz. It is understood that the Financial Agent of Rezaiyeh has been killed.
>
> These reports have just been received and are being forwarded for Your Excellency's knowledge with reference to our conversations.

Rising Insecurity

Dreyfus on February 2, 1942, four days after the signing of the Tripartite Treaty of Alliance (Dispatch 194, 891.00/1827):

> I have the honor to offer the following comments on Iran's important problem of internal security. Internal security in Iran has shown steady

deterioration since the invasion of the country on August 26, 1941, until at present it constitutes a major preoccupation of the Government. This condition has grown from several related causes, all of them resulting from the invasion of the country by the Russians and the British. It arose primarily out of the confusion and uncertainty in the period following the invasion. It was aggravated by the fact that tribesmen obtained possession of arms abandoned or sold by fleeing Iranian soldiers. It was abetted by the extremely bad morale of the people, deriving from decades of ruthless exploitation. It was heightened by the attitude of defeatism and impotency adopted by the Government which attended the abdication of Shah Reza, who had acted and thought for Iranians for twenty years. It was increased, finally, by the shortage of wheat and sugar, the two mainstays of Iranian diet, by the increase in the cost of living, by the economic depression and by the disruption of communications. The situation could have been controlled to some extent had the Iranian Government taken forceful action instead of expending time and energy in bemoaning its fate and playing politics. However, the decks now appear to be cleared for action with the Anglo-Russian-Iranian treaty signed and with a Government alert to the danger of the situation and already embarked on a policy of action. The consideration of the treaty, with its attendant jockeying for political advantage, uncertainty and obstructionism has, indeed, absorbed most of the energy of the Iranian officials in recent weeks. It is hoped with this impediment out of the way that the Government will be able to devote more time and thought to internal matters. The security situation has become particularly bad in the Rezaiyeh area. . . . In Khuzistan, under British occupation, security is good but it is reported that wheat for seed is scarce and that the police have not been paid. . . . Forceful and sustained action on the part of the Iranian authorities will be necessary if the greatest accomplishment of Shah Reza, establishment of security throughout Iran, is not to be lost. Action is being taken and I feel it is significant that Field Marshall Ahmadi, the strong-arm agent of Shah Reza in breaking the tribes in the 1930s, has been brought into the cabinet as Minister of Interior. The whole question is extremely important for Iran and also for the allied war effort, for breakdown in security in this country would make more difficult the shipment of supplies to Russia.

On March 19, 1942, Paul Alling, newly appointed Chief of the Division of Near Eastern Affairs, had addressed a memorandum to Assistant Secretary Adolph A. Berle and Under Secretary Sumner Welles (Memorandum, 891.00/1827):

It is thought that you may find of interest a brief summary of a despatch dated February 2, 1942 from the American Legation at Tehran discussing internal security in Iran. The summary follows. Internal security in Iran has shown steady deterioration since the invasion of August 28 (sic), 1941, and constitutes a major preoccupation of the Government. The already bad morale of the people, the confusion and disorder following the invasion, and the fact that tribesmen obtained possession of the arms from fleeing Iranian soldiers have all adversely affected the situation. The security situation has become particularly bad in the Rezaiyeh area. This situation was discussed in detail in a despatch of January 29.

In southern Kurdistan, Iranian forces operating with the assistance of the British are in action against the Kurds. The division engaged is not as strong as Iranian officers desire. Army officers generally believe that the Kurds must be kept in complete subjection, otherwise they become restive. Shortage of wheat both for food and seed has aggravated the situation. Iranian forces have been hampered by fear of pushing very far north lest the Russians incite and assist Kurds. The Soviets have, however, given consent for Iranian troops to proceed to certain restricted Russian-occupied areas. If the Russians enlarge somewhat the permission granted and cooperate, forcible action by Iranian troops should bring good results. Christians and Jews in the Rezaiyeh area are worried and have appealed to the British for guarantees of safety or visas for British possessions upon Allied withdrawal. The British Minister has assured them that the British and American Governments will do everything in their power after the war to see that minorities are protected. An American missionary, the Reverend Mr. Zekler, who wields much influence at Malayer, has been accused by the British of not using his influence to further the Allied cause. The Legation will discuss the matter with Mr. Zekler when occasion permits. In Khorassan Iranian troops are active and it is hoped the situation will improve. In Khuzistan under British occupation security is good but it is reported that wheat for seed is scarce and that the police have not been paid. Near Kermanshah the Kurds have been approached in a friendly way to determine their terms for surrendering arms. In Fars the Iranian troops have dispersed members of the Boir Ahmadi tribe. The Government has been courting the Kashkai tribes in an endeavor to win them over peacefully. The Minister concludes that forceful and sustained action by the Iranian authorities throughout the country is necessary. The Minister is hopeful that such action will be taken. The whole question is considered to be extremely important for Iran and also for the Allied war effort as a breakdown in security in Iran would make more difficult the shipment of supplies to Russia.

Steinhardt from Ankara on March 16, 1942 (Telegram 169, 891.00/1839):

> In conversation with the Iranian Ambassador this morning he stated that reports concerning disturbances in Iran were grossly exaggerated and that the situation was entirely in hand. He attributed whatever local disturbances may have taken place to "too much liberty since the change of Shahs or German money." He added that the Shah had not left Tehran and that the Queen who was visiting her brother in Cairo would return to Tehran tomorrow. Repeated to Tehran.

Dreyfus again on the deteriorating security situation in a report of May 6, 1942 (Dispatch 260, 891.00/1860):

> On the whole, the tribal and security situation in Iran may be described as unsatisfactory although only in Kurdistan has it gotten out of hand. Much of the blame for this condition lies with the Iranians themselves. Their inertia, their spirit of defeatism, their attitude of impotency, their childlike helplessness after the disturbances of August and the abdication of Shah Reza and their tendency to play politics to the detriment of efficient action have prevented the carrying out of an intelligent and forceful policy. The entire situation might, in fact, have been avoided had they kept their balance in September and used their large army to keep order in the country and regain possession of the arms thrown down by their soldiers. The task confronting them now is an enormous one and calls for leadership and intelligent dealings with the tribesmen, backed by forceful military action. They must, above all, get a grip on themselves and lift the morale of the population and of the army.

The dispatch, similar to that of February 2, 1942, ends on an optimistic note:

> The political atmosphere has been somewhat cleared by the signing of the treaty of alliance with Russia and Britain, by the extension of Lend-lease aid to Iran and by the approaching settlement of certain aggravating financial disputes with the British. It is hoped that the Iranians may now be willing and able to put their domestic ménage in order.

The treaty, extension of lend-lease, and financial disputes with Britain will be discussed in this and several following chapters. Dreyfus' optimism again proved unfounded.

Proposed Treaty of Alliance

Immediately after the advent of the new Foroughi cabinet, as noted, the British had set about arranging a formal treaty. Winant on September 23, 1941 (Telegram 4492, 741.9111/3): "Most Secret. Mr. Eden gave me this afternoon the text of a draft tripartite Anglo-Soviet-Iran treaty of alliance which his government proposes. He gave one draft this afternoon to the Soviet Ambassador for submission to his government." The Russians were in no hurry. Winant on October 3, 1941 (Telegram 4710, 741.9111/6): "Foreign Office states that status of proposal is that draft has been submitted to the Soviet Government through the Soviet Ambassador in London and that the Soviet Government is still studying it. Foreign Office has sent a reminder and requested early consideration and reply." Winant on October 8, 1941 (Telegram 4798, 741.9111/7):

> Foreign Office informed me this afternoon that they have still not heard from the Soviet Government regarding draft treaty with Iran. Sir R. Bullard, British Minister at Tehran, has, however, informed the Foreign Office that he communicated the text to the Iranian Government but his Soviet colleague has received no instruction from Moscow.

Dreyfus on October 13, 1941 (Telegram 186, 741.9111/8): "The British Minister informs me that the delay in presenting a final draft of a treaty to the Iranian Government has been caused by the Soviet Government which has not yet approved the proposed draft." Dreyfus on October 17, 1941 (Telegram 194, 741.9111/9): "The Soviet Ambassador informs me that his Government has given its approval of the draft of the treaty with Iran and that he and the British Minister are to begin negotiations jointly this morning with the Foreign Minister. Soviet and British troops are withdrawing from Tehran tomorrow."

The proposed treaty, similar to the Anglo-Persian Treaty of August 1919, was highly unpopular. Dreyfus on November 1, 1941 (Telegram 213, 741.9111/12):

> Reference my 201. Although Iranian committee appointed to consider treaty has not finished its study Foreign Minister informs me the treaty

> has been approved in principle and that Iranian counter draft will shortly be presented. The opposition which has developed in official circles and among the public to the treaty, particularly to any clause which would require Iran to fight for the Allies, has made it necessary for the Iranians to proceed carefully and to obtain support of various factions in Majlis. British Minister deprecates delay in signing treaty. He believes it could have been put through quickly had not Russian Government delayed so long in giving its approval. The historic and deep-seated feeling of hostility of Iranians towards Russia and Britain has been accentuated by recent events. This fact is confirmed to me by all observers including the Shah and British Minister. A high Iranian official informs me that in his opinion 80 percent of Iranians are pro-German. This friendly feeling towards the Germans is in my opinion based more on antipathy for Russia and Britain than on consciously pro-German sentiment. In any event I believe Iranians may be expected in case the German thrust toward Iran eventuates to give sympathy if not open support to Germans particularly if they come in the guise of liberators.

Dreyfus again on November 1, 1941 (Telegram 216, 741.9111/13):

> Referring to my no. 213, British Minister informs me the Foreign Minister has just notified him and the Soviet Ambassador that the Iranian Government accepts the treaty in principle and will make a formal reply within three days. Foreign Minister stated his Government will propose only two minor changes—they will request clarification on the clause on economic assistance to Iran and make certain reservations on the use of Iranian armed forces.

Steinhardt from Moscow on November 5, 1941 (Telegram 1882, 741.9111/14):

> The British Ambassador informed me yesterday that the negotiations for the alliance between Great Britain, the Soviet Union, and Iran were progressing rather slowly due to the fact that the British Foreign Office had several times amended its desiderata. I am reliably informed the Soviet Russian Government had thus far conducted its part of the negotiations in an entirely satisfactory manner.

Steinhardt on November 6, 1941 (Telegram 1892, 741.9111/15): "The Iranian Ambassador, who has been ill for the past ten days, told me yesterday that he hopes to leave for Tehran about November 10th in order to hasten the conclusion of the negotiations for the alliance between Great Britain, the Soviet Union and Iran." The Iranian ambassador was Mohammad Saed.

Dreyfus on November 8, 1941 (Telegram 223, 741.9111/17):

> Referring to my telegram number 222. The Prime Minister yesterday made an important statement to the press regarding the treaty. He prefaced his remarks by saying public statement was necessary to clarify public opinion and dissipate false interpretations. After discussing background of invasion, he stated that Iran should base its relations with its neighbors particularly with Great Britain and Russia on a spirit of comprehension and reciprocal understanding. The treaty he said had been studied carefully and he had consulted and sought the advice of parliamentary factions and eminent Iranians. He declared that it had seemed to him after careful study that collaboration and entente with Great Britain and Russia based on principles which guaranteed the interests of Iran were in principle useful, in view of the present situation, particularly since the statement published following the interview of the President of the United States and the Prime Minister of Great Britain concerning liberty and independence of the people of the world supported this point of view. Turning to the false reports being circulated as to the terms of the proposed treaty, he denied categorically that the Allies have demanded the right to interfere in the political or military affairs of the country and that the Iranian armed forces will be required to fight beside the Allies. He assured the public that the Iranian forces will be used only to maintain internal security and the Government does not intend to call up additional military classes. The Prime Minister's statement has been well received by the people most of whom had believed the widespread false reports. It should tend to quiet public opinion and weaken to some extent the opposition to the treaty mentioned in my recent telegrams.

Not many had been reassured by Foroughi. Dreyfus on November 12, 1941 (Telegram 225, 891.00/1804):

> Popular opposition to treaty and to government's policy of cooperation with allies is causing increasing uneasiness in Tehran. Opposition is being encouraged and incited by nightly broadcasts in Persian from Berlin which attack government in strong terms. This situation has given rise to a fresh surge of rumors as for example that disturbances are imminent and Cabinet will be forced to resign. Another current

> rumor is there will be popular demonstration and possibly disturbances when Shah opens Majlis tomorrow.

This was a reference to the opening of the 13th Majlis. On November 14, 1941 (Telegram 227, 891.00/1805):

> The demonstrations referred to in my 225 of November 12, 8 p.m. took place but were mild in character. Groups in front of the Majlis shouted disapproval of the Prime Minister, of the recent elections and of the British. The Shah in his speech yesterday at the inauguration of the 13th Majlis reiterated his desire in foreign matters for close collaboration with nations whose interests are allied to those of Iran and his intention in internal affairs to continue the program of social and economic reforms.

Approval of the Treaty

The new Majlis which had been chosen under Reza Shah had no legitimacy, but in keeping with tradition, the cabinet had resigned. Dreyfus on November 29, 1941 (Telegram 243, 891.00/1807): "The Foroughi cabinet resigned today. Foroughi is forming a new cabinet which will probably be presented to the Medjliss tomorrow." Dreyfus on December 3, 1941 (Telegram 247, 891.00/1813):

> Reference my no. 243. Foroughi is having difficulty in forming new cabinet which will be acceptable to Majlis and British. In prevailing confusion certain conservative leaders refuse cabinet positions while numerous opportunistic politicians are exerting great influence to gain power. Many candidates, many of them wholly unqualified, are being suggested for every cabinet position. The strings of this puppet show are being drawn by the British through their Legation and through Fateh of the oil company. . . . It is believed new cabinet be formed in a few days, possibly tomorrow.

Dreyfus adds:

> It seem probable that Dr. Sadiq, the only competent Minister of Education in recent years and a firm friend of the United States, will be forced out to make way for a more cooperative politician. There are indications this move is backed by British who seem in general to be apprehensive of increasing American influence in Iran and in particu-

lar to be displeased by at the sudden announcement in press that Dr. Sadiq has invited an American educational mission to come to Iran.

Dreyfus on December 4, 1941 (Telegram 248, 891.00/1810): "The new Foroughi Cabinet has just been announced and will be presented to the Medjliss today." Again on December 4 (Telegram 249, 891.00/1811):

> Reference my numbers 243 and 248, the new Cabinet was presented to Majlis this morning. Prime Minister in asking for vote of confidence explained that his Cabinet's program is essentially that of his former one and that the urgent needs of Iran at the moment are restoration of security and provision of food stuffs. The Majlis refused to consider question of vote of confidence until Cabinet submits a formal program. Prime Minister then announced the Cabinet would assume its full functions immediately and submit its full program later. New Cabinet appears to be strong and competent to deal with present situation. Strength however appears to be its prime virtue and individual standard of many of its members is not high. The unscrupulous and ruthless Ahmadi was included to put down tribal disorders. The inclusion of such a man, the dismissal of the Cabinet Ministers of Commerce and Posts, will not contribute to development of an enlightened democratic Government in Iran. . . . One of our missionaries commented that Cabinet "put Iran back twenty-five years."

Dreyfus adds:

> American relations have perhaps suffered with loss of our two good friends Sadiq and Hekmat and the entry into the Cabinet of Kazemi who was Foreign Minister at time of our breach of relations. New Minister of Education is a molla with whom our missionaries had difficulty some years ago over question of elementary education.

This was a reference to Mohamad Taddayon. The new cabinet had quickly approved the proposed treaty following the Japanese attack on Pearl Harbor on December 7, 1941, and the entry of the United States in World War II. Dreyfus on December 10, 1941 (Telegram 253, 741.9111/20): "The Foreign Minister informs me the treaty has been approved by the Council of Ministers and will be submitted to the Majlis within a few days. He stated that the procedure of ratification by the Majlis before formal signature was followed at British request."

Dreyfus on December 12, 1941 (Dispatch 167, 891.00/1818):

I have the honor to offer the following remarks regarding the new Foroughi cabinet which was presented to the Majlis on December 4, 1941. . . . The formation of the new cabinet, it should be noted, was a routine procedure occasioned by the adjournment sine die of the Twelfth Session (of the Majlis) on October 31 and the inauguration of the Thirteenth Session on November 13. . . . Foroughi, when he presented his cabinet to the Majlis on December 4 asked for but did not receive a vote of confidence, which was withheld pending the presentation of the government's program. This fact is rather important for it shows that the present government in unable to control the Majlis in the high-handed manner of its predecessors. The program was presented to the Majlis on December 7 and a vote of confidence was given the government on December 14. . . . All is not a bed of roses for the cabinet, the opposition having become both widespread and vocal. The press has taken the government to task recently on a number of subjects, particularly the lack of security, the shortage of food, the threat of censorship, dilatory action in putting reforms into effect, and dissatisfaction with various ministries. For example, the writer counted 19 editorials in the newspapers *Ettelaat, Setareh, Tajaddod-i-Iran, Iran, Ayandeh-ye-Iran* and *Kushesh* from December 1 to 10 which attacked the government, some mildly some violently, on these subjects. Of these, eight made strong objection to the imposition of censorship, which it is widely stated the government intends to introduce. . . . In conclusion it may be remarked that the cabinet is now faced with the onerous task of cramming the unwanted and unpopular treaty with Russia and Great Britain down Iranian throats. It is expected that this treaty will be initiated by the cabinet and presented within a few days to the Majlis for ratification. This procedure of ratification before signature will at least have the advantage as far as the cabinet is concerned of putting some of the blame for the treaty on the shoulders of the Majlis. There are those who believe that the second Foroughi cabinet was constituted only to take the brunt of the opposition to the treaty, after which it would make way for a new one.

Dreyfus on December 16, 1941 (Dispatch 168 and enclosure, 891.00/1819):

I have the honor to enclose the French text of a speech delivered by the Prime Minister before the Majlis on December 13, 1941, on the subject of foreign affairs. . . . Its particular purpose was to justify the government's attitude toward the allied powers, particularly in the matter of the treaty, which the Prime Minister stated will soon be presented to the Majlis for ratification. Although an Iranian observer in discussing the speech remarked that it was "a masterpiece self-justification and evasion of responsibility," it seems to me the Prime Minister was extremely clever in approaching the matter from the allied rather than the Iranian viewpoint in order to show the great necessity which impelled Russia and Great Britain. After developing the theme of the necessity for a treaty, the Prime Minister indicated clearly that he intends to have the treaty approved by the Majlis before it is signed by the Government, thus placing a part at least of the onus on the shoulders of the deputies.

Dreyfus on December 19, 1941 (Telegram 260, 741.9111/21):

The Foreign Minister informs me the Iranian Government would like to have the United States adhere after the signature of the Iranian-Russo-British treaty which has been initialed and which will be presented to Majlis in a few days. American adherence would, he says, would increase value of treaty in Iranian eyes tenfold. He added that he has not considered it opportune to broach the matter to the Allied representatives. I will forward a copy of the final draft by air mail.

Dreyfus on December 20, 1941 (Telegram 261, 741.9111/22):

Prime Minister reiterated to me today desire of Iran Government to have United States adhere to treaty. He explained that the Government's situation is precarious because of widespread dissatisfaction created by Russian occupation. He stated that Soviet propaganda, political activity and interference continue and that Russians feel they have a sphere of influence in Iran. He expressed opinion that Iran's position vis-à-vis the Allies might be improved were United States adhere to the treaty.

Dreyfus on December 30, 1941 (Telegram 267, 741.9111/23):

A strong editorial in *Ayandeh Iran* stresses the desirability and necessity of having the United States adhere to the treaty. It declares such is desirable because of Atlantic Charter and due to special confidence Iranians have in Americans. It states that the procedure is necessary because the United States is actually a party to the treaty, was consulted as to its provisions and will benefit from it by use of Iranian facilities in transport of war goods; America therefore has an obliga-

> tion to sign as an ally. The editorial is significant as marking the first suggestion in the press that America be brought into the treaty. The treaty meanwhile is meeting with stiff and growing opposition in all quarters including the Majlis. People are being strongly influenced by inciting and threatening Iranian broadcasts from Berlin. Iranians are generally adopting in the present crisis over the treaty the same unreasoning and unrealistic attitude which resulted in invasion in August. Leading officials and more intelligent elements while in most cases finding the treaty personally objectionable are more realistic and wish to force it through simply because they see no acceptable alternative. As a leading official put it "it is bitter but necessary medicine."

Eden was not amused at the suggestion of American adherence to the treaty. Winant on January 21, 1942 (Telegram 307, 741.9111/26):

> I have just received the following communication dated January 20, 1942 from the Foreign Office. "You may remember that I told you recently that the Iranians might be putting forward a suggestion that the United States should adhere to the proposed Anglo-Soviet-Iranian Treaty of Alliance. I have now heard from our Minister at Tehran that the Iranian Minister for Foreign Affairs recently put this suggestion to your Minister who replied that the object of the treaty was to regularize the situation between Iran and the two powers whose troops were in her territory and that the United States had nothing whatever to do with this. The suggestion was, however, revived on 10th January in a local newspaper which proposed that Mr. Bullitt, who was then in Tehran, should submit it to the United States Government. I imagine the State Department will share the views of your Minister at Tehran about the Iranian proposal which we have a shrewd suspicion was put forward with the Iranian object of postponing any action as definite as the signature of a treaty. In view of our earlier conversation I thought I would let you know what had happened; unless contrary to our expectations the Iranian Minister for Foreign Affair's suggestion appeals to the United States Government it would be a help to us if the idea were scotched as soon as possible." Signed Anthony Eden.

Dreyfus on January 15, 1942 (Telegram 11, 741.9111/25):

> Foreign Minister informs me that cabinet crisis has been caused by the refusal of the British Government to accede to request of Iranian Government for several small changes in the treaty. The most important of these which were to be handled by exchange of letters are (1) provi-

> sion against the use of Iranian forces outside the country without Iranian consent and (2) provision that Iran will not have to pay for useless or unnecessary construction or installation by Allies. He states that upon learning of this refusal Prime Minister wished to resign without delay but was persuaded to make a last endeavor through Iranian Legation in London to obtain British consent. He is certain if this fails Prime Minister will resign as he feels he cannot otherwise face Majlis which has demanded the treaty changes. British Minister confirms the refusal and states it appears to be based on belief by British Government that it has made numerous concessions while Iranians have indulged in delaying tactics. . . . Meanwhile situation in the north is deteriorating. The Kurds are reliably reported to have expelled the Governor of Rezaiyeh, killed a number of police, committed acts of brigandage and interfered with Government services. The Iranians allege this disorder is instigated by Soviets and profess themselves helpless to put it down because of absence of Iranian forces there and insufficient number of police permitted by Russians.

Dreyfus on January 25, 1942, describes the chaotic scene in the Majlis following an assault on Foroughi (Telegram 17, 741.9111/28):

> An incident of great political importance took place today at noon when a large stone was thrown at Prime Minister as he was addressing Majlis on occasion of second reading of Anglo-Soviet-Iranian treaty. The assailant who has been arrested but not fully identified ran at great speed from the spectators gallery and threw the stone with violence from range of only few yards which would indicate that his purpose was to kill. . . . On a point of order vote on ratification was postponed until tomorrow's session.

Details in a report of February 5, 1942 (Dispatch 200, 741.9111/50):

> The assailant, who was seated in the visitor's gallery, suddenly arose and ran with great speed toward the rostrum from which the Prime Minister was addressing the Majlis on the occasion of the second and final reading of the Anglo-Soviet-Iranian treaty. He threw a large stone at the Prime Minister's head with violence and at point blank range of only some three yards, which would indicate his intention of committing murder. As mentioned in my telegram, the Prime Minister was fortunate not only in dodging the stone but also in not having a cardiac collapse for he suffers from heart trouble which at any time may cause his death. The assailant was arrested at once. In the ensuing confusion

and tumult, several deputies, notably Messrs. Javan, Ettebar and Nobakht, exchanged insults and slaps in heated arguments over the treaty. The Prime Minister, after an interval, returned to the rostrum and made what is described as a courageous and eloquent speech in which he explained that he was recommending ratification of the treaty purely in Iran's best interests. He deplored as much as any other person, he said, the unhappy recent events which have taken place in Iran but believed the signing of the treaty was essential in order for Iran to draw the maximum benefit from the present admittedly unfortunate situation and to reduce to a minimum the harmful effects of invasion. I will reserve further remarks regarding the treaty for a separate despatch devoted to that subject. Before turning to the possible motives and significance of the attack, it will be of interest to set down what is known of the background of the assailant. The person accused of the attack, now under arrest and investigation, is Sheikh Ali Roshan, born in Kermanshah, said to be 50 to 60 years of age, son of deceased Haji Akhund Mulla Hossein. He is said to have taken an active part before 1922 in political parties in Kermanshah, and to have persuaded a friend, Abbas the Turk, to make an unsuccessful attempt against the life of Mo'aven-ol-Molk. Between 1922 and 1932 he is alleged to have worked among the Sanjabi tribe of Kurds for the purpose of inciting them against the Government. For this, he was arrested and confined to Qasr-e-Qajar prison in Tehran but was later released and exiled to Isfahan. As a result of the amnesty granted persons confined or exiled for political offenses, he returned only recently to Tehran. It appears that he has been without work and that he and his wife and children have suffered hunger and privation. The motive for the crime is not clear. . . . If the motive was to prevent the signing of the treaty, the assailant failed of his purpose, for the treaty was signed the next day by 80 votes to 8. If the motive was to discredit the Prime Minister, the crime was unsuccessful, for Foroughi gained rather than lost by it. If, however, the incident was staged by the communists, it might perhaps be described as a success in that it created a disturbance, called attention of the people to the unfortunate assailant, and served to accentuate class strife. Iranians generally deplored the crime. The newspaper *Iran* in an editorial of January 26 called it a "prelude to danger" adding that unless all Iranians joined in repudiating such action the country might come to be saddled with another dictator. Not all the press, however, took such a balanced view, at least one newspaper taking advantage of the opportunity to play politics. The irresponsibility and abuse of freedom of speech which a number of newspapers have revealed recently is illustrated by the following incident. The newspaper *Eqdam* printed an article shortly after the attack in which it was asserted that the

> Prime Minister had fainted and fallen, whereupon the assailant had grappled with him, a report probably based on misapprehension and given without malice. The President of the Majlis wrote to the editor of the newspaper to explain that the statements were untrue. Thereupon, the editor trained his guns on both the Prime Minister and President of the Majlis, both of whom are old and highly respected men, representing the very quintessence of Iranian culture. He ridiculed the President of the Majlis for the poor grammar in which his letter was couched. He then took the absurd stand, based on political considerations or pure vindictiveness, that since the assailant did not grapple with the Prime Minister he should be placed in liberty.

The treaty was approved by the Majlis on January 26, 1942, and formally signed on January 29, 1942. On February 4, 1942, Eden made a statement in the House of Commons (Dispatch 2875, 741.9111/49):

> I am glad to say that the Anglo-Soviet-Persian Treaty of Alliance, which was approved by the Persian Parliament on Monday, 26th January, was signed in Tehran on behalf of the three Governments on Thursday, 29th January. The Treaty entered into force on signature. The large majority by which the treaty was approved in the Persian Parliament shows that it has gained the free assent of the elected representatives of the Persian nation. It is a justification of the patience with which the long and sometimes difficult negotiations have been conducted by all concerned. I should like to take this opportunity of extending a cordial welcome to our new Ally. The full text of the Treaty is being laid as a White paper. Copies will be available to Honorable Members today. It will be seen that the Treaty provides for the grant of those facilities which the British and Soviet authorities have considered necessary for the prosecution of the war. It covers, for example, the facilities to be provided in Persia for the passage of troops and supplies, for the maintenance and improvement of the means of communication, and for censorship control. I should also like to emphasize, as is explicitly laid down in the Treaty, that His Majesty's Government and the Soviet Government undertake to respect the territorial integrity, sovereignty and political independence of Persia. They have no designs or ambitions which would conflict with this principle.

Although the treaty had been initialed on December 15, 1941, and formally signed on January 29, 1942, the State Department had received no information on its provisions. On February 6, 1942, W.G. Hayter,

First Secretary of the British Embassy, had called on Alling (Memorandum, 741.9111/41):

> Mr. Hayter said that following his conversation a few days ago with Mr. Murray concerning the failure of the British Government to keep us informed of developments in connection with the Anglo-Soviet-Iranian Treaty, he had taken the matter up with the Foreign Office and was now in receipt of a reply. According to this statement the Foreign Office had furnished Ambassador Winant with a first draft of the treaty in September 1941. Early in 1942 the final draft had been handed to the Embassy, but the Embassy had apparently inadvertently failed to forward a copy to Washington. Mr. Hayter said that he merely wanted to point this out and to show that the British Government had every intention of keeping us advised of developments. I said that there had been a considerable period between September and January when we had little or no news as to developments. He said the reason for this was that there had been no developments. The Iranian Government had pursued a policy of delayed tactics, and there was therefore nothing to report. He hoped, however, that the statement which he had made would convince us that the British had no intention of withholding information.

Dreyfus comments on the treaty on February 9, 1942 (Dispatch 205 and enclosure, 741.9111/48):

> Negotiations for this treaty began in late September but reached a final stage only in January. The treaty was ratified by the Majlis on January 26 by a vote of 80 to 8 with 5 abstentions and was signed by delegates of the three nations on January 29. This treaty is a by-product of British diplomacy. Engineered by the British, apparently for the purpose of placing their relationship with Iran on a formal and legal basis, the treaty was not pushed by either the Russians or the Iranians. The Soviet attitude may be described one of acquiescence while the Iranians adopted an attitude of obstruction. The treaty was, as I reported to the Department on numerous occasions by telegraph and despatch, extremely unpopular with the Iranians, who disliked negotiating with the invaders of their country. Iranian sentiment, as I have also called to the Department's attention frequently, has been pro-German, although I prefer to describe it as anti-British and Russian rather than as consciously favorable to the Germans. Iranians generally, in considering the treaty, showed the same unrealistic attitude which resulted in their invasion in August, preferring to base their actions on sentiment rather

than on realism. However, there was a marked change toward the end of the negotiations, many of the more intelligent Iranians having begun to realize that they had something to gain by regularizing their status with the allies and nothing at all to gain by obstruction. This viewpoint was well expressed by the Prime Minister in his eloquent speech in the Majlis after the attack on his life. . . . It is well for Iran that the treaty has been disposed of, for the atmosphere is now cleared somewhat and attention may be turned to pressing internal problems, which have gone unattended in the heat of the argument over this controversial matter. It is not to be expected that political dissension will cease now that the treaty is signed but at least one cause of discord will have been removed. There is an interesting American angle to this general question of the treaty. Weakening of opposition to the treaty among more intelligent Iranians may be attributed to a considerable extent to the entry of the United States into the war. The mentioning of the Atlantic Charter in the treaty was clearly an Iranian bid for American sympathy and an endeavor to place some responsibility for the treaty on American shoulders. Iranians wish for open American adherence to the treaty as a guarantee of eventual Russian withdrawal from the north but, if this cannot be obtained, would be satisfied with a statement by the American Government taking cognizance of the treaty and giving its express or implied blessing. Several newspapers have come out into the open to demand American adherence, holding that the United States has a certain responsibility in the matter because of the Atlantic Charter and because Americans will benefit from the use of Iran for the sending of war supplies to Russia. The Prime Minister forestalled an attempt in the Majlis to bring up the question of American adherence by informing a deputy that responsibility for negotiation of treaties is vested in the Government and not the Majlis. The Shah, as the Department is aware, addressed a telegram to the President informing him of the signing of the treaty. This telegram, sent on January 31, was notable in its outspoken declaration that the friendship of the President was the best guarantee of the execution of the terms of the treaty. The President's reply, received on February 8 and made public on February 10, has been generally well received locally. The Prime Minister informed me yesterday that he greatly appreciated the President's telegram and believed it would serve a useful purpose. He said, however, that he had hoped the President would be able to go farther toward a definite guarantee of the territorial integrity and independence of Iran. . . . Iranian newspaper comments on this American angle are summed up by the following extracts from *Iran* of January 30. Writing of the signing of the treaty and the aid which Iran expects to receive, this newspaper remarks: "Public opinion is waiting to see what assistance will be given. We wait for the Government and people of the United States to make ready with the great power of which they are disposed to help us in our political and commercial interests, since we adhere to the Atlantic Charter. It is necessary that the United States know that our historic nation is its friend and awaits its assistance. We hope that our relations will enter into a new phase of rapprochement with the countries signing the treaty as well as with the United States, which is one of the pillars of the Atlantic Charter."

Annex: Text of the Tripartite Treaty of Alliance

The text of the treaty was forwarded by the American Embassy, London, on January 24, 1942 (Dispatch 2694 and enclosure, 741.9111/36). The preamble reads:

> His Majesty The King of Great Britain, Ireland and the British Dominions beyond the Seas, Emperor of India, and the Union of Soviet Socialist Republics, on the one hand, and His Imperial Majesty the Shahinshah of Iran, on the other; Having in view the principles of the Atlantic Charter jointly agreed upon and announced to the world by the President of the United States of America and the Prime Minister of the United Kingdom on the 14th August 1941, and endorsed by the Government of the Union of Soviet Socialist Republics on the 24th September 1941, with which His Imperial Majesty The Shahinshah declares his complete agreement and from which he wishes to benefit on an equal basis with other nations of the world and; Being anxious to strengthen the bonds of friendship and mutual understanding between them and; Considering that these objects will best be achieved by the conclusion of a Treaty of Alliance; Have agreed to conclude a treaty for this purpose and have appointed as their plenipotentiaries. . . .

The initial treaty consisted of nine articles and two annexes. Annex 3 was added at Iran's insistence prior to its signature:

Article 1. His Majesty The King of Great Britain, Ireland and the British Dominions beyond the Seas, Emperor of India, and the Union of Soviet Socialist Republics (hereafter referred to as the Allied Powers) jointly and severally undertake to respect the territorial integrity, sovereignty and political independence of Iran.

Article 2. An alliance is established between the Allied Powers on the one hand and His Imperial Majesty the Shahinshah of Iran on the other.

Article 3. (1) The Allied Powers jointly and severally undertake to defend Iran by all means at their command from all aggression on the part of Germany or any other Power. (2) His Imperial Majesty the Shahinshah undertakes: (a) to co-operate with the Allied Powers with all the means at his command and in every way possible, in order that they may be able to fulfill the above undertaking. The assistance of the Iranian forces shall, however, be limited to the maintenance of internal security on Iranian territory: (b) to secure to the Allied Powers, for the passage of troops and supplies from one Allied Power to the other or for other similar purposes, the unrestricted right to use, maintain, guard and, in case of military necessity, control in any way that they may require all means of communication throughout Iran, including railways, roads, rivers, aerodromes, ports, pipelines and telephone, telegraph and wireless installations: (c) to furnish all possible assistance and facilities in obtaining material and recruiting labour for the purpose of the maintenance and improvement of the means of communication referred to in paragraph (b): (d) to establish and maintain, in collaboration with the Allied Powers, such measures of censorship control as they may require for all the means of communication referred to in paragraph (b). (3) It is clearly understood that in the application of paragraph (2) (a) (b) (c) and (d) of the present article the Allied Powers will give full consideration to the essential needs of Iran.

Article 4. (i) The Allied Powers may maintain in Iranian territory land, sea and air forces in such number as they consider necessary. The location of such forces shall be decided in agreement with the Iranian Government so long as the strategic situation allows. All questions concerning the relations between the forces of the Allied Powers and the Iranian authorities shall be settled so far as possible in co-operation with the Iranian authorities in such a way as to safeguard the security of the said forces. It is understood that the presence of these forces on Iranian territory does not constitute a military occupation and will disturb as little as possible the administration and the security forces of Iran, the economic life of the country, the normal movements of the population and the application of Iranian laws and regulations. (ii) A separate agreement or agreements shall be concluded as soon as possible after the entry into force of the present Treaty regarding any financial obligations to be borne by the Allied Powers under the provision of the present article and all paragraphs (2) (b) (c) and (d) of Article 3 above in such matters as local purchases, the hiring of buildings and plant, the employment of labour, transport charges, etc. A special agreement shall be concluded between the Allied Governments and the Iranian Government defining conditions for any transfers to the Iranian Government after the war of buildings and other improvements effected by the Allied Powers on Iranian territory. These agreements shall also settle the immunities to be enjoyed by the forces of the Allied Powers in Iran.

Article 5. The forces of the Allied Powers shall be withdrawn from Iranian territory not later than six months after all hostilities between the Allied Powers and Germany and her associates have been suspended by the conclusion of an armistice or armistices, or the conclusion of peace between them, whichever date is earlier. The expression 'associates' of Germany means all other Powers which have engaged or may in the future engage in hostilities against either of the Allied Powers.

Article 6. (i) The Allied Powers undertake in their relations with foreign countries not to adopt an attitude which is prejudicial to the territorial integrity, sovereignty or political independence of Iran, not to conclude treaties inconsistent with the provisions of the present Treaty. They undertake to consult the Government of His Imperial Majesty the Shahinshah in all matters affecting the direct interests of Iran. (ii) His Imperial Majesty the Shahinshah undertakes not to adopt in his relations with foreign countries an attitude which is inconsistent with the alliance, nor to conclude treaties inconsistent with the provisions of the present Treaty.

Article 7. The Allied Powers jointly undertake to use their best endeavours to safeguard the economic existence of the Iranian people against the privations and difficulties arising as a result of the present war. On the entry into force of the present Treaty, discussions shall be opened between the Government of Iran and the Governments of the Allied Powers as to the best possible methods of carrying out the above undertaking.

Article 8. The provisions of the present Treaty are equally binding as bilateral obligations between His Imperial Majesty The Shahinshah and each of the two other High Contracting Parties.

Article 9. The present Treaty shall come into force on signature and shall remain in force until the date fixed for the withdrawal of the forces of the Allied Powers from Iranian territory in accordance with Article 5.

In witness thereof, the above named plenipotentiaries have signed the present treaty and have affixed thereto their seals. Done at Tehran in triplicate in English, Russian and Persian, all being equally authentic, on the . . . day of 1941.

Annex 1. Text of notes to be addressed to the Iranian Minister for Foreign Affairs by the Soviet Ambassador and His Majesty's Minister. "With reference to Article 6 paragraph 1 of the Treaty of Alliance signed today, I have the honour, on behalf of the Government of the Union of Soviet Socialist Republics/His Majesty's Government in the United Kingdom, to assure Your Excellency that my Government interpret the provisions of this clause as being applicable to any peace conference or conferences held at the conclusion of the present war, or other general international conferences. Consequently they consider themselves bound not to approve anything at any such conference which is prejudicial to the territorial integrity, sovereignty or political independence of Iran, and not to discuss at any such conferences anything affecting the direct interests of Iran without consultation with the Government of Iran. The Government of the Union of Soviet Socialist Republics/His Majesty's Government will further do their best to secure that Iran will be represented on a footing of equality in any peace negotiations directly affecting her interests."

Annex 2. Text of notes to be addressed to the Soviet Ambassador and His Majesty's Minister by the Iranian Minister for Foreign Affairs. "With reference to Article 6 paragraph 2 of the Treaty of Alliance signed this day, I have the honour, on behalf of the Iranian Government, to assure Your Excellency that the Iranian Government would consider it contrary to their obligations under this clause to maintain diplomatic relations with any State which is in diplomatic relations with neither of the Allied Powers."

Annex 3. Text of notes to be addressed to the Iranian Minister for Foreign Affairs by the Soviet Ambassador and His Majesty's Minister. "1. With reference to Article 3 (2) of the Treaty of Alliance which has been signed today: the Allied Powers will not require of Iran the participation of her armed forces in any war or military operations against any foreign power or powers. 2. With reference to Article 4 (2): it is understood that there is no provision in the Treaty which requires that the Iranian Government shall bear the cost of any works which the Allied Powers carry out for their own military ends and which are not necessary for the needs of Iran. 3. It is understood that Annex 1 will remain in force even if the Treaty ceases to be valid, in accordance with the provisions of Article 9, before peace has been concluded."

Chapter 3

Soheily Cabinet, Rupture with Japan, and Extension of Lend-Lease to Iran

Dreyfus on February 16, 1942 (Telegram 43, 891.00/1826):

> It appears likely there will soon be cabinet changes perhaps of sweeping nature and possibly involving the Prime Minister. Ostensible reasons are general dissatisfaction with Government action in such matter as signing of unpopular treaty, shortage of food and other goods, soaring prices, unfavorable economic situation and lack of internal security and wide spread feeling that cabinet has failed to meet urgent needs of country in present crisis. A more obscure but equally important reason is unbridled ambitions of politicians who aspire to high positions. Foroughi who is still popular and respected may continue or may be replaced, probably by Qavam-es-Sultaneh or by Tadayyon. New Government would per force continue orientation towards Britain and Russia with emphasis on latter since Soviet influence seems lately to be increasing and British declining. Government I believe would necessarily continue well disposed towards United States.

Dreyfus on February 28, 1942 (Telegram 51, 891.00/1828): "Referring to my telegram no. 43, February 16, 4 p.m. the cabinet has resigned and Foroughi is now forming a new one." Dreyfus on March 2, 1942 (Telegram 53, 891.00/1829):

> New Foroughi Cabinet was approved by Majlis today by vote of 65 to 4 with 43 abstentions. . . . General impression is that cabinet is of weak composition and rests on poor foundation with little support in

> Majlis. Present very unsatisfactory political situation. . . . Scene in Majlis this morning was one of utter confusion. I consider it unlikely that anything constructive can be accomplished by this or any other Government until these self-seeking elements in Majlis are restrained.

On March 3, 1942 (Telegram 54, 891.00/1830):

> The Foroughi Cabinet resigned last night after only a few hours of existence. Foroughi felt that Cabinet position was too weak in view of Majlis opposition. Two most likely candidates for Prime Minister are Tadayyon who is favored by British and Qavam-es-Sultaneh whom I believe has Russian support.

The crisis had continued. Dreyfus on March 6, 1942 (Telegram 56, 891.00/1831):

> After several days of confusion and intense political activity Foroughi has consented to form another Government which should be completed in a day or two. His consent to form a new Government after steadfastly refusing was obtained by a delegation from the Majlis which called at his home to beg him to continue. The British continue to give Foroughi full support having favored Tadayyon merely because of Foroughi's withdrawal. Tadayyon I am pleased to report received almost no support in this crisis. Qavam was running strong and had a good chance of becoming Prime Minister had Foroughi stood fast in his refusal. The Majlis is said to have opposed the fourth and short-lived Foroughi cabinet because of the inclusion of politicians such as Hekmat who are unpopular because of their connection with the former regime. . . . The press has widely supported the Majlis in its stand against persons closely connected with Shah Reza and has taken Foroughi to task for his failure to accomplish anything substantial.

Dreyfus on March 7, 1942 (Telegram 57, 891.00/1832):

> Foroughi yesterday suddenly and without warning departed from Tehran leaving a letter to the Majlis stating that he was unable to undertake the formation of a new Government. Ali Soheily has been named Prime Minister by the Shah and I am informed that the Majlis in secret session expressed approval of this appointment by an overwhelming vote. Soheily is now forming his Cabinet.

On March 9, 1942 (Telegram 58, 891.00/1833): "Referring to my telegram no. 57, March 7, 4 p.m. Soheily presented his Cabinet to Majlis this morning. Vote of confidence was postponed until Majlis has time to consider Cabinet's program." Dreyfus on March 12, 1942 (Telegram 65, 891.00/1838):

> The Soheily Cabinet was given vote of confidence by Majlis this morning of 101 to one with two abstentions. Scene in Majlis was complete reversal of confusion and agitation of recent weeks even opposition speakers with dignity offering support. It is not unlikely Majlis has learned a lesson in democratic procedure by seeing the harm done by unreasonable and selfish opposition and by realizing the possibility of being dissolved. With full Majlis support, the press being friendly although reserved and with British and Russian encouragement Soheily is getting away to a good start. He indicated his intention of having Cabinet meet Majlis in frequent secret sessions to exchange ideas and advice. His program follows closely the Foroughi program given in despatch 167 December 12. I consider the Soheily Cabinet relatively high in ability, integrity and force. It is noteworthy in being headed by young Prime Minister and in including new blood in form of young and energetic career officials. Elimination of objectionable persons such as Tadayyon, Kazemi and Ahmadi, inclusion of new blood and more wholesome attitude on part of Majlis offer some hope of development of more stable democratic Government. As regards United States I have every reason to believe Cabinet will be most friendly.

Dreyfus on March 19, 1942 (Dispatch 228, 891.00/1858):

> I have the honor . . . to offer the following discussion of the Soheily Cabinet and its program and of the general political situation. . . . The Iranian crisis, in a general sense, dates from the invasion of Iran by the British and Russians in August, 1941, and the abdication of Shah Reza in September. The political confusion into which the country was plunged and from which it has not yet emerged derives principally from the violent change from dictatorial to democratic government, for which the country was ill prepared by experience or tradition. It was heightened by popular revulsion to the occupation of the country by the two powers traditionally regarded with suspicion and distrust. It is natural that self-seeking elements in the Majlis and elsewhere, without background training in democratic procedure, should take advantage of the situation for their own benefit. Small groups with various irons in the fire grew up in the Majlis, in many cases to seek their own

ends but in other cases to offer blind opposition. Small political parties were born only to pass into oblivion. The most interesting example of these abortive parties was the so-called "He" (meaning the Shah), headed by the Chief of Police. It is believed to have had the Shah's blessing, since he did not deny his connection, but it proved to be another fleeting fancy. Not all of the Majlis opposition was based on personal opportunism, however, for in many cases, as for example in the matter of the treaty, deputies were genuinely inspired to offer opposition in what they believed to be the best interests of Iran. The crisis entered a more aggravated stage on February 27 with the resignation of the Foroughi cabinet. This was brought about apparently by Foroughi's realization that the cabinet had lost support of the public, the press and the Majlis. Popular dissatisfaction with the cabinet was caused by several factors, among them a general feeling that Foroughi had accomplished almost nothing, desire for the elimination of Ahmadi and other military members of the cabinet for fear that a new dictatorship might arise, opposition to Hekmat and other politicians who were thought to be too closely connected with Shah Reza. . . . Foroughi, although under constant attack, maintained throughout his personal popularity. . . . He has now found a haven in his new post as Minister of the Court, where he can pass the remainder of his days as befits an Iranian scholar. The press, with the exception of *Ettelaat*, gave him little support. . . . In spite of dissatisfaction with Foroughi's accomplishments as Prime Minister, he was charged with the constitution of a new Government, which he presented to the Majlis on March 2. It became clear to him, because of the poor vote of confidence given him by the Majlis—65 to 4 with 43 abstentions—that his position was untenable and the new cabinet consequently resigned after a life of only a few hours. The crisis then entered a more acute stage and the heyday of political intriguers arrived. Tadayyon, supported by the British, was an active candidate for Prime Minister; Qavam-os-Saltaneh, backed by the Russians but distrusted by the British, was another. The British would, I think, have preferred Taqizadeh, but he was out of reach in London and also it was not certain he would accept. I must admit surprise (and relief) that Tadayyon was able to rally almost no support. Qavam was running strong and I believe would have been the next Prime Minister could he have obtained British support. . . . In this atmosphere of confusion and "dog eat dog," the Shah instructed Soheily to form a cabinet.

The choice of Soheily as Prime Minister came as something of a surprise for, while he was known as a competent and sincere man, he was not generally considered to be of sufficient stature and prestige for Prime Minister. It is widely believed that the Shah not only chose Soheily but also took advantage of the opportunity to impress upon a Majlis delegation the seriousness of the political situation, the need for national unity, the harm caused by unscrupulous political activity and even the possibility that the Majlis might have to be dissolved since it could not be said to represent the will of the people. Whatever transpired, it was a subdued Majlis which on March 12 gave the Soheily cabinet an almost unanimous vote of confidence of 101 voted to one with two abstentions. As the Director General of the Foreign Office put it, the Majlis appeared terrorized. In any event, the scene in the Majlis on March 12 was a complete reversal of the confusion which has prevailed there in recent weeks. . . . With full Majlis support, with British and Russian encouragement and with a friendly press the Soheily cabinet has got away to a good start.

Dreyfus on December 10, 1942 (Dispatch 402 and enclosures, 701.9111/755):

I have the honor to refer to my telegram No. 403 dated November 27, 1942 reporting the death in Tehran of Mohammad Ali Foroughi, Minister of the Court and Ambassador Designate to Washington. Foroughi had been suffering from cardiac complaint for more than a year but had been seriously ill for only a very short time. Born in Tehran in 1875 of a distinguished Iranian family, originally Zoka-ol-Molk, had a long and varied career. . . . While in recent years he was more in the public eye as a public servant, Foroughi's best claim to fame will probably rest in his writings, as poet and philosopher. Prior to his death, Foroughi had been subject to vicious attacks from almost every newspaper in Tehran, brought on partly by the size of the entourage that was to accompany him to Washington and the amount he had requested for travel expenses. As abuse followed abuse every phase of his public career was raked over and any possible trace of scandal brought out, elaborated and exaggerated. A few samples of this vituperation are enclosed. It was rather sickening to watch the same journals lavish sickly sweet praise upon him when the news of his death was announced. One paper, "Eqdam," however, had the courage to stick to its convictions and continued the abuse following Foroughi's death.

A state funeral was held for Foroughi on Sunday, November 29 and schools and public offices were closed as a sign of respect. A French account of the funeral, which was attended by me and the whole commissioned staff, is enclosed. It fails to describe the near riot which took place when the funeral procession was leaving the mosque. An enormous crowd, estimated as high as 50,000 thronged the two short blocks of the procession. Curious and emotional, the mob surges into the procession trampling one another and destroying any pretense of dignity that the ceremony might have had. The police charged them with whips, clubs, motorcycles, and horses and gradually forced them back. It is most fortunate that the crowd was in a good mood, for an ugly situation could easily have resulted.

Foroughi's acts in a public capacity have been fully covered by the Legation during his various tenures of office. As Prime Minister following the invasion in August, 1941, he probably did as much as any Iranian statesman could have done to keep his country going. His career was one of the most distinguished enjoyed by any Iranian in recent years—poet, philosopher, Prime Minister, President of the League of Nations, and finally named as his country's first Ambassador to Washington. Foroughi's last term as Prime Minister was as difficult as any Iranian has ever been called upon to cope with. The transition period from an absolute dictatorship to the present pseudo democracy was one that would have taxed the abilities, health, and courage of anyone. Foroughi lost his popularity by having the onus of the Tripartite Treaty fastened on him and by a natural reaction of the public which had been led to believe great things upon the change in government. It is interesting to note that Foroughi was one of the men responsible for putting Reza Shah on the throne and was his first Prime Minister upon his accession, and it was the same Foroughi who last year requested Reza Shah's abdication. Despite the recent vilification of Foroughi, the majority of thinking people in Iran realize the magnitude of their loss and that he was a statesman far above the usual men in public life in Iran.

Expulsion of Japanese Legation

Cable to Dreyfus on February 25, 1942 (Telegram 43, 701.9491/1): "Your no. 34, February 8, noon. Please make further inquiries of the Prime Minister as to Iranian intentions respecting continued relations with Japan." Another cable on March 6, 1942 (Telegram 57, 891.00/1830):

Your 51, February 28, 12 a.m. and 54 March 3, noon. As soon as possible after the formation of a new cabinet it is requested that you see the Prime Minister and discuss with him courteously but firmly the question of the continued presence in Iran of Japanese diplomatic and consular representatives. In that discussion you should point out that the presence of these officials is a grave danger not only to the interests of the United States and its associates in the war against aggression but also to Iran itself. In this latter connection you should stress the fact that fifth column activities of Japanese officials have played an important part in subjugating those countries in Asia which Japan has temporarily overrun. Accordingly you should express the strong conviction of this Government that the best interests of Iran require the prompt severance of relations with Japan. Please keep me promptly informed of developments in this matter.

Dreyfus replied on March 11, 1942 (Telegram 61, 891.00/1837):

Referring to Department's No. 57, March 6, I today discussed this matter with Prime Minister along lines suggested by Department. Soheily received my suggestion with apparent sympathy although he refused to commit himself to a definite line of action and promised early consideration by Cabinet. The Foroughi cabinet he revealed had discussed it but failed to take action because of confused internal political situation and due to example of Egyptian Cabinet which was understood to have failed in connection with expulsion of French Legation. He was of opinion that it would be difficult to get Majlis' consent to expulsion of Japanese because Japanese have managed to obtain some support among the Deputies. He made it clear that he values American friendship highly, desires to cooperate with us and will therefore seek a pretext to expel Japanese. He expressed regret that American Government has yet taken no action in matters which concern Iran so vitally, i.e., furnishing of food, supplies and advisers. He stated rather pointedly that he would be in a much stronger position in matter of expulsion of Japanese if he could go to Majlis with some concrete evidence of American help. I gained the impression that Soheily wants to be helpful but is afraid his fledging Cabinet is too weak to weather the political storm which might ensue unless he can discover a suitable pretext. It seems clear too that he thinks in terms of quid pro quo and wishes to be assured that tangible American aid will be forthcoming. After lapse of reasonable time I will again approach him on the subject.

On March 23, 1942, Viscount Halifax had spoken with Under Secretary Welles (Memorandum, 701.9491/25):

> The British Ambassador called to see me this evening at my request. The Ambassador brought up the question of the continued diplomatic representation of Japan in Tehran. He said that his Government had learned that Japan intended materially to increase diplomatic representation in that capital for purposes which, of course, were obvious. He requested that a further message be sent to our Minister in Tehran urging him to request again that the Iranian Government severe diplomatic relations with Japan, and that this Government use as leverage the economic assistance which the Iranian Government was requesting of us. I said I would be glad to have a further message sent to our Minister.

Cable to Dreyfus on March 28, 1942 (Telegram 79, 891.00/1840):

> British Government is informed Japanese plan increase in diplomatic staff at Tehran. Please again approach Iranian Government and urge severance of diplomatic relations with Japan. You may state that American Government attaches great importance to this question and our attitude toward Iranian requests for economic assistance will undoubtedly be affected by Iranian action in this respect.

Dreyfus on March 29, 1942 (Telegram 85, 891.00/1851):

> Referring to my 61 of March 11, 5 p.m., the Prime Minister informs me the Cabinet at last night's meeting formally agreed to expel the Japanese Legation. Japanese Minister will be informed of this action within the next few days. Referring to Department's 66, March 13, 6 p.m. and my 84, Prime Minister feels it would strengthen his hand in explaining this action to Majlis if he could make public the extension of Lend Lease aid to Iran.

Dreyfus on April 7, 1942 (Telegram 98, 891.00/1856):

> Prime Minister informs me Majlis in secret session today refused to sanction expulsion of Japanese Legation. This action was taken in spite of solemn pledge given me by Prime Minister as reported in my number 85, March 29, and his statement to Admiral Standley quoted in my number 95, April 4. Prime Minister states there is widespread dissatis-

> faction in Majlis with manner by which Russians and British are carrying out their treaty with Iran. Members complain bitterly that Russians are taking their cattle, that Poles are being dumped in Iran, that British are failing to provide food and are sending Iranian wheat to Iraq, that Russians are exploiting situation in northern Iran, that British are taking advantage of Iran in financial and other matters and that Iranians are being generally deceived and exploited. He added many feel that Japanese and Germans will soon be in Iran. British Minister in a note of April 4 to Iranian Government stated in strong terms that his Government regards expulsion of Japanese Legation as matter of utmost military necessity and that such action must be taken at once if Iran is to retain good will of British Empire and if goods are to continue to be furnished. In view of growing pro-Axis attitude of Iranians and their refusal to cooperate with British, tendencies which are now climaxed by refusal to expel Japanese Legation, we should, I feel, take a strong line and refuse to furnish advisers or economic assistance on Lend-Lease or any other basis until Iran shows more inclination to cooperate.

Dreyfus on April 8, 1942 (Telegram 99, 891.00/1857):

> Reference my no. 98, April 7. Prime Minister called me early this morning to tell me he is not satisfied with Majlis decision refusing to expel Japanese and that he is calling another secret session tomorrow in a final endeavor to obtain such action. Meanwhile British Minister has telegraphed London reporting this decision and requesting instructions.

Instruction to Dreyfus on April 10, 1942 (Telegram 85, 891.00/1857):

> Your 98, April 7 and unnumbered April 8, 10 a.m. Unless the refusal to expel Japanese Legation was reversed at meeting of Majlis mentioned in your April 8, 10 a.m., you are requested to convey to the Iranian Government immediately the substance of the following: The Iranian Government is well aware of the desire of the United States to assist Iran in every way possible, both now and in the future as it has done in the past. The United States Government is at present giving its best attention to Iranian requests for advisers and has been prepared to give sympathetic consideration to further requests of this character if presented. This Government is actively working on a program of economic assistance designed to meet the urgent needs of Iran. Evidence of this is provided by, among other things, the recent action making

Iran eligible for Lend-Lease aid. However, the United States cannot be expected to continue its efforts along these lines while Iran maintains friendly relations with the enemies of this country—relations which the Government feels are quite as dangerous to Iran as to the United States. Consequently, unless immediate and positive action is taken to expel all Japanese diplomatic and consular representation, the United States will be forced to reconsider and revise its entire economic policy toward Iran.

Dreyfus on April 12, 1942 (Telegram 103, 701.9491/20):

Prime Minister informs me he will notify Japanese Minister this afternoon that his entire Legation must leave Iran without delay. Majlis in secret session April 8 approved expulsion of Japanese but with provision that consent of Russians be obtained. This unnecessary injection of Soviets into picture was apparently another of the delaying tactics in which Iranians have been indulging in this matter. When Soviet Ambassador refused to make commitment in this regard British Minister made it clear to Prime Minister that he considered conditional Majlis approval unsatisfactory. Prime Minister therefore promises positive action today regardless of Soviet attitude. In view of this development I shall refrain from delivering the note suggested in Department's No. 85, April 10, 2 p.m. unless the Prime Minister fails to take the promised action.

Dreyfus on April 13, 1942 (Telegram 104, 701.9491/21):

Referring to my 103, April 12, Prime Minister last evening informed Japanese Minister that his Legation must depart within a week. Questions of means of exit now under discussion. Japanese wish to proceed to Turkey to which Iranians have no objection. British however do not approve dumping of further Axis diplomats in Turkey and are insisting that Legation return to Japan via Russia.

Dreyfus on April 23, 1942 (Telegram 120, 701.9491/23): "Referring to my No. 104, the Japanese Legation left Tehran this morning en route to Japan via Russia."

Memorandum of April 14, 1942, from Murray to Welles (891.00/1857):

I think we may assume from the attached telegrams from Tehran that our objective in Iran was accomplished and relations with Japan were

> severed without the necessity of delivering the rather stiff note of April 10. This is, I believe, all to the good, since the Iranian Minister is already pressing us to "reward" his Government for its behavior in this matter. . . . I sensed from a brief conversation with the Minister, following his conference with you, that he expects large Lend-Lease benefits to start to flow at an early moment as a result of his Government's acquiescence in our demand that relations with Japan be severed. I shall, of course, have to make it clear to the Minister that Lend-Lease status for Iran does not mean that the Iranian Government will necessarily be furnished with all it may ask for; that, on the other hand we are already rendering great assistance to Iran by facilitating the purchase in this country of sorely needed commodities. . . .

Immediately after the expulsion of the Japanese Legation, numerous Iranians were arrested for alleged pro-Axis activity. Cable to Dreyfus on April 15, 1942 (Telegram 91, 894.20291/1): "United Press despatch from Tehran and Axis radio report arrest last week of six prominent Iranians charged with Axis activities under direction of Japanese Legation. . . . Please telegraph whether this report accurate, reasons for arrest and possible effect on Iranian opinion." Dreyfus replied on April 18, 1942 (Telegram 111, 894.20291/2):

> Department's 91, April 15. Arrests in question were carried out over last week by Iranian authorities but at British request. British Minister informs me he demanded this action because of his pre-occupation at increasing pro-German sentiments and activities of many Iranians and because he hoped thereby to deter others of like persuasion. He stated he expected to leave matter of arrest and exile to Southern Iran entirely in the hands of Iranian authorities. However, because police action was so half-hearted and dilatory and because he has had to exert such strong pressure to obtain detention he now intends to send accused to Ahwaz where they can be kept under British surveillance. Russian Ambassador was kept informed and offered no objection. . . . Persons arrested are accused of pro-Nazi and anti-constitutional activities. I have discussed cases with British Minister and examined some of files. Evidence of guilt is sketchy, vague and circumstantial but I have not slightest doubt that all those arrested are at least pro-German and perhaps are actively working in German interests. Iranian reaction is unfavorable but relatively mild due partly to fact that Iranians are inured to arbitrary arrest and partly because they consider it only another British act which it is their fate to bear. Many Iranians feel that at least the accused should have been given hearing. While I believe the ar-

> rests will not have desired salutary effect but will only serve further to alienate Iranians, I should be reluctant to criticize British act. Iranians, while giving lip service to Allied cause, have frequently obstructed British and have offered little of the cooperation which their treaty obligations and official statements have given the Allies the right to expect.

The arrests had continued. Dreyfus on May 1, 1942 (Telegram 133, 891.00/1861): "Reference my 111, April 18. British Legation has handed police list of 24 additional persons suspected of pro-Axis activities with request they be investigated and kept under surveillance. Action is still secret and arrests may follow."

Iranian Request for American Advisers

Soon after the dispatch of an Iranian Economic Mission to the US, described in chapter 4, the Foroughi government had requested American advisers. Dreyfus on November 5, 1941 (Telegram 218, 891.51A/515):

> The Foreign Minister informs me he will shortly request the assistance of the American Government in obtaining for Iran American finance, health, municipal and perhaps other advisers and missions. His delay in making formal proposals is probably due to fact that Majlis which expires October 31 will reassemble November 13 at which time Government will be reconstituted. Iran is looking more and more toward United States for assistance and guidance and we should not, I feel, miss the opportunity to improve our position. I suggest in case formal overtures are made on this score that Iranian requests be sympathetically received. We must of course bear in mind growing possibility of German invasion of Iran which may prevent actual selection and arrival of such advisers. Even in event of invasion the preliminary steps taken now would facilitate the resumption of conversations after the war.

Dreyfus on January 17, 1942 (Dispatch 183, 891.51/542):

> I have the honor to enclose an English translation of a memorandum prepared in French by the Iranian Ministry of Finance setting forth Iran's commercial and financial position and describing the assistance Iran desires to obtain from the United States. . . . The statement of the Ministry of Finance was prepared in consequence of a conversation

held on January 8, 1942, between the Honorable William C. Bullitt and the Minister of Finance and other high Iranian officials. During the talk the Iranian officials, who were cognizant of Lease and Lend aid extended recently to Turkey and Egypt, expressed their desire to obtain similar aid for Iran. Iran is indeed, as suggested by the Minister of Finance, passing through a difficult period. It would seem desirable to prevent a commercial or financial breakdown of the country, particularly when it is partially under Allied occupation and when it is so important for transit of goods to Russia. There are those who will say that the Iranians are pro-German in sentiment and in any event are being purely opportunistic by turning to the United States now that they are cut off from their European markets. As to the first allegation, I have always taken the view that the admittedly strong leanings of the Iranians toward Germany are inspired by dislike and mistrust of the Russians and British rather than by any consciously pro-German feeling. As to the second suggestion, the fact that Iran may return after the war to her European markets should not deter us from pressing our present advantage and greatly strengthening our own position.

Memorandum of February 26, 1942 (891.51A/517):

Sir Ronald Campbell, Minister Counsellor of the British Embassy, called upon Mr. Murray this morning to acquaint him with the contents of a telegram received by the British Embassy from the British Minister at Tehran. This telegram stated that the Iranian Prime Minister and the Iranian Foreign Minister had discussed with the British Minister the possibility of securing the services of an American financial adviser who would also deal with the question of supplies. According to the telegram, the British Minister expressed his approval of this suggestion. The British Minister also thought it would be desirable to obtain the services of trained American relief workers to supervise the distribution of bread, sugar and cotton piece goods. He felt that such supervision would increase both the efficiency and honesty of the distribution of these products. Sir Ronald indicated that he was bringing these matters to the Department upon instructions from his Government and that the British Government supports these proposals.

Mr. Murray expressed his gratification of the interest of the British Government in the matter and stated that such an adviser could assist materially in solving financial problems confronting the Iranian Government and that trained American relief workers would prove extremely helpful in arranging for the equitable distribution of essential foodstuffs and clothing. He referred to incidents in the past when corrupt officials and speculators had cornered foodstuffs in times of famine. . . . Mr. Murray then referred to general conditions in Iran and stated that good men are being replaced in high office by reactionary, self-seeking politicians with unsavory reputations. He continued by saying that an American financial adviser would be unable to accomplish anything worthwhile if constantly opposed by such men. Men of this type in the Cabinet, he continued, would be unable to maintain law and order in the country. If law and order were not maintained by the Iranians themselves, the occupying forces would be obliged to devote themselves to internal police duties and the protection of supplies. . . . Mr. Murray then remarked that, although there might be anti-British sentiment in Iran, the British were highly respected in the Near East. He suggested that it would be helpful if the British Minister in Tehran were instructed to indicate to Iranians that the return to public office of disreputable politicians is harmful both to Iran and the cause of democracies. It was suggested also that similar suggestions might be sent to the American Minister at Tehran and that both the American and British Ministers might cooperate closely in regard to the matter. Sir Ronald stated that he would take up the matter with London.

Cable of March 3, 1942, to London (Telegram 912, 891.51A/515A):

The British Embassy has informed the Department of the concern felt in London over the deteriorating financial and economic situation in Iran and has inquired whether this Government would be prepared to lend its assistance in securing the services of an American financial adviser who would also assume direction of the importation of badly needed supplies for the civilian population, principally bread, sugar and cotton piece goods. The suggestion was also made that it would be highly desirable if some experienced American relief organization would supervise the distribution of above-mentioned supplies. The Embassy states that the matter has been discussed with the Iranian Government, who are anxious to see the above proposals implemented as soon as possible. The Embassy has been advised informally that these proposals will be given careful and sympathetic consideration. The Embassy was, at the same time, reminded, however, that an American financial adviser and relief organization could not perform their duties without the full support of competent Iranian officials; that, in this connection, the Department has noted with concern the recent deterioration in the Iranian political situation resulting from the regrettable emergence from

> political obscurity of reactionary politicians with unsavory reputations who appear to be slated for cabinet posts and other positions of influence. . . . It was also pointed out that, as a result of a probable breakdown in internal administration arising from the corruption and incompetence of such leaders, the occupying forces might well be obliged to expend considerable time and energy in the maintenance of law and order. The maintenance of such law and order was imperative if the safe transportation of military supplies to Russia was to be assured. The point was made that it is in the interest of both Iran and the United Nations that men of integrity and ability should assume posts of leadership in Iran, in order that the country may assume the role of a willing partner resisting aggression rather than that of a passive appendage. . . . Please seek an early opportunity to discuss this question with the Foreign office with a view to securing its cooperation. The strategic position of Iran at this time, as a result of Japanese successes in the Far East and the threat of German action in the Near East, is so obvious as scarcely to require stressing. The Department, therefore, trusts that the competent British authorities will concur with us in believing that no time should be lost in strengthening Iran's position as greatly as possible along the lines outlined above. Please keep the Department fully and promptly informed of developments.

On March 13, 1942, Dreyfus had cabled Washington on the need for economic assistance to Iran (Telegram 66, 891.51A/518):

> Following reply to Department's 55, March 4. (One) Economically Iran is suffering from loss of European markets, inability to secure shipping space for exports, disruption of internal life due to invasion and difficulty in obtaining much needed goods such as wheat, sugar, cotton goods, automotive products, tires, and medicines. A memorandum setting Iran's needs was handed Mr. Bullitt by Minister of Finance. Financially Iran's position is fairly good for although revenues have fallen, British are bringing in almost a million pounds a month. Rial has strengthened and further increase in value is contemplated. (Two) Politically present confused and unsatisfactory situation derives from violent change from dictatorial to democratic government for which country was ill-prepared and from popular reaction to virtual occupation of the country by two powers regarded as hostile. . . . The political situation in my opinion gives no immediate cause for alarm unless, of course, the threatened Axis thrust toward Middle East materializes. (Three) British position. British prestige already low when Iran was invaded has declined further. Factors which contributed to

this included: their unsuccessful war effort; interference in Iranian politics; pressure on Iran to sign an unwanted treaty; establishment through UKCC (United Kingdom Commercial Corporation) of virtual monopoly over Iranian trade and such acts as removing from Tehran radio station to Egypt a transmitting set badly needed here. British are now trying to prevent Iranians from altering rial value upwards. . . . British bid for American support in Iran may well be an attempt to bolster their own declining prestige. (Four) American position. American prestige in Iran is very high. Our aims should be first a short range objective of using Iran's strategic position for prosecution of war which aim nothing should be permitted to thwart, and, second, maintenance of our high prestige for constructive use in postwar period. . . . Iranians can hardly be expected to cooperate fully with two powers regarded with suspicion and distrust and if they are to be converted from passive appendage to willing partner it will only be through American sympathy and assistance. (Five) Conclusion. I recommend we give Iran our sympathetic support in this hour of need and furnish where possible the goods and advisers requested. I advise that any action suggesting force or open interference in internal affairs be avoided unless necessary for war effort. I recommend that we avoid if possible joining British in representations for fear we thereby lower our own prestige and share to some extent the historic onus which is certain to attach to British action in Iran. We must of course continue close collaboration and friendly relations with British officials in Iran in matters connected with war effort.

Dreyfus on June 9, 1942 (telegram 191, 891.01A/174):

Prime Minister told me yesterday "Government Majlis and people enthusiastic about United States advisers and are anxious to have them arrive." He has cabled Minister in Washington asking details about engaging Schwartzkoff in order to draw up contract but has had no reply. He is particularly anxious to have a financial commission which should be headed by a man of the highest caliber such as Millspaugh. He said Millspaugh who is being mentioned here might if available be considered but added his powers would be less than on previous visit because of present democratic form of government. Whoever is selected should use great care in selection of subordinates since there was considerable criticism of Millspaugh's assistants. Prime Minister also wants food and commodity expert who should arrive soon if to be of any value.

Dreyfus on June 11, 1942 (Dispatch 279, 891.01A/179):

> I have the honor to offer the following summary of Iranian press opinion concerning the desire and intention of the Iranian Government to engage American advisers and commissions in various fields of activity. Reference is made to my telegram No. 191, June 9, 1 p.m., which reported popular reaction in this respect and commented on the general subject. The desire of the Iranian people to have American advisers in many fields of endeavor has grown into a popular clamor in which people, press, Majlis, and Government join almost without dissenting voice. . . . To turn now to popular reaction to the employment of American advisers, it may be remarked that the subject is being widely discussed by the Iranian public as a result of the press publicity it is receiving and because of a secret session of the Majlis which is said to have approved fully of this course. All of the comments which have come to my attention have been favorable, most of them enthusiastically so.

The *Journal de Tehran* of June 11, 1942, has a long editorial entitled, "Iran and America." After praising the work of Morgan Shuster in 1911, and the work of Arthur C. Millspaugh during 1922-1927, the paper adds:

> but, as we said in the beginning of this article, it is not only for these reasons that Iran today turns her eyes toward America. Before the question of financial advisers arose, long ago, exactly in 1871, there was in Iran a terrible famine which took innumerable victims. At that time the Americans with the humanitarian sense which characterizes them, came to the aid of the victims and saved the lives of a large number of Iranians. This charitable gesture was again repeated during the famine of 1917. . . . And naturally these things are not forgotten easily.

The dispatch ends:

> American prestige in Iran is indeed at a peak. This is gratifying but at the same time a potentially dangerous situation. Much is expected of us in the way of furnishing advisers and economic aid; if we fail to live up to our reputation, or if we are unable to furnish the aid requested, permanent harm to our good relations with Iran may ensue.

Extension of Lend-Lease to Iran

On March 10, 1942, President Franklin D. Roosevelt had signed a Presidential finding on Iran (891.20/133). Cable to Dreyfus on March 13, 1942 (Telegram 66, 891.00/1837):

> On March 11 the President found the defense of Iran vital to the defense of the United States, thereby making Iran eligible to receive Lend-Lease assistance. For the present it is considered advisable to keep this development secret, except for the Iranian officials immediately concerned, and you are requested to see that no repeat no announcement on the subject is made in Iran. The Iranian Minister in Washington has been informed. With reference to your 61, March 11, you should take the first opportunity to emphasize to the Prime Minister that this action represents definite evidence of this Government's intention to help Iran. You may further state that arrangements are going forward with all possible speed to send wheat to Iran under Lend-Lease authority on a cash reimbursement basis. Action is being taken to requisition 20,000 tons, which is proposed to ship at the minimum rate of 2,000 tons monthly or greater quantities if the shipping situation permits. It should be noted that no effective action in this regard could have been taken by this Government prior to the designation of Iran as eligible for Lend-Lease, since no other Governmental machinery exists for such operations.

Dreyfus on March 17, 1942 (Telegram 73, 891.00/1840):

> The Prime Minister was very much pleased when I communicated the contents of the Department's 66, March 13. He said that he would like to be informed as soon as it can be made public as he wishes to give it the widest possible publicity here. He volunteered the statement that he is keeping in mind the matter of the expulsion of the Japanese Legation.

Meanwhile, on March 29, 1942, Soheily had presented to Dreyfus a long list of needed goods and desired quantities (Dreyfus, Telegram 84, 891.00/1850). Soheily's optimism was completely divorced from reality. It soon became clear that not even a tiny fraction of these requested items was likely to be made available to Iran.

On April 11, 1942, the State Department had informed the Iranian Minister that it was actively exploring the assignment of Iran to the Middle

East Supply Center (MESC) in Cairo, Iran's "designation" for Lend-Lease notwithstanding. The "action" mentioned in the first sentence of the cable to Dreyfus on April 15, 1942, refers to the expulsion of the Japanese Legation (Telegram 92, 701.9491/21):

> Your 104, April 13. Please express to the Prime Minister our gratification at the action taken and our conviction that it will prove to be in the best interests of Iran. For your confidential information, the Iranian Minister in Washington on April 11 communicated to Department a message received from the Prime Minister reporting discontent of the Majlis with attitude of Soviet forces of occupation and failure of British to fulfill commitments made regarding supplies et cetera. This was stated to be reason for reluctance of Majlis to authorize expulsion of Japanese. Iranian Minister further said that Prime Minister found himself in very difficult position and might be forced to resign if excessive British and American pressure should be exerted. In such a case, he personally feared conditions in Iran might become greatly disturbed. Minister was informed this Government could see no connection between British and Russian activities in Iran and question of Japanese representation. As a friend of Iran, United States would do everything it possibly could to persuade Russia not to take unwarranted action in Iran and would also do everything possible to facilitate fulfillment of British commitments to Iran, but we could not admit that this affected vital question of subversive Japanese activities.
>
> Minister was further assured that this government was working out details of assistance to Iran. In this latter connection we are discussing with British questions of over-all supply program for Iran to be tied in the general Middle East program. It would be helpful if you could report exact procedure now being followed by British in assessing Iranian economic needs and handling Iranian economic requests. Please report details of British organization and its relation to Middle East Supply Center Cairo and other British economic agencies. Please keep Department informed regarding arrivals in Iran of wheat and other supplies for civilian use. Questions of Anglo-Iranian exchange difficulties reported in your 97 April 6 Section 2 is under consideration by Department following presentation formal British request for American intervention. If possible, Department wishes to avoid exerting pressure on Iranian Government in this connection, and hopes to work out some more constructive solution.

On April 15, 1942, the First Secretary of the Iranian Legation had called on John D. Jernegan (Memorandum, 891.24/190):

> Mr. Davallou called and stated that, in the absence of the Minister from Washington, he had been instructed to bring to our notice the contents of a telegram which he had just received from the Prime Minister. Mr. Davallou referred to the conversation which the Iranian Minister had with the Acting Secretary on Saturday, in which the Minister pointed out the serious difficulties which the Prime Minister was encountering with the Mejliss in his efforts to bring about the expulsion of the Japanese Legation from Tehran. The Prime Minister had now instructed the Legation to state that it would assist him greatly in his dealings with the Mejliss if he could make public announcement of the fact that Iran had been found eligible for Lend-Lease by the United States. Mr. Davallou stressed again and again the importance which such an announcement would have in strengthening the position of the Prime Minister. I assured Mr. Davallou that I fully understood the point he was making and that I would be glad to bring the matter to the attention of the interested officials in the Department.

In a memorandum of April 16, 1942, addressed to Murray, Fred Winant and Acheson, Alling writes:

> Please note the attached memorandum of conversation with the Secretary of the Iranian Legation, regarding the desire of the Iranian Prime Minister to make announcement of the fact that Iran has been found eligible for Lend-Lease. As you know, we have been withholding any announcement of the extension of Lend-Lease to Iran until such time as a decision had been reached whether Lend-Lease aid should not be extended to Iraq and Saudi Arabia. It was our idea that if Lend-Lease aid was to be extended to the latter two countries, it would be possible to make a simultaneous announcement in regard to all three countries, that is Iran, Iraq and Saudi Arabia. Furthermore, the British have expressed the view that it would be preferable not to make an announcement regarding Iran until we are able to make a similar announcement regarding Iraq. If it appears likely that no early decision is to be reached regarding Lend-Lease for Iraq or Saudi Arabia, it seems to me that, with a view to supporting the present Iranian Prime Minister, we might consider the possibility of making an early announcement concerning Lend-Lease for Iran. It seems clear that the Prime Minister is in a rather precarious situation as regards his own Parliament, and in view

of his own friendly attitude towards the United States I believe it would be desirable to accord him the support which he requests and that this should be done at an early date.

Dreyfus on April 22, 1942 (Telegram 118, 891.24/180):

Prime Minister was pleased when I conveyed to him the message contained in first sentence of Department's number 92. He in turn asked me to express to Department his appreciation of the heartening information given by Department to Iranian Minister in Washington. He added that he would much appreciate immediate permission to announce the extension of Lend Lease to Iran. A public statement to this effect he thought would not only strengthen his political position but would also reassure certain elements in the Majlis who are beginning to ask when and how the United States intends to assist Iran. The specific questions raised in Department's number 92 are being investigated.

Jernegan on May 1, 1942 (Memorandum, 891.24/199A):

Mr. Early's office informed NE by telephone at 4.45 today that the President had signed the letter designating Iraq as eligible for Lend-Lease. The Iranian designation was made on March 11 but kept secret until the present. Simultaneous public announcement of the eligibility of Iraq and Iran will be made by the White House at 10.30 tomorrow, May 2.

Dreyfus on May 4, 1942 (Telegram 140, 891.24/186):

Prime Minister's announcement yesterday of extension of Lend-Lease aid to Iran made in a speech to Majlis was extremely well received by Deputies and public. He began his speech by saying that United States long in cordial relations with Iran has once again given practical demonstration of its good intentions toward this country. American advisers, he said, have rendered brilliant services to Iran. . . . He ended by saying he was sure the Deputies and all persons interested in Iran's welfare will welcome this good news which is sure to have important repercussions in economic affairs of Iran. Interrupted by frequent and enthusiastic cheers from Deputies. Extension of Lease-Lend aid should serve to strengthen our already cordial relations with Iran. However, actual harm may result if there is much delay in supplying Iran with much needed goods.

Dreyfus on May 13, 1942 (Dispatch 263, 891.24/201½):

> The Iranian press, I have the honor to inform the Department, has without exception commented most favorably on the President's announcement that lease-lend aid is to be extended to Iran. . . . All of the principle Tehran newspapers have carried leading editorials on the subject. Comments have been in all cases favorable and have expressed sincere appreciation not only of the extension of lease-lend but also for the many outstanding and unselfish services performed in Iran by Americans. . . . First comment was made by *Ettelaat* on May 3, which reported the Prime Minister's speech before the Majlis. . . . The same newspaper carried an editorial the following day, May 4, along much of the same lines, stressing Iran's need for wheat, sugar, automobiles, spare parts, tires, paper and medicines. . . . A note of sincere friendship and appreciation runs through these editorial comments and the same tone is noted in remarks made by private individuals. However . . . there is danger that actual harm will be done to our good relations with Iran if, after raising the hope of the Iranians, we are unable to deliver the goods. There is always potential danger in doing good deeds as Shakespeare suggested in his sound injunction of "neither a borrower nor a lender be." We should bear this in mind in considering the allotment of goods and shipping space for Iran.

Chapter 4

Iranian Appeals and British Counteractions in Washington

In October 1941, the Foroughi Government sent an economic mission to the United States headed by Allah Yar Saleh, former undersecretary of finance. Taghi Nasr, previously head of the Agricultural Bank, was his designated adviser. They arrived in New York on November 1, 1941. The Iranian Minister in a note of December 18, 1941, had informed the State Department of the mission's arrival (891.01B11/21). On February 24, 1942, Saleh had written to Murray (Note 1181, 891.48/303):

> You may be already informed that as a result of shortage in the supply of wheat my Government has been having difficulty in assuring the supply of bread in many cities of Iran. The United Kingdom Commercial Corporation which had promised to supply the needed amount of wheat has been unable to do so as a result of transportation difficulties. Due to these circumstances the Minister of Finance in Teheran discussed the matter with the Honorable William Bullitt, United States Special Envoy to the Middle East, and Mr. Bullitt was good enough to promise that upon his return to Washington he would try to make arrangements for the shipment to Iran of certain quantities of wheat which might be sent on board steamers bound for the ports of the Persian Gulf. I have now received a cable from the Minister of Finance, stating that the question of bread supply in many towns of Iran is becoming extremely acute and asking whether any decision has been taken on the subject of wheat shipment as discussed with Mr. Bullitt. I had in mind to go to Washington in order to discuss this matter with you personally but, as you know, it is nearly impossible to make reser-

> vations at any hotel in Washington, and the matter being of an urgent nature I decided that I should write to you while awaiting for hotel arrangements. No person realizes better than yourself the importance of this question in the situation in Iran. Bread being the chief food of the country, a shortage of it would naturally result in famine and I am confident that your Government would like to take any steps that are possible to prevent such a forthcoming condition. May I, therefore, request you to be good enough to see what can be done on this subject before it is too late and to inform me of your decision so that I can send a telegram to the Minister of Finance.

Two months later, nothing had happened. On April 14, 1942, Saleh had telephoned Alling (Memorandum, 891.24/185):

> Mr. Saleh telephoned from New York to say that he had received a telegram from the Minister of Finance reading as follows: "Please insist that wheat be shipped to Iran with the greatest rapidity." I told Mr. Saleh that we were going into the whole question of supplies for Iran, and we hoped that a satisfactory solution would be found in the very near future. He volunteered the idea that it would be well for our Legation at Tehran to concert with the Iranian Government authorities and with the British authorities in arranging a supply program. I told him I was very glad to have this suggestion and we would look into it.

On May 1, 1942, Saleh had a conference with Murray, Alling, Fred Winant and Jernegan (Memorandum, 891.24/202½):

> Mr. Saleh said that he was disturbed by an apparent tendency on the part of the Iranian Government to feel that no results could be expected from attempting to deal directly with the United States on the question of supplies. He has the impression that the Tehran authorities might shortly conclude that his mission in the United States was useless. This attitude, he believed, was largely due to the failure to obtain the wheat which he had been instructed to purchase and also to statements made by the British representatives in Iran to the effect that needed commodities could best be secured through the United Kingdom Commercial Corporation. . . . Mr. Murray . . . explained, as Mr. Winant had already done, that the difficulties in connection with the wheat had arisen because of the existence of a previously drawn-up British program of supply about which we had not been informed. On account of the very serious shipping shortage we were unable to insist upon the shipment of additional wheat, except for the 5,600 tons for

which arrangements were now in progress, but we were definitely watching to see that the British arrangement was carried out. Mr. Saleh was informed that our Minister in Tehran is keeping us informed regarding the situation, with special reference to actual arrival of wheat in Iran. Mr. Saleh said that he was exceedingly glad to hear this, since his greatest worry had been that the American Government was not itself investigating but merely accepting without question the assurances given by the British. He said for a time the British deliveries had been suspended entirely, which had caused the Iranian Government to lose all faith in British promises in this respect.

Mr. Murray then referred to the organization now being set up for handling Iranian supply requests, whereby a central supply council is to be established in Tehran with Iranian, British and American representation. This council will consider the needs of Iran and pass on its recommendations to London and Washington for final consideration. It was explained that this would afford the American Government triple opportunity to make sure that everything possible was being done to meet Iran's requirements. Mr. Saleh expressed himself as very pleased that such an arrangement was to be put into effect. . . . Mr. Saleh reiterated several times his belief that the United States should deal directly with the Iranian Government in matters of supplies, rather than to permit everything to be channeled through the United Kingdom Commercial Corporation. He said that Iran much preferred not to have to deal with the British and only acquiesced in their intervention out of necessity. For example, last fall he had attempted to obtain a quantity of tires. There were considerable delays, and finally the British had told the Iranian Government that the tires could be obtained through the UKCC and had persuaded the Tehran authorities to agree to a distribution of 40% of the tires to the UKCC for British use in Iran, 40% for the Iranian Government and 20% for Iranian civilian use. Despairing of getting the tires through the American Government direct, Tehran had agreed to this arrangement.

Cable to Dreyfus on May 5, 1942 (Telegram 115, 891.24/100):

Saleh called at Department May 1 and expressed uneasiness regarding possible discouragement of Iranian Government as result of failure to obtain wheat and other supplies from the United States. He said the British were telling his Government that supplies from the United States could only be obtained through the United Kingdom Commercial Corporation and he feared Iranian authorities in Tehran would conclude that United States is no longer interested in assisting Iran. In such a case Saleh thought his mission would probably be recalled. He thought it would be most unfortunate if we failed to do something positive and so gave the impression that we intended to leave Iran at the mercy of the British and Russians. Following is a summary of our oral reply to Saleh which you may use with Iranian Government as occasion offers:

> "The United States is decidedly not (repeat not) losing interest in Iran and has every intention of doing whatever is possible to assist in the relief of that country's difficult situation. The program of wheat purchases which Saleh was instructed to carry out could not be completed because the limited shipping space available was already taken up by a previously arranged British program for supplies to Iran of which this Government was unaware at the time negotiations with Saleh were begun. However, the Department intends to make sure that adequate supplies of wheat, within the limits of shipping possibilities, are in fact delivered to Iran whether from British or other sources. According to your reports and information received from British Embassy Washington, fairly substantial quantities of wheat are now being received and at least 30,000 tons are now at sea or in process of shipment from American ports to Iran. We felt that these quantities should take care of the most urgent needs for the time being and we would give further consideration to the question as soon as definite information regarding the coming harvest is available.
>
> "This Government, in conjunction with the British, is now setting up machinery to insure proper handling of Iranian requests for economic assistance. This includes formation of an Anglo-American-Iranian central supply council which will forward its recommendations to the Middle East Supply Center at Cairo, on which the United States will also be represented. The recommendations of MESC will be forwarded to Washington and London for final consideration. The United States will thus participate fully in determination of Iranian needs and supply possibilities and will be able to make its interest felt more effectively than in the past. This system will, it is believed, also make for greater speed and efficiency in every respect in dealing with supply problems. Saleh was told that this Government attaches great importance to his continued presence in the United States where it is felt he plays a

> very important role. In addition to the trade agreement negotiations, for which it is essential that he be here, he will undoubtedly be needed to supervise the actual procurement and shipment of goods scheduled by the supply council in Tehran and the MESC and to deal directly with the American agencies concerned in all matters connected therewith."

As the telegram indicates, the State Department had no knowledge of the workings of the MESC. In addition, Saleh was told that 30,000 tons of wheat was en route to Iran. Cable to Dreyfus on May 21, 1942 (Telegram 137, 891.24/200A):

> Saleh had received a telegram from his Government stating you have informed Iranian authorities that the United States has shipped 30,000 tons of wheat for Iran. There appears to have been a misunderstanding in this connection, since all wheat shipped from United States ports has been sent by the British, with the exception of 6,000 tons purchased by Saleh. The statement made in Department's 115, May 5 that at least 30,000 tons were at sea or in process of shipment from American ports referred to British shipments and to Saleh's purchase, not (repeat not) to any consignments made by this Government. Saleh is cabling his Government to correct this misunderstanding.

It turned out that the claim that the 6,000 tons of wheat (part of 20,000 tons) purchased by Saleh was on its way to Iran had no foundation in facts. Only 400 tons had been shipped and even that was sunk.

On May 13, 1942, Saleh had written to Wright Thomas at the State Department (Letter, 891.24/199):

> Yesterday, when Mr. Frederick Winant was good enough to call at my office here, I discussed with him the Iranian Government's order for the purchase in the United States of approximately $200,000 worth of medical supplies for shipment to Iran. I stated to him that, as a result of the war, Iran has not been able to import the medical needs of the country from other places, and I asked him if there was any possibility of obtaining export license and shipping space for the above order. I explained to him that I have not yet taken action in regard to the purchase of this material feeling that I should first make sure that it will be possible to ship the material to Iran once it is purchased. Mr. Winant asked me to write this letter to you as he will be absent from Washington for a few days, and he assured me that you will be good enough to

take the necessary steps to find out what are the present prospects of obtaining a license and shipping space for the above material. I shall appreciate any steps you may take on this matter, and I hope that you will be able to write to me at your earliest convenience.

On May 22, 1942, Saleh had written to Alling, Murray's successor as Chief of the Near Eastern Division (Letter and enclosures, 891.24/213):

> I beg to enclose herewith copies of two letters, dated May 15th and 22nd, which I have written to Mr. Frederick Winant of the Division of Exports and Defense Aid in regard to the needs of Iran. Ever since we discussed this subject at the office of Mr. Wallace Smith Murray on Friday, May 1st, particularly after the official announcement that Iran had been placed in the list of lend-lease countries, I have been receiving cables from Teheran in which the Ministry of Finance points out the urgent need of Iran for various materials and asks me to take action for their early shipment. I have not been able to give a definite answer to these cables, in view of the fact that I have been awaiting the decision of the State Department as to the procedure to be followed by us in the matter of applying for license and shipping space. It now seems that the situation, particularly in the matter of the extreme need for trucks and tires, is becoming acute. . . . Like many other countries of the world our eyes are upon the United States. The immediate needs of Iran are so insignificant compared with the huge American effort and production that Iran believes it will be possible for you to relieve us from our present predicament, even if you were to spare a very limited portion of your assistance for Iran. I would, therefore, appreciate very much if you could once more bring to the attention of the State Department the question of Iran's needs, and to communicate to me at your earliest convenience the decision of the State Department in this matter.

Saleh's letter to Fred Winant, dated May 22, 1942, is an interesting document. The announcement on the extension of lend-lease to Iran had greatly raised hopes. The letter reads:

> In my letter of May 15, 1942, I explained about various articles that are needed in Iran, and I requested you to advise me at your earliest convenience of the new procedure in regard to obtaining licenses and shipping space for these goods. Since I mailed that letter, several tele-

grams have been received from the Ministry of Finance in Teheran. The question has again been brought up as to whether, now that Iran is officially on the list of lend-lease countries, the American Government will directly furnish the Government of Iran with shipping space, and whether facilities have been made under the present circumstances in regard to the issuing of licenses for Iranian needs. Special attention has been called to the following subjects:

Tires and Tubes; Trucks and Passenger Cars. Particular anxiety has been expressed in regard to the needs of Iran for tires and tubes. It seems that the American Legation in Teheran has obtained from the Iranian Government the figures concerning needs for passenger and truck tires, as well as passenger cars and trucks. It is stated that a large portion of the means of transport in Iran has been placed out of service as a result of lack of tires and spare parts. My attention has been called to the fact that, with the exception of the only trans-Iranian railway system, all of the domestic transportation of Iran is accomplished by motor vehicles. Camels, mules, and donkeys which carried a large portion of Iran's loads during past times have, in recent years, mostly disappeared, having given their places to motor vehicles. A situation has, therefore, been created wherein Iran depends entirely on motor vehicles for a major portion of its transportation. The need for transportation of war material to Russia and other Allied activities have brought about the appropriation of a considerable part of existing trucks, at the same time when Iran has not been furnished with any additional supply of trucks and tires for civilian purposes. The question of transportation in Iran has, therefore, reached an acute stage, as a result of which the economic condition of the country is daily becoming critical, so that in case urgent action is not taken to furnish Iran trucks and tires, it is feared that famine will break out all over the country, and a situation will be created which will be impossible to remedy. The Iranian Government, therefore, hopes that with the closest ties of friendship fortunately existing between Iran and the United States, and with the assurance that the Government of the United States desires to assist Iran in every possible respect, some urgent action will be taken to furnish Iran with certain quantities of trucks and tires. The Ministry of Finance in conclusion suggests that a part of trucks and tires that the Allies now own in Iran, or trucks and tires that are on the way between the United States and Iran, which may have been destined principally for Russian and British activities, be now placed in the hands of the Government of Iran in order to ameliorate the immediate situation.

Wheat. Notwithstanding the fact that certain quantities have been imported into Iran through the good offices of the British Government and certain quantities have been imported from Russia, and a shipment of 30,000 tons (according to the American Legation in Teheran) has recently been made from American ports, the shortage of wheat must still be met by the shipment from America of further quantities, as the last crop of wheat in Iran was actually 300,000 tons short of ordinary years. Therefore, the quantities that have reached Iran or that are on the way to Iran, will not be sufficient. I would, therefore, venture to ask that you be good enough to take further action so that our office here may be able to ship the remaining wheat which we purchased from Laval and Company, and which is ready for shipment. (As you know, a license for 5,750 tons of this wheat has already been issued.)

Sugar. The need for sugar has again been emphasized and it is explained that although certain quantities have been imported through the UKCC it is believed that the UKCC will not be able to furnish the remainder of Iran's needs in sugar. In my previous letter (dated May 15, 1942) I mentioned that we have negotiated with the Dyer Sugar Export Corporation for 1,100 tons of cube sugar. In your telephone conversation yesterday, you stated that while it might be possible to obtain license for granulated sugar, it would be impossible to obtain one for cube sugar. In this connection, we have talked with the Dyer Sugar Export Corporation which explains that the particular quantity of cube sugar prepared by them for shipment to Iran is a type that is not consumed in America but is especially prepared for exportation. The Dyer Sugar Export Corporation feels that in case the necessary explanation is given the authorities concerned will be willing to issue a license on this particular sugar. It, therefore, asks us to furnish the name of such authority so that it can explain the matter directly. I shall, therefore, appreciate it if you inform me of the name of the official to whom the necessary explanation must be given. In this connection, may I add that this 1,100 tons of cube sugar is a portion of the sugar that the Dyer Sugar Export Corporation had prepared last year for exportation to Iran. The Corporation had actually obtained a license for the exportation of that sugar, but as a result of later developments, the license expired and the shipment of the material became impossible.

Paper. Iran is in need of a minimum of 500 tons of paper, which I believe is mainly for the use of newspapers. In this connection, it is explained that the Iranian Government had placed an order for 1000

> tons of paper with the UKCC. The UKCC has, however, advised that it will be impossible to deliver more than 200 tons while the Ministry of Finance emphasizes that at least 500 tons will be needed in addition to the 200 tons accepted by the UKCC.
>
> Medical Supplies. Another material that has been mentioned in the recent telegram from the Ministry of Finance is medical supplies. As I wrote to Mr. Wright Thomas on May 13 on your suggestion, I had formerly received orders for approximately $200,000 worth of medical supplies. As a result of the answer received from Mr. Thomas, I am trying to prepare a list of articles that are actually needed, and as soon as that list is ready, I shall forward it to you. I am mentioning this here in case you may want to take it into consideration when making arrangements for Iranian needs.

Soon after, control of imports for Iran was assigned to the Middle East Supply Center in Cairo and its Tehran branch, the Central Supplies Committee, dealt with in chapter 7. State Department instruction to Dreyfus on June 6, 1942 (Telegram 145, 891.24/201A): "We have advised Saleh that all Iranian supply requests not already in process of approval should be submitted first to the Central Supply Committee at Tehran. He is also informing his Government." The above notwithstanding, on July 23, 1942, Saleh had written to Orsen Nielsen of the Division of Defense Materials (Letter, 891.24/229):

> This is to remind you of my talk over the telephone with you a few days ago on the question of two hundred trucks and accessories needed for the Iranian Army which the Government of Iran desires to obtain under lend-lease. As I must send an answer to the cable from the Ministry of Finance, I shall appreciate any information that you may be able to give me on this subject. P.S. Did you hear anything further from the British authorities in regard to our wheat? If you are good enough to let me know the names of the British authorities concerned about this matter, I shall also try to get in touch with them.

Nielsen's reply of July 27, 1942:

> With reference to your letter of July 23, 1942, I am glad to be able to inform you that the 200 trucks and accessories are receiving active consideration. Your Minister in Washington is maintaining close contact with the Department regarding this matter. The British Supply

Council in Washington has not as yet received further information from London with respect to the 9,600 tons of wheat. Mr. Alan (sic) Christelow is handling the details at this end.

On August 17, 1942, Saleh had submitted an aide mémoire to Under Secretary Welles. He first gives a brief outline of American-Iranian relations up to World War II, his arrival in the US on November 1, 1941, pointing out that "in the matter of shipping American material to Iran my mission has been a total failure," and describes economic conditions in Iran:

> As a result of war and particularly the events of August 1941, Iran was faced with a very serious economic situation. The Iranian railway and nearly all other means of transportation were appropriated by the Allied powers for the purpose of transporting war materials to Russia. The shortage of grain and the impossibility of distributing food material in the country as a result of lack of means of transport threatened Iran with famine. The Iranian Government instructed me to buy wheat in the United States and ship to Iran immediately. With the approval of the State Department I purchased 10,000 tons of wheat, for which the State Department promised shipment. Only 400 tons of this was actually shipped (and that was sunk). The remainder still lies in New York and we are compelled to pay $6,000 a month for warehouse charges. British authorities later agreed to exchange a part of this wheat for a similar quantity that they had afloat and we were advised by the State Department that we should sell the remainder. The exchange has not yet taken place and there is no market at the present time for selling wheat in America. Our efforts to send the needed quantity of tires and tubes as well as trucks did not bring forth any result. A similar situation has existed with regard to various other materials, such as sugar, matches, medical supplies, etc.

Saleh then comments on the workings of the Middle East Supply Center (MESC) and its branch in Tehran, the Central Supply Committee (CSC):

> When the name of Iran was officially placed on the Lend-Lease program the hope of the Iranians rose, but we later found out that we could not send to Iran even things for which we had paid for or we were willing to pay for in cash. A system was established whereby we had to make our requests to a so-called Central Supply Committee in

> Teheran. If the Committee approved of our request the matter had to be taken up with another committee in Cairo and later through the United Kingdom Commercial Corporation in New York. The establishment of this system necessitated various formalities and delays. The result of all this has been that I have not yet heard of any of our applications having been approved by these committees. Consequently, conditions in Iran are becoming acute. The State Department knows very well of disturbances that have been taking place all over the country. It also knows of the existing discontent and unrest among Iranians which has resulted in the lack of stability of Government. The result of all these conditions is that the people of Iran are hungry and no Government can remain in power unless it provides food for them.

He notes that the Government of Iran had requested various American advisers and the State Department had consented:

> It is my duty to call your attention to the fact, however, that these American advisers will not be successful in their work if the Government of the United States does not decide promptly to furnish Iran with certain very needed materials, for what can a Supply Administrator do in Iran if he has no wheat at his disposal to send to hungry people, or if given the necessary quantities of wheat, what can he be expected to do if he does not have the necessary trucks with which he might distribute his wheat in a vast country like Iran? A similar question might be asked in regard to an Administrator for Sanitation who had not in his possession any medical supplies to meet immediate demands of the country. A lack of success on the part of these advisers at such an anxious time in Iran would reflect upon their entire work and upon the future of Iranian-American relations. I would, therefore, request that the Government of the United States give urgent attention to this matter and supply Iran with at least some of the material it badly needs. The present procedure is, I believe, not suitable to the present emergency. It is already very late and I therefore beg that something be done before it is too late. I cannot suggest what procedure should be adopted but I do believe that no immediate result will be achieved unless a decision is taken by the higher authorities of the United States Government.

The memorandum ends with this poignant remark: "It is impossible to explain to Iranians how no shipping can be provided for some of the immediate needs of Iran while the people of Iran constantly observe that

American material is being unloaded in the Persian Gulf and carried through Iran to Russia."

Cable to Dreyfus on August 19, 1942 (Telegram 217, 891.5018/5A):

> In an interview with Under Secretary August 17 Saleh stated that Iran is facing a critical situation due to food and transport shortage and that despite all assurances given during the past months no supplies to remedy this condition have been received. Please telegraph available information on the following points: 1. What steps are being taken to relieve the food shortage? Do you consider situation so serious that Department should press for shipment of wheat despite shortage of shipping space? 2. Do you believe wheat shortage could be relieved without imports if essential transport and distribution were improved? 3. What steps are being taken, through Central Supplies Committee or otherwise, to relieve transport situation? British have repeatedly informed us some 44,000 tires were being sent to Iran (in addition to the 24,230 requisitioned on Iranian behalf and now about to be shipped from this country). Have any of these tires been received and distributed for civilian use? Are spare parts and accessories being obtained to place in service large number trucks previously reported laid up? Are additional trucks being obtained from any source? 4. What is the status of proposed transport committee? 5. Please cable summary of Iranian requests so far presented to CSC, action taken by Committee and action taken by MESC on any recommendations forwarded by CSC. Do you consider CSC and MESC are functioning efficiently with respect to Iran?

Dreyfus' recommendations contained in his reply of August 26, 1942, were to have unfortunate consequences. As indicated in chapter six, his optimism was possibly a result of the establishment of an Allied-Iranian Road Transport Board which was expected to solve Iran's critical transport problem. The correspondence between the Iranian Prime Minister, Ahmad Qavam, and the British Legation mentioned in the cable is given in chapter 13. The cable reads (Telegram 271, 891.5018/6):

> Department's 217, August 19. Following answers to Department's numbered paragraphs. One. Wheat. See my number 251 August 5. It is doubtful if there is an actual wheat shortage in Iran. The problem is primarily an internal one of collecting in rural areas and distributing to urban areas wheat crop which has just been harvested. Iran is normally

self-sufficient in wheat and this year's crop is on the whole fair. The Government has been delinquent in locating the wheat and making hoarders disgorge and hence a serious shortage in urban centers has developed. Other than take strong measures to correct this internal situation the Iranians prefer to have Allies ship 100,000 tons of wheat which will cause prices to fall and hoarders sell. British Legation in a note to Prime Minister August 19 takes stand that Allies have fulfilled their obligation by providing Iran with 80,000 tons of wheat which carried them over to the harvest, that since present harvest is good the country should have sufficient wheat for all for the greater part of the coming year and that before turning to Allies Iran should take energetic steps to collect wheat and apply hoarding laws. On Iranian side it may be said that collection is extremely difficult under present circumstances and it may be impossible with the best of good will to obtain control of a large portion of the crop. For example the crop in Azerbaijan is excellent and should help in supplying the urban centers with 350,000 tons a year they need but it is not expected Soviets will permit surplus to be exported. My recommendation is that we support British stand and insist that Iranians take necessary measures to help themselves before asking us to provide vital shipping space for imports but that we keep an open mind as to necessity for later shipments if these measures fail to remedy the situation. Two. Transport and distribution are important phases of wheat problem but it is believed they can be satisfactorily dealt with if basic problem of finding and obtaining control of wheat can be solved. Three and Four. Active steps are being taken to solve transport problem. Iranian Government has employed Birkle, formerly UKCC Manager here and a transport expert, as director of transport and is now forming after much delay the transport board outlined in my 242, July 27. Iranian Government has obtained possession of part of the three thousand tires mentioned in my 242 but will need considerable stocks in near future. The 44,000 tires imported by British, part already received, are strictly for use of UKCC in war transport and cannot be released for civilian use. UKCC has some 17,000 tires in stock and it may be possible for them to lend tires to transport board against eventual return from 24,230 allocated to Iran. Spare parts are being received to place laid up trucks in service. It is hoped that above measures will result in substantial improvement in transport picture. Five. CSC . . . Iran Government has now called in all outstanding orders (those placed before June 21) and is in process of classifying and submitting them to CSC. So far two commodity groups (16,000 tons of sugar, 398 tons of tea and 150 tons of paper) have been presented to CSC which immediately approved them substantially as presented and passed them on to MESC whose action is as

> yet unknown. . . . It is my opinion that CSC and MESC are functioning energetically and efficiently with respect to Iran. Delays have been caused by Iranians first in approving import licensing system; second, in publishing notices; and third, in examining and transmitting outstanding orders to CSC. Summary. Saleh's statement that Iran faces critical situation is true but his inference that blame therefore lies entirely with Allies is unfair. It has been very difficult to get Iranian cooperation and there has been great delay, confusion and inefficiency on part of Iranian Government. Both British Minister and I have had to press Prime Minister repeatedly in above matters and our efforts are just now beginning to bear fruit. It will never be possible to satisfy Iranians fully in matter of (supplies) since they are unable to appreciate basic fact of acute shipping shortage.

Soon after sending this cable, Dreyfus must have come to regret having expressed such opinions. The consequences for Iran were tragic, but this is just what the State Department wanted to hear. Murray's memorandum to Welles on August 28, 1942 (891.5018/8):

> I refer to your conversation on August 17 with Mr. Allah Yar Saleh, head of the Iranian Trade and Economic Commission, at which time he left with you a memorandum setting forth Iran's need for civilian supplies. In accordance with your instruction, I have looked into the present status of the civilian supply program for Iran. You have undoubtedly already seen the attached telegram No. 271 from our Minister at Tehran, in which the Minister gives his opinion that the wheat shortage is largely the fault of the Iranian Government. He recommends that we insist upon better control of domestic wheat supplies and advises against shipment from abroad at this time. In view of the acute shortage of shipping space, I am inclined to agree with the Minister's views, especially since we expect to dispatch to Iran within the next week or two a competent American adviser to assist the Iranian Government with its food and general supply difficulties. We hope that this man, Mr. J.P. Sheridan, will be able to straighten out many of the internal troubles which have contributed to the present situation. Accordingly, we have drafted the attached telegram to Tehran, supporting the Minister's recommendation. In the light of the Minister's report, I do not believe that we should take any further action at present. The procedure which has been worked out for regular, coordinated handling of Iranian supply needs through the Middle East Supply Center is now beginning to function, and there is as yet no reason to believe that it will not prove satisfactory.

The telegram to Tehran mentioned by Murray is dated August 29, 1942 (Telegram 227, 891.5018/6):

> Your 271, August 26. Department approves your recommendation and authorizes you to join British in insisting that Iranians take all possible steps to effect efficient control and distribution of domestic wheat supplies before requesting further imports. In taking this action we have in mind imminent departure of Sheridan, who should be of great assistance in straightening out internal organization. Kidd, who should be able to help with work of transport board, was to leave London August 27 for Tehran via Cairo.

With the above instruction, the American government could not escape responsibility for the lamentable conditions that followed. Moreover, Joseph P. Sheridan turned out to be unsuited to the task.

Iranian Note to Casey

Dreyfus was forced to change his tune on October 31, 1942 (Dispatch 366 and enclosures, 891.00/1954):

> I have the honor to enclose a copy of a letter from the Foreign Minister, October 24, 1942, and an Aide-Mémoire enclosed therewith, the latter having been prepared for the information of Minister of State Casey on the occasion of his recent visit to Tehran. I commend this Aide-Mémoire to the Department's earnest attention, since it represents a faithful representation of the Iranian Government's position vis-à-vis the allies and includes many of the Iranian complaints and claims to which I have drawn the Department's attention in telegrams during the past few months. While the Iranians have, as they often do, overstated their case somewhat, I feel there is a great deal of justice in their complaints that their food, railways, transport facilities and general economic situation have been exploited or depleted by the allies for their own benefit.

Foreign Minister Saed's note of October 16, 1942, to Casey is given in entirety, with emphasis in the original:

> The Imperial Iranian Government desire first of all to express their sincere appreciation of the assistance that the British Government have so far rendered to Iran. If, however, they should deem it necessary to

persist in their justifiable request for further indispensable economic help, it should not be regarded in any respect by the British Government as implying a lack of recognition on the part of the Iranian Government of the assistance thus afforded them.

The principal requirements of the Iranian Government are essentially concerned with the supply of foodstuffs, and the attention of the British representative in Teheran has been repeatedly called to the scarcity of food that is experienced and to the difficult and unpleasant situation arising therefrom. In the second place, the means of communication which, owing to its close connection with the transportation of food has also from time to time been the subject of a number of representations. It is hoped that the British Government will agree that neither of these two requests can scarcely be considered as extravagant or unreasonable. Obviously the present difficulties of Iran in respect to the above questions are in no small degree due to the events of last August with the entry of the forces of the Allies into Iran and their being stationed in the country. The Allied troops, whose exact number though unknown to the Iranian Government has never apparently been fewer than 50,000, have acquired for their use a considerable quantity of local food supplies. In addition to this, a large number of Polish nationals, whose number can be estimated at between thirty and forty thousand, are living in Iran and their livelihood naturally constitutes an additional drain on the food supplies of the country. Furthermore, a large quantity of foodstuffs finds its way out of Iran either by being smuggled out of the country owing to the prevailing situation referred to above which on the frontier makes complete control impossible; or *in some cases by being directly purchased and exported by the Allies.* It is not possible to determine the exact quantity of foodstuffs thus taken out of the country as the observance of the usual declaration of such goods at the Customs is often refused. *However, the scarcity of food which is prevailing throughout the country and is daily growing in intensity is a clear indication of a considerable quantity of food supplies that is continually flowing out of the country.* Finally, workmen numbering about 70,000, who should normally be at work on the land, have been occupied in rail and road construction for the Allies. Consequently these men are not only unable to contribute to the production of food for the nation, but their livelihood is to some extent a further burden on the country's food resources. It will thus be observed that the actions of the Allies have, directly or indirectly, adversely affected the food situation in the country.

With regard to the country's means of communication, as has repeatedly been pointed out, apart from the fact that a number of cars and lorries amounting to 473 were requisitioned or otherwise lost at the time of occupation of Iranian territory, the United Kingdom Commercial Corporation have now in their service a large part (about 1500 – amounting to practically 40%) of the entire fleet of lorries in the country, thereby leaving available a relative small number out of all proportion to the transport requirements for the necessary distribution of wheat, etc., throughout the country. The UKCC, not being content with this, claim for themselves the exclusive right to distribute the quantity of tires and spare parts apportioned to Iran by USA. On the other hand, although the UKCC have for some time past promised their assistance in the matter of executing orders placed by the Iranian Government for tires and spare parts, they have so far not only rendered no assistance in this respect, but they have on the contrary availed themselves of a great part of these orders. Moreover, the Trans-Iranian Railway, as well as the Tabriz Railway, is under the control of the Allies and serve to carry their supplies. It is therefore hoped that it will be appreciated that the request of the Iranian Government to be enabled to meet their own transport requirements is not asking for a gratuitous favour, but rather an expectation of a return for the benefits which the Allies are deriving from the entire resources of the country.

The Iranian Government and people accordingly expect that the Allies will fulfill their promises of assistance to relieve the economic position of the country as stipulated in the Tripartite Pact. The assistance so far rendered by the Allies during the past ten months falls short however of the vital needs of Iran. If, in view of the foregoing, the Iranian Government have felt themselves justified in persisting that their reasonable requests be complied with, can they be justly charged with lack of appreciation of the assistance so far rendered? Should not the Iranian Government in their turn regret that the assistance so far received in turn for the many benefits the Allies have undoubtedly derived from Iran be so insignificant?

The suggestions that the Iranian Government have been tardy in securing the available stock of the country's grain, that the price offered for wheat has been low and that the officials have not been efficient in collecting the stocks would not seem to conform to facts. As a matter of fact the price of wheat has been raised by 150% during the past year in the various parts of the country, but as the agents of the Allies, without their observing the regulations, have purchased monopoly and non-monopoly goods, the price of all kinds of commodities has risen abnormally and the owners, in expectation of still higher prices, are reluctant to dispose of their goods to the Government. It therefore follows that the difficulty in collecting the available stocks of wheat in the country is also to a certain extent due to interference on the part of the Allies' agents.

The Iranian Government desire to emphasize that in making their representations they have been careful to refrain from exaggeration or extravagance and have never put forward any unreasonable claim. On the contrary they have always been mindful of the prevailing transport difficulties, and what requests they have so far made have been with regard to the international situation and the minimum needs of the country, and they have therefore endeavored to make them as moderate as possible. Accordingly, the Government and the people of Iran look forward to the Allies, taking into consideration the economic situation of Iran, the deterioration of which has been principally due to their operations; and further, having due regard to the promises they have made in this respect in the Tripartite Pact, to take immediate steps to comply with the requests of Iran. If the anticipated fulfillment of these requests is not forthcoming at the appropriate time, the situation in Iran will be liable to deteriorate and the consequences will inevitably devolve unfavorably on both Iran and the Allies.

I trust that His Britannic Majesty's Government, after giving due consideration to the foregoing statements, will see their way to meet the earnest wishes of the Iranian Government and I feel sure that the sympathetic consideration of the very important and, I should say, vital matters contained in the above communication would be most highly appreciated by my Government.

British Counteractions in Washington

British agencies in Washington, with the consent of the State Department, had sabotaged Saleh's efforts to obtain supplies for Iran. On March 25, 1942, the British representative on the Board of Economic Warfare (BEW), had telephoned Jernegan (Memorandum, 891.24/199):

Mr. Williamson called me at the suggestion of Mr. Peurifoy, DE, with regard to an application for export license filed by Laval & Co., Inc., 2 Broadway, New York, to cover 735,000 bushels of Manitoba wheat consigned to the Iranian Ministry of Finance. Although the application

> does not state, Mr. Williamson thought, and I agreed, that this purchase was undoubtedly made by Mr. Saleh, head of the Iranian Trade and Economic Mission in the United States. (It appears that 735,000 bushels is roughly 20,000 long tons or 24,000 short tons, which is approximately the figure Mr. Saleh is understood to have had in view for his initial purchase.) Mr. Williamson explained that the British Ministry of Food in London has in effect a program of wheat supply to Iran. Under this plan shipments of Canadian wheat averaging 17,000 tons monthly have been made to Iran. For the month of April only 14,500 tons are scheduled, although if shipping space is available the quantity may be increased to 20,000 tons. These shipments are made through the ports of New York and Baltimore, being handled by three main firms in those cities, one of them being Laval & Co. . . . Mr. Williamson does not know the exact basis upon which the Ministry of Food's program was worked out, but he thinks it was based upon calculations of the needs of Iran taken in combination with available shipping. He admits that it may be inadequate for Iranian needs and that any additional wheat that might be sent from this country would probably be very helpful. (Incidentally, he thinks that wheat may be going to Iran from other sources as well as from Canada at present.) Upon learning today of Laval & Co.'s export license application, Mr. Williamson communicated with the Ministry of Food's wheat agents in Montreal and asked them to check with London on the matter. Accordingly, they are cabling London this afternoon and will inform Mr. Williamson immediately upon receipt of a reply. I was unable to learn exactly why Mr. Williamson felt it necessary to take this action, except that he seems to feel that shipments by Saleh might possibly upset the general Ministry of Food program in some way. He also said that he had been informed that the shipping situation was bad and had been surprised when Mr. Fred Winant told him that space was believed to be available for Saleh's proposed initial shipment early next month. On hearing this, he had requested the Joint Shipping Board in New York, or its representative there, to check and advise him. I told Mr. Williamson that, as he already knew from Mr. Winant, the Department is anxious to see Saleh's shipment go forward, and he said that he agreed entirely. He said he could see no reason, other than lack of shipping, for limiting wheat going to Iran. He promised to let me know as soon as he received word from Montreal.

On March 26, 1942, Williamson had telephoned Jernegan (Memorandum, 891.24/186):

Mr. Williamson said that Montreal has received an answer to its cable of yesterday to the Ministry of Food in London, regarding the wheat which Mr. Saleh wants to ship to Iran. The substance of London's reply was to the effect that it hoped the shipment would not be permitted. If additional supplies were needed in Iran, the Ministry would make every effort to provide them. Mr. Williamson repeated what he had said yesterday to the effect that his information indicated that almost no shipping space was available for Saleh's shipment, despite the assertion made by Saleh that the Isthmian Line had promised him 4,000 tons of space on a ship sailing April 5. Mr. Williamson asked that the State Department check with the War Shipping Administration on this matter, since, as he pointed out, the ship involved is American and is not subject to British control. He made the definite statement that the British program of sending wheat has been actually in operation for two or three months, and that the January and February shipments actually amounted to about 28,000 tons each. I suggested that it might be useful for all interested persons in the British and State Department organizations to get together and discuss the Middle East food situation, as there seemed to be a great deal of misapprehension. Mr. Williamson agreed and said he would try to arrange something of the sort within a few days, when he would have full information. I mentioned that early this month the British Embassy had suggested that we should help out the Iranian situation by supplying, among other things, bread. He expressed great surprise at this.

Cable to Dreyfus on April 1, 1942 (Telegram 80, 891.24/178A):

Confidential. Department informed that British Ministry of Food has program contemplating shipment of approximately 17,000 tons Canadian wheat monthly to Iran consigned to "Irano-British Trading Corporation" for consumption by civilian population and Allied Military Forces. Please telegraph available information on following points: One. Has execution of any such program begun? Two. Is it satisfactory to the Iranian Government? Three. On what basis is distribution made? Four. Is Iran at present importing wheat from any other source for its own needs? In what quantities? Five. Estimated imports required to satisfy minimum Iranian needs? Six. Do you consider that Ministry of Food program, if carried out, would eliminate necessity for other imports of wheat? In any discreet inquiries which you may make in this connection, you should avoid giving the impression (a) that the United States is thinking of leaving question of Iranian food supply entirely in British hands, or (b) that we doubt good faith and good intentions of either Iranians or British. Reference Department's 66, March 13, for your confidential information, it has been found that Canadian wheat can be purchased in open market more cheaply than American. Consequently, Saleh has purchased about 10,000 long tons Manitoba wheat and is trying to arrange shipment small quantity next month. Lend-Lease machinery not repeat not involved but this Government is giving active assistance in obtaining shipping space and expediting export license.

Dreyfus replied on April 6, 1942 (Telegram 97, 891.24/179):

Following answers to numbered paragraphs of Department's No. 80, April 1. (One) British Minister assumes the 17,000 tons referred to by Department consists of 8,000 tons wheat and 8,800 flour (half of latter for Polish army in Iran) to be delivered in April only. None has arrived but first consignment is expected shortly. (Two) Iranians allege that British promises of 8,000 tons monthly not being fulfilled only about 6,000 being received. British express annoyance that Iranians would prefer Allied seamen to risk lives to bring wheat rather than make local hoarders disgorge. (Three) All above wheat for Iranian Government which is responsible for distribution. (Four) British state they have furnished Iran 40,000 tons since August mostly from India. They are now sending 3,000 tons monthly to East Iran from India. Iranian Government has purchased some 6,000 or 7,000 tons from Soviets and 10,000 tons bought in the United States by Saleh. (Five) British and Iranians do not agree on minimum needs. Latter place minimum needs up to end of July at 60,000 tons of which 20,000 immediately. They further estimate they will need to import 100,000 tons from July 1942 (harvest time) to July 1943. British believe that promised April deliveries plus whatever they can send in May plus other Iranian purchases should tide Iran over until new crop comes in. British Minister informs me confidentially that in his opinion very little wheat need be imported after new crop comes in and that small amount needed might be obtained in Iraq where there should be surplus. (Six) Although Iranian estimate of 60,000 tons needed up to July seems high it may be that British estimate is too low and that some wheat from the United States will be required. No estimate of needs after July can properly be made until new crop comes in. Iran although normally self-sufficient in wheat may have to continue importing as sowings this year were subnormal due to disturbed conditions.

The telegram concludes with the following:

> This matter of economic assistance for Iran must be approached carefully since it involves not only our relations with Iran but also the British and hence our war effort. British as the Department knows have had great difficulty with Iranians and have had to use question of supply of essential goods as a weapon to obtain some degree of cooperation. . . . I have consistently recommended avoidance of undue pressure on Iranians and advised against joining British in representations to Iran Government unless such action essential to war effort. I feel that present Iranian intransigence toward British is potentially harmful to war effort and I recommend we work in close harmony with British in question of supplies for Iran. While British themselves are somewhat responsible for their bad relations with Iran we cannot escape fact that Iranians by refusal to cooperate with our Allies are creating potentially harmful situation. Our economic policy with regard to Iran should dovetail with that of British in order to avoid placing our Allies in disadvantageous position and to prevent appearance of backing Iran against the British.

A year later, Dreyfus must have had ample reason to regret having given such advice.

Dreyfus follows up on April 25, 1942 (Telegram 124, 891.24/184):

> Referring to the Department's no. 92, April 15, 7 p.m. Since Legation's last report (see telegram 97, April 6) 7,059 tons of wheat 6,000 tons of sugar and 1,500 tons of flour have been imported bringing total wheat imports since September 1, 1941 to 51,208.81, and sugar imports same period 27,381 tons. The British Legation states that in addition 13,905 tons of wheat of which 7,350 is from Australia had just arrived or is now arriving. A further 3,200 tons is expected before May 1 and a last installment of 14,000 tons is expected in May and June.

The above indicates that British wheat imports for the eight-month span of September 1, 1941 to April 30, 1942, amounted to 65,113 tons, or an average of 8,140 tons per month. This did not even meet the needs of the occupation armies, the 70,000 laborers employed by the Allies, 40,000 Polish refugees, and 100,000 oil company employees, let alone provide for the civilian population.

On April 16, 1942, John S. Dent of the British Embassy in Washington had written to Fred Winant, Office of Export Control (Letter, 891.24/236):

> Dear Winant, I think you may be interested in the gist of a telegram which I have just seen which our Minister in Teheran dispatched to London on April 4th. He informed London that the State Department had informed your Minister in Persia that a representative of the Persian Government in the United States purchased 10,000 tons of Canadian wheat and that your Government was assisting him to ship it. H.M. Ambassador stated that he had explained to your Minister that independent efforts to obtain space for wheat would embarrass our arrangements for supplying the country and would tend to encourage the Persians in the tiresome attitude they have taken up on the subject of currency. He continued "to enable U.S. Ambassador to reply to detailed questions from his Government about the needs of Persia for wheat and about supplies to Persia from all sources I have furnished him with full information." I think you will be pleased to see that our representatives on the spot are getting into close touch on this subject and that it will be easy for them to discuss in future problems about Persian supplies. If you have occasion to telegraph to Teheran for information as is likely to happen if the Persians here continue to ask you for assistance you can rest assured that your Ambassador is in a position to ascertain without difficulty what arrangements we have made and what opinion is held by British representatives in Persia.

Having sabotaged Saleh's wheat shipment, the British had also succeeded in preventing other imports. On June 30, 1942, Allan Christelow of the British Supply Council in North America, had written to Winant (Letter and enclosure, 891.24/225):

> Dear Fred, I regret that we have done so slipshod a piece of work for you on Iranian sugar and on the other list of Iranian requirements which you handed to John Dent some time ago. I hope you will make it clear to the State Department that responsibility on delays rests not on London but on myself for, most unfortunately, nothing was done to report these cases during the month I was ill. Furthermore, I would be grateful if you would also point out that London has given speedy service when cases have been put to them. They did so in the case of newsprint and the first shipment of sugar, while the confusion over the wheat cannot, I think, be ascribed to them. In case of the miscella-

neous list of requirements which you gave to John Dent we have now received a reply, a paraphrase of which I enclose. Any delay in London's answer, other than that ascribed to my own inefficiency, should be attributed to the difficulties of communication with the Middle East and of checking a list of orders (none too clearly described) presented to them for the first time against a list of requirements for similar articles. Yours sincerely, Allan Christelow.

The mentioned telegram from London contains the following:

We have cabled the Middle East asking MESC for their opinion on the various requirements which you recently reported to us. We have not yet heard from MESC but we think that the State Department should be informed that the orders notified to us appear to duplicate items already sent to Iran by UKCC. For example, we have in the past three months alone shipped over £70,000 worth of medical supplies to Iran from the UK. We have also shipped 100 tons of baling wire for baling Iranian cotton and MESC feels that this will amply cover this year's requirements. UKCC have also placed orders in the US for chemicals required by the Iranian match industry, and we should be grateful if proper checks in order to avoid unnecessary duplication of orders and unnecessary burdening of the cable facilities between here and Teheran. In case of the matches we believe that adequate supplies for Iran will be available from India, and that this comparatively short haul should be preferred. We will cable you views of MESC as soon as we receive them for communication to State Department.

The next day, July 1, 1942, Christelow had written to Jernegan (Letter, 891.24/226):

I have instructed Mr. Geolot, our liaison officer in BEW not to protest the shipment of 1,100 tons of sugar for the Iranian Government when the export license is referred to him. . . . May I express the hope that IETC (Iranian Economic and Trade Commission) will be given clearly to understand that no further shipment from the US will be permitted unless they have the prior authorization of MESC, procurement in such cases being only through the established channels. I think you will agree with me that this sugar can be given only a very low shipping priority since Russian supplies and the requirements of our own military must have first claim on shipping space on a clearance capacity from the Iranian ports. The British Merchant Shipping Mission tell me that the clearance capacity allotted to Iranian requirements is only

> about 10,000 tons per month and that this amount would probably remain constant, since any increase in capacity would probably be used for sending increased amounts of war material to the Russian front. This clearance capacity covers goods arriving in Iranian ports from all loading areas, including those arriving from the United States.
>
> I think the best thing we can do is to make it quite clear to the Iranians that the total clearance tonnage which could be allotted to them is strictly limited and that if they obtain an extra 1,100 tons of sugar they will merely be depriving themselves of an equivalent capacity for other articles. It should also be made clear that even if the Iranians are confined to a clearance capacity of 10,000 tons the shipment of sugar from the United States is nevertheless a waste of shipping space, since the 1,100 tons should be provided on a short haul whenever supplies are available from short haul sources, leaving the US tonnage to carry those goods which can be procured only from the United States. If the sugar is allowed to go may I suggest that its approval should be conditional on distribution through the usual UKCC channels.

On July 18, 1942, Alling had informed Christelow that his "suggestions" had been duly conveyed to the Iranians:

> I refer to your recent telephone conversation with Mr. Jernegan of this Division and to your letter of July 1, 1942 regarding the 1,100 tons of sugar purchased by the Iranian Trade and Economic Commission. We were advised on July 7 that an export license had been granted for this shipment. In accordance with your suggestion, Mr. Saleh of the Iranian Trade and Economic Commission was informed that we would not object to the allotment of shipping space for the sugar, but that there was an over-all limitation on the amount of space available for civilian supplies for Iran from all sources and that, consequently, if the sugar were shipped it might later be necessary to refuse space for some more essential commodity which could only be obtained from the United States. Mr. Saleh said that he would take this into consideration in determining whether or not to proceed with the shipment.
>
> As Mr. Jernegan told you, we feel that for political reasons it would be desirable to have this particular sugar go forward, and the American shipping authorities with whom we have been in contact indicate that it should not be difficult to fit it on vessels whose main cargoes are of a different character. We are making it clear to Mr. Saleh, however, that no further sugar shipments from the United States will be consid-

> ered unless previously approved by the Central Supplies Committee at Tehran and the MESC.
>
> In the light of the cable from London which you enclosed with your letter of June 30 to Mr. Winant, we are taking no action on the informal Iranian requests for medical supplies and baling wire.

The subsequent critical shortage of medical and pharmaceutical supplies as well as sugar is described in chapter 9.

Chapter 5

Currency and Exchange Dispute with Britain and Paucity of Oil Revenues

Reference was made by Saleh to a financial accord with Britain in which after making concessions, Iran received nothing in return. In effect, while restricting imports, the British had forced Iran to print massive amounts of money to meet Allied war needs, resulting in hyperinflation. Dreyfus on September 24, 1941 (Telegram 163, 891.5151/208):

> Since the end of Iranian resistance to the British forces the local British Legation has been endeavoring to persuade Iranian authorities to establish for military expenditures stable rate of exchange of approximately 175 rials to the pound sterling. . . . The Ministry of Finance has held hearings on the subject and certain Iranian bankers have held out for a rate of 120 rials to the pound sterling. . . . British, after having financed their forces for some time by borrowing from Imperial Bank, have now demanded establishment of a new rate immediately and it is generally believed that such action will be taken within a day or two.

On September 29, 1941 (Telegram 172, 891.5151/209):

> Referring to the Legation's telegram no. 163 . . . the Iranian Council of Ministers established a new official exchange rate of 35 rials to the dollar. . . . The effect on the Legation's local staff will be little short of calamitous since each dollar paid in salaries will be diminished by ten rials. A new cost of living statement is in preparation and recommen-

dations for cost of living allowances and adjustments in salaries of Iranian employees will be made shortly.

Matters had rested until the spring of 1942.

First Currency Crisis

Dreyfus on March 28, 1942 (Telegram 82, 891.51A/521):

Referring to the Department's telegram no. 75, March 23, 11 p.m., the inability of Iran to dispose of foreign exchange because of lack of transportation facilities (see my 66, March 13, 4 p.m., paragraph one) and heavy sterling sales by British here estimated at a million pounds monthly have created tendency to raise rial value. This tendency is supported by a group of merchants represented in Majlis and by part of press. The "devaluation of pound" referred to by British is in fact raising of the rial value and would necessarily effect the dollar as much as sterling. The increase contemplated by those supporting revaluation is reported to be from present 140 rials to as much as 100 rials per pound. United States Government operation expenditures might therefore be increased by as much as 30%. Any effort to prevent revaluation would undoubtedly and with some reason be resented by Iranian officials as unnecessary and unjustified interference in their internal affairs in a matter not essential to our war effort and would contribute little toward transforming Iran from a "passive appendage" into a "willing partner" as suggested by the Department in its telegram no. 58, March 4, 9 p.m. I therefore do not recommend association with the British in this matter. A financial counselor has been added to the British Legation staff in order to prepare the British case. The threat to the Iranians that economic help or shipping space will be withheld in the event of revaluation is a very powerful weapon in British hands and will probably prove successful in preventing such action.

Dreyfus again on March 28, 1942 (Telegram 83, 891.515/76):

As the legal limit to the note issuance has been reached in Iran a critical situation has arisen. The currency shortage threatens to create an impasse in financial transactions especially for the British who must convert as much as a million pounds sterling monthly to defray expenditures in sending wages for their manifold war operations here. The British Minister informs me that the condition is so serious that he has

> been forced to issue an ultimatum to the Prime Minister that unless the government agrees to take steps at once to relieve the currency shortage the Imperial Bank and all its branches in Iran will close on Monday. This will probably result in a run on the Mellie Bank and would soon create widespread economic disturbances throughout the country. It is believed that the government realizing the gravity of the situation will take emergency measures to increase the note issue as requested by the British.

Dreyfus on March 30, 1942 (Telegram 87, 891.515/77):

> Iranian Government has given assurances to British Minister that legislation will be passed by tomorrow midnight raising legal limit of note issue to 2,700,000,000 rials, an increase of 700,000,000 rials. The Government appears to have become financially convinced of necessity for such action and proposes to authorize a larger increase than the British had suggested. British Minister informs me branches of Imperial Bank will not close today but will do so Wednesday unless legislation is enacted. He states he is satisfied with proposed increase and believes it will relieve the situation at least for the present. This still leaves unsolved the question of revaluation of rial.

Dreyfus on April 2, 1942 (Telegram 93, 891.515/78): "Referring to my telegram no. 87, March 30, 4 p.m. The law authorizing issuance of additional 700,000,000 rials was passed and situation with regard to currency is becoming normal."

Immediately after the passage of the currency law, a new dispute had arisen. Dreyfus' telegram of April 6, 1942, discussing wheat supplies for Iran, given above (Telegram 97, 891.24/179), also contains the following:

> British relations with Iran have arrived at a critical stage as result of present dispute over issue of currency and exchange control. Iranians finally increased note issue by 700 million rials but refused to issue currency against sterling holdings because of lack of confidence in both British and sterling. Instead new issue is backed by gold and crown jewels. Of the 700 million authorized 300 are for Government and remaining 400 are for exchange transactions an amount which will suffice British for only two months. Situation was altered and impasse reached because of Government order of April 1st directing banks to buy no more foreign exchange. Consequently British can at present

> obtain rials by overdrawing at Imperial Bank. This supply of credit will be exhausted in about ten days after which extensive war effort may have to be suspended for lack of rials. Iranians would like to have the 400 million rials used as a floating fund to supply British rials against importation of goods from sterling area. British refuse to bind selves to such a scheme and accuse Iranians of bad faith and virtual blackmail. British believe solution lies in (one) issuance of currency against sterling holdings, and (two) maintenance of exchange control which, if abolished, would, in view of growing Iranian foreign currency holdings, result in disastrous drop in pound and dollar. Memorandum setting forth British view is being forwarded by mail.

Dreyfus on April 7, 1942 (Dispatch 242 and enclosure, 891.24/183): "I have the honor, with reference to my telegram no. 97, dated April 6, 1942, to enclose the memorandum setting forth the British attitude with regard to the present dispute between the British and Iranians over the issue of rial currency and the rial-pound exchange rate." The memorandum, dated April 3, 1942, is entitled "Note on currency Situation in Persia." It reads:

> For a long time the currency supplies in Persia have lagged behind the country's needs. Recently currency had become even scarcer because of the promotion of important road, railway and harbour works in the country, mainly by His Majesty's Government, all directed towards the Allied War effort in the Middle East, and especially towards expediting the delivery of supplies, mainly American and British, to Russia. These works are paid for in Persian money at the prevailing standard rates. The rials have been obtained by the sale of sterling to the Exchange Commission at the controlled rate of Rials 140 equal one pound sterling. About two weeks ago the Exchange Commission informed the Imperial Bank of Iran (the British Government's banker in Persia) that, owing to the acute shortage of local currency, it could no longer undertake to deliver rials to the Bank against sales of sterling by His Majesty's Government. The Commission even found itself unable to deliver an amount of 170 million rials against purchases of sterling already effected by the bank for the Persian Government and of which a settlement was long overdue. On 27th March the situation was that the cash reserves of the Imperial Bank of Iran had dwindled to a little over 100 million rials, of which 50 million had to be ear-marked against urgent war requirements of the British Government, leaving only about 50 million available against liabilities of about 350 million rials. The cash reserves situation of the Banque Mellie Iran (the National bank)

was even more acute. A currency crisis was therefore in sight. Such a development in the situation had been foreseen by His Majesty's Legation, who had frequently and vigorously drawn the attention of the Persian Government to the necessity of obtaining statutory authority for an increase in the note circulation. (The legal limit was 2,000 millions, and His Majesty's Legation suggested that an addition of at least 500 millions was needed to meet the situation.) The question was, however, shelved for a month during the cabinet crisis, and another valuable week was lost by the new Government when the Mejlis adjourned over the No Ruz holidays.

When, therefore, a critical situation developed on 27th March, His Majesty's Minister found it necessary to ask the Prime Minister to take the following steps: (a) Legislation to increase the note-issue by at least 500 millions to be passed through all its stages not later than March 31st. (b) A minimum sum of 200 million rials in local currency to be delivered to the Imperial Bank of Iran before noon on March 30th. The Prime Minister was informed that if the situation was not met in this way it would be necessary for His Majesty's Government to take other steps, one of which would involve the cessation of payments of local currency by the Imperial Bank of Iran to its ordinary depositors. (This step was necessary because the Imperial Bank of Iran had undertaken, at the request of His Majesty's Minister, to conserve all the rials in its Treasury for the urgent war needs of His Majesty's Government). After several meetings of the Persian cabinet and secret cessions of juntas of the Mejlis, the Prime Minister informed His Majesty's Minister on the morning of March 30th that a Bill to increase the note issue by 700 million rials would be passed through the Mejlis on the following day, and that he would do his best to get the new notes issued immediately after the Bill had become law.

The Bill was duly passed by the Mejlis on March 31st, but in the following form: (a) The note issue is increased by 700 million rials to be covered by the value of the Crown Jewels. (b) The Banque Mellie is authorized to place the whole additional sum at the disposal of the Government in the form of an additional credit to be used as: (i) as to 300 millions for the internal purchase of monopoly goods, and (ii) as to 400 millions for transactions of foreign account. The Mejlis added two amendments as follows: (a) The period of the credit will be limited to 18 months, and (b) Within one month from now, the Government must present to the Mejlis a law amending the present enactments relating to Exchange Control. The Government has since made arrangements for the delivery to the Imperial Bank of Iran the 170 million rials owed from previous sterling transactions that they had previously been unable to settle. The passage of the Bill and the delivery of the notes to the Imperial Bank of Iran will ease the immediate currency situation but the form which the Bill takes and the policy which the Persian Government has indicated its intention of pursuing is likely to result in a fresh crisis in a few weeks' time.

During the discussions that have taken place between His Majesty's Legation and the Persian Government on the currency situation the Persian Government have manifested a strong disinclination to hold sterling balances; not only do they wish to cease to add to their sterling balances, but they are even seeking to liquidate in one way or another those that they already hold. They sought during the earlier stages of the note-issue discussions to extract from His Majesty's Government (in return for granting an increase in the note-issue) an understanding that His Majesty's Government would consent to a conversion of all or part of their existing sterling balances into gold or silver, and that His Majesty's Government would guarantee to deliver goods from the Sterling Area over the next twelve months to the value of our sales of sterling. His Majesty's Government declined to give any undertakings of the kind. Persia already holds adequate stocks of the precious metals, and His Majesty's Government found itself unable to associate itself with a conversion policy based on a mistrust of the pound sterling. As regards goods, His Majesty's Government was unable to give a guarantee which the general war situation might make it impossible for it to fulfill.

The situation is further complicated by the fact that the Government is seeking to bring about a drop in the value of the pound, and rumors have been put round the bazaar that the controlled rate is to be abolished and the rate allowed to go free, or alternatively that the rate of 140 is to be reduced to 120 or even to 100. As His Majesty's Government is now spending in Persia on war activities at the rate of about 200 million rials a month, any alteration in the rate, against sterling, is a matter of serious consequence, and His Majesty's Government could not consent to a reduction in the rate on any grounds other than the presentation of a convincing case that the present rate overvalued the purchasing power of the pound in terms of rials. No such case has as yet been made by the Persian Government.

On the day that the Currency Bill was presented to the Majlis, the Minister of Finance asked the Financial Adviser of His Majesty's Legation to call on him. The Minister of Finance explained the proposed provisions of the Bill, and went on to say that a corollary to it would be what he called his "Financial Plan." It was, he said, the intention of the Government to cease purchasing sterling from His Majesty's Government. In order that our need of rials might be met, however, he proposed to use the 400 millions provided by the Bill for transactions on foreign account to establish a "Floating fund" on which we could draw for our local currency needs. The Fund would be sustained by the value in rials of any goods imported into Persia by the Persian Government from the Sterling Area. The prices in rials at which such goods would be credited would be fixed by the Sterling area exporter, thus getting over for the present any difficulty about a rate of exchange. Further, it was, he said, the intention of the Government to abolish Exchange Control, and to allow the sterling/rial rate to go "free." He argued that as His Majesty's Government's requirements in rials would be met by the "Floating Fund" arrangement, it would cease to be a matter of consequence to His Majesty's Government what happened to the rate when it went free. The Financial Adviser informed the Minister of Finance that His Majesty's Minister could not acquiesce in any arrangement that would fail to secure to His Majesty's Government all the rials that it needed *against sales of sterling*, and further that he should in no circumstances commit the Persian Government to the policy of abolishing Exchange Control. The Bill was passed in the form described without any promise by the Government, at all events in public, that Exchange Control would be abolished, although the rider on the subject added by the Majlis (may) well have been inspired by the Government in secret session.

Even if the principle of a "Floating Fund" were acceptable to His Majesty's Government, an amount of 400 millions would meet our war needs for not much more than a couple of months. Rials are needed at the rate of about 200 million a month; imports by the Persian Government from the Sterling Area could not keep pace with the drain, especially as Lend/Lease aid, if granted, would diminish Persia's need to buy essentials from the Sterling Area. The Fund would therefore be exhausted in a matter of months. The effect of removing Exchange Control in present circumstances would be to lead to an immediate and perhaps substantial fall in the pound; but once the initial shock had been absorbed, the pound would tend to rise again, for the bazaar will always want to import more goods than it can export, and there would therefore be a demand for sterling. But the Government could intervene in the market, using its holdings of sterling in the manner of an Exchange Equalization Fund, and so manipulate the rate of exchange to suit itself.

> Late on the afternoon of 1st April, the Persian Government instructed the Banks to cease to make any further purchases of foreign exchange. This step was taken without any notification of His Majesty's Legation; it is the first move towards putting into operation the "Financial Plan" of the Minister of Finance. Such a financial policy on the part of the Persian Government will inevitably lead to embarrassment to the Allied war effort in the Middle East, and the Persian Government must be persuaded or induced to adopt a line more consistent with its obligations under the Treaty of Alliance, and with the policy of defense against aggression. Many other problems arise out of the financial relations between His Majesty's Government and the Persian Government, but no progress can be made with their settlement until the major issues of currency and rate of exchange have been disposed of. His Majesty's Legation, Tehran. 3rd April 1942.

The currency dispute had placed the American government in a difficult position. While admitting that the Iranian position was "just and reasonable," it could not abandon the British. On April 9, 1942, the Financial Division of the State Department had produced a report on the dispute (Memorandum, 741.9111/60):

> Telegram 97 from Tehran under the date of April 6, 1942 indicates that the dispute between Iran and Great Britain with respect to the sale of rials for pounds sterling has reached an impasse which may have undesirable effects on the war effort in Iran. Recent telegrams from Iran show that the Government of that country reluctantly agreed to raise the legal limit on note issues from two billion rials to two billion seven hundred million rials as a result of strong British pressure and that the Iranians wish to revalue the rial upward from 140 to the pound sterling to 100 to the pound sterling. Telegram 97 informs the Department that in addition the Iranian Government wishes to reserve 300,000,000 of the 700,000,000 rial increase in circulation for the use of the Iranian Government and to allot only 400,000,000 for sales against foreign exchange. Apparently the British have been purchasing rials at a rate of £1,000,000 monthly or approximately 140,000,000 rials monthly so that if there is no change in the attitude of the Iranian Government the British might soon exhaust the 400,000,000 rial quota for exchange operations. It should be noted, however, that since April 1 the impasse between the British and Iranians seems nearly complete since on that date an order was issued directing Iranian banks to buy no more foreign exchange. The British are apparently obtaining rials by overdrawing at the Imperial Bank and Dreyfus states that this source

will be exhausted in about ten days after which war work may have to be suspended for lack of local currency.

According to Tehran's 97 the Iranians would like to have the 400,000,000 rials used as a floating fund to supply British rial needs against the importation of goods from the sterling area. In other words the Iranians are apparently very reluctant to increase further the monetary circulation against purchases of sterling in a situation in which the sterling must accumulate in their hands because of British unwillingness or inability to liquidate the sterling by exports from the sterling area. Dreyfus also indicates that the Iranians have refused to admit sterling as reserve for the note issue because of a lack of confidence in both the British and the pound itself. As reported by Dreyfus and indicated by Mr. Stopford's letter of March 17, 1942, the British apparently consider the Iranian attitude unreasonable and uncooperative. The British position seems to be that there should be no appreciation of the rial in terms of sterling and that rials should be freely issued against sales of sterling by the British. The British accuse Iran of bad faith and virtual blackmail and have so far refused to bind themselves to the Iranian scheme for linking the amount of rials sold to the British to the importation of goods from the sterling area.

In the letter from Mr. Stopford to Mr. Livesey referred to above the British requested us to join them in putting pressure on Iran to accede to the British demands. After requesting a report from Dreyfus the Department advised Mr. Stopford that the Department did not consider that our intervention with the Iranian authorities with regard to this matter would be advisable at this time. In his telegram 97, however, Mr. Dreyfus states that while he has consistently recommended avoidance of undue pressure on Iran and advised against joining the British in representations unless such action appeared essential to the war effort, he feels that present Iranian intransigence toward the British is potentially harmful toward that effort and recommends working in close harmony with the British in questions relating to supplies for Iran. It should be noted that Section One of telegram 97 relates to supplying Iran with wheat. It is not clear whether Dreyfus has in mind primarily facilitating the supply of Iran wheat and other necessary commodities in order to gain the cooperation of that country or whether he has in mind that if we follow too liberal a policy in supply matters we may largely destroy the chief bargaining lever which the British have against Iran. That the latter interpretation may be the correct one is suggested by telegram 1697 of April 8 from London reporting informal conversations of Casaday and Penrose with Keynes. According to the London telegram the British feel the concessions to Iran would merely be followed by further demands and that a firm stand must be taken on the present issues. The telegram states that in view of the recent announcement of Lend-Lease aid to Persia the British would appreciate Anglo-American cooperating in dealing with the matter.

Possible courses of action which the Department may wish to follow in this situation appear to be: (1) The Department could adhere to the position it took in the letter to Stopford and simply decline to intervene in the matter leaving it to be settled by Great Britain and Iran. (2) The Department could follow a policy of strongly supporting the British position in attempting to coerce Iran into compliance therewith. (3) The Department could undertake to discuss the question thoroughly with the British and attempt to mediate the existing impasse.

With respect to the first policy the possibility that continuance of the impasse may impair the war effort in Iran suggests that this policy may be inadvisable. From Dreyfus' report there also seem to be strong considerations against the second policy. From the economic point of view the Iranian case is not without merit. Iran can hardly be blamed for not wishing to have its note issue rapidly expanding against reserves of a currency such as sterling subject to rigid exchange control and readily convertible into neither goods for import nor gold. The British demand is essentially that Iran inflate its currency until the present rate between the rial and sterling can be obtained without difficulty. In my opinion the Iranian position on purely economic grounds is reasonable and just in spite of the British attitude indicated in London's 1697 that one motive behind present Iranian demands is a desire to create opportunities of post-war enrichment for highly placed persons in the governing group.

On the other hand the British are strongly opposed to any depreciation of the sterling in terms of the rial since such depreciation would set a different ratio of exchange between the dollar and sterling in Iran from that in other countries. The British also apparently fear setting undesirable precedents which might lead to similar demands from other Middle Eastern countries. It is apparently for this reason that the British are also opposed to sending gold to Iran to purchase rials. It is possible that the British also feel that Iran should be willing to make sacrifices against the Axis and feel that Iran is not providing the cooperation envisaged in the treaty of alliance between the United Kingdom, the

> Soviet Union and Iran. As against such a position Iran can of course cite Article 7 of the treaty in which "the Allied Powers jointly undertake to use their best endeavors to safeguard the economic existence of the Iranian people against the privations and difficulties arising as the result of the present war." Moreover the treaty in its preamble takes cognizance of the principles of the Atlantic Charter. There is some doubt as to how consistent with the Atlantic Charter coercion of a small "captive" country such as Iran to compel it to adopt measures against its economic interest would be. It would appear that the United States from the standpoint of the war effort and the principles of the Atlantic Charter might find it advisable to attempt to mediate the dispute.
>
> I have a feeling that the next step might well be a frank and full discussion of the whole question with the British who may be better informed on the whole situation in Iran than the State Department at present. It may be that some expediting of furnishing supplies to Iran by the British and by ourselves may induce Iran to adopt monetary policies more in line with what the British desire. A considerable inflation in Iran will be inevitable under the circumstances but the effects of the inflation may be modified to some extent by provision of more adequate supplies. If shipping or other considerations make imperative continued severe restrictions on the amount of supplies going to Iran the attitude of that country might be modified to some extent if the monetary circulation were expended against dollars or earmarked gold rather than what are in effect blocked paper pounds. Again some compromise of these two suggestions might be possible. While the inflation might proceed apace in Iran regardless of whether the rials were issued against gold or sterling, the psychological effect of having the note issue backed by gold rather than sterling might appeal to Iran. . . . It would appear that this whole question is so largely political and so broad, covering the supply aspects as well as monetary and exchange matters, that the Department should attempt to keep a strong voice in the matter rather than to allow it to become a question for direct settlement between our Treasury and the British Treasury.

On April 20, 1942, two British officials called on Murray and Assistant Secretary Berle (Memorandum, 741.9111/68):

> At Mr. Berle's request, Mr. Bewley and Mr. Hayter of the British Embassy called to discuss the disagreement which had arisen between the British and Iranian Governments as a result of the reluctance of the Iranians to purchase sterling exchange and authorize the expansion of

Iranian currency circulation to meet the needs of British operations in Iran. Mr. Berle referred to the substance of the British aide-mémoire left with Alling by Mr. Hayter on April 11, 1942, in which inquiry was made as to whether this Government would be willing "to cause strong representations to be made in Tehran for the supply to British authorities of local currency needed for our common purposes against sterling and indicating that failing this, Lend-Lease arrangements must be held in abeyance." Mr. Berle also referred to the British suggestion that we bring pressure on the Iranians to meet the British demands by threatening to freeze Iranian balances held in this country. Even if the measures suggested by the British were practical on political grounds Mr. Berle felt that they would be useless as instruments of pressure upon the Iranians for the simple reason that the amount of Iranian funds in this country is very small and that a threat to withhold goods under Lend-Lease from the Iranians would hardly be an impressive argument when no such goods have thus far gone forward. Furthermore, if we decided to send goods to Iran under Lend-Lease it would be for our own specific advantage, which we would not be willing to forego for reasons now being put forth by the British. Turning to the political considerations involved, Mr. Berle felt that a dangerous internal situation might be created if we joined with the British to use the "mailed fist" on the Iranians, which would only serve to drive them further into Axis hands. It had to be remembered that the maintenance of security in Iran for purposes of transit to Russia was of vital concern to us all and that it would serve no useful purpose to take any action which would contribute to a deterioration of the internal situation of the country and thus bring about a greater drain on British military forces to police the country and preserve order. Both Mr. Bewley and Mr. Hayter said they fully agreed with Mr. Berle in that regard.

Turning then to a practical solution which we wished to present to the British, Mr. Berle observed that the present British demands on the Iranians entail certain very distinct disadvantages for Iran and that the Iranians are not unreasonably unwilling to build up further blocked sterling balances. The Iranians are, on the other hand, apparently ready to sell rials for gold or dollars. In response to the British inquiry as to whether we would endeavor to obtain local currency for the British Government against dollars, Mr. Berle stated that the question of increasing the British supply of dollars was now being canvassed by the Treasury and he understood that negotiations were in progress with the British on that subject. He therefore wanted to put forward the proposal for British consideration as to whether they might not be prepared to pay in dollars for the Iranian currency needed in Iran. We, in turn, would endeavor to find some means of insuring the maintenance by the British Government of adequate dollar balances that would more than meet their needs in Iran. This proposal seemed to be entirely agreeable to Mr. Bewley and Mr. Hayter, and Mr. Bewley said he would put it up at once to his Government by telegraph and give us a reply at the earliest possible moment. . . . Reference was then made to the question of purchasing certain Iranian military supplies, particularly army trucks. It was felt that there would be no difficulty in making these purchases under Lend-Lease for the British if the need arose. It was pointed out, however, that it would be unwise to deplete too greatly the Iranian supply of trucks since they are apparently needed at the present time for the transporting of food and troops necessary for internal security in the country.

After the conference, I communicated with Mr. Harry White of the Treasury and informed him of the discussion that had taken place with the two British officials and of the suggestion which Mr. Berle had made as a possible solution of the monetary difficulty being experience by the British in Iran. Mr. White was very pleased to receive this information as he said he was going into conference this afternoon on the related problem of assuring adequate dollar balances for the British. He said he would appreciate being informed as soon as possible as to the reaction of the British Government to the proposal made by Mr. Berle.

Cable to Dreyfus on April 25, 1942 (Telegram 102, 891.24/179):

Department has informed British that this Government considers it inadvisable to apply economic pressure on Iran in connection with Anglo-Iranian exchange and monetary dispute. It is felt that such measures should be employed only as a last resort, since under existing circumstances they might only serve further to exacerbate Anglo-Iranian relations and perhaps bring about the fall of the Soheily cabinet without achieving the desired end. Therefore, as it is understood that the Iranian Government is not averse to increasing its reserves of dollars or gold, this Government has proposed that the British should meet their expenses in Iran by selling dollars, convertible into gold if desired. In turn, the United States would undertake to keep in view the loss of dollars such payments to Iran would entail in considering measures for maintaining a satisfactory British dollar position. British Embassy in Washington is consulting London with regard to this proposal.

Anglo-Iranian Monetary Agreement

Inevitably, the British had prevailed. Mathews from London on April 29, 1942 (Telegram 2269, 891.5151/228):

> I discussed with Sir Maurice Peterson and also with Waley of the British Treasury this morning the point of view set forth in the Department's telegram 1811, April 25, 11 p.m. Sir Maurice said that the British are willing to accept our point of view as to the inadvisability of applying economic pressure on Iran in connection with the Anglo-Iranian exchange dispute. He agreed that it might be dangerous to take any steps which might result in an overthrow of the present Iranian Government which he describes as "perhaps not all that could be desired but about the best that can be hoped for under the circumstances." He added: "We have no desire to bully the Iranians, but sometimes it is useful to have a little bullying in the air. It worked quite well in getting the Japanese Legation out of Tehran." Waley, however, did not look with much favor on the question of utilizing dollars to cover British expense needs in Iran. He said that negotiations seem to be proceeding favorably in Tehran whereby the Iranians will accept sterling and whereby quarterly a certain percentage of their sterling balances will be made available to them in gold. He said that the British Treasury is now discussing with our Treasury the question of our making gold available for that purpose and he was wondering whether the Department's telegram no. 1811 was in the nature of a reply to recent telegram the British Treasury sent to Washington. I said that I did not believe so and that he would probably hear directly from our Treasury people. In conclusion Sir Maurice said that order seems to be relatively well maintained in Iran now and that the British fully share our view that nothing should be done which might interrupt the supply line to Russia at the present time.

Dreyfus on May 3, 1942 (Telegram 137, 891.5151/229):

> Referring to my no. 127, April 29, noon. British Legation acting under instructions and Iranian Government have reached tentative and informal agreement along following lines: (One) Iranians to guarantee supply of rials to be issued against sterling holdings. (Two) British to convert sterling into gold to meet Iranian dollar imports. (Three) British to convert 35% of remaining Iranian sterling holdings to gold. (Four) Exchange rate to be fixed at 32 rials per dollar and 128 per pound. Council of Ministers last night approved plan but requested

> alteration of exchange rate to 124. British Minister has telegraphed foregoing to London and awaits final instructions.

Dreyfus on May 14, 1942 (Telegram 154, 891.5151/230):

> British and Iranians have reached informal financial agreement along lines given in my 137, May 3. Rial would be pegged at 128 for buying and 130 for selling. Sterling exchange would be free but dollar would still be controlled. British would guarantee conversion of sterling into gold for Iranian dollar purchases and in addition it is expected that 40% of unused sterling balances into gold. . . . It is expected that new exchange rates will go into effect in a few days and that formal agreement will be signed shortly thereafter. Agreement will be presented after signature to open session of Majlis but Prime Minister expects no difficulty in obtaining ratification.

On May 15, 1942 (Telegram 158, 891.5151/231): "Referring to my no. 154, May 14, 11 a.m. The Ministry of Finance yesterday issued an order setting exchange rate at 128 rials per pound for buying and 130 for selling." On May 27, 1942 (Telegram 170, 891.5151/233):

> Reference Nos. 137, May 3, 154, May 14, and 158, May 15. A formal financial agreement was signed last night by Prime Minister for Iran and British Minister for Great Britain. Its terms are identical with those given in my No. 154, full text being sent by air mail. This agreement was expeditiously and fairly negotiated and is advantageous to Iranians and British.

Dreyfus on June 5, 1942 (Dispatch 276 and enclosure, 891.5151/237):

> I have the honor to enclose a copy of a financial agreement between Great Britain and Iran signed at Tehran on May 26, 1942. The agreement, as I indicated in my telegram No. 170, dated May 27, 11 a.m., was fairly negotiated by the British and contains clauses advantageous to both parties. The British obtain the assurance that they will be able to obtain rials for their essential war needs in Iran at a reasonably favorable exchange rate of 128 rials per pound. This rate may not be altered unless there is a change in the dollar-pound cross rate. The Iranians, on the other hand, are permitted to convert sterling into gold

> for payment of dollar imports and obtain the important right to convert in addition 40 per cent of their unused sterling balances into gold. The agreement was negotiated expeditiously and in an atmosphere of calm friendliness, in contrast to recent British negotiations with Iran, particularly those concerning the treaty and expulsion of the Japanese Legation, which were based to some extent on firm pressure.

Contrary to Dreyfus' opinion, the "accord" constituted a complete surrender by Iranians. While Iran continued to accumulate sterling, it could not convert its sterling holdings into imports. The result was unchecked inflation. Moreover, the accord set the stage for another financial dispute in the fall of 1942, discussed in chapter 14.

Financial Crisis

A year later, the Iranian government was on the verge of financial collapse. Dreyfus on May 10, 1943 (Telegram 484, 891.51/564):

> My 429, April 26. Millspaugh requested I reiterate to Department the absolute necessity of obtaining a dollar credit of $30,000,000 if Iranian Government is to be saved from complete financial collapse. He does not disguise fact that the credit would have inflationary effect nor deny possibility of recurrence of similar crisis next year. However, it would buy a year's time strengthening Government, make it possible to collect revenues and give the stability necessary to carry in Government the price stabilization and other plans. He finds that the many pressing obligations of the Government will not, as he had hoped, permit reduction of this year's deficit. In addition he feels that unless Government salaries are increased a general strike and disorder may eventuate. He states that an important factor in the financial crisis is the unwillingness of Russians to postpone their financial demands or place them on reasonable basis. As example Russians are demanding 32,000,000 rials as part payment for the 25,000 tons wheat (my 382, April 13) although wheat has not been delivered and despite fact they themselves owe Iran Government some 60,000,000 rials for grain they purchased in Azerbaijan. British are pressing him for payment of about 554,000 pounds for grain purchased. He believes that alternative to granting of this credit would be financial collapse and eventual withdrawal of his mission.

Dreyfus on June 25, 1943 (Telegram 661, 891.51/570):

> My 608, June 11. Millspaugh has written letter to Prime Minister calling attention to seriousness of Iran's financial situation and urging Majlis approval of income tax law, bill for issue of Treasury bonds and approving contracts for six Americans for his mission. Prime Minister has promised to present letter Sunday to secret session of Majlis in hopes of breaking the Majlis attitude of intransigence and indolence which has prevented action on numerous important pending bills. Millspaugh again urges overriding necessity of Allied loan but now states amount required is $50,000,000 which will enable him to grant essential increases in Government salaries and make it unnecessary for him to turn to Allies later for a second loan. Current financial situation is desperate and deficit for present and next month will probably be more than $10,000,000. He urges, therefore, that immediate advance of part of loan will be necessary if Government is to meet its obligations. In addition he is requesting Anglo-Iranian Oil Company to advance at once oil royalties of 4,000,000 pounds due during the coming year. British Legation views Millspaugh's position sympathetically and I am sure will recommend that British grant loan alone if United States will not participate. Millspaugh states that for obvious reasons it would be better to have American or Anglo-American loan. Soviet Ambassador still holds unrealistic belief that Iran does not need a loan. British Minister and I are discussing question tomorrow.

As described in chapter 6, the Iranian government could not come up with $2.5 million needed to pay for some 100 Lend-Lease trucks sent its way.

The paucity of oil revenues was the main reason for the financial plight. As noted in chapter 1, Iranian oilfields and the large refinery in Abadan were of critical importance to the Allies. Iranian oil was the principal source of fuel to the Allied forces in the North Africa and Pacific theatres, and even large amounts were sent to the Soviet Union. Iranian oil also became the main source for the Allied forces in the Mediterranean and European theatres. From 1941 to 1945, 67 million tons of petroleum products were exported from Iran by the Anglo-Iranian Oil Company. The financial terms for Iran, however, were extremely disadvantageous.

Up to 1940, payment to Iran was tied to output. In August 1940, the regime of Reza Shah Pahlavi negotiated a supposedly "temporary" agreement with the British government and the Anglo-Iranian Oil Company altering the basis of royalties. Under the new agreement, payment to Iran for 1941 and 1942 was fixed at £4 million per year regardless of production. The agreement also provided for the conversion of £2 million per year to dollars for deposit in American and Swiss banks.[1] As Reza Shah desired to transfer his personal wealth from London to New York, it was very advantageous to him.[2] This temporary agreement was subsequently extended to the end of the war. Dreyfus on June 9, 1943 (Dispatch 577, 891.6363/801):

> I have the honor to refer to my despatch No. 561 of May 26, 1943, enclosing answers to a questionnaire on the general situation concerning oil exploitation in Iran and to quote the following translation of an item appearing in the local newspaper *Ettelaat* on June 3: "After the numerous discussions which took place in 1319 (1940) between the Persian authorities and the southern oil company about the royalties on the southern oil during the present war, it was arranged that for the two years 1941 and 1942 AD the company should pay four million pounds as royalty; but from the beginning of 1943 (Dey 1321) the idea of the company was that in view of the economic crisis the share of the oil royalties ought to be paid in accordance with the provisions of the 1933 agreement. Finally, as a result of the discussions and measures which have been taken it has been agreed that from 1943 until the end of the present war the figure for the Persian Government's royalties from the Anglo-Iranian Oil Company shall definitely be this same four million pounds." The *Nur-i-Iran* of June 4 printed the foregoing, proceeded by the statement: "that the royalty was fixed by the agreement of 1933, but after the beginning of the war the consumption and export of oil as of everything else fell considerably and the means of transporting oil products became so limited that its effects were even felt in the interior of the country; consequently the oil royalties due to Iran fell considerably." It also added a phrase describing the royalties which would be due under the 1933 agreement as "of course, a very small amount."

Iran oil exports stood at 8.7 million tons in 1941 and by 1945 it had reached 18.3 million tons, but Iran received the same amount in royalties. Exports during 1941-45 were 67 million tons and royalties £20 million, or about $1.50 per ton and a mere pennies per barrel. As described in chapter 25, in a conversation with Assistant Secretary Berle, General Patrick J. Hurley, adviser to President Roosevelt, had bluntly stated that while Iranians were dying of starvation, the Anglo-Iranian Oil Company was reaping fabulous profits and had declared a 20% dividend in London. Moreover, the situation greatly resembled that of World War I when the British had ceased payment of oil royalties on some flimsy excuse. In both wars Iranian oil had been obtained practically for free.

Notes

1. Majd, Mohammad Gholi. *August 1941: The Anglo-Russian Occupation of Iran & Change of Shahs*. Lanham: University Press of America, 2012. 130-135.

2. Majd, Mohammad Gholi. *Great Britain & Reza Shah: The Plunder of Iran, 1921-1942*. Gainesville: University of Florida, 2011 Reprint Edition. 305-330.

Chapter 6

The Transportation Crisis and the Establishment of Road Transport Board

It was made clear in chapter 4 that of the pressing problems facing Iran, the transport crisis was the most serious. The seizure of Iran's trucks by the British and the Russians and the inability to import vehicles, tires and spare parts were the cause. To discuss tires for Iran, on April 29, 1942, Jernegan and four officials of the Office of Lend-Lease Administration (OLLA) met with Swiggett and Christelow of the British Purchasing Commission (Memorandum, 891.24/194):

> Dr. Orchard called a meeting at his office in order to discuss two requests for tires for Iran, one being a British requisition for 24,230, and the other an informal request made by Mr. Saleh, Chief of the Iranian Trade and Economic Commission, for 94,000 tires. Mr. Swiggett explained that the British authorities had laid down a program to meet the estimated essential needs of Iran which called on the shipment of approximately 68,000 tires for the year 1942. This figure was based on an estimate that 8,000 were needed to put into service trucks laid up at the start of the year for lack of tires, and that 5,000 would be needed monthly as replacements and for new trucks being sent into the country by Great Britain and the United States. Some 46,000 tires out of the total of 68,000 contemplated have already being shipped or are in process of purchase and shipment. The pending requisition for 24,230 constitutes the last installment on this program. According to Mr. Swiggett and Mr. Christelow, the British Government feels that all tires sent to Iran should be kept under the control of

the Allied authorities acting through the United Kingdom Commercial Corporation, in order to insure their use only for transport services essential to the war effort. . . . Mr. Christelow and Mr. Swiggett are not informed as to the exact details of the control exercised by the United Kingdom Commercial Corporation, but they believe that only a part of Iranian motor transport is at present directed by UKCC, the remainder being in the hands of independent Iranian firms or in the hands of the Iranian Government. Their objective, however, is to eliminate this independent section of the transport machinery by preventing supplies of tires to any operators who do not work in cooperation with the UKCC. The theory behind this is that the minimum needs of the country can be met more efficiently under Allied control and that essential war transportation can be better maintained in this way. Consequently, the British Government requests that its requisition for 24,230 tires be approved for shipment to the UKCC, which proposes to allocate these tires for use as follows: 40% for transportation of supplies to Russia, 40% for Iranian governmental and military uses, and 20% for Iranian civilian use. The British feel that this will take care of the needs of Iran during the current year and that, therefore, the Iranian request for 94,000 tires should be denied. It was pointed out that there is to be constituted very shortly a central supply council in Tehran on which will be represented the Iranian Government, the British services and the United States, and it was suggested that if the Iranian Government still feels that it requires more tires it could present its request to this central supply council which would be in the best position to pass on the question. Dr. Orchard said, however, that if the British tire requisition is approved, the short supply situation might make it difficult to approve any later Iranian requisition, even though passed by the Central Supply Council and the Middle East Supply Center. Dr. Orchard said that Lend-Lease would like to have the views of the State Department on the political question of whether we would adopt the British policy of restricting all tire shipments to the UKCC or should insist upon making an independent allocation to the Iranian Government for use by that Government as it might see fit. I said that I would consult the interested officers in the Department and would try to let him have an answer within the next few days.

Cable to Dreyfus on May 5, 1942 (Telegram 113, 891.24/194):

British have presented requisition to Lend-Lease for twenty-four thousand two hundred and thirty tires, which constitutes final lot of total sixty-eight thousand tires scheduled by British for shipment to Iran in

1942. This latest requisition is to be consigned to UKCC which proposes to allocate tires forty per cent for transportation to Russia, forty per cent for Iranian governmental and civilian uses and twenty per cent for Iranian civilian use, all under direction of UKCC. British consider their program of sixty-eight thousand sufficient for Iranian needs this year and further believe tires should be distributed and controlled entirely by UKCC in order to insure most efficient use in furtherance of war operations and maintenance of essential Iranian economy. They therefore request approval their requisition and denial any independent Iranian request which may be made. Please telegraph urgently your views on following, bearing in mind Anglo-American participation in local supplies committee and MESC and at the same time Department's desire to maintain American prestige on its present high level and keep American-Iranian relations on as direct a basis as war controls will allow: 1. Whether British program of sixty-eight thousand tires sufficient for minimum needs Allied military and Iranian civilian transport this year; 2. Advisability of leaving distribution of tires and consequent indirect partial or total control highway transportation in hands of UKCC. If possible please report number of trucks now operating in Iran, differentiating between those under British, Russian and American control and those controlled by Iranian Government and private citizens.

Dreyfus replied on May 10, 1942 (Telegram 147, 891.24/195):

Department's number 113, May 5, 8 p.m. One. Following estimate of motor vehicles in Iran compiled by Legation after consulting Iranian Government, private sources, and UKCC. (A) Trucks now operating 4,000, laid up for lack of tires and parts, 1,500. This includes all Government and private trucks except Russian and British military. UKCC have about half of those 4,000 trucks under contract and in addition are expecting arrival soon of some 2500 Lease-Lend trucks for their use. (B) Buses, 600. (C) Passenger cars now operating, 3,000, laid up 1,000. (D) Motor cycles, 400. Almost all of the above vehicles are in private hands. Two. Estimate of tire needs: Although 12 tires per truck per year (mortality rate is high due to bad roads) and 2 per each passenger car, it would appear that British estimate of 68,000 fairly reflects minimum needs for Allied military and civilian use. Iranian Government is unaware that orders for 68,000 tires have been placed; they themselves having ordered only 24,000 through UKCC. If 68,000 tires actually arrive in Iran and are distributed roughly along the lines suggested by UKCC, I am of the opinion that Iran's minimum needs would be met. Three. Distribution: This is delicate and controversial point. The UKCC wishes to control distribution of tires because (1) they do not trust Iranians to do it honestly (2) they believe they can do it more efficiently and (3) it would be an excellent economic weapon. The Iranians ardently desire to have tires delivered directly to them and to control distribution. Iranian Government has recently given to UKCC virtual control over tire imports because they had become convinced that only the UKCC wielded sufficient influence to obtain tires. Thus the 24,000 tires were ordered through UKCC. Now however that Lease-Lend aid has been granted Iran, the Iranian Government would be most displeased if control over tires was placed in hands of UKCC. I should be most reluctant to see tire control vested solely in UKCC because (1) it would aggravate Iranians and some of the blame might be placed on us (2) it would increase the stranglehold which the UKCC is gradually acquiring over Iranian economy. In addition I do not see why British should have the credit for this transaction which might well be handled as Lease-Lend to Iran. On other hand I do not have confidence in ability or honesty of Iranian Government to make equitable distribution. The best solution would be the sending of Lease-Lend representative or commission to control matters of this kind. The Iranians would welcome such an official and the British could hardly object since they have frequently suggested that the Iranians engage an American to supervise distribution of essential goods. The next best solution would be distribution of these by a mixed commission of Iranians, British and Americans, a procedure to which the Iranian Government has indicated it would agree.

Dreyfus on May 29, 1942 (Telegram 175, 891.24/201):

I concur in Department's suggestion that tires be consigned to this Legation or Central Supply Committee and distributed under Committee's supervision although this procedure will be bitterly opposed by UKCC. . . . UKCC is insisting on obtaining monopoly on import and distribution of tires, trucks, and spare parts in order to control all road transport. This coupled with control of other imports through MESC and British control of railways would complete their strangle hold on Iran economy. British Commercial Secretary, on return from MESC meeting in Cairo, without consulting this Legation or Iranians, delivered to Iran Government a note setting forth quotas for six months and told Minister of Finance verbally that Iran must accept the quotas or receive nothing. These quotas provide for no trucks for Iran and that tires and spare parts importation and distribution be mo-

> nopoly of UKCC. I am forwarding a copy of this note and enclosures by air today. I have discussed matter at length with Prime and Finance Ministers who are indignant at British attitude and leave no doubt that they will refuse to accept the tire and truck procedure suggested. While they wish to receive tires and trucks themselves, they are willing to deliver percentage to be agreed on to trucks for vital war work. Remainder they wish to distribute but are willing to submit to control by an American expert or any committee we suggest. They complain with reason that British already control 90% of railway capacity and more than half country's trucks are laid up or under contract to UKCC. This leaves Iran without sufficient transport and fully at UKCC mercy. Result will be depletion of Iran's road transport.
>
> I consider the British attitude in general and the UKCC position on tires and trucks in particular to be highhanded and completely lacking in consideration for Iranians. The result of such procedure could only be to embitter British Iranian relations, which have recently been improving, and to reduce greatly our own high prestige. I do not propose giving Iran more than the bare minimum needs. I do propose however to hear the Iranian side and keep an open mind until the matter can be seriously discussed by the committee. I have therefore asked the Ministers of Finance and Commerce to comment freely and fully on the British note. I feel frankly that the British are endeavoring to turn Iran's unfortunate position to their advantage and to our disadvantage. I don't for example see why UKCC should get 2,500 Lease Lend trucks while Iranians receive not one or why distribution of any commodity should be turned over to a foreign agency against Iranian wishes. While my relations with British Legation have been excellent I realize that they may be harmed by my opposition in this matter and that I lay myself open personally for attack. This will not deter me although will make every effort to be tactful and friendly.

The note from the British Legation concerning Iran's MESC import quota mentioned in the above telegram is given in chapter 7. On June 19, 1942, the Iranian Minister, Schayesteh, had presented a note to Under Secretary Welles requesting 80,000 tires and 1,000 trucks (Verbal Note 619, 891.24/211):

> The matter of food and distribution of supplies in different parts of Iran has become more and more difficult, the main reason being the lack of transportation facilities. Iran . . . depends entirely upon transportation by motor truck. From the beginning of the war the export of

cars, trucks and tires has been reduced to a very small quantity. During the last year exportation has been practically zero. Moreover, the need for transportation of war materials and other Allied activities have brought about the appropriation of a considerable part of existing trucks. The question of transportation in Iran has, therefore, reached an acute stage, as a result of which the economic condition of the country is daily becoming critical so that in case urgent action is not taken to furnish Iran with trucks and tires, it is feared that famine will break out all over the country, and a situation will be created which will be impossible to remedy. One other aspect which is not less important is that for maintaining order in the country it is necessary to have sufficient trucks for the expeditious movement of the gendarmerie, police and military forces to cope with uprisings. If the Government is unable to send quickly the necessary force to places of unrest, unruly activities will increase. Such a situation would certainly not benefit the program instituted by the United States Government at this time for that part of the world.

The Iranian Government and its people have shown by their cooperation their friendship toward the United States in these difficult times. Upon the official announcement of the President of the United States that Iran is a beneficiary of the Lease-Lend Act, the hopes of the Iranian people have risen in regard to receiving the necessary supplies from the United States. We are sure that the United States Government desires to give Iran every possible aid and we understand the difficulties facing this country in regard to tires, but it is my duty to draw the attention of the United States Government to the fact that if quick action is not taken in this matter, a situation will be created in Iran which cannot be easily remedied. The need of Iran, which has been estimated very carefully, is for one thousand trucks and eighty thousand tires and tubes. The question was presented to the proper authorities in Washington months ago but nothing definite has resulted. The United States has been for long years, and is especially now, the only source of supply for trucks and tires for Iran, and there is no doubt of the immediate need of the country for these commodities. Therefore it will not be necessary to refer that question to the Supply Committee in Teheran or the Central Supply Committee in Cairo. A decision should be taken here in Washington to authorize the exportation of that quantity of tires and tubes directly to Iran, but if it is really impossible to do so, the Iranian Government should be notified of the fact so that it can explain the situation to the people of Iran.

The "Central Supply Committee in Cairo" refers to the Middle East Supply Center. On June 20, 1942, Alling had written to Assistant Secretary Dean Acheson (Memorandum, 891.24/207):

> Mr. Welles called me to his office yesterday and handed me the attached note which had been given him by the Iranian Minister. Mr. Welles asked me to get in touch with you urgently and ask that the request of the Minister be studied with a view of giving him a definite answer not later than Tuesday or Wednesday of next week. In this connection I invite your attention to telegram no. 204 of June 18, from the Legation at Tehran. In this telegram Mr. Dreyfus recommends that immediate steps be taken to make tires available to the Iranians. He also recommends that heavy and light trucks be furnished to them to equip them to move troops and bring in the harvest and other essential goods. He suggests that a portion of the Lend-Lease trucks now arriving in Iran be earmarked for immediate delivery to the Iranian Government. As you know, the difficulty in making direct aid available to the Iranians is due to the system employed by the UKCC, which controls the distribution of goods in Iran. As pointed out in a recent memorandum to you, we are becoming greatly concerned at the growing tendency of the UKCC to obtain a stranglehold on the Iranian economy. We are at your disposal to discuss this question at your convenience.

On July 2, 1942, the substance of the reply to Schayesteh's note of June 19, 1942, was cabled to Dreyfus (Telegram 180, 891.24/195):

> On June 19 Iranian Minister here personally presented request to Under Secretary for 80,000 tires and 1,000 trucks, stressing their urgent necessity for maintenance of Iranian economy. Department replied July 1 as follows: 1) This Government understands dependence of Iranian economy upon motor transport and intends to do everything possible, consistent with war effort, to see that Iran receives minimum essential supplies of tires and trucks. 2) Department informed that British Government has in process of shipment, or actually en route, about 44,000 tires. British have further submitted Lend-Lease requisition, which has been approved, for 24,230 tires and tubes for Iran. American Minister Tehran has reported this order was placed at instance of Iranian Government. (Your 147, May 10). 3) Iran should receive, therefore, about 68,000 tires during current year and American Minister Tehran has indicated this should be sufficient for period of one year. 4) United States and Great Britain have recently formed Tehran Central Supplies Committee to consider Iranian import requirements in conjunction with

similar Iranian committees. If Iranian Government considers further supplies of tires are necessary, United States would consider request made through Central Supplies Committee. 5) Department would like further information with respect to trucks. American Minister Tehran reported that in May about 1,500 trucks in Iran were laid up for lack of tires and spare parts. Attention should first be directed to placing those trucks in service. However, United States would be willing to consider Iranian request for trucks made through CSC. Iranian Legation was further informed orally that Department contemplates sending to Iran an American representative to supervise the distribution of supplies from the United States. (It is expected that a United States Commercial Corporation man will be selected for this work. He would be in addition to American food and supply adviser requested by Iranian Government.)

On July 1, 1942, the First Secretary of the Iranian Legation had called on Jernegan (Memorandum, 891.24/231):

I handed Mr. Davallou an aide mémoire embodying our reply to the note the Iranian Minister had left with Mr. Welles on June 19 requesting 80,000 tires and 1,000 trucks. Mr. Davallou expressed some doubt whether the 68,000 tires supposed to be on order or in process of shipment to Iran would be released by the British for the use of the Iranian Government. . . . I told him that we contemplated sending a special representative to Iran to look after the distribution of supplies from this country and that the representative would be in a position to make sure that the Iranian Government received its proper share of everything sent. I further told him that the exact division of the latest order for 24,230 tires, which is now being processed by Lend-Lease, has been left open and that the Iranian Government undoubtedly would have an opportunity to present its views when the decision is made.

Dreyfus on July 7, 1942 (Telegram 226, 891.24/215):

I appreciated helpful attitude outlined in Department's 180, July 3. However, Department's attention is called to the fact that credits for 24,230 tires were formally transferred to UKCC by Iran Government since latter felt itself impotent to obtain tires. Thus, entire 68,000 are consigned to UKCC, which states openly it will not give one tire or truck to Iranians to distribute, but rather it will dole them out as it sees fit. A deadlock has now been reached in my relations with UKCC and

Transport Subcommittee of CSC over tires and trucks. . . . My attitude remains unchanged. I feel British are treating Iranians in high-handed manner and that they are unfair in assuming Iranians are incapable of distributing tires equitably under foreign supervision. Moreover, if we thus oppose UKCC and CSC, we are placed in position of suggesting workable alternative. Since time is important, would it not be possible to send immediately the official mentioned in the last paragraph of Department's 180. This official might be able to reorganize and supervise the tire distribution and transport service already set up in Ministry of Finance. Further, if Iranians are to get any of the 68,000 tires, steps will have to be taken to consign part to the Legation or earmarked for the Iranian Government rather than all to UKCC. Iranian transport problem is urgent and present problem of moving harvest and goods cannot be solved by delivery of tires after several months. I am confidentially informed UKCC have 14,000 tires in stock, but since these are reserved for essential war work, there is little hope of any being turned over to Iranians.

I have suggested to Iranian Government that the immediate problem might be met by using the plenary powers they now hold in transport field to requisition tires which have found their way into the black market, where they sell for up to $2,000 each, and hands of hoarders and to requisition trucks now not doing essential work. The Iranian Government has been weak in these internal matters and should be required to help itself before turning to us. I should appreciate a frank expression of the Department's opinion concerning merits of this dispute and as to its possible solution. Since drafting above, I have talked at length to Finance Minister who said he was grateful for information contained in Department's no. 180 which he used to good advantage in Majlis today in supporting Government's position. He expressed great irritation at treatment being given Iran by British. He especially resented recent case in which British military "stole" 3,000 tires which arrived for Iranian Government (part of tires originally shipped on *Steel Navigator*). He needs these tires badly and intends to make strong representations to British Government. He added that the Automobile Section of his Ministry is already equipped to handle problems of tire distribution and transport and that he would welcome an American to supervise it.

Dreyfus's telegram 226 had elicited a memorandum dated July 10, 1942, from Alling to Murray and Acheson (Memorandum, 891.24/215):

As you are aware, the question of properly distributing American supplies sent to Iran for civilian use has become increasingly pressing in recent weeks. The British authorities dealing with the matter, both here and in Tehran, have consistently maintained that all important items, such wheat, sugar, tires, trucks, spare parts and the like, should be handled only through the United Kingdom Commercial Corporation. In the case of tires and trucks and other elements of motor transport they have insisted upon a complete monopoly by the UKCC and apparently do not even consult the Iranians regarding their needs. On the other hand, the Iranian Government bitterly resents British control over these articles, which are vital to the badly-strained economy of the country, and has protested repeatedly that the British are not giving sufficient attention to Iranian requirements. Our Minister at Tehran considers that there is much merit in the Iranian contention, and both the Minister and the Department have been trying to reconcile the conflicting positions. However, the attached telegram no. 226 July 7, from Tehran reports that Minister Dreyfus has reached a deadlock with the British authorities in Iran on this point.

This Division feels strongly that the importance of the point at issue is far greater than might appear from the relatively small quantities of tires, trucks and other supplies likely to be involved. Our recent telegraphic reports from Tehran show clearly that the political situation in Iran is deteriorating rapidly and a breakdown that might result in chaos is seriously threatened. We fear, therefore, that unless some solution for conflicting British and Iranian demands is found, in such a way that the Iranian Government and people can be convinced that everything possible is being done to take care of their essential needs, the repercussions might be far-reaching and very damaging to the Allied political and military position in the Middle East. As you will recall, at a recent meeting in Mr. Acheson's office it was decided that a United States Commercial Corporation representative should be sent to Iran to supervise distribution of American supplies. . . . As a second step, the Division believes it advisable that the entire question be discussed frankly with some high-ranking officer of the British Embassy here, preferably by Mr. Acheson or one of the other executive officers of the Department, in order that our point of view may be clearly understood and an agreement on policy reached here, in London and in Tehran.

Cable to Dreyfus on July 8, 1942 (telegram 182, 891.24/215A):

We assume General Greely has given you substance of his telegram of July 3 to War Department stating Iranian Army unable maintain internal order because of lack of motor transport. He states this is serious threat to Allied supply line and recommends be allocated immediately 200 lend-lease trucks now in Iran. Department would appreciate your comments together with following information if readily available: 1. What lend-lease trucks now in Iran could conceivably be directed to Iranian Army? 2. To whom are they destined at present? 3. For what purpose does the present consignee plan to use them? If you or Greely have a particular shipment in mind, please give sufficient information to enable its identification by Lend-Lease here.

Dreyfus replied on July 11, 1942 (Telegram 229, 891.24/216):

Greely had in mind either (1) Russian lend-lease trucks being assembled in Iran and flowing into Russia in large numbers or (2) British lend-lease trucks consigned to UKCC for war work in Iran. I agree with Greely that Iranian transport is seriously depleted. This is partly result of predatory and monopolistic policy of UKCC who have been frequently called to Department's attention. Iran Army has only 181 trucks of which less than 30% are serviceable with result that it cannot even move fodder for horses. Similar situation is developing with regard to civilian transport. Iranian Army has asked British military for 1000 trucks but it is believed not more than 150 will be forthcoming. British here have informed both me and Iranian Government that in agreement with Washington Iranian military needs can be obtained only through British military. I am informed that UKCC is expecting some 4,000 Lend-Lease trucks of which a few hundred have arrived. None of these trucks nor those destined for Russia are suitable for Iranian transport but would be better than nothing. Iran needs eight ton trucks with six tires and one differential rather than these combat trucks with ten tires and three differentials and small load capacity. The small Dodge trucks, however, would be of considerable value. The Iranian transport problem is immediate and urgent and cannot be fully solved by shipment of tires and trucks in the future.

Dreyfus on July 20, 1942 (Telegram 236, 891.24/220):

Reference my no. 226, July 7. Relations between Iran Government and UKCC over matter of tires is approaching breaking point. At a meeting Saturday attended by delegates of Ministry of Finance, UKCC and Minor a high Iranian official found it necessary in describing UKCC activities to use such expressions as abuse of confidence, dishonest and unfair treatment. He took violent exception to what he called theft of tires by British (my 226) and said that strong and formal representations will be made to British Legation on the subject. Specific question now at issue is disposition of 24,230 tires ordered by Iran Government credits which were delivered to UKCC. Iran Government insists that UKCC acted only intermediary for obtention of tires for government while UKCC state tires are theirs and that they will retain and distribute them. Result of UKCC viewpoint if carried out would be to place Iran Government at UKCC mercy. General British attitude in this and other matters is one of destructive criticism of Iranian competence and honesty rather one of constructive suggestion, a condition of mind which has contributed in no small degree to British unpopularity here. . . . I feel that due largely to UKCC obstruction and deception we are fiddling while Rome burns. Iranians are in a desperate position for road transport and will be unable to move crops without outside help. I venture to suggest following specification (one) that we approve distribution of tires and trucks by Ministry of Finance under CSC direction (two) that we suggest return of tires belonging to Iran Government which requisitioned by British Military, a political act instigated by UKCC (three) that we consign the 24,230 tires to Iran Government in care of this Legation or CSC (four) that American expert to supervise distribution of American goods be sent to Iran without delay in order to assist in this matter and (five) that representations be made to British Government with a view to obtaining UKCC cooperation with Iranian Government in place of its present attitude of obstruction.

Allied-Iranian Transport Board

The British had relented. Dreyfus on July 22, 1942 (Telegram 240, 891.24/221):

Reference my 238, July 20. Sir Frank Nixon London Director of UKCC now in Tehran, has intervened personally in difficulties between UKCC and Iran Government. Called on me yesterday to explain his action and viewpoint. He admitted that great mistakes had been made by UKCC in Tehran, especially in riding rough shod over Iranian susceptibilities, and that he now plans to correct these errors. He has begun by reorganizing the Company, dismissing some, transferring others,

> and taking two of the most objectionable out of jobs where they have contact with Iranian officials. He has called on Dr. Amini, a leading official of the Ministry of Finance, to apologize for his employees and to offer cooperation in future. He states he and his new transport manager favor establishment of Allied Iranian Committee to supervise distribution tires and trucks and that they will give all possible consideration. In view of above I recommend we await further developments before making representations I suggested in (five) of my no. 238.

Dreyfus on July 27, 1942 (Telegram 242, 891.24/222):

> I am glad to report UKCC shows signs of abandoning obstructive tactics in favor of friendly cooperation and that negotiations are proceeding in more cordial atmosphere. UKCC yesterday formally informed Ministry of Finance that it consents to immediate delivery of the 3,000 requisitioned tires. American and British Legations have prepared memorandum which will be delivered to Iran Government tomorrow suggesting solution along following lines; (1) a transport committee will be set up in Ministry of Finance headed by Iranian official with rank of Under Secretary. American and British representatives will sit on the committee and no objection will be raised to Russian inclusion if desired. Duties of committee would be (a) to organize and supervise Iranian transport, (b) submit to CSC Iranian request for tires, trucks and parts, (c) supervise tire distribution and consider gasoline rationing, (d) prepare legislation to give effect to its findings and (e) explore possibility of increased use of animal transport. (2) UKCC would restrict transport activities to (a) goods to Russia (b) British military needs and (c) Polish military and civilian needs. UKCC has expressed approval of plan and offered cooperation. I feel certain Iranians will be pleased to accept plan perhaps with some modification. This arrangement if successfully carried out will I believe go far toward solving Iran's transport problem. Iranians would receive as many of the tires and trucks consigned to UKCC as the committee, on which they would be heavily represented, believe necessary. British Minister has already telegraphed for British expert to serve as technical member of committee and he suggests we do same. Meanwhile British Commercial Secretary and Minor will sit on committee.

The proposed transport board and the reduction in the transport activities of the UKCC was a step in loosening its grip on Iranian road transport. Dreyfus on September 10, 1942 (Telegram 287, 891.5018/7):

> Transport Board mentioned in my 271, August 26 has been organized and held first meeting. It is headed by Ali Motamedi, young man of good record and reputation, and includes delegates for police and finance departments. British Legation is represented by its Commercial Secretary and this Legation by Minor, both of whom will serve until suitable experts can be obtained. Committee considers nationwide registration of motor vehicles in different categories is necessary before it can proceed with tire and gasoline rationing or other essential duties. It has requested authority of Council of Ministers to proceed therewith without delay.

The above-mentioned telegram 271 of August 26, 1942, was given in full in chapter 4, and its relevant part is reproduced here:

> Active steps are being taken to solve transport problem. Iranian Government has employed Birkle, formerly UKCC Manager here and a transport expert, as director of transport and is now forming after much delay the transport board outlined in my 242, July 27. Iranian Government has obtained possession of part of the three thousand tires mentioned in my 242 but will need considerable stocks in near future. The 44,000 tires imported by British, part already received, are strictly for use of UKCC in war transport and cannot be released for civilian use. UKCC has some 17,000 tires in stock and it may be possible for them to lend tires to transport board against eventual return from 24,230 allocated to Iran. Spare parts are being received to place laid up trucks in service. It is hoped that above measures will result in substantial improvement in transport picture.

As noted, it was this unjustified optimism that had prompted Dreyfus to advise the State Department that there was sufficient wheat in Iran.

It had taken the crisis in the fall of 1942 to spur further action. Dreyfus on December 4, 1942 (Telegram 414, 891.24/313):

> A transport decree drawn up by the informal committee mentioned in my telegram 242, July 27 has been approved by Council of Ministers and promulgated. . . . A formal transport board consisting of one delegate each of Iran (Iranian delegate the President), Russia, Great Britain and two of United States (Kidd and Minor) will be set up at once. This decree gives committee full control over Iranian transport and makes it illegal for trucks to operate except under way bills of Iranian transport board, UKCC or Soviet Transport Agency. It repre-

> sents substantial step forward in solving Iran's important transport problem.

Dreyfus had forwarded the transport decree along with his comments on December 9, 1942 (Dispatch 401 and enclosure, 891.24/336):

> I have the honor, with reference to my telegram No. 414 of December 4, 1942, to enclose a copy of a decree of the Council of Ministers dated November 21, 1942, which prescribes basic regulations for the operation of motor vehicles in Iran. This decree, which has the force of law, was passed under powers derived from the Anti-Hoarding Law of June 14, 1942. It is a foster child of the allies, having grown out of a joint suggestion made to the Iranian Government by the British and American Legations. This suggestion, as reported in my telegram No. 242 of July 27, 1942, was made by the two Legations in parallel notes of July 28, 1942, which outlined a constructive solution of Iran's troublesome transport problem. This initiative was based on allied desire to help Iran in this matter of transport, which is also the key to other perplexing problems, such as security and food. It also has for its aim to insure precious tires and vehicles which might be sent to Iran from the United States would be carefully used for essential purposes. . . . A second decree of the Council of Ministers, required by Chapter Six of the enclosed decree, will soon be published setting forth the composition of the formal committee. This committee, which will have its first meeting tomorrow, will be composed of the following: President and Iranian Representative - Ali Motamedi; British representative - Sir Arthur Parsons; Soviet representative - to be named; American representatives - Harold B. Minor and Philip C. Kidd. Two American representatives were suggested by the British Legation because tires and vehicles will come from the United States and to prevent a deadlock in voting by four members; since the Iranians clearly approved of this arrangement, I saw no reason to object. Besides elaborating this decree, the informal committee accomplished two substantial things. At its request, the Iranian Government required a re-registration of all vehicles in Iran, broken down into various categories of trucks, busses, taxis, Government cars, and private automobiles. . . . I will report these important figures as soon as they are available. Secondly, the committee was able to start the nucleus of a transport organization in the Ministry of Food, under the direction of Mr. C.E. Birkle. Other useful things have been done such as the firm action of the committee in requiring the UKCC to return 90 buses to the streets of Tehran, buses which had been contracted to transport Polish refugees and which

were being held for an emergency; also the board, backed by the Legation, was able to require the British Military authorities to return to the Iranian Government 3,000 tires requisitioned arbitrarily (see my telegram No. 242, July 27).

The present transport position is roughly as follows: The UKCC has under contract some 1,700 of Iran's best and largest trucks; Iransovtrans, the Russian transport organization, has about 400 trucks under contract; and the remainder of the several hundred trucks in the country are doing either private work or are owned by various Iranian Government agencies. The prime purpose of this decree is to bring all trucks in Iran, except those contracted to UKCC and Iransovtran, under the central transport organization. Trucks, in fact, cannot operate in Iran except with a way bill or special license of one of these three organizations. The present fleet of the Iranian Government is clearly insufficient. The committee's plan in this regard is as follows: When the registration is completed and the decree takes effect, all trucks not under contract to the two above-mentioned bodies, will be blanketed into the Edareh Barbari Rah (Road Transport Department), the Government organization. These will then be allotted first to Iran's vital needs, such as hauling of wheat and sugar beets, operation of mines, etc., and secondly to hauling of all private goods. If the number of trucks thus obtained is insufficient to meet current needs, the committee will call upon UKCC and Iransovtrans to surrender some of their fleet or, since it seems unlikely they will do so, arrange for the importation of trucks from the British army or from the United States. Already the British army has agreed to release 50 trucks which will shortly come forward from Egypt.

The committee begins its work under satisfactory conditions. It is headed by an Iranian of ability and integrity, it is supported by the Iranian Government which recognizes its importance to Iran and it has the blessing and support of the British and American Legations. There would seem to be only one possible fly in the ointment and that should be extracted with a little tact and resolute dealing. The Department will recall my series of telegrams during the last six months dealing with the harmful tactics of the UKCC in endeavoring to monopolize Iran's transport for its own benefit with little regard to the needs of the country or the susceptibilities of the people. Our efforts in this regard have not been in vain, the monopolistic power of the UKCC having been gradually reduced until it has now been eliminated by the taking over of the direction of its transport facilities by the British military.

> While the UKCC transport organization continues to function, its direction is entirely in the hands of the British army, priorities and loadings being directed by the army officer in charge of movements control. The danger which now lies ahead is that the British army may follow in the monopolistic footsteps of its UKCC predecessor. The first meeting of the members of the Iranian transport group with the British army on this question were quite satisfactory, the army offering full cooperation in every phase of activity and promising that the fleet of the UKCC will under no circumstances be increased. There have, however, been numerous straws in the wind in the last few days to indicate that this attitude is changing. The army appears now to prefer to have the UKCC contract vehicles and allocate them to Iranian civil transport and to have their organization receive the new and used trucks now coming forward and to pass them on to the Iranian transport board as they see fit. This trend, if it is not to be nipped in the bud, would probably grow to include the allotment of tires also by the British army and, in fact, to get motor transport in Iran back into the unsatisfactory position of several months ago. In my opinion, the British army should be required to confine its activities to carrying essential war goods and leave the Iranian transport organization to work out its own destinies. If the board, set up largely at our suggestion, should fail, it will be an allied failure; this we must do everything in our power to prevent. Should my endeavors in this regard meet with untoward difficulty, I shall not fail to inform the Department immediately and fully.

Matters were unlikely to run smoothly, as shown by the delivery of 50 Lend-Lease trucks from Egypt. Lend-Lease's Kidd from Tehran on January 24, 1943 (Telegram 84, 891.24/359):

> For Stettinius Office of Lend-Lease Administration. From Kidd. Following telegram has been sent to Cairo January 24, 4 p.m. From Kidd to Winant. One. 48 Lend-Lease trucks arrived Tehran consigned to Hobson of Middle East Supply Center. En route the remaining two broke down. At my request Hobson had the British Army deliver them to me. 43 of these have been transferred to the Iranian Government and the remaining 5 will be transferred as soon as United States can make the necessary repairs. With the agreement of Mr. Dreyfus I transferred the trucks subject to subsequent determination of conditions and terms in view of the emergency need. Two. Trucks for Iraq and Iran are arriving without spares. I have been informed that 30% spares accompany Lend-Lease trucks so I assume the remainder are held by

> British army. Please investigate this at once as spares are urgently needed. In the meanwhile I am trying to secure repair parts here in order to put the trucks into operation. Three. I can see no justification for consigning Lend-Lease trucks to British Ambassador at Baghdad and to Hobson Middle East Supply Center agent Tehran. This results in delay double handling and confusion. Suggest consign deliveries in future to me in care of British movement control Baghdad and in care of Persian Gulf Service Command here. Four. The program of 80 trucks a month for Iran and Iraq should be continued with no interruption. Monthly allocations made at Cairo should be regarded as only tentative and subject to my revision in consultation with British authorities. I shall of course act only with the agreement of the American Ministers at Baghdad and Tehran. Repeated to Baghdad and Stettinius.

Winant replied on January 30, 1943 (Telegram 210, 891.24/358):

> For Kidd from Fred Winant: One. Transfer of trucks to Iran subject to subsequent determination of terms of sale has my concurrence in view of urgent need. Two. Understand spares for trucks soon to be furnished. Three. Trucks in question were taken from British military stores and delivered by British drivers to their diplomatic offices, from which official release to the Lend-Lease representative was to be made. Question of future consignments being discussed with appropriate officials. Four. Allocation trucks for Iran and Iraq made by Anglo-American MSTOB transport committee of MESC monthly, and basis of availability and most urgent requirements. Relative need of each country specifically set, therefore loop will not be formed for all vehicles going Iraq and Iran for affixation quotas by representatives there; however if trucks which ordinarily would go to Iraq will be withheld due lack control or insufficient need, they will be reallocated other territories by committee and Iran's relative requirements will be considered. . . . Repeated to Washington for Stettinius.

Moreover, most of the 24,000 tires intended for Iran had been diverted to "other territories less favorably fixed," thereby perpetuating the transport difficulties. Cable from Cairo on January 25, 1943 (Telegram 165, 891.24/357):

> Following is our January 24, 5 p.m. to Tehran: For Kidd from Winant. "One. Tires for Persia. According to records here, as of November 30 United Kingdom Commercial Corporation had 35,000 tires in stock in Iran under PAIC (Persia and Iraq Command) control. This is consid-

ered six months' supply for United Kingdom Commercial Corporation and civil requirements. It is now understood that 24,000 more tires are coming out consigned to United Kingdom Commercial Corporation for distribution by Combined Supplies Committee. It is recommended here that approximately 18,000 be delivered to other territories far less favorably fixed. Major Hobson will discuss with you on arrival home. Please advise views regarding proposed diversion. Two. Trucks. Please advise status of negotiations on 50 Lend-Lease trucks and make no firm commitments without authority from me." Repeated to Office of Lend-Lease Administrator.

Continued Road Transport Crisis

The tire situation is described in a cable of April 29, 1943, from George Washington, Kidd's successor in Tehran (Telegram 365, 891.24/421):

From Washington for Stettinius. Department's 159, April 1. One. PGSC (Persian Gulf Service Command) has furnished following secret information: (a) PAIC (Persia and Iraq Command) as of January 1 had a total of about 402,000 tires on hand and about to arrive including United Kingdom (Commercial) Corporation stocks. They have made arrangement with PGSC for about 265,000 to be kept for British military operations. PGSC receives remaining 137,000. (b) PAIC need for 265,000 tires retained not questioned by PGSC as they were procured in United States for British military use, as distinct from aid to Russia program. (c) PGSC will receive 1,260,000 tires and 121,000 tubes plus 11,000 tires to arrive late from United States. PGSC must supply its own and United Kingdom Corporation aid to Russian needs. (d) PGSC is requesting immediate attention for its requisition and emphasizes its anticipation of running short of tires.

Two. In Iran civilian tire stocks amount to about 3,000; in Iraq less than 5,000 including recent shipment from United Kingdom to Iraq of 2,000. Majority these stocks are of unusable sizes which matter Middle East Supply Center is studying. In both countries control of issuance is very strict. Three. For Iranian civilian use we expect to receive 24,000 Lend-Lease tires. Although none have yet come to Tehran, understand part of this has reached gulf. Also expect shipment of 2,000 for Iraq, said to be en route and we hope to approval of requisition for 6,000 more for Iraq (Cairo's 563, March 23 to Department). Four. In Iraq and Iran civil tire position is acute. No help can be expected from United States Army. Appear to be no American or British officers here who can supply information on exact tire position of PAIC (except that given above). . . . Repeated to Winant in Cairo.

Dreyfus' report of May 3, 1943, gives an update (Dispatch 545, 891.24/443):

I have the honor to render the following report on the work of the Allied-Iranian Road Transport Board which supervises the operation of motor transport in Iran. The purpose of this despatch is to bring up to date the story of the efforts of the Iranian Government, with the assistances of the allies, to organize and operate Iranian civil road transport. The last chapter of this story was given in my despatch No. 401 of December 9, 1942. . . . Responsibility for Iranian civil road transport, including such matters as operation of trucks, allocation of tires, and control of government owned passenger cars, is by law placed on the Road Transport Board. This organization, as outlined in my previous despatch, was set up as a result of conversations between the British and American Legations and the Iranian Government. Its raison d'être was first the necessity of close control of precious tires and trucks in view of the world shortage, and second, the need for organizing Iran's road transport, which was depleted and demoralized because the allies had taken over practically all large and serviceable trucks for transport of war supplies to Russia. The Road Transport Board, a policy making and supervising body, does not endeavor actually to operate road transport. For this purpose, an organization known as Edareh Barbari Rah (Road Transport Office) was set up in the Ministry of Food under the direction of Mr. C.E. Birkle, a British subject who was formerly transport manager for the UKCC. This latter organization actually operates Iran's road transport under the supervision and direction of the Road Transport Board. The Road Transport Board consists of the following five members: Mr. Ali Motemedi, Iranian Chairman; Mr. Noel Cumberbatch, Commercial Secretary of the British Legation; Colonel Krasnov for the Russian Embassy; Mr. Harold B. Minor, Second Secretary of the American Legation; and Mr. George Washington of the Office of Lend-Lease Administration.

The work of the Road Transport Board, in spite of many political and operational difficulties, is going forward steadily and satisfactorily. When the board was organized last year, Edareh Barbari Rah had no trucks with which to begin its task; today, it has 750 privately owned Iranian trucks under contract. In addition, the Edareh Barbari Rah now has a total of 342 lease-lend trucks in operation. This makes a total of some 1100 trucks doing Iranian civil transport of both government owned and private goods. The contracted trucks are operated through six Iranian contractors who make agreements with the individual truck owners under conditions laid down directly by the Edareh Barbari Rah and indirectly by the Road Transport Board. One of the principle conditions is that tires are issued on a rental or loan basis and reclaimed when the truck no longer is under contract or when the tires are no longer serviceable. It is generally calculated that one new tire must be issued for every 4,500 kilometers of work done. Every tire application, whether for truck or passenger car, must be specifically approved by the Road Transport Board at one of its regular meetings. Passenger car tires are issued only to government owned cars doing essential work and to practicing physicians. The second category of vehicle, government owned lease-lend trucks, are used for essential government work, especially the hauling of wheat and other food supplies. Some are allotted to Government departments for the use of mines and essential industries. These lease-lend trucks are flowing into Iran overland from Egypt at the rate of about 50 a month. The flow has been temporarily stepped up to some 100 a month in order to build up a government owned fleet capable of gathering the wheat harvest which will soon come in. Tires are flowing into Iran in sufficient quantity to meet the needs of the country if only one can keep the Middle East Supply Center from obtaining possession of some of them for diversion elsewhere. Some 20,000 tires, almost entirely truck sizes, enough to last Iran for perhaps a year, have arrived or are about to arrive at Persian Gulf ports. As to passenger car sizes, only a few hundred are expected, so that severe restrictive measures will have to be taken to control their use on essential government owned cars. . . .

One of the Road Transport Board's first task was to carry out a re-registration of all motor vehicles in Iran in order to be in a position to gauge the problem it was tackling. The results of this registration are as follows: passenger cars including taxis – 4,476; trucks – 3,556; busses – 584; and ambulances – 17. . . . It is generally estimated that before Iran was invaded a year and a half ago there were some 5,500 trucks and 6,000 passenger cars in operation. The difference between these pre-war figures and the present registration figures represents vehicles which have been "cannibalized" for parts or which have died of old age. The 3,556 trucks now registered are distributed roughly as follows: under contract to UKCC for hauling war goods to Russia – 1,600; under contract to Iransovtrans for the same purpose – 450; under contract to the Iranian Government – 750; laid up, voluntarily out of service, or doing illegal work – 756. The Board hopes to be able to put some at least of these 756 under contract in the near future. It also hopes to obtain all or part of the vehicles now in the hands of the UKCC when the American army takes over the road transport division of that organization and imports a sufficient number of trucks to take care of this vital work. In any event, Iran is faced with a troublesome truck problem since almost all of the 3,556 trucks in the country are so old that they will have to be replaced within a year or two. It is hoped, therefore, to obtain a constant flow of large and small trucks to build up the permanent fleet which is so essential to the economy of this country.

Relations between the Road Transport Board and the British Army, which has taken over responsibility for the road transport work of the UKCC, have been good in recent months. However, the British Army and the UKCC are fading out of the civil transport picture as the American Army takes over full responsibility toward Iranian civil transport. I will follow this question closely in coming weeks and keep the Department informed of trends and developments. Relations between the Board and the MESC are also good. The MESC seems to feel that better control of tires and trucks is being exercised in Iran than in any other Near Eastern country and for this reason Iran's applications for tires and trucks have received favorable consideration.

The Road Transport Board and the Edareh Barbari Rah are not popular in political circles in Tehran. This is due largely to the two circumstances, first, a certain amount of resentment that passenger car tires are not issued for use on private vehicles and, second, dissatisfaction engendered by certain politicians and merchants who are prevented in making war profits out of transport. There has been as a result of these two points, considerable criticism of the Edareh Barbari Rah in the Majlis and press. Conversations are now taking place with a view to meeting the views of these critical elements as nearly as may be possible. While under normal conditions I should be most reluctant to take part in an effort which meets with criticism on the part of the Iranians, under the circumstances it seems to me we have no alternative. Tires must be carefully issued and properly controlled because of their shortage and a system such as has been instituted appears to be essential to the carrying out of this objective. Also it must be remembered that the opposition is almost entirely destructive and emanates from persons interested in making huge war profits out of transport. We have at least the comforting thought that we are rendering substantial aid to

> the economy of the country. Indeed, without the control we have instituted it seems unlikely that Iran could have obtained from the allies either tires or trucks. It is most fortunate, especially now that the harvest is about to be collected, that Iran has a fleet of contracted and government-owned vehicles capable of handling a large part of the country's essential transport. It should not be thought, however, that Iran's road transport problem is solved. At least a 1,000 more trucks are required before all Government and private goods can be efficiently moved and several thousand will be needed to enable the country to replace its fleet of aging vehicles.

The precarious transport situation was further aggravated by the financial position of the Iranian government and its inability to pay for the few Lend-Lease trucks sent its way. Dreyfus on May 30, 1943 (Telegram 558, 891.24/441):

> For Stettinius and Fred Winant, OLLA, from Richard May and George Washington. "One. Iranian Government has now received 391 Lend Lease trucks priced at $2500 each and MESC plans to allocate up to 400 additional trucks during the next 4 months. Latter will be priced at $3,000 each as per recent advices. We also expect to deliver Lend Lease tires at the rate of 2500 per month as needed. Total Iranian commitment to OLLA for stated period will this total upwards of $2,500,000. Two. Discussions with Millspaugh have convinced us that Iranian Government finances are exceedingly precarious, and that cash payment for these Lease Lend goods would either be a practical impossibility or would bring the Government close to financial collapse. . . . Three. The maintenance of civilian economy of Iran appears to us to be vital to efficient operation of aid to Russia program. Particularly essential is continued supply of trucks and tires for cereals collection and food distribution. Accordingly we recommend that no steps be taken at present to insist on immediate payment. . . . Lease Lend deliveries of trucks and tires will not be suspended and immediate payment will not be demanded. . . ." I am in full accord with the foregoing. Dreyfus.

The acute shortage of transport on the eve of the harvest is shown by a cable to Dreyfus on June 11, 1943 (Telegram 286, 891.5018/26A):

> Iranian Minister has requested Department's support of his Government's representations to the United States military authorities

for assistance in expediting movement north of 7,600 tons dates and 17,000 tons of other food supplies and essential material now piled up at Ahwaz because of reported shortage of transport facilities. While Department appreciates difficulties due to military requirements and has so informed Iranian Minister, it would welcome any information you may have on the subject and authorizes you to exercise your good offices in effort to avoid any unnecessary spoilage of these essential foodstuffs.

Chapter 7

Iran and the Middle East Supply Center

Established in April 1941 as part of the Ministry of War Transport (MWT) for the avowed purpose of supplying the civilian needs of Middle Eastern countries under British occupation, the United States became a participant in early 1942 and had approved the assignment of Iran to the MESC framework of import quotas and shipping permits, designation of Iran for Lend-Lease notwithstanding. Imports outside the MESC system became impossible.

Dreyfus on April 23, 1942 (Telegram 119, 891.24/182):

> My 118, April 22, 5 p.m. Discussions with the British Legation and Jackson, head of MESC have elicited following: (1) Hitherto there has been no centralized British agency for dealing with Iranian economic needs. . . . (2) Jackson proposes that a central supply committee be formed in Tehran to handle all matters of economic aid to Iran, the committee to be composed of one representative from each of the following organizations: Iranian Ministry of Finance, Iranian Ministry of Commerce and Industry, British Legation, American Legation, Imperial Bank, UKCC, MESC and possibly Ministry of Economic Warfare. It is proposed that all requests for economic assistance for Iran be made through this committee. Local merchants or importers will obtain import licenses from Iranian Ministry of Finance or Ministry of Commerce and Industry which will forward them to the committee. These Ministries will likewise put forward the requests of their government. The committee will decide which commodities should not be supplied and will recommend quantities in case of commodities to be

> supplied, the American and British Legation delegates to decide on the latter point. The committee will also recommend method of handling requisitions i.e. whether the normal commercial methods in the case of private purchases, by government purchase in the case of bulk articles such as cereals, sugar and tea, or by Lend-Lease. Three. The Central Supply Committee will forward all recommendations to MESC which will classify requisitions as to priority in the case of commercial purchases, will arrange through British Ministry of Food for supply of government purchases and sale by UKCC to Iranian Government, and will forward Lease-Lend requests to Washington. (It is contemplated Lease-Lend will be the exception, to be used only when normal commercial purchases or government purchases cannot be arranged.) It is proposed in future to eliminate all independent purchases by Iranian Government. Four. Distribution will be as follows: an import license system will be established by Iranian Government for private imports. Government purchases and Lease Lend material will be delivered only to the Iranian Government. It is proposed that a rationing system be adopted by the latter with the participation of the Supply Committee. Five. Shipping space will be arranged as follows: merchants possessing import licenses will forward these through Central Supply Committee to MESC which after according priority will in turn forward them to Ministry of War Transport representative in area from which goods are coming. Government purchases will be handled directly by Ministry of War Transport. Lease Lend will be shipped through United States Maritime Commission. Whereas under proposed plan, the American representative would be outnumbered five to one in relation to the British, it is believed that a centralized agency to control economic aid is essential and that the advice of the Imperial Bank, the UKCC, and the British Ministry of Economic Warfare might be useful. It is recommended, therefore that the proposed plan be accepted. . . .

State Department replied on April 30, 1942 (Telegram 106, 891.24/182):

> Your 119 of April 23. Department has decided upon formal participation in the Middle East Supply Centre. There will be military and civilian representation. A member of the Legation in Cairo will serve as interim representative for civilian supplies until a representative is sent out from here. Your cable closely reflects opinion here as to organization and functions of Central Supply Committee in Tehran. . . . In view of the above the Department designates you the American representative on the Central Supply Committee in Tehran and requests that

> you associate yourself with your British colleague with a view to immediate joint action on that Committee.

The MESC system is described in a British Legation note to the Iranian government. Telegram 175 was given in chapter 6 in the context of tires for Iran (Dreyfus, Dispatch 272 and enclosures, 891.24/205, May 29, 1942):

> I have the honor, with reference to my telegram no. 175, May 29, to enclose the memorandum prepared by the British Legation and delivered to the Iranian Government outlining the procedures to be followed in making imports into Iran under regulations drawn up by the MESC and setting forth the quotas for the period July-December 1942. As indicated in my telegram under reference, this memorandum was prepared by the British Commercial secretary immediately on his return from the MESC in Cairo and without consulting either this Legation or the Iranian Government. It represents the opinion of the British Legation based, it is supposed, on the MESC deliberations and conclusions. This memorandum and its enclosures were delivered to me only yesterday and the urgent necessity of placing them in the Department's hands without delay precludes my making analytical comments at present.

The British note is dated May 24, 1942:

> At the present time every available ton of shipping under the control of the Free Nations is required for the transport of munitions and men to the many spheres of war. For this reason the amount of shipping which they make available for the carriage of goods for civilian needs is being progressively decreased, and in order to assure that this minimum amount of shipping brings the maximum benefit to friendly nations, the British and United States Governments have instituted a system of control with the aim of preventing the carriage of luxury goods and organizing the supply of essential goods. This control is operated by the Ministry of War Transport in London, in co-operation with the US Government and for the sake of convenience a central office of this ministry has been set up in Cairo to deal with the requirements of the Middle East States. This central office, called the Middle East Supply Centre, has for some time collected from a number of Middle East countries information as to their minimum requirements, and has arranged the shipment of these requirements from overseas where they

could not be obtained from neighbouring countries. It has now been decided to extend the facilities of this organization to Iran.

From experience it has been found that a system of import licensing is essential for the purpose, and it is desired that the Imperial Iranian Government should now institute such a control on the following lines: Quotas for the majority of commodities have been drawn up on the basis of Iran's previous import statistics and will serve as a basis for the issue of import licenses. A commodity index will also be furnished to the Imperial Government showing what commodities are likely to be shipped from the various countries of supply; what commodities can be supplied only from Government to Government owing to their being centrally controlled; and what commodities are not available owing to their short supply or to their luxury nature.

Merchants should be instructed to approach the licensing Department of the Imperial Government, who would accept applications within the quota already established in cases where there is a definite need for the goods in question. It should be borne in mind that shipping will not be available for any other goods, and applications may be rejected at this early stage if they exceed the quota or if it is clear from the commodity index that the goods will not come forward. Moreover, the applicant should produce evidence that he has received a firm offer from his consignor and intends to do business: otherwise it is clear that the country may not receive the full quota of goods. Having accepted suitable applications, the Import Licensing Department should forward them (and such evidence of good faith as the importer has produced) with an English summary, the form of which will be supplied, to the Tehran branch of the Middle East Supply Centre. This body, which is called the Tehran Central Supplies Committee and has its office in the Commercial Secretariat of the British Legation, will examine the applications and will return them to the Import Licensing Department with information as to which items can suitably be licensed in the light of the latest information received from the Middle East Supply Centre. The approved items will then be licensed under a continuous series of numbers by the Imperial Licensing Department, who will send the final summary of import licenses, as issued and numbered, to the Central Supplies Committee for immediate recommendation of shipping space.

Fortunately the Imperial Government have considerable experience of import licensing and by the amendment of current regulations should

> very soon be able to institute the above system. . . . In publicizing the institution of the system the Imperial Government will no doubt make it clear to merchants that no goods will come forward from overseas without such import licenses. Orders placed by the Imperial Government with foreign firms have not so far been mentioned. Although it is clear that they will receive special treatment they should be included in the import license summaries mentioned above and when agreed should be covered by a numbered import license which should be issued by the licensing department to the purchasing Ministry, so that there may be no doubt about their being recommended for shipment.

Difficulties had arisen from the first meeting of the CSC. Dreyfus on June 9, 1942 (Telegram 192, 891.24/203):

> Reference my no. 175, 4 p.m., May 29. Central Supply Committee has held first meeting and appointed permanent subcommittee and transportation subcommittee which also had first meetings. Committee is endeavoring to induce Iranian Government to introduce effective July 1 import licensing system which is considered necessary to proper functioning of MESC. Iranians will I believe consent to system of import licenses but they object to small quotas established. (See despatch no. 272, May 28). However committee prepared to discuss quota increases if adequate reasons advanced. Confidential. There is danger that British are endeavoring to use committee to further British trade. In addition to selfish attitude of UKCC which I have reported, the following serves as an example. Yesterday agent of Socony Vacuum complained to me he cannot continue to import lubricants because committee have given Anglo-Iranian Oil Company a monopoly for importation from England. I explained to Hobson (sent here from MESC Cairo to head Central Committee Commission) that under no circumstances should the Committee be used as a trade or political football and he agreed to consider question of lubricants at next meeting. UKCC are still intent on obtaining monopoly on import and distribution of tires, trucks and parts. Prime Minister told me he is unwilling to submit to UKCC control and he said confidentially that the Soviet Ambassador feels similarly. Prime Minister said he hopes soon to obtain from Majlis plenary powers for control of both food and transportation. For the Prime Minister's information I should appreciate following details with regard to Lease-Lend. (One) Is a formal agreement with Iran contemplated and (Two) How will Lend-Lease fit into MESC picture.

State Department replied on June 19, 1942 (Telegram 162, 891.24/203):

> Your 192, June 9, last three paragraphs. One. Formal Lend-Lease agreement with Iran is (repeat is) contemplated and will be drawn up in due course. Confidential: It is proposed to conclude agreements with United Nations before beginning negotiations with other countries. Two. Lend-Lease will probably be handled on same general basis as other Government orders. Requests would be channeled through Central Supplies Committee and MESC before presentation to Lend-Lease Administration here. Exact manner of delivery in Iran has not yet been decided. Confidential: Question of Lend-Lease delivery and distribution in Iran is under consideration here and decision will probably depend largely upon ultimate composition of Tehran Central Supplies Committee and the attitude adopted by the British regarding use of that committee to supervise supply distribution. . . . In talking with Prime Minister, you should emphasize American participation in MESC. An officer of the Department will shortly proceed to Cairo to head our representation on that body.

Dreyfus on June 18, 1942 (Telegram 204, 891.24/207):

> Referring to my 192, June 9, Iranian Government has now agreed to institute import licensing system and is naming a committee to meet with CSC to work out details. They agreed with reluctance because they are displeased with Allied treatment in matters of supplies particularly with quotas established (see my despatch 272, May 28). Iranian displeasure with Allied treatment arises from following: (1) Allies have not lived up to promises to provide essential supplies to Iran; (2) Allies fail to take into consideration fact that Iranian reserves have been depleted to great extent by Allied armed forces and Polish refugees; (3) transport facilities of Iran are being depleted by Allies. Railway is being used 80% by Allies; United Kingdom Commercial Corporation has taken over all heavy and large part of light trucks and now propose to give Iranians no trucks or tires thus placing them at mercy of British; Iranians are unable now to move troops and soon will be unable to move wheat, beets, and other goods. Iranian officials growing more critical of us on grounds that while we promise to assist them in economic sense nothing actually is done. They make a point particularly of their right to receive tire and trucks because British have depleted their transport facilities. There is much merit in Iranian case and I recommend immediate steps be taken to make tires available to them along lines suggested in my no. 175, May 29. I also recom-

> mend that heavy and light trucks be made available to Iranians as soon as possible to enable them to move troops (now being handicapped by immobility in action against the tribes) and to move the harvests and other essential goods. These tires and trucks to be of value must arrive soon. I suggest therefore that a portion of the Lend-Lease trucks now arriving in Iran be earmarked for immediate delivery to the Iranian Government. If we do not take some action soon to fulfill our promises of aid to Iran, the incipient wave of criticism of United States is sure to grow.

On June 18, 1942, the State Department had expressed great surprise at the changed composition of the CSC and its permanent subcommittee from what it had been previously reported by Dreyfus (Telegram 158, 891.24/205):

> Your despatch no. 272, May 28. We note that British Minister's letter of May 27 to you lists one American and seven British members of Central Supplies Committee and that apparently Iranians are not represented. Your telegram 119, April 23 proposed a committee of American and British Ministers and representatives of Iranian Ministries of Commerce and Finance, with other British representatives acting in an advisory capacity only, and it was on this basis that Department authorized your participation. (See Department's 106, April 30.) Department's suggestion that tires and other American supplies be distributed under supervision of Central Supplies Committee was made on understanding that Committee would be joint Anglo-American-Iranian body. If this is not the case, we may have to reconsider our attitude. Please telegraph exact composition of committee as now functioning and whether any changes are contemplated.

Dreyfus replied on June 25, 1942 (Telegram 214, 891.24/210):

> Department's number 158, June 18, midnight. There was, as Department indicated, considerable deviation from original understanding of Legation as to constitution of CSC. I was as shown in despatch 272, presented with a fait accompli as to quotas and organization of committee and the Iranians also were not consulted. I have not accepted this arrangement as final but have been in constant negotiations with Iranians and British to find some suitable plan. Delay in arriving at agreement has been caused principally by Iranian reluctance to accept licensing system because of what they consider inadequate quotas and because Iranians did not appoint representatives to discuss question.

The matter has now been settled along following lines, if Department agrees thereto: The CSC will consist of eight persons as indicated in the British note attached to despatch 272 but it has been agreed that in all matters considered, the opinion of the British and American Ministers will be the deciding factor. This I believe takes care of our preoccupation about being out voted seven to one. At the first meeting of CSC on May 29, two subcommittees were formed: (One) permanent subcommittee for doing routine work of CSC consisting of delegates of following MESC (chairman) American Legation, UKCC, MEW (Ministry of Economic Warfare), Imperial Bank of Iran and British Legation. (Two) transport subcommittee to consider transport problems and supplies, consisting of Anglo-Iranian Oil Company official as chairman, American Legation, UKCC, MESC, MEW, Transportation Directorate and British Legation. Minor represents Legation on both committees and sits with me unofficially on CSC. Question of having Iranian delegates on CSC proper was given serious consideration but it was consensus of opinion that discussion of vital war work such as shipping position and supplies to Russia made this undesirable. Since I insisted on Iranians being heard, the Iranian Government was invited to form a committee of its own to meet with permanent subcommittee. After much delay following strong committee of five was named: Director General of the Ministry of Commerce, Director General of Customs, head Imports Department, official of Ministry of Commerce and head Foreign Transaction Department.

Committee met with our permanent subcommittee on Monday in atmosphere of cordial understanding and another meeting will be held today. Iranian committee agrees in principle to institution of licensing system although details have yet to be worked out. They have taken immediate steps to ascertain outstanding orders placed abroad by Iran merchants and action on this preliminary phase is expected soon. I believe formation of this committee meets our desire to have Iranians fully heard. I might say that Minister of Finance expressed his satisfaction with this arrangement—Iranians do not care about machinery but are interested only in results. Although a good atmosphere now prevails I must warn Department that great difficulty will be encountered soon since Iranians are dissatisfied with quotas and finally consented to cooperate only on promise of reconsideration of many items. I am in a difficult position between intransigent British on one hand and grasping Iranians on other. It seems likely the increasingly difficult shipping situation will preclude any possibility of radical readjustment upwards of quotas. However, Iranians should be given satisfac-

> tion on matters of tires and trucks (see my 175, May 29). The only present discordant voice is that of UKCC which not only wishes to monopolize Iranian transport and distribution of tires and trucks but seems reluctant to submit to CSC on grounds that it is a governmental agency. I have been, and intend to continue to be, adamant on this point—nothing can be accomplished unless CSC is supreme in matter of supplies to Iran. UKCC apparently does not want to give up its private trade which is lucrative for present and holds promises for British trade for future. I do not object to UKCC trade if British Government desires that procedure but I insist that UKCC submit to CSC as would any other trader. If they do not I would suggest we counter with reservation of right to proceed outside CSC with Lend-Lease goods. I might add that UKCC are receiving four thousand Lease-Lend trucks and intend that none be allotted to Iranians.

Dreyfus on September 18, 1942 (Dispatch 349 and enclosure, 800.24/462):

> I have the honor to enclose a memorandum concerning the organization and operation of the Tehran Central Supplies Committee, the branch in Iran of the Middle East Supply Center. It is hoped that this memorandum, prepared by the chairman of the permanent or working subcommittee of the Central Supplies Committee, will give the Department a better idea of the set-up and operation of the Middle East Supply Center. The Central Supplies Committee is functioning actively, and I believe, as efficiently as the difficult local conditions allow. The main committee meets once a month to pass on matters of policy, while the permanent sub-committee meets every few days according to the work to be done. A chemical and industrial development sub-committee, set up for the purpose of assisting the Iranians to develop their own mines and industries, meets once a week. . . . The transport sub-committee has been able to set up a joint Anglo-American-Iranian Transport Board (see my telegram No. 287, September 10) which will control all transport in the country and is now engaged in registering the motor vehicles of the country as a necessary preliminary step. All of the committees have their headquarters in the Commercial Secretariat of the British Legation. Major Hobson and Captain Amos of the Middle East Supply Center, assisted by two secretaries and a chemical expert, give their entire time to this work. Experts in various lines, such as rubber, agriculture and pharmaceuticals, as well as officials of the Middle East Supply Center, visit Tehran at intervals to advise their fields. Mr. Winant, American representative to the MESC has not yet visited Tehran

> but is expected in the near future. The principle work of the committee, that of passing on applications for imports, is proceeding after considerable delay on the part of the Iranians, who accepted the import restrictions with reluctance and put them into effect with lethargy. All outstanding orders, that is those placed before June 21, 1942, have been assembled by the Iranian Department of Commerce in their various categories and passed on to the committee. These are now being considered and will very soon be completed and passed on to the loading areas. New applications, under the quotas for the six month period July to December, will then be considered.

The enclosed memorandum is entitled, "Organization and Work of the Central Supplies Committee in Persia in Relation to Import Licensing Procedure." The Central Supplies Committee had grown to 11, two Americans and nine British: US Minister, First Secretary of US Legation, British Minister, British Military Attaché, British Commercial Secretary, Director of Transportation, Manager of the Imperial Bank of Iran, and representatives of MESC, UKCC, Ministry of Economic Warfare, and Ministry of War Transport. The working or permanent subcommittee had five members, four British and one American: representatives of MESC (Chairman and author of the memorandum), UKCC, Ministry of Economic Warfare, Commercial Secretary of the British Legation, and First Secretary of the US Legation. The memorandum also further clarifies the procedure the Iranian government and merchants had to follow in order to obtain an import license:

> Persia was recently brought within the Middle East bloc of countries whose needs for civil supplies are planned and coordinated by the MESC. In order to give effect to MESC policy and procedure in this country the first step taken was the formation of a Central Supplies Committee to implement a similar method of import licensing control to that operative in other countries of the Middle East bloc, and thereafter to deal with all supply and transport problems in connection with the civil requirements of this country. . . . A working Sub-Committee under the Chairmanship of the Middle East Supply Centre Representative deals with all the routine work in connection with import licensing and the main problems relating thereto. . . . The actual import licensing procedures which has been instituted is as follows: Merchants wishing to import goods into Iran make an application for an import license direct to the Ministry of Commerce and Industry (in no circumstances to the Central Supplies Committee or the UKCC) on a standard

> form. . . . The applications are considered by the Ministry on the basis of their essentiality for the country or, where quotas have been laid down, on the basis of agreed quotas. The Ministry of Commerce then forward their recommendations in duplicate to the Permanent Sub-Committee. The Permanent Sub-Committee then "vets" these recommendations again and allots import license number to each order for which shipping is recommended. The import license numbers allotted to the items approved are advised to the Imperial Government by returning the duplicate import license application summary; at the same time similar information is passed to MESC Headquarters, Cairo, for final "vetting" and thereafter on forwarding to the loading areas concerned. In order to assist the Ministry of Commerce with these import license applications the Ministry has been supplied with a combined Commodity Index and Quota List which shows the agreed quotas for the current half year and also indicates the source from which supply can be obtained. . . . In the case of Iranian Government or UKCC orders only application for import license numbers is made direct to the Central Supplies Committee on the standard application form. Details of UKCC orders approved and allotted import license numbers are advised to the Iranian Government so that the quantity of any commodity involved may be deducted from the agreed quota.

The Central Supplies Committee was renamed as the Combined Supplies Committee, and the permanent working sub-committee was renamed the Executive Committee (Dreyfus, Dispatch 427, 800.24/557, January 5, 1943).

With the help of MESC, the UKCC had gained control of Iran's foreign trade. Dreyfus on January 4, 1943 (Telegram 6, 891.24/338):

> UKCC continues to handle following imports: (a) Commodities centrally pooled under control MESC Cairo including cereals, sugar and tea; (b) other commodities under special control including motor vehicles, parts and tires; (c) Various commodities which UKCC contend cannot be handled as expeditiously through private trade channels. Most Iranian industries are owned and operated by government. Purchases are made through Supply Department of Ministry of Commerce which must use UKCC USCC or private importers as Iranian Government is not prepared to handle imports. As a matter of general principle I favor leaving imports as much as possible to private channels. However, private traders have encountered so many obstacles such as inability to obtain export permits and shipping space that it is becoming increasingly difficult to carry on private trade. For example, Ira-

> nian Government early last year delivered to UKCC credit and documents covering 24,230 tires ordered by private Iranian dealers because neither the importers nor Iranian Government was able to obtain allocation of shipping space. UKCC was able to obtain permits and space and tires are now arriving.

Dreyfus on January 13, 1943 (Telegram 43, 891.24/346):

> Department's 15, January 7. Kidd recommends, and I concur, that imports from the United States now handled by United Kingdom Commercial Corporation can and should be handled by United States Commercial Corporation except that bulk commodities centrally pooled under MESC should continue to be handled by United Kingdom Commercial Corporation.

Dreyfus-Winant Controversy over MESC

While relations between the American army in Iran and the MESC had soured, those between Dreyfus and Fred Winant in Cairo had reached breaking point. Dreyfus on January 24, 1943 (Airgram-3, 891.24/373):

> General Harrison recently visited Tehran on a mission to investigate into relations between (American) military authorities and MESC. In a meeting attended by him, General Connolly, Lend-Lease representative and myself, it was consensus of opinion that MESC is so obstructive, bureaucratic and mindful of British post-war considerations that military operations are hampered and supply of civil goods for Iranian needs is made unnecessarily complicated. General Connolly made it clear that he is compelled to acquiesce in this state of affairs because he is temporarily dependent on British here but that he does not intend to do so after his organization is operating fully. Particular dissatisfaction was expressed with new MESC policy of pooling wheat (see my telegram No. 12 of January 6, 1943) and American army officials are considering importing own wheat for their forces. It was agreed at meeting that Iranian problems being sui generis cannot be handled from Cairo; as proof of this it was observed that the British have finally set up a separate Persia-Iraq Command. Opinion was expressed that MESC is the political instrument of Casey and that its ultimate object is to gain control for British of post-war trade in Near East.

There is much to be said for foregoing attitude. I am coming to opinion that MESC complicates and obstructs supply problems and makes it extremely difficult to obtain direct and positive action. Some examples of this are: the question of typhus vaccine which was handled by MESC so that Iranians were completely let down; pooling of wheat shipments in southern Iran; consignment of Lend-Lease trucks to British Embassy at Baghdad which determined number to be sent here on basis (of) its relations with Iraq; approval of importation of battery radio sets from United States and electric ones from England; interference in Iranian internal affairs such as mines and industries and endeavors to place British experts in Iranian departments against the desires of Iranians; refusal to allow imports of luxury items of high value and small shipping space which would use some of Iran's surplus foreign exchange; unfriendly attitude of British MESC delegates in dealing with Iranians; MESC representatives do not always consult American members or advise Legation of action taken; MESC representatives in Cairo seldom visit Iran and then only for a day or two at a time; Iranian Government officials complain bitterly at the low quotas set by MESC (it was a tactical blunder to permit Iranians to know that quotas existed and would have been better to permit them to assess own needs and furnish whatever parts of their demands possible in light of supplies of goods and availability of shipping space); merchants feel that MESC was created to prevent import of merchandise. All things considered it would seem that this entire matter of supplies for Iran could be handled more expeditiously and with more consideration for Iran's needs and susceptibilities by an allied committee acting independently in Tehran. The above is given for the Department's information and background, not with the suggestion of any immediate action. Copy sent to Cairo.

Stung by criticism of the British and MESC, Fred Winant in Cairo had sent a long response on January 27, 1943 (Airgram-10, 891.24/375):

Reference is made to airgram No. A-3, dated January 24, 1943, addressed to the Department by the American Legation in Tehran concerning the MESC's position with regard to civilian supplies for Iran. My reply will be divided into two parts: (I) dealing with the general allegations contained in paragraph one of airgram under reference, and (II) dealing with the more specific allegations in paragraph two of the airgram.

On the so-called general allegations, Winant writes:

> 1. That "MESC is so obstructive, bureaucratic and mindful of British post-war political considerations that military operations are hampered. . . . " If the Persian Gulf Command of the US Army in the Middle East felt that military operations were being hampered because of the action of any organization, it would seem that such a situation should have been called to the attention of the Commanding General of the US Forces in the Middle East - General Maxwell, who has been the responsible military authority for US Army operations in Iran. As General Maxwell has been a member of the Executive of MESC, any complaint against that organization could have been investigated immediately at the top level. As neither General Maxwell nor Colonel Claybaugh, his representative to MESC, has ever raised such an issue, I can only surmise that no such complaint has ever been presented here. . . . 2. Regarding Minister Dreyfus' statement that supply of civil goods for Iran has been made unnecessarily complicated, I can only say that the procedure for Iran is similar to that of other territories, and although it is admitted that the result of the system does not curry popular favor it is not necessarily the fault of the system. The simple facts of the case are that we are engaged in an unpopular business. Moreover, if there is any constructive criticism of our methods we would be the first to receive and act upon it. 3. As the comment regarding the pooling of wheat is repeated under specific example in paragraph two of airgram it will be dealt with in Part II of this reply. 4. That the highest British military authorities decided to set up a separate Army Command for Iraq and Iran seems hardly to bear on the question of civilian supplies for Iran. Frankly, I do not know the reasons for such a change. If I were to guess I would say that the change was involved with military and strategic considerations in the operation of British land forces. . . . 5. As to the opinion that "MESC is the political instrument of Casey and that its ultimate object is to gain control for British of post-war trade in the Near East," I wish to point out that MESC was started in April 1941, whereas Mr. Casey did not reach the Middle East until May 1942. In this connection I wish to add a personal observation to the effect that any connivance of this sort, whether for short or long range is entirely foreign to Mr. Casey's nature and that through my relations with him I feel that any such accusation is entirely unfounded. As to post-war objectives of MESC I have no reason to suspect the material motives of the British from my association with them todate. . . .

The matter of typhus vaccine in Part II of the reply is dealt with in chapter 8:

> 1. "The question of typhus vaccine which was handled by MESC so that Iranians were completely let down." Request of Minister Dreyfus for one million doses of typhus vaccine led authorities here to believe that a dangerous situation had developed in Iran. Immediately arrangements were made to dispatch by air 1,000 doses, to be followed by another 1,000 doses from London. Department in Washington arranged for 100,000 doses to be flown to Cairo for forwarding to Tehran. In meantime Colonel Sams, Surgeon general of US Middle East forces flew to Tehran to make a personal survey. Colonel Sams conclusions were that there existed no epidemic in Tehran or elsewhere in Iran and that the danger of an epidemic there was no greater than in other territories of the Near East, that the request for 1,000,000 doses was purely precautionary to avoid possible epidemic; and that therefore the 100,000 doses coming by air from the United States should be retained in Cairo as nucleus of central pool for protection of whole area. I might add that decisions in this matter were confirmed by Washington authorities, and in this connection reference is made to Department's 1686 of December 26. . . . 2. "Pooling of wheat shipments in Southern Iran." This system is necessary in view of the fact that most wheat shipments are in broken stowage with a comparatively small amount aboard each ship, and generally are spread among several of the ports. In order to coordinate properly the distribution of this wheat in order of priority, a form of pooling arrangement has been devised. . . . 3. "Consignment of Lend-Lease trucks to British Embassy at Baghdad which determined number to be sent here (Tehran) on basis of its relations with Iraq." The trucks in question were made available for civilian use in Iran and Iraq from British military stores under an allocation made by the Anglo-American Motor Vehicle Allocation Committee of MESC in Cairo. They were driven overland from the Red Sea area by British military drivers and delivered to their Embassy and Legation there to be turned over to Lend-Lease representatives who were to negotiate with the respective Governments for the terms of the sale. The British Embassy at Baghdad, of course, did not determine the number to be sent to Tehran. That was determined by the Motor Vehicle Allocation Committee long before the trucks were delivered. . . . 4. "Approval of importation of battery radio sets from United States and electric ones from England." This matter was brought up some time ago in an airgram from the Teheran Legation, and in my reply dated December 22, 1942, I explained that the policy of the MESC was to allow the importation

of radio sets only as "special case" items for specific propaganda purposes, and for hospitals, etc., and that the choice of the supplying country will be left to the import licensing authorities. I am therefore unable to understand why this misunderstanding still exists. 5. "Interference in Iranian internal matters such as mines and industries and endeavors to place British experts in Iranian departments against desires of Iranians." We know of no instance where MESC has attempted to place British experts in Iranian Departments against the desires of Iranians, and would appreciate more specific information from the Teheran Legation regarding this comment. . . . We have not been aware of any "interference" in Iranian internal matters. From information available in Cairo it does not seem that the Iranians have complained to the British of such interference and advice as to their specific complaint to the Teheran Legation would be appreciated. 6. "Refusal to allow imports of luxury items of high value and small shipping space which would use up some of Iran's surplus foreign exchange." This, of course, is in general true and reflects the usual policy of the MESC for all of the area. With available shipping sufficient only for a small fraction of the normal imports of the countries it is difficult enough to provide the bear (sic) necessities, and furnishing such necessities is our real objective and responsibility. 7. "Unfriendly attitude of British MESC delegates in dealing with Iranians." We are not aware of this condition but are immediately looking into the situation. Certainly the policy of MESC is to cooperate fully with the territorial Governments and there should be no deviation from this rule. 8. "MESC representatives do not always consult American members or advise Legation of action taken." I am surprised to hear this complaint now. By letter of November 12, Minister Dreyfus mentioned the lack of information on matters pertaining to the Center. I immediately instituted corrective measures and under date of December 7 Mr. Dreyfus wrote me: "Your request through Jackson to have Hobson give us copies of MESC telegrams and bulletins bore immediate fruit and they are being furnished us regularly." 9. "MESC representatives in Cairo seldom visit Iran and then only for a day or so at a time." The reply to this complaint is that at the present time we do not have Americans available to send to the territories for an appreciable period. . . . 10. "Iranian Government officials complain bitterly at the low quotas set by the MESC." This is quite natural and is not unusual in any other Middle Eastern country. The fact is, of course, that the low quotas are necessitated by the exigencies of war. The most recent cut which is being made by the highest and most competent authorities in London and Washington undoubtedly will be received with much com-

> plaint. . . . 11. "Merchants feel that MESC was created to prevent the import of merchandise." This is a correct assumption. One of the objects was to prevent the importation of non-essential goods and to establish a method of assuring that the most essential goods are received. Regarding Minister Dreyfus' suggestion that an allied committee acting independently in Tehran would better handle supply matters for Iran, my answer is simply a restatement of the reasons for the establishment of MESC: to coordinate civilian requirements for the entire area in order to get the greatest possible benefit from the limited shipping space available, taking into consideration the overall conditions of the units of the territory. Through a central organization the relative needs of the respective countries can be appraised in a manner of equality and balance that would be impossible under a decentralized system.
>
> I believe we all realize that if the MESC is to effectively function in the elimination of non-essential imports and the establishment of programs within the many times reduced shipping space it is bound to incur some unpopularity in the several territories, especially by individuals whose interests would be inclined otherwise. . . . As will be seen by my foregoing analysis of complaints of Minister Dreyfus, almost all allegations are without adequate factual support. The fact that he has seen fit to file with the Department an attack on MESC of such a sweeping character without first making an effort to discuss the case with me may well be due to the existence of circumstances which are not evident in the airgram and with which I am not familiar, particularly since Minister Dreyfus arrived in Cairo on January 24, the day on which his airgram was dispatched. . . . I am retaining a copy of this airgram which I shall deliver to Minister Dreyfus when he passes through Cairo in a few days on his return trip from Luxor.

The justification Winant gave for "pooling" wheat shipments in southern Iran was his claim that shipments arrived in small quantities and at different ports. That this was a bogus argument can be seen from a conversation on February 4, 1943, between William C. Armstrong of the Office of Lend-Lease Administration (OLLA) and Jernegan (Memorandum, 891.24/372):

> Mr. Armstrong called me on February 4 to ask whether the Department would have any serious objection to shipping the entire monthly quota of wheat for Iran (or rather that part which is to be sent in American vessels) in a single ship. He explained that 7,000 tons would make a complete shipload, which would greatly simplify loading here

> and unloading in the Persian Gulf. It would also avoid the inevitable arguments involved in getting space set aside on ships allocated for the transport of supplies to Russia or for American troops in Iran. It was true, of course, that a certain risk was incurred in putting everything on one vessel, but sinkings en route to the Persian Gulf had been light recently. The proposal was favored by War Shipping Administration, General Spalding and OLLA, and it would be adopted unless the Department had some serious objection. After consulting Mr. Murray, Mr. Alling, and Mr. Merchant, I called Mr. Armstrong on February 5 to say that we had no objection, provided it were understood that if the ship were sunk it would be replaced. Mr. Armstrong said that this would be done, in the sense that the necessary additional space would be provided the following month.

Dreyfus replied to Winant's remarks on February 17, 1943 (Telegram 185, 800.24/585):

> For Winant. Referring to your airgram 10 of January 27 to Department. I very much regret that you considered my airgram an attack on Middle East Supply Center and that you did not discuss matter frankly with me when I was in your office January 26. Only purpose of my airgram was to report the sense of an important meeting and to give facts as I saw them. This whole matter I am happy to state has been clarified by McDuffie's 10 day visit to Tehran. Steps have been taken to effect closer liaison between Allied Legations and Middle East Supply Center and open and frank discussions which took place have done much to improve mutual understanding. I also note from your February 15 to Kidd that strong American representation on Middle East Supply Center in quarters removed from British Legation has been decided upon. You are perhaps not aware that this Legation played an important part in organizing Middle East Supply Center branch in Tehran, was the main instrumentality in obtaining Iranian compliance with Middle East Supply Center procedure and has taken most active part in Middle East Supply Center deliberations. Permit me to assure you that this Legation intends to continue to offer heartiest cooperation with Middle East Supply Center in its important war work. However, I am sure you will admit my right and duty to express my views in frank and constructive manner particularly when aimed at correcting abuses and effecting better cooperation. Such a course usually results, as it already has in this case in improved relations. Repeated to Department.

British policies and MESC practices received strong support in important American quarters. On March 5, 1943, W. Averell Harriman had written a "Personal and Confidential" letter from London to Assistant Secretary Dean Acheson (Letter, 891.24/422):

> I have read Fred Winant's letter to you dated January 28 enclosing a copy of Minister Dreyfus' airgram and a copy of Fred's reply, both of which he enclosed with his letter to me. I want to support the position Fred has taken in this matter. In the light of my experience in the Middle East and Iran I believe that Fred is handling the situation out there well. He has a very large area to cover and considering the number of people he has working for him, I believe he is doing a first-rate job. I can personally testify to the good relations between Fred and his British colleagues in Cairo.
>
> I share Fred's view that the unhealthy Anglo-American situation in Teheran is most disturbing. My impression is that the UKCC people in Teheran have not been first-rate and have not handled matters well. The British Government people, both in London and Teheran, recognize this and are trying to improve the organization. It does not seem to me, however, that there is a sufficient basis for condemning British Government's motives. The Minister, Mr. Bullard, although a hard hitter, I found could be dealt with on an equally straightforward basis. In my negotiations in regard to the taking over the operation of the Persian railroad I met with initial resistance on the part of the British, particularly on military grounds. However, after analyzing the points of difference we reached what I consider a reasonable agreement. After all, if the British were primarily concerned in the post-war situation as Dreyfus intimates in his correspondence, they never would have let us operate the railroad which is the key to the Persian economy. I think part of the difficulty in Iran is the fact that our people find it hard to realize that Persia is, in effect, occupied by the British military. It is perfectly clear that, from a military point of view, it is a British responsibility. I do not believe that it is difficult for us to work out our problems with them if we are prepared to recognize theirs. I think, also, some of our people pay too much attention to the complaints of the Persians who are actuated by mercenary motives all down the line. I am strongly in favour of leaving Iran in the MESC area.

Alling's note to Acheson and Rostow (Memorandum, 891.24/422):

> With reference to Mr. Harriman's underlying letter to Mr. Acheson, this Division feels that we should regard the Fred Winant - Dreyfus controversy over the MESC as a closed issue, at least for the present. As you may recall, Minister Dreyfus, after his return to Tehran from his leave in Egypt, cabled that satisfactory readjustments in MESC Iranian operations were being made and that he did not object, in principle to the MESC. Consequently, whatever merits of the original complaints from Tehran and Fred Winant's reply, it would appear that no action is required at this time.

Growing Dissatisfaction with MESC

With famine and the spreading typhus epidemic in the spring of 1943, Dreyfus had again turned on the MESC. On April 7, 1943 (Dreyfus, Dispatch 511 and enclosure, 891.24/431):

> I have the honor to enclose the quota schedule established by the Middle East Supply Center for importations into Iran for the semester ending June 30, 1943. I shall take advantage of this opportunity to set forth in some detail my views on the status and operation of the Middle East Supply Center in Iran. The enclosed quota schedules are not confidential and may be used by the Department as it sees fit. I have labeled this despatch strictly confidential because I fear that the views I have set forth might, if made known, disturb the friendly spirit of cooperation which I have at great pains established between my Legation and the MESC. The Department is aware of Mr. Winant's strong reaction, as given in the Cairo Legation's Airgram No. 10 of January 27, 1943, to the criticism of the Middle East Supply Center contained in my Airgram No. 3 of January 24, 1943. While it is precisely this kind of family and allied squabble I desire to avoid, I feel that I would be delinquent in my duty were I to fail to bring my views frankly to the Department's attention. As a matter of practical operation, meanwhile, I take the view that the MESC is "a poor thing but mine own" and I assure the Department that it will have this Legation's full support. I might add that, as a result of the frankness of both Mr. Winant and myself, the atmosphere has been considerably cleared. Mr. McDuffie was sent to Tehran, the first visit here of any length of an American representative of MESC, and the modus operandi that he worked out has resulted in improvement. I should also like to stress that my remarks are not intended to reflect on Mr. Winant or any of the other American members of the MESC in Cairo. They are working very hard to make the MESC a success and deserve support, not condemna-

tion, but I doubt whether they are aware that the organization is being used as a political vehicle.

MESC operation is cumbersome, slow and bureaucratic. With its handmaiden, the UKCC, it operates over Iranian commerce an effective monopoly which is beginning to bring criticism from the Iranians as well as skeptical eyebrow lifting on the part of the Russians. Although it is intended to serve a war purpose in controlling imports and saving shipping space, it has all the earmarks of economic and political infiltration, at least on the part of the British. Although I know that the United States has no trade or political motives whatsoever in this matter, we must accept our full share of responsibility for MESC action. It seems to me impracticable to operate a supply system for Iran by remote control from Cairo. The overriding desire of MESC is conserve shipping space. I do not for a moment contend that shipping space should not be saved; on the contrary, I agree that imports should be reduced to rock bottom. This, however, should be done in keeping with our often repeated commitments, and those of the British, to see that Iran's minimum needs are met. It is valueless, for example, for Cairo to say arbitrarily, as it did, that Iran's yearly quota of light globes is established at 60,000, when the Iranians had asked for one million. An endeavor should be made by impartial persons to arrive without delay at Iran's minimum needs in this or any other item and then to see that the goods come forward without delay if the supplying center agrees that the request can be met and if shipping space is available. Iran, as the Department knows, is a problem peculiar to itself and cannot be considered in the same light as other countries, either politically or from a supply viewpoint. Dr. Atkins of the Millspaugh Mission states that in South America the problem is handled in a direct manner by a local committee in each country which assesses the country's needs and passes the orders along to the United States, where it is decided whether the goods can be supplied and whether shipping space is available. This would be, it seems to me, the logical solution for Iran's supply problem. It would not only be more efficient but would also reduce the almost interminable delays being experienced in getting licenses approved and goods actually shipped. Take pharmaceuticals as an example of this slow routine. About a year ago, Mr. Saleh and Professor Oberlin, then in the United States, bought and prepared a much needed lot of pharmaceuticals for shipment from the United States to Iran. Before they could get the shipment off, however, MESC procedure was begun and it was decided that this shipment could come forward only as part of an Iranian bulk indent. The matter was tackled in typical MESC manner, by a pharmaceutical subcommittee, which was required to seek out all kinds of information as to Iranian drug stocks and needs, statistics which are impossible to obtain in Iran. The order was bandied around from subcommittee to the main Combined Supplies Committee, a sort of "short first to second play" and it was not until a few weeks ago that final agreement was reached. Then a new game began, the play now being Tehran to Cairo to London. I am informed that the bulk intend has been approved in Cairo, with what cuts I do not know, and has been forwarded to London. The final play, London to Washington, will now take place. In the meantime drugs are needed and Saleh's order in America is awaiting shipment. This is certainly an inefficient way to handle a supply problem. Nor will shipping space, the main desideratum of MESC, be saved by the end of this procedure.

The MESC has two methods of approach, one for a friend and one for the Iranians. The Anglo-Iranian Oil Company, for example, are in the first category and they hardly bother to consult MESC. For example, the AIOC have just increased their ration of bread for laborers from the established 800 grammes a day to 1,000, informing the MESC after the action that their demands for cereals will be increased accordingly. I do not criticize the AIOC for its action as I believe that 1,000 grammes of bread a day for a laborer in Iran is really a minimum, but no one suggests a similar increase for Iranian workers outside the AIOC! The MESC has rightfully disapproved the import of whiskey and other spirits for Iran but notwithstanding this decision it has approved an AIOC demand for four bottles of whiskey a month for each European employees of AIOC and certain other amounts for AIOC clubs. Other requests of AIOC, as for example one for the import of 250,000 yards of cotton piece goods from India for use in bartering with Iranians to obtain cooking fats, are treated with special consideration. Requests for cars for allied diplomats are usually approved but, with the exception of one car for the Shah, similar requests of the Iranian Government are refused coldly. The Iranian Government requested that 35 Buicks which somehow managed to arrive in Iran in the name of a merchant be delivered over to it for the use of the American advisers but they were instead divided between the UKCC and the American and British armies. There is amazing discrimination between Iraq, a British dominated country, and Iran, a presumably independent country. Although Iran's population is four times that of Iraq, the Department will note from the enclosed schedules that Iraq is allotted almost double the Iranian tonnage. This is due only partially to the fact that

Iran is to some extent supplied by its own industries. The MESC has been endeavoring to divert to other countries some 16,000 of the 24,000 tires destined for Iran. It is almost heartbreaking for me to have to combat this kind of tactic. The Department is well aware of the gigantic struggle in which I was engaged last year to protect Iran in the matter of tires. Only last week the MESC, Cairo, wished to divert from Iran to Iraq 500 passenger car tires which had arrived at a southern port, notwithstanding the fact that Iran's passenger car tire stocks are completely exhausted. They were requested not to insist on the transfer.

The MESC policy of peaceful penetration of the Iranian Government, by endeavoring to worm their officials into positions, exert influence and obtain information, has for its ostensible purpose obtaining information to aid in imports control and suggesting means of utilizing local industries to the fullest extent. Whatever its purpose, this policy is resented by Iranians. As examples of this penetration, they have managed to introduce Mr. Simmons into the Department of Commerce, with MESC salary and without formal consent of the Iranians, to supervise the Iranian end of import licensing. Mr. Barnett, a MESC mining expert, interferes in all sorts of matters having to do with mining and chemicals. Mr. McDowell has just arrived to take charge of MESC transport work and the British are trying to introduce him into the Road Transport Board. Major Jarvis is investigating into the textile industry. Visiting experts in agriculture, pharmaceuticals, mining, etc., come to Iran frequently to obtain information and tell the Iranians what they must do to obtain goods. At present the MESC is requiring the Iranian Government to make a complete inventory of customs houses. The MESC, without the approval of the Iranian Government, is looking for a British miller for the Tehran central bakery. The Industrial Committee, now being set up, will go into all phases of Iranian industrial life. MESC has, as will be seen, outgrown imports control and has penetrated straight into the heart of Iranian civil and business life, always under the implied or even direct threat that any obstruction will result in imports being cut off.

The tool of the British in carrying out the trade aspects of MESC is the UKCC, which has by now obtained what amounts to an effective monopoly of Iranian import trade. The UKCC method of approach is simple. It ascertains what the Iranians need and offers to obtain it, an offer readily accepted because of the urgent need for the goods in question. The UKCC, being a powerful government agency with an inside track can in almost all cases obtain the goods without delay. Most MESC supply telegrams contain a clause that the goods will be obtained by the UKCC. I understand that the channel for all approved MESC orders is through UKCC, New York. The UKCC is the only channel for the import of controlled items, which consist of wheat, flour, corn, millet, barley, rice, other cereals, sugar, tea, coconut oil, olive oil, fertilizers, nitrates, newsprint, cigarette paper, lubricating oils, greases, pig iron, motor vehicles, radio, telephone apparatus, and phosphate. In addition, it competes with merchants in the import of most other goods and, being in a favored position, almost monopolizes Iran's commerce. There follows examples of UKCC trade penetration.

1. The UKCC imported for the British pharmaceutical trade a large order of English drugs, without MESC consent and in spite of the fact that Saleh's order of drugs is still being held up in the United States. This import, which must be attributed solely to the desire of the organized English pharmaceutical trade to sell trademarked British goods in Iran, caused considerable surprise in Tehran commercial circles. It has now been agreed that the order will be sold to the Iranian Government. 2. The UKCC is trying to get British Blackstone motors for the Iranian textiles mills. 3. The UKCC is importing a limited quantity of sports goods for the Middle East. 4. It is now suggested that the UKCC be the only channel for the import of steel products into the Middle East. 5. The UKCC are, without an order being placed, receiving 800 bicycle tires for distribution in Iran. 6. The UKCC has imported into Iran £17,000 worth of diamonds, although my suggestion that similar goods of high value and small bulk should be encouraged to help the currency situation was refused by the MESC. 7. The UKCC is importing 3,000 tons of the 7,000 tons of cotton to be imported this year. At a MESC meeting the UKCC representative stated that UKCC ought really to import all of the cotton because they could do it more efficiently and cheaper.

UKCC is truly a dangerous commercial colossus. There are many indications that the British use MESC to further British trade in Iran. They do not, as far as I can observe, endeavor to cut the United States out of the market or actually divert orders in any case from the United States to Great Britain. Action is more subtle and indirect methods are found. Their aim would appear to be divide the trade with the United States, a good stroke of business since before the war they had practically none of the Iranian market. Examination of the attached schedules will show that the United States is indicated as the source of supply principally for rubber, automotive vehicles, chemicals, paper, metals and machinery, which must in any event come from the United States. It seems to me that a disproportionate part of the goods come from Great Britain. The Department is undoubtedly aware that MESC policy provides for obtaining all possible goods in India and other nearby places in order to save shipping space.

An important case in which the MESC has operated to the detriment of American interests in Iran was that of typhus vaccine. Dr. Neuwirth had drawn up a program, at Iranian request, which called for inoculating a part of Tehran's population against typhus as an unusually high incidence was expected this year. As the Department knows, the vaccine was held up by the MESC in Cairo. The high incidence of typhus has developed as expected but now it is too late to carry out the plan even if the vaccine were to be received. Dr. Neuwirth reported to me on March 21 that there are about 10,000 cases of typhus in the Tehran area and that deaths increased from 9 in the week ended February 12 to 23 in the week ended March 4. The epidemic continues to grow. Regardless of the merit of the typhus vaccine dispute, the American Government committed itself to a course of action which it failed to carry out solely because of MESC interference. I mention the matter here to show the impossibility of handling these Iranian questions by remote control from Cairo.

General Connolly expresses full agreement with me as regard the cumbersome and bureaucratic methods of MESC, which do not permit the swift decisions so necessary in military matters. He is determined, therefore, not to submit to MESC jurisdiction but intends to import his supplies direct from the War Department. He is, for example, importing his own wheat from the United States because he does not agree to the MESC wheat pool. MESC procedure has not been well received by the Iranian merchants or the Government. The average merchant believes that MESC was set up to prevent the importation of goods. As one observer put it, either he does not know the complicated procedure, in which case he is unable to find his way through the maze of regulations, or knows it too well, in which case he believes it is useless to bother. Mr. Baylis, who is in charge of MESC quotas in Cairo, expresses surprise to Mr. Washington, Lend-Lease representative, in a recent conversation that only eight import license applications were received from Iran in January. To me this is not surprising, knowing the inadequacy of the quotas for Iran. Mr. Simmons, British representative of MESC and head of the Tehran Imports Licensing Sub-Committee, recognizes the inadequacy of these quotas and is agitating for their revision upwards. He stated, in reply to my inquiry as to why the Iraq quotas are so high compared with the Iranian, that in Iraq there are influential British and Iraqis who are willing to fight for their country's rights while in Iran there are no such champions and in addition the Iranians are so demoralized by the invasion that they will not stand up for themselves. The Iranians, as the Department is well aware, are a peculiar people who cannot always be dealt with on the same basis as other nationalities. This is not, I am afraid, recognized by MESC officials in Cairo.

As I have suggested above, the Russians are becoming ever more aware of this Anglo-American trade domination and infiltration of MESC so-called experts into key positions. Undoubtedly their growing economic pressure on Iran is in partial reply. Only yesterday Sheridan came to me with an amazing story to the effect that the Russians are insisting that the Foreign Office accept the appointment of a Soviet engineer at the Tehran silo. If this is done, it may be the thin edge of the wedge looking to Soviet control of bread making and distribution in Tehran, an important political and economic weapon.

The above in intended for the Department's confidential background information and is not intended as sabotage of MESC. I fully realize that I am "a voice crying in wilderness" in representing MESC in the above light and I hope that my remarks will be taken in the spirit in which they are intended. There are many who will say that these arbitrary methods of MESC are essential in times of war. I do not agree. I sincerely believe that a procedure of this kind does far more harm than good. The best example of this is wheat. Had the allies not taken almost all of Iran's trucks for their own use, last summer's harvest could have been gathered more efficiently and security might have been maintained, which in turn might have reduced wheat importation this year to much less than the huge figure of some 55,000 tons. MESC has been primarily a British organ but it has recently been converted to an Anglo-American affair. As American influence in MESC grows, American responsibility for it will increase. I am confidentially informed that MESC will soon send an American to Tehran, who after some time will take charge of their work here. We must be prepared to accept the added responsibility this entails. Our adviser program is apparently not outside the scope of MESC. Mr. Washington came back from Cairo with reports that the MESC is dissatisfied with Mr.

Sheridan and would welcome his removal. In the meantime, they are nosing into his plans for collection of wheat for next year.

In conclusion, it seems to me that Iran is the ideal proving ground for the Atlantic Charter. It is perhaps time to indulge in some honest introspection to see if American action in the past and plans for the future measure up to the ideals of the Atlantic Charter. Personally, I sincerely believe that our actions and intentions in Iran in all matters where we have operated unilaterally as Americans may be weighed in the balance and not found wanting. I cannot say as much for British action in Iran. It is, therefore, the more unfortunate that we should be linked with in responsibility for the MESC. We should, it seems to me, operate as free agents and not in conjunction with a power traditionally unfriendly to the Iranians and little concerned with seeing that Iran is given fair treatment. MESC and UKCC procedure in dictating to a helpless people, in treating the Iranians as inferiors, and in operating an organized trade monopoly are a far cry from the democratic ideal. On the other hand, I am not sufficiently naive to think that the Iranians are always right or to accept their viewpoint without reservation. Iranians are at best, a difficult, obstructive and stubborn people who criticize freely and complain with or without cause. Weighing all factors, however, I feel that they have considerable cause for complaint at the treatment they have received from the allies. MESC action will not contribute toward betterment of this situation. For the future, it is hoped that some system can be devised which will be more acceptable to the Iranians and which will meet their requirements more quickly and effectively. The logical, and admittedly drastic, solution would be to exclude Iran from the jurisdiction of MESC and to control supplies through a less cumbersome allied committee. This would, of course, require agreement with the British. In any event, the MESC should certainly be confined to war time imports control and should not be permitted to penetrate, as some of the more ardent MESC officials contemplate, into post-war rehabilitation.

In another classic dispatch dated April 29, 1943, Dreyfus further discusses the causes of Iran's economic ills (Dispatch 540 and enclosure, 891.51/565):

I have the honor to enclose a copy of a letter from Dr. Millspaugh outlining in some detail the causes of Iran's financial and economic ills and suggesting certain remedies. A resume of this letter was given in my telegram No. 429, April 26. This letter merits careful reading. Dr.

Millspaugh has come to understand in a comparatively short time the fundamental causes of Iran's financial and economic difficulties. He faces issues with realism and proposes remedies with courage. He works with speed and self-assurance, making decisions quickly and with breath-taking boldness. His task, however, is gigantic. Working as de does without adequate staff, he is confronted with many complex problems which have been allowed to drift until solution is extremely difficult. He must face, too, the stubborn opposition of political and business elements which are still thinking in terms of fat profits and political gains. Dr. Millspaugh deserves our full support in his almost single-handed struggle to prevent Iran from plunging over the financial and economic precipice on which it is hovering. While all of the points raised by Dr. Millspaugh deserve our careful consideration, there are two in particular which seem to me to be especially worthy of our study. There are, first, the question of the consumption of Iranian products by allied forces in Iran and, second, the related matter of importing from abroad more adequate supplies of all kinds. I have frequently called to the Department's attention the Iranian complaint that their country has been pillaged by the allies, and its road and rail transport taken over for allied use. Iranians frequently protest also at the inadequate import quotas permitted by MESC and allege that this is an important contributing cause of high prices and inflation. I have often remarked that there is much justice in these complaints and in despatch No. 511 of April 7 I pointed out how the operation of the Middle East Supply Center has had, in my opinion, harmful political and economic effects on the life of the country. It is gratifying and encouraging that Dr. Millspaugh appears to appreciate the justice of the Iranian complaints and the necessity for remedial action.

There seems to me little doubt that part at least of Iran's woes arises from the fact that it has been thoroughly exploited for allied benefit and well pillaged of produce. This is a claim which the allies continue to refute with some heat. Evidence, however, is abundant: huge purchases of meat, eggs, vegetables and other foods by the British and Poles; purchases of wheat, barley and rice by the Russians in the north; exploitation of shoe, textile and other factories by the Russians in Azerbaijan; contracts by the British for blankets from the Isfahan textile mills; the contracting of most of Iran's good trucks by the UKCC and Iransovtrans for carrying allied war goods to Russia; the exploitation of the trans-Iranian railway by the allies, allowing Iran a tiny and insufficient tonnage for civil use; purchases of cattle; contracts for operation of Iranian arms plants; etc., etc. But when the Iranians, calling attention to the fact that they are giving these things for allied benefit, request the importation of goods from abroad they run up against the restrictive policy of the Middle East Supply Center. This organization, set up to save shipping space, went about its task in a whole-hearted manner with little consideration for the real needs of the country or for the possible consequences of its severe restrictions. A pitifully small amount of goods has been imported recently into Iran with the exception of products in which the allies are themselves interested and with the important exception of wheat which was handled by special agreement. Now is the time to break this vicious system and insist that goods flow into Iran in quantities sufficient to take care of the needs of the people and to help to counter the present inflationary trend. I noted with interest the press report that in the few months after the invasion of North Africa we sent to that area some 126,000 tons of goods. What a contrast to the treatment of Iran!

Desperate situation requires courageous and drastic remedies. I suggest, therefore, that we either operate in Iran outside the MESC or that, alternatively, we require that organization to permit an adequate flow of goods into this country. It would be necessary also to overhaul the heavy and bureaucratic procedure of MESC so that applications may be handled more expeditiously. Under present operation, the procedure is so complicated and heavy that merchants are discouraged from applying. In addition, as in the case of pharmaceuticals, the time between the making of an application and the arrival of the goods is far too great. The MESC, it should be remarked, appears to be convinced that the severe restrictions they have imposed on imports into Iran during the last year have had harmful effects. Mr. Jackson, Cairo director of that organization, stated to me in a recent conversation that, whereas the problem of MESC has been to restrict importations, conditions have so changed that the problem now appears to be one of finding goods to keep the country going. Whether they will really take steps to correct this abuse remains to be seen.

As to the question of consumption of goods in Iran by allied forces, Dr. Millspaugh suggests the setting up of a committee, under the control of his assistants, to coordinate and supervise all demands of the allies for goods or services. It should be observed that the American forces are not severe offenders in this regard since they have brought with them almost all of the food and other goods they require. These are matters vital to the internal economy of Iran. They are also questions to which we must give serious consideration if we are to live up to our pledges to assist this unfortunate country.

Dreyfus on July 3, 1943 (Airgram-19, 800.24/1016):

> Reference my despatch No. 511 dated April 7, 1943, I was alarmed at newspaper report that Foreign Secretary Eden made statement in House of Commons to effect that British Government is bearing in mind the possibility of making use of the Middle East Supply Center in long term development schemes for the Middle East. It is my hope that there is no intention of imposing this type of paternalistic fascism on helpless independent nations in postwar world. The MESC was established to coordinate supply problems and save shipping space. On these terms and because of absence of any other control I have given and will continue to give my full support and cooperation to MESC. However, its extension into postwar era, at least as far as independent nations are concerned, would in my opinion be a fatal blunder. Iranians have come to look upon MESC as an instrument for allied political and economic domination; the Russians view it with suspicion as Anglo-American trade penetration. The MESC is psychologically unprepared to assume leadership in postwar rehabilitation or development because its approach is based on denial of sovereignty and assumption of the corruption and incompetence of independent nations. Its operation is a negation of the principles of the Atlantic Charter. Under excuse of necessity of saving shipping space and controlling supplies it has penetrated straight into the heart of Iranian life. Its so-called experts are to be found in almost every field and more are always on the way. It has become a kind of Government within two Governments with the reins securely in the hands of the Minister of State Casey in Cairo. I do not recommend that we withdraw support from MESC as an emergency wartime agency. However I do urge that sovereign nations not be placed at its mercy for development or rehabilitation in the postwar world but be given a freer hand to solve their own problems with the sympathetic support of the United Nations through some such agency as the Office of Foreign Relief and Rehabilitation Operations.

Iranian Note on MESC

On July 13, 1943, Schayesteh had submitted a note to Secretary of State Cordell Hull (Note 817, 891.24/598):

> Upon instruction of the Minister of Foreign Affairs of Iran, I have the honor to draw the attention of Your Excellency to the difficult situation in which my country is placed as regards imports of essential requirements. In accordance with the desire of the Government of the

United States and The British Government, a Combined Supply Committee was established at Teheran to study the civilian requirements of Iran and to fix quantities which could be supplied to her within the limitations of the tonnage space available. This Committee's decisions, however, are not final. Its recommendations are presented for approval to the Middle East Supply Center in Cairo, which in turn presents its views to London and Washington. I may state that Iran is represented on the Combined Supply Committee in Teheran but is not represented on the Middle East Supply Center in Cairo. The method of procedure of these Committees is very cumbersome and slow. Several months pass before an application is approved and many more months until a license is issued. Even then nothing can be done until mail service is received in Washington, which takes several more weeks. It will thus be seen that with difficulties of securing supplies and of obtaining shipping space, almost a year will elapse before the goods reach their destination. Thus, during the year of 1942 a quota of 35,000 odd tons was fixed for Iran, of which 20,850 tons was subsequently cancelled, leaving a balance of 15,000 tons, the greater portion of which has not yet been shipped, and the quantity which may eventually reach Iran is problematical.

As I feel sure that Your Excellency is determined to see that my country is dealt with justly, and that such a concept of fairness and justice is a fixed policy of your government, permit me to state frankly that my countrymen feel that they have not received just treatment in this respect. The difficulties connected with the shipping situation during the past year and the early part of this year are fully patent to us, and while admitting that the military requirements are paramount, we feel that of the total quantity of civilian supplies allocated to the Near East a fair proportion has not been allocated to us. For example, I am given to understand that during 1942 about 100,000 tons of space was allocated to the Near East from this country alone, out of which only an infinitesimal quantity reached Iran, although from the point of view of her population and standard of living, Iran is entitled to a larger share than other Near Eastern countries. Apart from this, the Military forces of three of the Nations responsible for the prosecution of the war are in Iran, and the Government and people of my country are sincerely cooperating with the United Nations. For these reasons the people of my country expect, subject to the availability of supplies and to the shipping situation, to receive just and fair treatment in respect to the essential civilian requirements of the country. I regret to state that to the contrary this has not been the case.

For example, an American Army doctor who was loaned by the American Government to the Iranian Ministry of Health ascertained the existence of typhus in my country and foreseeing its spread recommended that one million doses of typhus vaccine be dispatched to Iran. The Cairo Committee at first approved 5,000 doses and subsequently increased it to about double this quantity. Actually, 100,000 doses of typhus serum for Iran were dispatched by air from the United States, but the consignment was held up in Cairo and not permitted to go forward by the Middle East Supply Center. The Supply Center sent a representative to Teheran to inquire about the spread of typhus in Iran and reported that typhus was at that date not prevalent. Therefore the Cairo Committee thought fit to hold the serum in Cairo at its own disposal. This decision had unfortunate results which are no doubt well known to you. Typhus has spread in Iran and thousands have succumbed to it who might have been saved if the serum had not been held up in Cairo.

Your Excellency will probably be surprised to hear that the Middle East supply Center intends to allocate only 20,000 tons to Iran for 1943 although the minimum necessary is 300,000 tons. It is obvious that such a reduction in civilian requirements creates conditions which cannot but have an unhappy result. I will not ask Your Excellency to rely solely upon the information which I receive from my country but I would like you to make a personal inquiry of every American who has been in Iran during the year 1942 and who has witnessed the suffering of my unfortunate countrymen. Apart from the appeal to the humanitarian point of view, the people who are collaborating so eagerly with the United States and whose cooperation is so valuable at this time are expecting better treatment.

In view of the seriousness of the situation, my Government asks me to request Your Excellency to give special consideration to the matter, and bearing in mind the recent improvement in the shipping situation to direct that the whole question of the quantity to be allocated to Iran should be gone into anew and a tonnage commensurate with her requirements and the improved shipping situation be allotted to her. Furthermore, that the procedure of the Combined Supply Committee of Teheran and the Middle East Supply Center in Cairo be revised with a view of speeding up the process of getting the necessary supplies to their destination. Please accept, Sir, the assurances of my highest consideration.

Schayesteh's note had been communicated to the American Embassy in London with instruction that a copy be given to the Foreign Office. Report of September 27, 1943 (W.J. Gallman, Dispatch 11386 and enclosures, 891.24/505):

> With reference to the Department's instruction no. 3132 of September 9, 1943, I have the honor to enclose a copy of a letter dated September 25, 1943 from the Foreign Office, together with copies of notes exchanged between the Foreign Office and the Minister of Iran in London concerning supplies for Iran.

The letter from R.M.A. Hankey:

> Dear Gallman, Very many thanks for your letter of the 18th September, in which you enclosed copies of correspondence between the Persian Minister at Washington and the State Department regarding supplies for Persia. It is very useful for us to have information about any representations which the Persian Government may make to the United States Government on this subject, since we naturally receive similar representations from the Persian authorities ourselves. The Persian Minister in London raised the question of Persian import quotas at about the same time, though in less detail and in a less formal manner. In this connection, you may be interested to see the enclosed copies of correspondence between M. Taqizadeh and Sir Maurice Peterson.

Taqizadeh's letter to Peterson is dated July 7, 1943:

> My dear Sir Maurice, You will remember that in the course of the conversation I had with you on June 16th in connection with the complaint of the Iranian Government concerning the quota allotted to Iran by the Middle East Supply Committee (sic) for the year 1943, you were kind enough to promise to convey the views of the Iranian Government on this matter to the Supply Committee. I now write to say that I have received a further communication from Teheran wherein the Iranian Government express their extreme anxiety about the inadequate quota allotted, which would only meet a small fraction of their requirements. I am therefore approaching you again on this subject to see if anything can be done to bring about a reconsideration of this matter by the Supply Committee. The Iranian Government feel that the 20,000 tons put aside for the 1943 quota would hardly meet 10% of the essential needs of the country. I shall therefore be most grateful if

you will be so good as to use your good offices to do something to relieve the anxiety of the Iranian Government in this respect.

Peterson had replied on July 30, 1943:

My dear Minister, I am now able to reply to Your Excellency's letter of the 7th July (608-7-7) about the Iranian Government's quota for imports during 1943, as I have received a reply from our Legation at Tehran to the enquiry which I made as a result of our conversation on this subject on the 16th June. You will remember telling me on 16th June that 7,600 tons of dates and 17,000 tons of other foodstuffs had been waiting at Ahwaz for some time and ought to be moved soon, as they were perishable. I now learn that a large proportion of these dates had been imported from Iraq as a speculation. Although the Iranian Ministry of Food would prefer to devote the carriage of such commodities as sugar and tea the space on the railway which is available for civil goods, large quantities of dates have been and are being transported to Tehran, as a result of the strong influence wielded by the merchants who have imported them.

As regards the more general question of import quotas, I find that the July-December 1942 quotas were not cut as you suggested during our talk on 16th June. It was found in practice that the quantities of tea and sugar allowed far exceeded the amounts needed, particularly in the case of sugar. It was also found unnecessary to import the full quotas of certain commodities such as base metals and machinery, as adequate stocks were discovered in the country. Our Legation at Tehran have confirmed that the import quotas for the period January-June, 1943, totaled approximately 20,000 tons, which was the figure you gave me on 16th June. In your letter of 7th July you suggested that this figure represented the import quota for the whole of the year 1943, but this may have been due to an error. This comparatively low figure is due, firstly, to a reduction in the tea and sugar quotas in view of the local production and the discovery of large stocks held by the Iranian Government, and secondly, to a revision of the quotas for base metals and machinery as a result of the experience in the previous six months. These figures exclude all consignments of wheat, flour and oil and also trucks which have recently reached Iran. Including wheat and flour, the volume of civil supply sent by rail during the period January-June, 1943, is no less than 43,500 tons.

In respect of the six months July-December, 1943, the quota allotted to Iran totals approximately 40,000 tons. This figure also excludes cereals, motor trucks and oil. The increase over the quota for the previous six months is mainly in respect of heavy chemicals, cotton piece goods, tea and sugar. A further allocation of 10,000 tons has been made for cereals. There is now a sufficient reserve of cereals in Tehran for it to be possible to cease sending wheat from the south. As a result, it should be possible in future months to use the full monthly allocation of over 8,000 tons for civil goods to lift other imported goods and to accelerate the clearing of imports which have accumulated at the southern ports. We hope the Iranian Government will take adequate measures to ensure that full benefit is derived from the harvest. You will see from the above that this will have important effects for the supply of other products.

Chapter 8

The Middle East Supply Center and the Typhus Vaccine

The failure of the MESC to deliver the typhus vaccine to Iran was mentioned in chapter 7. More details follow. Cable to Dreyfus on November 25, 1942 (Telegram 342, 158.919/23A):

> Iranian Legation here has been instructed urgently to procure one million doses of typhus vaccines to meet new typhus outbreak in Iran. Please consult Colonel Neuwirth and report whether this vaccine is needed and if so whether urgency of situation warrants shipment by air. Please give all readily available information on reported epidemic.

Dreyfus replied on November 29, 1942 (Telegram 408, 158.919/24):

> Department's 342, November 25. It is understood MESC, Cairo, has taken steps to obtain this million doses vaccine. To avoid duplication copy of this telegram being sent Winant with request he inform Department of any action taken. Neuwirth says no typhus yet but situation potentially dangerous and immediate prophylactic measures are essential. Number of reported cases since November 1, fifty-one. Number of deaths reported same period, two. It is expected cases will increase greatly with coming of winter. Neuwirth is of opinion situation is sufficiently serious to justify shipment by air. He suggests that weight might be saved by shipping it in liter bottles.

Dreyfus on December 1, 1942 (Telegram 411, 158.919/25):

> Reference Legation's telegram no. 408, November 27 (29), 11 a.m. Following for Surgeon General from Neuwirth. Iranian Government wishes to purchase in the United States 100,000 doses of typhus vaccine not (repeat not) 1,000,000 as previously suggested. I recommend this amount be shipped by air in 100 bottles of liter each.

Cable to Cairo on December 3, 1942 (Telegram 1548, 158.919/24): "For Winant. Tehran's telegram 408, November 29 to Department. Please report immediately whether MESC is taking adequate steps to procure and despatch typhus vaccine for Iran. Please indicate where and through what channels it is planned to purchase vaccine." Winant replied on December 5, 1942 (Telegram 2142, 158.919/26):

> Department's 1548, December 3, 8 p.m.; Legation Tehran 408, November 29, 11 a.m. Following from Fred Winant. In matter of typhus vaccine MESC has done following: One. Supplies to Tehran about two weeks ago 1,000 doses. Two. Telegraphed MWT, London, under date December 1, stating Iran's requirement of one million doses and outlining general situation. Three. Requesting immediate release available supply meet requirements and asking that 1,000 doses forwarded by air. Telegram did not suggest channels of purchase. As yet no reply from London. Reference Time Magazine November 9, under medicine, will Minister Tehran advise confidentially possibilities of typhus vaccine from local Pasteur Institute under Colonel Neuwirth? Repeated Tehran as personal for the Minister.

Dreyfus on December 11, 1942 (Telegram 432, 158.919/27): "Following telegram has been sent Legation at Cairo. 2142 to Department. Neuwirth advises only small quantity of typhus vaccine can be produced in Tehran due to lack of facilities and shortage of eggs."

On December 8, 1942, Jernegan had telephoned Colonel John Franks, Director, International Division, S.O.S., War Department (Memorandum, 158.919/32):

> Colonel Franks said that he had already set in motion machinery to begin air shipment of 100,000 doses of typhus vaccine. He would make all arrangements in this connection and would assume responsibility for the arrival of the vaccine at Cairo, where it would be delivered to General Andrews with instructions to forward it on to Colonel

> Neuwirth at Tehran. I said that this seemed entirely satisfactory and suggested that the Department and OLLA felt it would be well, after the shipment got started, to instruct Lend-Lease representatives concerned, Fred Winant and Philip Kidd, to make arrangements with the appropriate Iranian authorities for payment and to notify the proper people in MESC. Colonel Franks agreed and pointed out that General Andrews is also represented on the MESC. He seemed to feel there need be no trouble of any kind with respect to procedure. Colonel Franks said he would show the Department the telegraphic instructions he planned to send to General Andrews and we could send parallel instructions at the same time to Kidd and Winant. Colonel Franks remarked that the War Department had previously received a request for 1,000,000 doses of this vaccine through Dr. Mote of the British Supply Council and had sent a query to General Andrews. However, in view of the cable we had received from Colonel Neuwirth and the urgency which State and G-2 attached to the matter, he had decided to go ahead with 100,000 doses without further delay.

Cable to Cairo on December 16, 1942 (Telegram 1624, 158.919/26):

> For Winant. On December 13 War Department shipped one hundred thousand doses typhus vaccines for Iran by air from Miami. Shipment was consigned to General Andrews at Cairo with directions to advise General Connolly and communicate with Colonel Neuwirth at Tehran for shipping instructions. Please inform proper MESC authorities and consult with Andrews to ensure speedy forwarding of shipment to Tehran for delivery by Neuwirth to Iranian authorities under such distribution safeguards as may seem necessary. Upon receipt of advice from Neuwirth that the delivery has been arranged, Iranian Minister Washington will be requested to present appropriate requisition under Lend-Lease cash reimbursable procedure. Consideration will be given shipment of further quantities by sea if you and Neuwirth so recommend. War Department says it will be impossible to continue large shipments by air and suggests program of regular steamer shipments for Iran should be prepared immediately. OLLA has been consulted and concurs. Repeated to Tehran.

The vaccine was held up by the MESC in Cairo. Cairo's telegram of December 19, 1942 (Telegram 2220, 158.919/28):

Department's 1624, December 16, 10 p.m. Following from Fred Winant: "Colonel Sams, Chief Surgeon of United States Army Forces Middle East, returned yesterday from personal survey in Tehran. His report corroborates recent report received at office of Minister of State. Advice, from these two sources, especially the recent findings of Colonel Sams provides more current authoritative information for determining suitable course of acting. Summed up, the present typhus situation appears as follows: One. There is no (repeat no) epidemic in Tehran or elsewhere in Iran. Two. Danger of such epidemic in Tehran and elsewhere in Iran is no greater than in any of other territories or areas, in fact perhaps less than in, for instance, Egypt. Three. Requirements of Tehran for one million doses of vaccine was a precautionary measure to avoid possible epidemic. If precautionary approach is adopted, similar requirements will develop six months hence. Although sympathetic to principle, medical supply authorities question practicability of such course in one territory in view of scarcity of vaccine for whole area and potential urgency for vaccine in any part of area in case of epidemic. Four. Chief Surgeon for United States Army Forces, Middle East, has telegraphed the Surgeon General that in his opinion the 100,000 doses on its way by air, should not (repeat not) be forwarded to Tehran but rather be retained here as central pool for protection of whole area. I suggest that Department contact Office of Surgeon General and on review of situation telegraph me if instructions contained in Department's telegram under reference should be amended in light of current advice."

Cable to Dreyfus on December 26, 1942 (Telegram 394, 158.919/28):

Department's 378, December 16. By telegram of December 16 Winant at Cairo reported opinion of Colonel Sams, Chief United States Army medical officer Middle East, that typhus danger Iran no greater than elsewhere in area. Sams recommends, and Winant indicated concurrence, that 100,000 doses vaccine be held at Cairo as central pool. After consulting Lend-Lease and Surgeon General's office, Department has replied to Winant as follows: "Your 2220, December 19 and Department's 1624, December 16. For Winant. In view your report, War Department has cabled General Andrews that he may hold at Cairo the 100,000 doses vaccine already sent. He is authorized to use this quantity as a central pool for protection of whole area whenever and wherever need arises. Department and OLLA concur in this decision and you may disregard instructions transmitted in Department's

> 1624. It is hoped that future shipments medical supplies will be consigned to you for ultimate distribution in accordance with MESC directives and in consultation with qualified American medical men. Please submit recommendations as soon as possible with respect to typhus vaccine needed to form adequate pool for Middle East."

Winant replied on December 28, 1942 (Telegram 2267, 158.919/29): "Department's 1668, December 26, 8 p.m. Following from Fred Winant. 'Provisionally it is believed that an additional 100,000 doses typhus vaccine will provide adequate central pool for Middle East and that this second shipment of vaccine come out by steamship.'"

Dreyfus on December 31, 1942 (Telegram 466, 158.919/30):

> Department's 394, December 26. Colonel Neuwirth urgently requests Department endeavor have competent authorities alter decision to pool typhus vaccine in Cairo and gives following explanation: One. Typhus vaccine is for prevention not (repeat not) treatment. To pool it awaiting an outbreak is as logical as hoarding arms while a battle rages or food while there is famine. Two. This vaccine was requested to fulfill following specific program to immunize large part of persons in poor quarter of Tehran during month of January. Incidence of typhus is high here from February to April due to fact poor do not bathe or take off clothing because of cold weather and hence become lice ridden. Greater incidence is expected this year because of increased suffering and poverty. Three. Since injections and immunization take much more than a month vaccine must come forward to Tehran at once unless this worthy program is to be abandoned. I associate myself with Colonel Neuwirth's request. It seems to me that the effects of our encouraging the Iranians along public health lines, promising assistance in obtaining typhus vaccine and then letting them down in the middle of their program are far more harmful than if we had refused aid in the beginning. Repeated to Cairo.

Response on January 4, 1943 (Telegram 9, 158.919/30):

> Department is informing Army Surgeon General of contents your 466, December 31, but it is doubted that War Department will be willing to act unless favorable recommendation is received from Colonel Sams and Frederick Winant. For your guidance in future cases of this sort, it is desired to point out that Department has been handicapped in this matter by lack of specific information regarding purpose for which

> vaccine was desired and by conflicting requests and reports received from Neuwirth, Iranian Legation here, British Supply Council here, Winant and Colonel Sams. Since General American-British policy now calls for handling all supplies for Middle East through MESC, it is preferred that all requests should reach us after approval by that body, and Department must have detailed information to substantiate any request which does not conform to MESC recommendations. In any case, it is suggested that special requests be sent first to Winant and that, if possible, agreement be reached with him before definite recommendations are transmitted to Washington. If practicable, your views and Winant's should be forwarded before Iranian Legation here is instructed to present formal request. Repeated to Cairo for Winant.

Winant on January 9, 1943 (Telegram 50, 158.919/31): "Department's no. 9, January 4, 10 p.m., to Tehran Legation. Following from Fred Winant: 'As Typhus Commission now in Cairo I shall await its findings before replying to last paragraph of telegram under reference.'" A follow-up telegram to Dreyfus on January 20, 1943 (Telegram 40, 158.919/30):

> Department's 9, January 4. United States of America Typhus Commission, headed by Admiral Stephenson, is understood to be now in Cairo preparing to survey typhus situation in Middle East. War Department is instructing commission to investigate question of best allocation of vaccine and is prepared to accept recommendations. You or Colonel Neuwirth may wish to communicate with Stevenson (sic) in this regard.

As predicted by Neuwirth, a serious typhus epidemic had broken out in the winter and spring of 1943, a documentary account of which is given in chapter 23. Neuwirth was soon after removed from Iran by the War Department. Dreyfus on March 27, 1943 (Dispatch 497, 891.20/205):

> I have the honor to inform the Department that, under orders received from the War Department, Lt. Colonel Abraham A. Neuwirth, who has been on detached duty as informal adviser to the Iranian Ministry of Health, will depart next week for the United States where he has been assigned to duty with troops. I cannot permit Dr. Neuwirth to depart without expressing to him and Department my deep appreciation for the work he has done for Iran. . . . Dr. Neuwirth's unflagging

> energy, his cheerful cooperation, his keen interest in public health in Iran, his sympathetic understanding of the unfortunate Iranian masses, and his tenacity in the face of opposition and difficulties have won him a high place in the regard of Iranians and Americans alike. . . . The Iranian Minister of Health in a note of recent date informed the Legation that he has been highly satisfied with the assistance rendered by Dr. Neuwirth in the furtherance of public health in Iran and expressed his appreciation and gratitude. He added that Dr. Neuwirth has been requested to carry out while in the United States certain measures connected with public health work in Iran.

Dreyfus on March 29, 1943 (Telegram 323, 891.1283/10):

> My 200, February 22, Lt. Colonel Neuwirth has been ordered by War Department to return to United States for duty. Millspaugh and Minister of Health desire to have Neuwirth remain in Iran to take charge of newly formed government corporation for the purchase, manufacture and distribution of pharmaceuticals. They suggest that Department endeavor to obtain War Department's consent. The initiative in above suggested appointment did not come from Neuwirth but he expresses willingness to accept. Considering that Neuwirth is highly qualified for this important work and is already familiar with its background I favor this appointment and request Department take steps to obtain consent of War Department. Since Iranians intend in any event to seek an American to fill this position Neuwirth's appointment would avoid long delay in finding another suitable candidate and obtaining air priority for his travel.

State Department replied on April 5, 1943 (Telegram 173, 891.1283/10): "Your 323, March 29. Department has supported your recommendation, but War Department feels Neuwirth is not (repeat not) fully qualified for position and prefers that he return to the United States."

The operations of the American Red Cross (ARC) in the context of the Polish refugee crisis, is described in chapters 10 and 11. Here suffice it to say that, similar to the MESC, the ARC had also turned a deaf ear to Iran's request for typhus vaccine. On June 24, 1943, Richard F. Allen, Vice Chairman, Insular and Foreign Operations of the American Red Cross, had written to Assistant Secretary Breckinridge Long (Letter, 891.48/339):

> In the absence of Mr. Davis, I am pleased to acknowledge receipt of your letter of June 16, 1943, in regard to the position of the American Red Cross with respect to relief operations in Iran. . . . With respect to the question of emergency needs for medical supplies, we were recently requested by the Red Lion and Sun Society of Iran to provide one million typhus vaccines. This request was presented to Mr. Bailey of our Cairo office who recently visited Iran. When it was discussed in Cairo with the Middle East Supply Council (sic), of which Mr. Frederick Winant is the American Representative, our Cairo representative was told that the provision of typhus vaccines for civilian population was not contemplated and that importation of these vaccines for civilian residents in Iran would seriously affect the controls over medical supplies maintained by the Middle East Supply Council. . . . We have, therefore, informed our representative in Cairo that we are not in a position to approve this request.

Renewed Iranian Attempts to Obtain the Vaccine

Fearing a typhus outbreak in the following winter, Iranians had again attempted to obtain a supply of vaccine. Cable instruction to Cairo on September 9, 1943 (Telegram 1315, 158.919/32A):

> For Moffat from Winant. Department and other Washington agencies have been approached by New York exporter Orlove who requests urgent clearance of ten thousand vials each of typhus and typhoid vaccine for consignment to Iranian Minister of Health. Orlove claims letters and cables from friends and officials in Tehran indicate widespread typhus in Iran, particularly in outlying districts. Department has stated its belief that any necessary Iranian requirement will be met promptly by shipment from Cairo in view of current central medical supply supervision and presence in area of General Fox, who is currently informed of improved vaccine supply situation in this country. Please investigate quickly and advise.

The reply from Cairo is dated September 14, 1943 (Telegram 1657, 158.919/33):

> Reference Department's 1315, September 9. For Fred Winant from Moffat: "(1) Believe most effective distribution of typhus and typhoid vaccine can be obtained by release of all supplies from centralized stocks under control of MEMAC (Middle East Medical Advisory Com-

mittee). Understand at present there is inadequate organization in Iran for proper distribution or inoculation program and it is considered best for releases to be made by MEMAC as needed. (2) 65,000 doses typhus vaccine recently sent to Iran for specific need. With supplies here and those coming forward for MEMAC controlled pool, shipment mentioned in your telegram not considered essential. (3) MESC and U.S. Army agree."

Unable to ship, Orlove had transferred his vaccine supply to an Iranian. Cable of September 20, 1943, from Cairo (A-171, 158.919/34):

From Moffat: Intercepted telegram September 3 from Morteza Khosrovschahi New York to Mohamed Khosrovschahi Teheran reads as follows: "Have available 10,000 typhus and 10,000 typhoid vaccines can ship through war shipping administration please cable if these vaccines are urgently needed and if no objections we consign them to Ministry of Health. . . ." Our telegram 1657 September 14 3 p.m. outlines our position regarding such shipments.

On November 9, 1943, Schayesteh had submitted a formal request (Note 1689, 158.919/36):

The Imperial Legation of Iran presents its compliments to the Department of State and has the honor to inform them as follows: Mr. Morteza Khosrovschahi, of 165 Broadway, New York City, intends to make a gift of 4,000 vials of typhus vaccines to the Iranian Ministry of Health and has asked this Legation to request that an export license be granted him for this shipment. The Legation of Iran, therefore would appreciate it very much if the Department of State would be so kind as to take the necessary steps in order that this export license be granted to Mr. Khosrovschahi, as these vaccines are very badly needed in Iran.

On November 24, 1943, the State Department cabled Cairo (Telegram 1809, 158.919/33):

For Landis from Winant. Department is confronted with note from Iranian Legation supporting export application of Morteza Khosrovschahi for 4,000 vials of typhus vaccine on gift basis to Iranian Ministry of Health. Khosrovschahi states on application "this shipment is a donation by me to people of Iran. I confirm that I do not receive any compensation whatsoever against this shipment. . . ." At hand is Cairo's telegram 1657, September 14 and Airgram A-171,

> September 20, as well as other data indicating clearly that most effective distribution of vaccine is through centralized schemes under control of MEMAC, in all of which Department concurs. In particular instance, however, you will appreciate extreme difficulty of denying application. . . . The Iranian Legation is advised further that this is not to be interpreted as establishing a precedent. Please explain to MEMAC and MESC. . . . Unless urgent message is received to contrary, we shall be obliged to proceed along lines indicated. This message repeated to Tehran as Department's 589.

Cairo was not about to let the shipment go through. Its cable of December 1, 1943 (Telegram 2196, 158.919/37):

> For Winant from Short and Landis. Reference your wire 1809. General Fox is sending the following cable to Bayne Jones. "Urgently request that no export authority be given to Morteza Khosrovschahi for typhus vaccine shipment to Iran regardless of whether basis for authority is gift or any other pretext. Before you permit anyone to break down our complete control over all supplies of typhus vaccine, we hope you will consider evidence we are sending you. . . . Black market operations with American typhus will become possible if we permit any breach in our control." In view of the above, recommend that you do not permit export application of Morteza Khosrovschahi until you receive supporting evidence of inadvisability being forwarded by Fox to Bayne Jones. .

State Department reply on December 7, 1943 (Telegram 1901, 158.919/37):

> For Landis from Winant. Thank you prompt telegram #2196. In view of urgent request on part USA Typhus Commission for complete responsibility for handling all US typhus vaccine and improved situation on vaccine supply we have denied export application of Morteza Khosroschahi and have so informed Iranian Legation. Information we have received of greatly increased quantity of vaccine for use in Near East is highly satisfactory.

The reply of December 18, 1943, to the Iranian note (158.919/36):

> The United States Government is deeply concerned with the typhus problem in Iran and other countries and, by order of the President, the United States of America Typhus Commission was established and

> made responsible, under the direction of the Secretary of War, for all anti-typhus measures. Brigadier General Leon A. Fox is Field Director of the Commission, with headquarters at Cairo, and it is understood that he is now in Iran in connection with his mission. Under present conditions the Commission considers it necessary to control all supplies of typhus vaccine from the United States, and it has established a central pool in the Middle East, to which very large amounts of vaccine have recently been sent. For this reason, applications for exports through other channels have been denied for some time past. In spite of the established practice of denying typhus vaccine export applications, the Department of State and other government departments concerned made a careful and sympathetic study of the possibility of favorable action in the proposed gift shipment of Mr. Khosrovschahi, but considered it unwise to make any exception to the rule. It is desired that Iranian requirements be supplied from the central pool through the agency of the Cairo office of the Typhus Commission, and it is stated that there is available for the Iranian health authorities sufficient vaccine for any reasonable immunization program.

The critical vaccine shortage is revealed in Ford's report of January 17, 1944. Given that a dose consisted of 3 cubic centimeters, it is revealed that of the 137,000 doses sent to Iran, only 40,000 doses remained at the onset of the typhus season in late January (Dispatch 798, 891.24/623):

> Of the 410,000 cubic centimeters of anti-typhus vaccine received in this country from Lend-Lease stocks in Cairo, 290,000 cubic centimeters have already been distributed for the inoculation of certain groups agreed upon by the Medical Advisory Committee and by the Iranian Ministry of Health, and more or less approved by Brigadier General Leon A. Fox of the United States Army on his visit here last month. . . . The Legation has been informed, in this whole connection, by one of the representatives here of the Office of Foreign Economic Administration, who has just returned from a visit to Cairo, that General Fox had concluded that the vaccine sent here had very probably been wasted, and that, in the circumstances, he was opposed, for the time being at any rate, to the shipment of further supplies of Lend-Lease vaccine to Iran. Copy to Mr. Landis, Cairo.

Iranian Approach to UNRRA

The Iranians had next tried the newly established United Nations Refugee Relief Administration (UNRRA). On January 10, 1944, a Counselor at the Iranian Legation had written to Governor Herbert H. Lehman, Director General of UNRRA in Washington:

> My dear Governor Lehman: Referring to the conversation which I had the honor to have with you in Atlantic City, in which I explained to you the health and sanitation conditions in Iran created by the present war, I also drew your attention to the lack of pharmaceutical drugs and medical instruments, and you were so kind as to give me the assurance that UNRRA will be helpful to our country in this connection, of which I informed my Government. I have now received a cable from the Iranian Ministry of Health stating that because of the typhus disease which is widespread in the entire country, the health authorities in Iran are in very urgent need of ambulances and portable machines for disinfection and for large and small sterilizers which can be transported from house to house. Instruments for surgery and equipment for hospitals and medicines, especially pharmaceutical goods, are completely lacking in our country. I shall appreciate it very much if you would kindly give me an answer as to how soon you will be able to ship to our country this material which we need badly. Looking forward to your renewed kind cooperation in this urgent matter, and with kind personal regards, I am, sincerely yours, (signed) Dr. A.A. Daftary.

On March 1, 1944, Iran's request to UNRRA was discussed at a meeting of American and British officials. State Department representatives included Fred Winant, George V. Allen, and Harold B. Minor. The USA Typhus Commission was represented by Colonel Bayne-Jones. The seven British participants included Dent and Christelow. Given Winant's presence, not only there was no mention of the 1942 typhus vaccine debacle, there was even a denial of the 1943 typhus epidemic (Memorandum, 891.24/645A):

> The meeting was for the purpose of discussing the request made by the Iranian Government to UNRRA for medical supplies to combat typhus. . . . The following points were brought out: 1. Supplies of typhus vaccine for the area of responsibility of the Middle East Supply Center are handled through a MESC pool in Cairo from stocks made available free of charge by the USA Typhus Commission. These au-

> thorities have been seriously concerned with typhus conditions in Iran, even though there has been no abnormal incidence of this disease during recent years. During 1943 450,000 ccs of typhus vaccine (one dose = 3ccs) were shipped to Iran out of the MESC pool. Of this amount, 250,000 ccs were in storage in Iran as of December 1943. An additional amount of 300,000 ccs has been cleared for shipment to Iran for the Iranian Army as soon as a formal request is made for it. . . . In addition, the Russian authorities have done considerable immunization work in the northern part of Iran. 2. The Typhus Commission and MESC are willing and able to release additional supplies of typhus vaccine to Iran if better controls were adopted. In an effort to improve the methods of distribution and public health, the Iranian Government has recently arranged for the services of two competent United States citizens. Dr. Avery, Dean of the Boston University Medical School, is now en route to Tehran to act as Adviser to the Ministry of Health and Mr. Stokeley, formerly of Parke Davis & Co., has been taken on to act as Director of the Iranian Pharmaceutical Institute. It is hoped that after the receipt of reports from these persons, further supplies of typhus vaccines can be released on the assumption that control and distribution measures will be improved. 3. With respect to medical supplies other than typhus vaccine, serious efforts have been made by the United Nations' authorities, specifically MESC, to meet Iran's requirements. At the present time it is claimed that substantial supplies of medical equipment and pharmaceuticals exist in Iran. In 1943 the Iranian Government was asked by MESC to prepare a statement of one year's requirements of medical supplies of all types, including those referred to in the letter from the Iranian Embassy to the Director General. Although the estimates prepared were rather large, they were substantially accepted by MESC and procurement has been commenced on bulk indent covering medical supplies of all types for one year. 4. There was general agreement among those present who had direct connection with this problem that special efforts had been made to take care of the requirements of Iran for medical supplies and that UNRRA should not in any way interfere with the functions now being performed by MESC; Colonel Bayne-Jones was particularly insistent on this point.

A copy of this memorandum had been forwarded to Tehran on March 6, 1944, with follow-up instructions on March 28, 1944 (Instruction 359 and enclosures, 891.24/647B):

> Reference is made to the Department's instructions nos. 345 and 351 of March 6 and March 15, 1944, respectively, concerning the efforts of the Government of Iran vis-à-vis the Department and UNRRA for assistance in obtaining supplies allegedly necessary for combating typhus in Iran. The request made by the Iranian Legation here to UNRRA (a copy of which is enclosed herewith for the Legation's information) was considered on March 3, 1944 by the Central Committee of that organization (which committee is composed of representatives of the United States, United Kingdom, Soviet Union and China). . . . Owing to the conflicting nature of the evidence as to the extent of typhus in Iran and as to the availability of medical supplies, it was decided by the Central Committee that further facts were needed before a decision could be made as to whether UNRRA should undertake to render assistance to Iran. It was felt that under the circumstances the most satisfactory way to obtain the additional information would be to request the representatives in Tehran of the five interested governments to prepare an agreed statement of facts as to these matters. . . . The Department and the other agencies of this Government feel that UNRRA's assistance should be extended in this case only if there is any useful function which it can perform in respect to typhus control. UNRRA is primarily an instrument of rendering relief to areas liberated from enemy occupation and its entrance into Iran (aside from possible activities in connection with assistance to refugees) could be justified only in the event of emergency epidemic conditions. Furthermore, in the UNRRA Agreement and Resolutions the principle has been firmly established that UNRRA's activities will be carried out through the existing war-time supply and allocation machinery of the United Nations. . . . It is requested that you work closely with the representatives of MESC in the preparation of the requested statement of facts.

Nearly two months later, Richard Ford, chargé d'affaires after the recall of Dreyfus, reports that he had not heard from the Iranians in the matter. They had apparently given up. In his interesting report of May 8, 1944, Ford reveals that the American health adviser, Dr. Avery, had found an innovative way of tripling the number of those "inoculated" (Dispatch 937, 891.24/670):

> I have the honor to acknowledge the receipt of the Department's instruction No. 359 of March 28, 1944, concerning the steps currently being taken by the Iranian Embassy in Washington vis-à-vis the Department and UNRRA with a view to enlisting their assistance in ob-

taining shipments of drugs and pharmaceuticals, and medical and surgical supplies and equipment for use in Iran. The Legation has studied the Department's instructions carefully and, as soon as it hears from the Iranian Government in the matter, it will assign a member of its staff to meet the representatives of the other Governments concerned with a view to preparing an agreed statement of facts along the lines laid down by the Central Committee of UNRRA in its meeting of March 3, 1944. . . . As for typhus, while there has been an admittedly large number of cases reported this year to the Iranian health authorities, Dr. Bennett F. Avery, the new American Director General of Public Health in this country, has felt it safe to predict that the situation this year will not reach epidemic proportions, or approach that of last year. This subject has been dealt with more fully by the Legation in its despatch No. 925 of April 29, 1944, entitled "The Typhus Situation in Iran." When the despatch just referred to was written, 83,140 cubic centimeters of the Lend-Lease vaccine remained undistributed from the stocks received in this country last year from Cairo. Since writing the despatch, however, 10,000 cubic centimeters of this vaccine has been sent to the Medical Committee in Shiraz, thus leaving a balance presently on hand of 73,140 cubic centimeters. As the expiry date on this vaccine is approaching, Dr. Avery has decided to use all of it at once in inoculating the poorer classes in such typhus centers as Tehran, Pahlevi, Resht, Semnan, Gorgan, Meshed, Kashan, Isfahan and Abadan. By limiting the inoculations to one cubic centimeter per person, some 73,000 persons will, it is hoped, be provided with a considerable degree of immunity from the disease.

Chapter 9

The Supply of Pharmaceuticals and Sugar: Case Studies in the Functioning of MESC

Similar to the transportation crisis, the importance of the medical and drug shortage is indicated by the volume of documents contained in the records. The MESC's dilatory measures and the resulting shortage of pharmaceuticals was referred to in the previous two chapters. The delaying tactics were part of an attempt to increase the British share of the market. Dreyfus on November 11, 1942 (Telegram 370, 891.24/286):

> Tehran representative of MESC insists that large annual pharmaceutical orders be placed through London in accordance with procedure agreed upon between British and Americans. I have been unable to obtain from Winant any satisfactory guidance on the subject. Iranians wish to order direct and only from United States. I see no reason why Iranians should not be permitted to order this and other goods where they desire providing shipping space is not wasted. I should appreciate receiving Department's urgent instructions as to proper procedure since pharmaceutical order long delayed is now under consideration.

The reply of November 19, 1942 (Telegram 329, 891.24/286):

> Your 370, November 11, 4 p.m. . . . Department does not understand insistence of Tehran representative of MESC in this matter for the reason that United States, United Kingdom, South Africa, and India are listed by War Cabinet as supply areas for pharmaceuticals, but

> quite apart from this Iranians should understand that shipping and supply situations may not always permit them to obtain materials from country of their choice. For your confidential information only, there is a plan under consideration under which medical supplies would go forward direct to the governments of the countries in the MESC area, after requirements had been screened by the MESC, in quantities sufficient (the supply situation permitting) for current requirements plus a small reserve for possible emergency.

In the margin it is stated: "Substance read to and approved by Allan Christelow on phone."

Establishment of Pharmaceutical Institute

As stated in the above cable, plans for the establishment of a government near monopoly on drugs was contemplated. As part of this plan, importing through private channels was prevented. Cable to Dreyfus on April 6, 1943 (Telegram 168, 891.24/423A):

> Anglo-American Colonial Co., Ltd. 401 Broadway, New York has had orders since last October from Habiboolah Mottahed, Shiraz, Iran covering medicines valued at $15,000. Company states that customer has had difficulty in obtaining approval of Combined Supply Committee in Tehran, for necessary import license. Company states funds are in New York for payment of merchandise when shipped.

Dreyfus replied on April 12, 1943 (Telegram 377, 891.24/424): "Department's 168, sixth. Middle East Supply Center have ruled Iranian Government should be sole importer of pharmaceutical products and Iranian bulk indent has already been made. Import license applications of private traders must therefore be refused."

Soon after, a Pharmaceutical Institute was established. As in the case of the Road Transport Board, it made matters worse. The combination of the MESC's slow pace and the bureaucratic inefficiency of the Pharmaceutical Institute created a nightmarish situation in the pharmaceutical market. Dreyfus on April 26, 1943 (Dispatch 531 and enclosures, 891.1283/4):

> I have the honor to enclose translations of (1) a law of March 9, 1943 (18 Esfand 1321) authorizing the establishment of an Iranian Pharmaceutical Institute and (2) regulations approved by the Council of Min-

> isters on April 19, 1943 (Farvardine 30, 1322), for the organization and operation of this Pharmaceutical Institute. This newly created organization is faced with the difficult task of regulating and controlling distribution of pharmaceuticals. The necessity for the setting up of such a body was obvious, taking into consideration the short world supply of drugs, the difficulties of ordering and shipping, and the overriding necessity of effecting orderly distribution and price control within the country. The Iranian Government was encouraged to take this step by the Middle East Supply Center which takes the position that pharmaceuticals may be imported into Iran only if satisfactory steps are taken to control prices and distribution. The Middle East Supply Center has ruled that consideration will be given only to pharmaceutical orders placed by the Governments of Near Eastern countries and that bulk indents covering a full year should be prepared by each Government. In compliance with this ruling, the Iranian Government has prepared its bulk indent, which has been approved by the Combined Supplies Committee in Tehran and forwarded to the Middle East supply Center in Cairo. As indicated in my despatch No. 511 of April 7, 1943, on the operation of the Middle East Supply Center, there has been almost interminable delay in passing and forwarding this comprehensive drug order, a fact which may conceivably result in drug shortage in Iran some time this year. I mention this fact since, should such a shortage occur, it will certainly be attributed by Iranians to British-American lethargy. The Iranian Pharmaceutical Institute faces a colossal task which can be carried out only under the direction of a competent guiding hand. For this reason the Iranian Minister of Health has asked the Foreign Office to seek, through the Ministry of Foreign Affairs, the assistance of the American Government in obtaining the services of an American citizen to head this organization.

Iranians were desperate. On May 4, 1943, Schayesteh had written to Alling (Letter, 891.48/338):

> I wish to thank you for your sympathetic attitude and appreciation of our problems in these difficult times – problems which threaten the very existence of the people of Iran. In the course of our conversation yesterday you suggested that I should make a concrete and workable proposal with regard to the Medical requirements of Iran. After a full consideration I put forward the following plan: 1) An estimate to be made by American specialists of the weight and tonnage of the minimum annual requirements of drugs and other medical and surgical supplies for the fifteen million population of Iran. 2) Whatever pro-

portion of the total requirements can be spared by the United States of America to be supplied from this country. 3) The necessary shipping space to be allocated on a monthly basis. 4) The purchases in this country to be made under the supervision of an American Government Agency or the American Red Cross. Payment for each consignment to be made by the Iranian Government in cash. 5) Distribution in Iran to be under the supervision of the American Red Cross to prevent any profit to intermediaries. You will notice that this plan fits in with the general policy of fixing the minimum requirements of each country and the maximum tonnage which can be allocated. The present system of applying to the Central Supply Committee in Cairo for an import license in respect to each and every item to be imported is impracticable for such urgent and vital necessities as drugs, and that is why I propose that a definite quota be fixed for drugs to be supplied from this country and the necessary tonnage allocated for its shipment. It is clear that Iran must import her drugs and medical requirements and it is obvious that a great proportion of such requirements must be supplied from the United States. During the last year the lack of sufficient supplies from the United States has been the cause of the present grave shortage and has resulted in suffering to my countrymen and loss of valuable lives. I hope you will give your support to this plan and recommend it to the proper authorities; I feel sure it will go a long way towards the amelioration of the present unhappy conditions.

Alling's reply of June 4, 1943, reads in part:

The Department fully realizes, of course, the importance to Iran of these supplies, and careful consideration has been given to the plan you suggest. However, as you are aware, Iranian medical requirements have been under consideration by the existing American-British supply organizations in Tehran and Cairo for some time, and it has now been learned that a bulk order for a year's supply of these goods has recently been approved by the Middle East Supply Center. The portion of this order which is to be filled in the United States is expected to arrive in Washington in the immediate future and will be given prompt and sympathetic attention. It is believed, therefore, that Iran's needs in this line will be adequately met, in so far as the items involved are available in this country, through the procedure already in effect. From a practical point of view, the Department feels that the institution of a new procedure at this time would, even under the best of circumstances, cause substantial delay. Since the bulk supply order in question will cover requirements for a year I believe that we will defer consideration of procedure for future orders pending the full organization of the newly-created Iranian pharmaceutical Institute and the installation of its executive director.

Although the pharmaceutical bulk intent had been supposedly approved in March 1943, continued British attempts to get a larger share of the Iranian market had caused additional strains and delays. Dreyfus on July 5, 1943 (Dispatch 603 and enclosures, 891.24/470):

> I have the honor to report certain developments of possible interest to the Department in respect to the Iranian Government bulk indent for pharmaceuticals. Although this order was finally passed by the local Combined Supplies Committee, after some months of seemingly unreasonable delays, and placed with the Middle East Supply Center in Cairo in March, it has only recently been forwarded, for reasons which are not yet clear. Even then, part of it was allocated to the United Kingdom rather than to the United States, as was originally requested, to be filled from an order already destined to Cairo from London. The replacement by British substitutes of certain propriety drugs, especially ordered from well-known American manufacturers is a source of puzzlement and irritation to certain Iranian physicians who have reported to the Legation that the drugs from the United Kingdom will not meet their needs or requirements. Several British orders have come forward to Iran consigned to the United Kingdom Commercial Corporation without the approval of the local Combined Supplies Committee but when discovered they have been accepted by the latter, covered by their consent and the imports included have been deducted from the bulk intent. This irregularity has been called to the attention of the committee by the Legation representative. An attempt to introduce British drugs into the local market in place of American items ordered and preferred by Iranian doctors may well be behind these importations.
>
> Evidence to support such a suspicion might be taken from statements made to me by Sir Reader Bullard, the British Minister, during the course of a recent conversation with him in my office. He asked to come to see me and appeared much agitated during the conversation. He practically accused the Legation of connivance in an attempt which he claimed he had evidence to show was being made by Colonel Neuwirth to import American drugs without the knowledge or consent of the Combined Supplies Committee. In order to clarify the position of the Legation in this matter, I authorized Mr. Paxton, my represen-

tative on the Executive Committee of the Combined Supplies Committee, to read and have incorporated in the minutes a statement, a copy of which is enclosed, to the effect that the Legation continued to maintain its consistent stand that no drugs should be imported into Iran except with prior Middle East Supply Center approval and that it would vote against subsequent approval of imports which have not received such approval in advance.

In the conversation mentioned, my British colleague brought forth his desire for British representation in the Iranian Pharmaceutical Institute. Though I informed him, at the time, that this was a matter for decision by the Iranian Government and that the American representative on that body was an official of that Government, he seemed too agitated to react reasonably to my suggestion that he approach the Government on the matter. Therefore, in order to make doubly clear the Legation's position in this regard, I authorized Mr. Paxton to include in his statement at the meeting a reaffirmation of the Legation's position in this regard. It is contained in the last paragraph of the statement enclosed. At the meeting referred to it was proposed by the United Kingdom Commercial Corporation representative that the function of that body, as consignee for the British share of the drugs in the bulk intent, be taken over by an Anglo-Iranian Pharmaceutical Company (AIPC). This was opposed by the Legation representative and by the Iranian Government representative, an American member of the Millspaugh mission, after discussion had revealed that it was hoped to control the handing over of the drugs ordered to the Iranian Pharmaceutical Institute, item by item, rather than as a single unit once it had been approved for release by the authorities at Cairo. Also it appeared obvious that the proposed company would be less easily controlled by the British Government than would the United Kingdom Commercial Corporation. Although everyone else was in favor of the proposal it was thus referred to me. The next morning, Mr. Minor, after a conference at the British Legation on another subject, was approached by the British Minister and several of his staff with a draft telegram, a copy of which is enclosed, which the British Legation proposed to send after having obtained my concurrence. I wrote a letter to the British Minister, a copy of which is enclosed. Under date of June 29 my British colleague gave me an answer, a copy of which is also enclosed. It will be seen that, as a result of my suggestion, the British Legation has abandoned its proposal for an Anglo-Iranian Pharmaceutical Company. This, I believe, is a definite accomplishment as no motivation for its establishment seems likely other than "reasons of trade policy" to satisfy the desires of British drug salesmen, several of whom are now in

Tehran, presumably for the purpose of pushing British trade in drugs through such an organization. However, as I anticipated, once this idea was brought into the open, the British repudiated any such intention.

The other two points dealt with in the draft telegram and the letters were satisfactorily disposed of: the question of British representation on the Iranian Government Pharmaceutical Institute remains for decision of the Iranian Government, which appears unlikely to consent to British participation in it; the formation of an Anglo-American Pharmaceutical Company appears, as I wrote, both unnecessary and useless at present and its value in the future remains problematical and has been abandoned by the British. The charges against Neuwirth seem to have fallen to the ground without substantiation, on further investigation, as it now develops that he did nothing in any way irregular but, though he tried, apparently at the request of the Iranian Government, to interest American drug exporters in supplying the local demand, at the same time he informed the American firms that they would have to clear their imports through the Allied control in the usual way.

MESC Request for an Inventory of Pharmaceutical Products

Richard Ford, chargé d'affaires after the recall of Dreyfus, in a report of January 17, 1944 (Dispatch 798, 891.24/623):

I have the honor, with reference to the Legation's despatch No. 603 of July 5, 1943, on the subject of the Pharmaceutical Bulk Intent for the Iranian Government, to inform the Department as follows with respect to the progress so far made by the Imperial Pharmaceutical Institute in arriving at a determination of the quantities and kinds of drugs now held in stock in Iran, and with regard to the disposition so far made of the supplies of anti-typhus vaccine received in this country from Lend-Lease stocks in Cairo. Certain shipment of drugs, some representing orders from the United Kingdom under the Iranian Government's Pharmaceutical Bulk Indent, and some representing certain previous orders, have arrived in Iran consigned to the United Kingdom Commercial Corporation and, after some delays and difficulties, have been cleared through the Iranian customs, and placed at the disposition of Imperial Iranian Pharmaceutical Institute. As it had become clear some time ago, however, that any further shipments under the Bulk Indent would not be sanctioned until an accurate inventory had been made of the supplies of drugs already in this country, the Medical Advisory

Committee of the Middle East Supply Center in Tehran has for some time past been endeavoring to the best of its ability to get the Pharmaceutical Institute started on the work of preparing such an inventory. This inventory was also required for another reason; namely, that there was a reluctance on the part of the Institute to commence the distribution of its supplies on anything near the required scale until it was definitely known what stocks were actually in the country and immediately available, and what replacements could reasonably be expected from abroad. Many annoying delays were experienced, due in large part to the inertia of the Institute's temporary director, an Iranian who, there is reason to believe, stood to gain financially by delaying the taking of the inventory with a view of holding up, for as long a time as possible, the distribution of Government drugs at controlled prices. This official was finally replaced by another, who has shown himself, so far at least, to be much more disposed to get things done. However, without thoroughly competent direction, such as would be supplied by the employment of a qualified American executive, the Institute cannot hope to function as efficiently as it should. It is unfortunate that so many delays should have been encountered in taking advantage of the Iranian Government's authorization for the employment of a qualified American to take over the direction of the Institute, but it is hoped that the approaches now being made by the Department will insure the arrival here of a competent man.

The inventory, at any rate, has at last been started, and it was originally estimated that it would be completed by March fifteenth. Certain unforeseen difficulties have arisen, however, in the taking of the inventory, due to the fact that large quantities of the drugs on hand have been found to be the property of the Ministry of Health. These drugs were purchased some time ago by the Ministry of Health in accordance with an act of the Majlis which provided that the drugs be distributed to the poor free of charge through the various Government hospitals and clinics. This situation has complicated the taking of an inventory, as the Institute's drugs are intended to be sold at a profit. At a meeting held on January 8th, under the informal chairmanship of Dr. Millspaugh, arrangements were made for two employees of the United Kingdom Commercial Corporation, both of whom have knowledge of pharmaceuticals, to review the arrangements under which the inventory is now being taken, and to submit a report containing their recommendations for expediting its completion. Should they consider it necessary or desirable, moreover, they are prepared actively to assist the members of the Institute's staff in the physical taking of the inventory. It is to be hoped, therefore, that, despite the difficulties which have

> arisen, the inventory will be completed by the date originally set.
>
> While a start has been made in the distribution of the Institute's supplies, little has actually been accomplished thus far. Some drugs, it is true, have been distributed through the two Institute drug stores in Tehran, and some have been sent to various factories, American and British mission hospitals, and certain Government hospitals, all situated outside of Tehran. The supplies distributed, however, have by no means met the demand and, as a result, the Institute has come in for a certain amount of criticism. Plans developed by the Medical Advisory Committee, moreover, for the distribution of the Institute's supplies through a number of especially licensed pharmacies, in addition to the Institute's own stores, have run into a snag. The pharmacies originally recommended for licensing have now all refused the Institute's offer on the grounds that the penalties provided in the licensing contract licensees found violating the price control features of the licensing agreement were too severe. The Medical Advisory Committee is at present considering what action might be taken to surmount this difficulty, but a conclusion in the matter has not been reached. It must be said, therefore, that the problem of insuring adequate distribution of the Institute's drugs at controlled prices remains yet to be solved.

While awaiting the outcome of an inventory, the MESC had continued to refrain from establishing Iran's pharmaceutical 1944 import quota (Ford, Dispatch 846 and enclosure, 891.24/643, February 16, 1944). Even the American Mission hospitals faced a critical situation. Drugs ordered in January 1943 had not reached them by April 1944. Ford on April 14, 1944 (Telegram 253, 891.24/651):

> Legation informed by American Presbyterian Mission here that certain difficulties have arisen in United States over licensing or shipping of approximately two and one-half tons miscellaneous drugs and pharmaceuticals ordered by Board of Foreign Missions early in 1943 for use of five mission hospitals in Iran. Shipment is covered by MESC transport license no. 587 issued February 7, 1943. Mission states it is entirely out of certain badly needed drugs and its drug supplies generally are running dangerously low. Considering importance of work being done by mission hospitals in Iran it seems highly desirable that if at all possible steps be taken to resolve existing difficulties to end that shipment may be sent forward at early date. Legation would appreciate information on status of matter and of any action contemplated so that it may inform Mission authorities here.

On March 2, 1944, Schayesteh had again written to Alling (Letter, 891.24/645):

> My dear Mr. Alling: In my letter of May 4, 1943, No. 378, I explained to you the critical shortage of drugs and medical supplies in Iran. You were kind enough to inform me in your letter of June 4, 1943, that every consideration had been given this matter by the appropriate authorities and that a bulk order for a year's supply was ready to be shipped to Iran. You also stated that you believed that Iran's needs in this line would be adequately met. I am now in receipt of a telegram from Iran informing me that some medical supplies have reached other Near Eastern countries but that they know of no definite shipment having reached Iran. The price of the simplest drugs is extremely high and the situation remains very critical. I would appreciate it very much if you would let me know the quantity of drug which has been assigned to Iran and the amount which has reached there. In the event that nothing substantial has yet been sent, I am sure the Department will do what is necessary to expedite these greatly needed supplies.

Ford on April 18, 1944 (A-14, 891.24/659):

> Reference Department's instruction No. 351 of March 15, 1944, regarding Iranian stocks of drugs and pharmaceutical supplies. It is believed Iranian Minister's letter of March 2 was based on instructions from the Foreign Office here which were in turn based upon statements made in a broadcast received from London to the effect that additional supplies of drugs had been made available to certain Middle Eastern countries among which Iran was understood by the Foreign Office not to have been mentioned. . . . Legation has been following drug situation here closely with a view to submitting comprehensive report as soon as all information has been obtained. While all of this information has not yet become available, for example it is not known what is contained in the approximately 2,300 cases of drugs and pharmaceuticals now in the customs here pending delivery to the Pharmaceutical Institute, Legation believes, and Stokely confirms, that the supplies of drugs and pharmaceuticals now in this country, or en route, should be adequate to meet Iran's requirements for a considerable period of time. Distribution, rather than supply, is the main problem here at the present time so far as drugs are concerned.

Ford on April 24, 1944 (Dispatch 916 and enclosures, 891.24/663):

I have the honor to refer to the Department's instruction No. 351 of March 15, 1944 regarding the situation in Iran so far as supplies of drugs and pharmaceuticals are concerned, and to amplify the information contained in the Legation's airgram No. A-14 of April 18, 3 p.m. as follows. The inventory of the Institute's drugs and pharmaceuticals, so long in the course of preparation, has at last been completed. . . . It should be noted, however, that the inventory does not present an exactly true picture of the Institute's stocks at the present time since the figures given are those of December 31, 1943, and since there has been some distribution made since that time. . . . It is believed, however, that the inventory may be regarded as being substantially correct as the stocks released since the first of the year have been relatively small. It appears that there are approximately 2600 cases of drugs and pharmaceuticals now held in the customs, largely at Tehran, pending delivery to the Pharmaceutical Institute. . . . Of the total of around 2,600 cases, some 900 were shipped to Iran from the United Kingdom some time ago in the opium barter deal. The Institute is slowly taking delivery of these cases. The balance, approximately 1,700 cases, consists of drugs and pharmaceuticals, the title to which still rests with the United Kingdom Commercial Corporation. The UKCC insists upon receiving payment for these drugs before releasing them to the Institute, and as Dr. Millspaugh has so far been unable to find the money (approximately 21,000,000 rials) necessary to pay for them, delivery has not yet been effected. . . . In addition to the drugs held in the customs for eventual delivery to the Pharmaceutical Institute, there are around 100 shipments in the customs, perhaps even more, consigned to private merchants. There is no way of telling at the moment just what drugs are comprised in these shipments, or to just what extent these drugs will affect the supply position in Iran. These shipments, which include one from Palestine valued at £15,000, were all ordered prior to the establishment of the Institute with its effective monopoly on imports. By the time that the drugs had arrived in Iran, however, the Institute had been set up and, until just recently, it had come to no decision as to what should be done about the shipments. It has now been decided that the shipments should be released to the importers against their signed undertakings to sell them to the public at controlled prices. While little, of course, can be done to see that the importers live up to their undertakings, it was believed better to accept the importers' undertakings for what they are worth, and to have the goods moved out of the customs into the normal channels of trade.

Eleven of these shipments have already been released under this arrangement, and others are in the process of being released. The Legation is enclosing, as enclosure No. 2, a list of the drugs comprised in the 1943 Bulk Indent. This list has been approved by all of the authorities concerned, and it is understood that some of the drugs included in the list are already at sea en route to Iran. Those not yet shipped are either awaiting shipment, or are in the process of being procured. There are also enclosed, as enclosures Nos. 3 and 4, respectively, lists of dental and surgical supplies and equipment. The items on these lists are expected shortly since their procurement and shipment were approved prior to the approval of the Bulk Indent proper.

As was reported by the Legation in its despatch No. 811 of January 24, 1944, the Iranian Government stands committed to the purchase of 3,000,000 rials worth of drugs from the Russians. With its despatch No. 880 of March 14, 1944, the Legation enclosed a list of the drugs which the Russians have offered to the Iranian Government under the terms of the purchase agreement. The Iranian Government has not yet decided what drugs to take, or what to do with the drugs after it takes them. The Pharmaceutical Institute does not want to handle any Russian drugs as Mr. Stokely, its director, knows nothing about them, has no confidence in them, and feels that they would in all probability be difficult to move. Consideration is being given at the present time to a proposal that they be taken over by the Government (not by the Institute), and auctioned off immediately at a public sale. There is still no information as to the quantities, prices, or sources of the drugs being offered.

There is, understandably, no definite information as to the stocks of drugs and pharmaceuticals held in Iran in the pharmacies, or in the merchants' warehouses. From information received from time to time, however, it would appear that most of the standard drugs may usually be obtained provided that the customer can afford to pay the exorbitant prices asked for them. . . . In view, however, of the size of the Institute's present stocks, the number of the cases of drugs still in the customs, and the quantities of drugs comprised in the approved 1943 Bulk Indent now coming forward, it would not appear, either to Dr. Avery, to Mr. Stokely, or to the Legation, that it should be necessary to import into Iran during the next quota year any very large quantities of any of the drugs on the so-called essential list, except perhaps in the case of a few drugs where the existing, or potential, stocks happen to be either low or entirely nonexistent.

As noted in the previous chapter, in his report of May 8, 1944, Ford had commented on Daftary's letter to Governor Lehman (Dispatch 937, 891.24/670):

> Dr. Daftary has stated in his letter to UNRRA that Iran lacks pharmaceutical drugs, that typhus is widespread in the country, that the Iranian health authorities are in urgent need of "ambulances and portable machines for disinfection and for large and small sterilizers which can be transported from house to house," and that "instruments for surgery and equipment for hospitals and medicines, especially pharmaceutical goods, are completely lacking" in Iran. Considering the stocks of drugs and pharmaceuticals now held by the Imperial Iranian Pharmaceutical Institute, the stocks held at present in the customs pending delivery to the Institute or to private importers, and the stocks comprised in the 1943 Bulk Indent now in the process of being shipped, it is not believed that Iran is badly off at all, so far as supplies of drugs and pharmaceuticals are concerned. . . . Dr. Daftary is probably on firmer ground when referring in his letter to Iran's needs in surgical and hospital supplies and equipment. While some surgical equipment is coming forward under the 1943 Bulk Indent (see enclosure No. 4 to despatch No. 916 of April 24, 1944), the quantity is not large, and it is assumed that further supplies will be required to meet the needs of the country's hospitals and clinics during the forthcoming year. The Ministry of Health is engaged at present in obtaining information from the various hospitals regarding their present stocks of surgical and hospital supplies equipment, and concerning their requirements in goods of this kind for the quota year beginning July 1, next. . . . As the Ministry has just started its work of assembling the background data required, it is not possible for the Legation at this time to furnish the Department with any very helpful information as to Iran's present supply position in goods of the type in question. Copy to Mr. Landis, Cairo.

John D. Jernegan, now Second Secretary of Legation, on June 16, 1944 (Dispatch 973 and enclosure, 891.12A/6-1644):

> I have the honor to enclose a copy of a report submitted by Dr. Bennett F. Avery, the new American Director of Public Health, to the Iranian Minister of Health under the date of May 12, 1944. . . . The Legation is pleased to say that it regards Dr. Avery as constituting a most welcome addition to the force of American advisers in Iran. Having lived for many years in the Near East, he has not been shocked, as so many

> of our advisers have, by the conditions one meets with over here. His temperament is such, moreover, that he has not become discouraged by the immensity of the problem before him, or by the difficulties encountered in Iran in trying to accomplish even the simplest sort of thing. . . . In addition to handling his own work in an efficient manner, he has found the time to be of considerable assistance to his American colleague, Mr. Harvey V. Stokely, in connection with the latter's work of organizing and directing the operations of the Imperial Iranian Pharmaceutical Institute. While not expecting the impossible, the Legation does feel that Dr. Avery gives every promise of being able, given continued support from the Government, to accomplish a great deal in reforming the country's health services, and in improving general health conditions throughout the country.

Despite these optimistic reports, the drug situation remained dire. Cable to Ford on July 14, 1944 (Telegram 426, 891.24/7-1444):

> The Iranian Minister in Washington has been pressing the Department, under instructions from Saed (Prime Minister), to obtain further shipments of pharmaceuticals to Iran. The Department has pointed out that according to our information there are 2,600 cases of pharmaceuticals in warehouses in Iran, including 2,000,000 tablets of aspirins, one of the items alleged by the Minister to be scare. The foregoing serves to emphasize one of the pressing problems in Iran, as understood by Landis and the Department, is the distribution of such commodities as sugar, tea, cotton piece goods and especially pharmaceuticals. It is of course futile to send scarce commodities to Iran, using much needed shipping space, only to have goods deteriorate in warehouses while the Iranian public suffers acute shortages. The Department has decided, therefore, that as immediate and effective a distribution as is possible of such commodities as pharmaceuticals and perhaps others should be made, even if recourse must be had to private trade channels and at some risk of the less effective distribution. Please bring this view to the attention of the appropriate authorities such as Millspaugh, Avery, Stokely and the MESC, and urge that a system be devised which will permit prompt distribution of these commodities. Please report to Department steps taken and results achieved.

Russian Pharmaceuticals

As noted, Iran had accepted to buy Russian drugs. Ford on March 14, 1944 (Dispatch 880 and enclosure, 891.24/648):

> I have the honor . . . to enclose a copy, in translation, of a list of drugs which the Russians, under the terms of the agreement, have now offered for sale to the Iranian Government. The Russians have not, so far, informed the Iranian Government of the quantities, or of the unit, or total prices of drugs included in the list. It will be recalled, however, that the agreement under reference provided for the purchase by the Iranian Government of Russian drugs in the total amount of three million rials, and it is possible that the Iranians are intended to select items from among those offered in quantities sufficient to make up this amount. . . . The American director of the Imperial Iranian Pharmaceutical Institute, Mr. Harvey V. Stokely, has informed the Legation that he is exceedingly reluctant to burden the Institute with any Russian drugs at all, that he knows nothing about them, has no confidence in them, and that his Iranian assistants have told him that they are not well regarded by Iranian doctors and pharmacists, and would, consequently, be very difficult to move. The Institute, nevertheless, has informed Mr. Bernard Lamb, the Administrator General of the Millspaugh Mission's Section on Price Stabilization, that it might be able to use certain quantities of eleven of the drugs mentioned in the Russian list, provided that the prices asked were reasonable, and that it was satisfied that the drugs were of good quality. . . . While the Iranian Government is committed to the purchase of Russian drugs to the value of three million rials, a great many of the details of the transaction (prices, sorting and so on) were left vague in the purchase contract, and were to be made the subject of later agreement between the two Governments. Mr. Lamb, who appears to be handling the matter on the Iranian side, has not, as yet, come to any decision as to the reply to be made to the Russian offer. The Legation will follow developments closely, and will report them to the Department as they occur.

News of the proposed Russian drug sales to Iran was not well received in Washington. On May 8, 1944, an official of Foreign Economic Administration (FEA) had telephoned Harold Minor now at the State Department (Memorandum, 891.24/671):

> Mr. Moore telephoned today to inform me of the results of the investigation made by FEA concerning the quantities and types of pharmaceutical supplies being furnished the Soviet Government under Lend-Lease. His report was in response to my request of several weeks ago and was based on Tehran's despatch no. 880 of March 14, 1944, which enclosed a list of pharmaceuticals the Soviet Government has offered to the Iranian Government under the terms of the Rice-Miscellaneous

Goods Agreement made between the Iranian and Soviet Governments. Mr. Moore said that his inquiry reveals that only six of the drugs offered by the Russians to Iran are being supplied to the Soviet Union under Lend-Lease. The quantities of five of these are exceedingly small. . . . The sixth item was urotropine, which is being furnished in huge quantities but is used for the manufacture of munitions rather than for medical purposes. Mr. Moore expressed the opinion that we would have a very weak case if we bring to the attention of the Russians the fact that they are offering Iran pharmaceutical supplies similar to those being furnished Russia under Lend-Lease.

Ford on August 15, 1944 (Dispatch 1067 and enclosures, 891.24/8-1544):

I have the honor . . . to enclose a list of the drugs which the Iranian Government finally agreed to take over from the Russians. The quantities and prices are also shown. . . . The purchase of these drugs, as well as of certain Russian manufactures, was provided for in an agreement between the two countries which was reported to the Department in my despatch No. 811 of January 24, 1944. The drugs listed in the enclosure, valued at Rials 3,026,832.50, have all been paid for by the Iranian Government. Due, however, to a somewhat confused situation caused by recent personnel changes in the Millspaugh Mission, the Iranian Government has not yet taken delivery of the shipments. The drugs are at present lying in Russian warehouses at Bandar Shah, Pahlevi and Tehran, and storage charges are accumulating daily. The Government has now taken steps, however, to obtain delivery of the drugs at an early date with a view to disposing of them as quickly as possible at public auction.

Iran's Sugar Import Quota

The reduction on various pretexts in Iran's 1943 quota of sugar imports was noted in the correspondence between the Iranian Minister in London and the Foreign Office given in chapter 7. Millspaugh had subsequently protested to the MESC the reduction in the sugar quota. It was ultimately futile, but Millspaugh's lucid statement of the case is very valuable. Ford on May 10, 1944 (Dispatch 947 and enclosures, 891.24/5-1044):

I have the honor to inform the Department that the Iranian Government has, for some time past, been dissatisfied with the quota fixed by the Middle East Supply Center for sugar imports into Iran. It was felt that, in setting upon 60,000 tons as Iran's annual requirements of sugar, MESC had used a population figure considerably below the actual population of the country, had not given due weight to the quantities of sugar imported into the country in past years, had not properly taken into account the need for sugar for industrial and other purposes, and, in general, had failed to pay sufficient attention to the peculiar position which sugar occupies in the life of the average Iranian. The general feeling of dissatisfaction with the situation was increased considerably recently when the Iranian Government became aware of the fact that the import quota agreed upon by Cairo for the current year was only 41,000 tons instead of the 60,000 tons which it had previously thought were to be allowed. The misunderstanding on the part of the Iranian Government arose from the fact that it had not, until recently, realized that MESC, in arriving at an import quota, had deducted the estimated local production from the figure of 60,000 tons which it had set as Iran's total requirements for the year. Considerable apprehension has been felt in Government circles, also, over the non-arrival so far this year of any sugar from foreign sources. A shipment consisting of 6,500 tons, however, is due to arrive at Khoramshahr today (May 13), with this shipment and the others which are scheduled to follow, it is believed that apprehension on this point will be to some extent allayed.

Dr. Millspaugh has set down the views of the Iranian Government with respect to the sugar question in a letter of May 8, 1944 to Colonel D.R. Hobson, the MESC representative in Iran. Dr. Millspaugh's arguments are believed by the Legation to be in the main sound and well thought out, and it is felt that, should the world supply position permit, some upward revision of Iran's quota might well be given consideration by the various agencies concerned. A copy of Dr. Millspaugh's letter to Colonel Hobson is enclosed. The Legation is also enclosing, as of possible interest in this connection, a table showing Iran's production of sugar during the season which ended several months ago. While the figures shown give no indication of the costs of production, the Legation understands that, without allowing for any profits by the refineries, the production costs averaged in the neighborhood of $0.23 a pound. Plans for next year's production of sugar, it may be added, have been worked out by the Ministry of Commerce and Industry. These plans provide for the growing of sugarbeets on approximately 30,000 hectares (74,130 acres) of land located in the vicinity of one or another of the seven sugar refineries. Contracts have already been let covering practically the whole of this acreage.

Millspaugh's letter of May 8, 1944, to Colonel Hobson:

My purpose in writing this letter is to present to the Middle East Supply Centre and others concerned a general statement of the sugar situation and problem from the standpoint of the organizations under my direction, which represent the Iranian Government in matters of supply. It is believed that such a general statement is needed and may be a useful means of bringing about the necessary coordination and harmony with respect to objectives and operations. It is desired that this letter should be treated as a formal statement of requirements and as an application for supplies mentioned therein.

We do not question the soundness at this time of centralized control of the purchase and allocation of sugar. We assume, however, that this control will be based on the facts regarding world-supply and the necessity of allocating shipping space, and that, in the exercise of the control, all of the countries will be treated alike with respect to individual rations, and consideration being given to the special conditions, customs and needs of Iran. We do not favor, and within the limits of our powers, we do not intend to permit the importation of sugar in uncontrolled shipping. Our regulations provide for the control of sugar imports. We have at present time, I am informed by the competent officials, a small amount of about 1,000 tons of merchants' sugar in the Customs. This was in the main ordered and some of it moved before our Price Stabilization Regulation No. 122/34 went into effect. Because of the high price of this sugar, it would not be advisable for the Iranian Government to purchase it. I have therefore authorized the release of this sugar to the merchants. Any sugar privately imported which was ordered after the above-mentioned Regulation went into effect will be taken by the Government at the Government price. In order to further prevent private traffic in sugar, I am issuing a new regulation prohibiting the transport of sugar within the country of privately-owned sugar except in reasonable quantities for private use.

Some confusion seems to exist with reference to the proper sugar quota for Iran. The present quota allowed by MESC for imported sugar is 60,000 tons annually, or 5,000 tons monthly. An impression seems to exist in the minds of MESC representatives in Tehran that the domestic production should be deducted from this quota. For reasons stated hereafter, we disagree with this view. An impression also seems to exist that the domestic production of Iran is 25,000 tons annually. The 1322 (1943/44) production of beet-sugar in Iran was 21,560 tons. This is the figure that must be taken in estimating our production during the current year. Any other figure would be the merest guess. Nevertheless, if the actual production exceeds this figure, as we hope it will, the quantity in excess may be considered in a recalculation of the total quantity available to meet the requirements of this country. We do not believe that the potential production of this country can be considered in fixing the quota. Various factors influence the realizing of potentials at this time. It is not logical, in my opinion, to say that our productive processes are inefficient. Of course, they are inefficient. A part of the inefficiency is due to the war and the pressure of Allied activities and policies on the country. Iran should make every effort to achieve efficiency in operations and maximum production; but it should not be penalized if it is unable, under present circumstances, to reach a hypothetical goal set by MESC.

With respect to the proper sugar quota for Iran, we are convinced that the minimum total requirements of Iran are considerably in excess of 80,000 tons. Sugar is one of the most essential articles of food for the people of Iran. It is a basic food, important for its nutritional value and not as a food supplement as is the case in most European and North American countries. Also its distribution and price is an important factor in the economic life of this country. A quantity of sugar totaling 97,000 tons (Customs figures) was imported in 1318 (1939/40), the same year in which Iran had a domestic production of beet sugar in the Government factories of 30,000 tons, a total available supply of 127,000 tons.

The annual requirements of sugar should be estimated on a basis of 12,000,000 population, the figure used on estimates of all other items. The existing quotas are based on a population of only 10,000,000. On a basis of 12,000,000 population, the import quota, if delivered in full as promised, together with the domestic production of the current year, making a combined total of 80,000 tons, would appear sufficient to allow approximately 550 grams per month per capita. This, of course, is not true in fact, because no allowance has been made for industrial or other uses which are recognized as factors in sugar quota allotments or rationing in other countries.

Furthermore, no allowance is made for the allocation of sugar to sugar-beet growers, a measure which will be necessary this year to insure the maximum of domestic sugar production. Nor has any allowance been made for the application of the sugar-barter scheme to grain-collection. MESC is fully informed of the grain prospects in Iran this year. The full collection of the harvest is necessary not only for the welfare and security of this country, but also for the economizing of the shipping space of the Allies. We do not desire or intend to use the sugar-barter scheme unless it is absolutely necessary to collect the surplus grain of the peasants. If the barter scheme is put into operation, it may call for an additional amount of 800 tons; and MESC does not need to be reminded that the barter scheme will work only if the sugar is in the country and is actually available at the interior distribution points. It will also be quite evident that sugar used in barter cannot be controlled. Much, if not all of it, will go into the black market. Sugar which in this way goes into the black market should not be deducted from the country's proper quota. The reason is that, because of the meager quota allocated to the country and the resulting insufficiency of the ration, this sugar will go into a limited, special and privileged market to those who can pay the free-market price. It will not be distributed to the masses.

Finally, in estimating the quota for Iran, no allowance is made by MESC for special institutional uses, for official entertainment purposes, for restaurants and tea-houses, or for the military. It appears that the Polish refugees in Iran receive a ration of at least 900 grams. Our considered opinion is that the individual ration should be at least 600 grams per capita per month, or a total quantity for the entire population of 86,400 tons per year. For the uses I have mentioned above, we estimate an additional quantity of 14,000 tons. The total minimum requirements, therefore, are estimated at about 100,000 tons. On this basis, the import quota should be 80,000 tons annually, or approximately 6,700 tons monthly.

Figures compiled about a month ago, after considerable study, indicate approximately 30,000 to 33,000 tons of sugar stocks within the country at the present time. Of this quantity, 20,000 tons represent the domestic production of the current year, and, of the balance, 4,000 tons at Bushire and 1,500 tons at Bandar Abbas owned by the Government is not, due to transportation difficulties, readily usable in full in our present 3 months sugar distribution program. There may be some addition as to the total of sugar stocks indicated. This will be determined when we receive the inventory reports from all the local kharbars throughout the country. Added to this, owned privately, which may be sold in the illicit or free market, but this has no value to us in our program of general distribution to the people of the country. During the last six weeks about 5,000 tons have been distributed.

We desire to record our conviction and earnest desire that not only should the full amount of 80,000 tons be allocated for import this year, but also that it should be imported regularly according to schedule. In 1943 only 42,000 tons (Customs figures) were brought into Iran, and, during the first quarter of 1944, none of the quota allowed was delivered. It is understood that MESC allocates only 4,500 tons, instead of 5,000 tons monthly. I am informed that the imports are still far behind even this inadequate schedule. I am informed that it is the view of the MESC representatives in Tehran that the importation of the full quota should be conditional on the adequacy and progress of distribution within the country. I do not question the long-run soundness of this view; but, in my opinion, it would be impracticable and premature to apply that policy at the present time. We have distribution now organized on sound and practicable lines. Sugar is actually being moved and distributed in constantly increasing quantities.

The success of distribution depends in the main on the following: 1. The possession of an adequate stock in the country at all times. 2. Transportation. 3. Honest distribution to the ultimate consumer. Iran requires more inventory than other countries that are smaller in area or population or which have more rapid distribution systems. To prevent distribution coming to a full stop and remaining at a standstill for a long period, imports must always be considerably ahead of actual distribution. Unless imports arrive on schedule in sufficient quantities, it will be impossible for us to plan warehousing and movements or carry through the intermediate stages of transportation process. It appears to me that MESC is not fully aware of the importance of the question of honest distribution to the ultimate consumer. This is not only a question of administrative organization and personnel, but it is also a question of control, free-market prices, and hoarding tendencies. The present insufficient ration obviously helps to create and perpetuate a black-market. The black-market price has risen recently. Among the causes of this rise were the Japanese invasion of India, rumors of changes in the quota, and the cessation of imports. If imports are actually restricted, we may expect a further rise in black-market prices, with increased tendencies to hoard and speculate. Such a situation also naturally increases smuggling. The effects on distribution is apparent. Bribery and corruption are stimulated, and the distribution of sugar to the areas impossible. The present policy of MESC, therefore, defeats the very end of distribution which MESC sets up as a condition precedent of imports. MESC, it is understood, demands an inventory of stocks in the country and reports of actual distribution. It does not seem to realize that, while we can make these reports right now on stocks, and movements, and distribution, these reports will for some time be incomplete. We have been trying for over a year to establish a general system of financial accounting and reporting in the older administrations, we have not yet succeeded. Moreover, reports in this particular field will always suffer from a time-lag, due to the slowness of communications and, in many cases, the inefficiency of personnel.

To insure the success of both control and distribution, it is necessary, in my opinion, that MESC should immediately adopt an increased quota as above recommended and should promptly provide for the import of sugar on schedule. The result will be to give us the physical prerequisites of planned and efficient distribution and also the means of controlling prices, inflation, hoarding, and distribution to the ultimate consumer. If, later on, it appears that stocks in the country are increasing beyond reasonable limits, imports can be easily reduced. The important thing at the moment is not to stop the flow into the country or even to create an impression that the flow may be stopped. It is highly essential that the United Kingdom Commercial Corporation should bring in white sugar instead of brown, or yellow sugar. The delivery of 7,000 tons in two shipments by the UKCC in November and December consisted entirely of brown sugar, the sale of which was strongly objected to by the people generally, the Prime Minister and the Council of Ministers. MESC and UKCC were advised of these objections. Iranians, by deeply rooted customs, are primarily users of white sugar, preferably in lump form. MESC is urged to give its attention to this matter. . . .

It is my hope that, following the receipt of this letter, officials and representatives concerned may meet with me for a discussion of the various points that I have herein mentioned.

On May 12, 1944, Alian Christelow of the British Civil Secretariat in Washington had written to Fred Winant at the State Department (Letter, 891.24/5-1244):

With reference to our conversation about sugar for Persia. May I draw your attention to Mr. Jourdain's remarks on page 6 of S.M.E. (44) 1st Meeting, of which I believe you have a copy. Mr. Jourdain's statements that it was suspected that there were large quantities of sugar in Persia which had not been distributed, were, I believe, well justified. You will also note that MESC was endeavouring to build up a 3-month stockpile and you will no doubt appreciate the importance of such stocks being under centralized control.

Not surprisingly, attempts to get more sugar for Iran were to no avail. On June 10, 1944, John P. Dawson, Director, Combined Agency for Middle East Supplies, had written to A. Perlman, INCO, 6 Broadway, New York (Letter, 891.24/6-1044):

> Dear Mr. Perlman: we have sought for some weeks to secure a final decision as to the possibility of exporting sugar to Iran. As you know, requests have been made by various importers in Iran including the Iranian Government, addressed to numerous suppliers in this country. The difficulty that principally prevents the approval of any export licenses for sugar shipments to Iran is the supply situation for sugar, which has been growing less rather than more favorable in recent months. We have consulted the War Food Administration and other authorities concerned with the control of sugar exports and have been informed that in their judgment shipments to Iran would be wholly unjustified in view of the shortage of supplies here and the existence of supplies from local production in Iran and from the Island of Mauritius. The whole subject has been very carefully reviewed by the Iranian authorities and by American officials, who are convinced that the supplies now available in Iran from nearby sources are adequate to cover essential requirements. I regret the delay in replying to your letter of May 10, but it has been necessary for us to secure a full report from the field and to consult the supply authorities in the United States before a final decision could be reached.

Iran's Production of Beet Sugar, 1943/44 (Metric Tons)

Factory	Sugarbeets	Refined Sugar	Granular Sugar
Kahrizak	6,357	411.324	502.703
Keredj	17,236	568.328	2,120.701
Shahabad	4,193	176.156	474.350
Shazand	11,017	468.202	1,093.086
Miandoab	23,011	963.356	2,263.272
Marv-Dasht	43,560	1,575.909	4,124.696
Abkuh	48,965	1,977.119	4,877.642
Totals	155,060	6,140.394	15,456.450

Total Sugar Produced: 6,140.394 + 15,456.450 = 21,596.844 tons
Source: Millspaugh's letter of May 8, 1944, to Hobson of MESC.

Chapter 10

Influx of Polish Refugees from Russia

As Iran was plunging into famine in the spring of 1942, Polish refugees from Russia had begun arriving in northern Iran. The flow which had continued until the summer of 1943 had brought at least 150,000 Polish civilians and soldiers into the country. The soldiers had moved on, but most of the civilians had remained until the end of the war. The relative magnitude of this number can be seen from the fact that the 1940 population of Tabriz, Iran's second largest city, was reported to be 213,000, while the population of Tehran was reported at 521,000. In a report of June 1, 1942, Maurice Barber, the American Red Cross (ARC) representative in Tehran, gives the following background information (Dreyfus, dispatch 262 and enclosure, 840.48 Refugees/2977, June 12, 1942):

> On February 6th, 1942, Mr. Ralph Bain, Director of the American Red Cross Middle East, left Cairo for Tehran, via Baghdad, in order to plan and make arrangements for the distribution of approximately 320 tons of ARC supplies—consisting principally of flour, beans, milk, clothing and blankets which had left Suez via British tankers and which was destined for Polish refugees supposed to be coming from Russia to Iran. In Baghdad, Mr. Bain visited General Wheeler, Head of the US Military Mission there. . . . General Wheeler courteously promised that American Red Cross supplies would be granted priority along with United States military supplies. Thanks to the helpful cooperation on the part of General Wheeler, ARC supplies sent this way have

reached Tehran in the shortest possible time and in excellent condition. . . . Mr. Bain interviewed the Polish Minister to Iran, the Delegate of the Polish Red Cross in Iran, Mr. Andre Walczak and other members of the small Polish local community and a few Polish refugees who had reached Tehran from Russia. In addition Mr. Bain had numerous interviews with British and Polish authorities. From all these sources, Mr. Bain learned of the terrible suffering of Polish refugees in Russia—many of whom had been in concentration camps for two years and among whom the death rate was exceedingly high—especially among women and children and all of whom were in a state of utter destitution from exposure, malnutrition and disease. It soon appeared to Mr. Bain that the question of Polish refugees coming to Iran was very vague and no one knew when, if ever, any adult Poles would be allowed to come out of Russia. Indeed, every indication pointed to the fact that the Russians would allow no Polish refugees to leave Russia, except 400 small children who were to be sent to Isfahan (Iran) and 500 more children which India had agreed to take. "Children would not talk" was alleged to have been the Russian attitude. In view of this situation the composite hope was to get aid to the Polish refugees who had finally reached the region of Ashkabad, which is about 30 miles from the Iranian border. In this connection, Mr. Bain sent an urgent appeal to ARC National Headquarters, for permission to send some of the ARC supplies—which were to be turned over to the Polish Red Cross in Tehran—to Russia. Meantime, the Polish Red Cross was authorized by Mr. Bain to use such ARC supplies as needed for Polish relief in Tehran and, in particular, for the Polish refugee children en route to India and those scheduled to be sent to Isfahan.

Meantime, also Mr. Bain made a thorough study of the relief needs among the Iranians and, as a result thereof, made tentative plans for the distribution of the aforesaid 320 tons of ARC supplies and also of an allotment of medical supplies contemplated to be sent from Cairo for distribution among poor Iranians—under the control of an ARC distributing committee in cooperation with the Red Lion and Sun—*provided* Washington Headquarters did not approve of the sending of ARC supplies for Polish refugees in Southern Russia.

On February 25th Mr. Bain returned to Cairo. By this time no Polish refugees had arrived in Iran from Russia and actually none was expected and the situation was status quo. Washington had acknowledged Mr. Bain's cable and had stated that the proposal of sending ARC supplies to Polish refugees in Russia was being cleared with the

> Russian authorities in Washington and in Kuibyshev. On March 9th, I arrived in Tehran and proceeded to make the necessary contacts with the British, Polish and Iranian authorities.

Barber from Tehran to Bain in Cairo on April 13, 1942 (Dreyfus, dispatch 249 and enclosure, 840.48 Refugees/2918):

> After months of refusals to allow Polish adult civilians to leave Russia, the Soviets apparently decided suddenly to dump thousands of them into Iran due perhaps to the lack of food in Russia and the fear of disease. Without warning, I was officially informed on March 25th by the local British authorities and by Mr. Karszo-Siedlewsky, the Polish Minister, that in two days 800 Polish women and children from Russia would arrive in Pahlevi, that in a few days thereafter another 1500 would arrive, and that a total of about 15,000 were expected in a week's time.

Barber describes the arrival of the first batch in Tehran:

> In the afternoon of March 29th. . . . I went to the Machinegun Barracks at Dowchan Tapeh with Mr. Walczak, Polish Red Cross Delegate where about 20 Polish women and 10 children had already arrived. A few of them were ill. . . . Later in the day of March 30th, Colonel Neuworth (Neuwirth) and I visited the Polish Refugee Camp where, on that day, had arrived 172 Polish children, 25 women, 2 nurses, 8 sisters and 2 officers. There had developed several cases of infectious diseases and both Col Neuworth and I became alarmed. There were absolutely no facilities for hospitalization or isolation. . . . Pandemonium reigned as hundreds more refugees streamed into the camp, packed like sardines on trucks from Pahlevi. Every facility was lacking, the confusion was terrible and the pitiable state of the sick children deplorable and very moving. To add to the confusion Polish troops were arriving along with the civilians. As of March 30th, 6000 Polish effectives had already arrived in Tehran. . . . By now over 1000 women and about 700 children had arrived in Tehran from Pahlevi in a tragic state. Cases of diseases were multiplying and the situation was becoming more serious. I took Lieut. Commander Laing, Medical Attaché to Admiral Stanley and he confirmed the fear expressed by Col Neuworth and me in connection with the danger of epidemics.

Dreyfus on April 3, 1942 (Dispatch 239 and enclosures, 840.48 Refugees/2885):

I have the honor to enclose copies of two telegrams dated April 2 and April 3 and excerpts from two letters dated March 29 sent by Mr. Maurice Barber, representative of the American Red Cross in Tehran, to Mr. Ralph Bain, Director of American Red Cross Middles East, Cairo, concerning the problem of Polish refugees arriving in Iran. These enclosures will give the Department a better picture than I could possibly portray of the magnitude of the problem of relief of the Polish refugees now pouring into Iran and of the work being done by the Red Cross and others. Relief of these unfortunates has been made the more difficult by inadequate preparation for their reception and by the fact that the Soviet authorities, after much procrastination as to whether they will permit the Poles to come to Iran at all, are now suddenly dumping them at the more rapid rate than had been expected and without regard to the facilities which are available for their reception. The strong adjectives, such as "appalling," used by Mr. Barber are not careless exaggerations. Conditions among these poor refugees are indeed pathetic. Excellent work is being done by Mr. Barber in obtaining and distributing supplies. Others, too, are actively engaged in helping in this great task, among them Dr. Neuwirth USMC, of the Greely Mission, the British authorities, the Polish Legation and the American Mission Hospital at Meshed. It is hoped that by their combined efforts it will be possible to give care and comfort to the 15,000 civilians, mostly women and children, and to the 45,000 soldiers who are arriving. It is expected that 40,000 additional soldiers may arrive in the not too distant future.

Mr. Barber told me yesterday that more active measures will have to be taken for hospitalization of the children if epidemics of typhoid, cholera, smallpox, and typhus, all of which are prevalent among them, are to be avoided. He reported that there is one case of meningitis. He described the conditions among these sick children as pitiful, with typhus, typhoid and other patients lying on cotton mattresses on the floors of the improvised rooms. I learn from other sources that numbers of them have arrived dead, one officer having seen 10 dead in a contingent of about 70. Mr. Barber is of the opinion that this relief work is the most urgent work to be done by the Red Cross in the entire Middle East. I will keep the Department informed of the developments.

The above-mentioned telegram from Barber in Tehran to Bain in Cairo is dated April 2, 1942:

> Nearly 1000 Polish women and 700 motherless children arrived suddenly Tehran and arriving 500 or more daily. Condition unbelievably pitiful and deplorable. Furnishing clothes, blankets, food and medicines to Pahlevi where refugees arrive with practically nothing, to Kazvin where sick children are left and to colony here where many children infected with cholera, typhus, dysentery and typhoid. All terribly undernourished. . . . Was officially informed yesterday approximately 15000 more women and children arriving within week. . . . Now obvious that condition Polish refugees Russia tragic. Thousands are dying from exposure, hunger and disease and everything should be done all sides to rush aid to perhaps greatest civilian emergency of war.

The follow up telegram dated April 3, 1942:

> General Anders, just arrived from Russia, told me yesterday that 50 percent of Polish children in Russia have already perished. . . . Send 10000 more blankets, some sheets and all clothing possible, especially women's, children's and clothing code, also meningitis serum and diphtheria antitoxin. . . . Meningitis and smallpox now present among Polish children Tehran.

Barber's letter of March 29, 1942, to Bain, also refers to transport difficulties and the desperate shortage of medical supplies:

> Local and personal transportation is difficult. There are very few cars or taxis for hire and the rates are exorbitant. Droshkees (carriages) are slow and the distances great. . . . Medical supplies are practically unobtainable here. Those that are obtainable are sold at prices between 500 and 1000 per cent higher than in normal times. . . . The need of medical supplies in Iran is plainly very urgent and the distribution of those to be donated by the American Red Cross should do much to relieve suffering among the poor.

Letter of April 4, 1942, from an American resident of Rasht, "Uncle Jim," to Irene Goldis of Newdale, Manitoba, Canada, intercepted by the American Censor (MID-Iran, 2050): "Just now sixty thousand Poles, fifty thousand men and ten thousand women and children are passing through Resht. They came from Russia and the British Government is fitting them out and arranging transport to take them to their different destinations."

In a report of April 12, 1942 (Dispatch 247 and enclosures, 840.48 Refugees/2902), Minor encloses copies of two letters, both dated April 5, 1942, from Barber in Tehran to Bain in Cairo and to Norman H. Davis, ARC Chairman in Washington. Letter to Davis:

> Today the number of wretched Polish refugees evacuated from Russia to Tehran has risen to 5000—mostly women and children all of whom have arrived here in less than a week. Within the next ten days, 10,000 more are expected. In addition there are thousands of Polish soldiers arriving from Russia along with the refugees. These Polish refugees present the most pitiable civilian emergency of the war to date. The refugee debacle in France, starvation in Spain were child's play in comparison. They arrive in Pahlevi on the Persian side of the Caspian Sea with literally nothing and in a state of utter destitution and starvation. I am busy day and night rushing clothing, blankets, food and medicines to Pahlevi and supplying the colony here with the same commodities. The fact that the American Red cross has these supplies in Persia at this time is providential and you can be confident that through our efforts we are saving hundreds of lives among these valiant people who have for so long been terribly undernourished and suffering from exposure.
>
> The other day a woman refugee in the camp here who was clothed in an American Red Cross flannel-dressing-gown and shawl and who was particularly active cleaning, dressing and feeding the children, suddenly broke down crying. The Polish Bishop asked her what the matter was. She replied that her own two children had died of starvation in Russia just three weeks ago and that her husband is still in a concentration camp in Siberia. "If only my children had lived for this freedom" she sobbed. . . . Last week a prominent member of the Polish community in Tehran went to the border to meet a family of five brothers and sisters whose parents he knew intimately in Poland and who were being evacuated from Russia where the mother had died and the father had been concentrated. The mother had been an unusually strong and robust woman and this family friend asked the eldest child how it happened that their mother had died. The boy replied slowly that she had sacrificed all of her own allotted food for her five children to keep them alive and that she had died of starvation.
>
> The sick children are haunting shadows, literally skin and bones, there are many cases of Typhus, Typhoid, Cholera, Dysenteria, Scarlet Fever, Meningitis, and Small Pox among both the women and children

> and the situation, in this respect, is very serious. However hospital facilities have been finally secured and the situation is now under control. In this connection too American Red Cross medical supplies are playing a very important part. Col Newworth (sic), medical officer attached to General Greely U.S.A. here has been of great assistance in organizing for the care of the sick. Both the American Minister Mr. Dreyfus and General Greely have been most sympathetic, cooperative and exceedingly helpful in connection with the administration of American Red Cross Relief in this awful holocaust. The condition among the Poles in Southern Russia is perhaps more tragic. They are dying by the thousands. Fifty percent of all Polish children in Russia have already perished from starvation, exposure and disease. . . . I did not mean to make this letter so long and please forgive me—but I have never in my life been more moved than I have been by the tragedy of these Polish refugees in Russia and now in Persia.

Dreyfus on April 24, 1942 (Dispatch 249 and enclosure, 840.48 Refugees/2918):

> Conditions in the camps are steadily improving although disease is rampant. It will be observed that there are almost 400 cases of typhus and Dr. Neuwirth of the Greely mission reports that there are some 16 deaths a day at the two camps. Dr. Neuwirth has inoculated all of the Greely mission and members of the staff against typhus with the limited amount of serum which he brought from the United States and is now working with the Pasteur Institute in an endeavor to make sufficient quantity to inoculate most of Tehran. Dr. Neuwirth deserves commendation for his unselfish and gratuitous work in this connection.

In a letter to Bain dated April 28, 1942, Barber writes (Dreyfus, dispatch 259 and enclosure, 840.48 Refugees/2919):

> What a week-end! 94 lorries arrived at the warehouse at 3 p.m. and were offloaded, checked and warehoused at 11 a.m. the following morning. . . . All supplies are guarded day and night by Polish soldiers. . . . There is much interest among the Iranians about the 1700 pounds of medicals for distribution to the Iranian population. Please let me know as soon as possible what these are, how they are being shipped and how they are marked.

He adds:

> All Polish refugees now in Tehran will probably be sent to Carej within a few weeks where, it appears, suitable arrangements will be made for them all. The Persian authorities are anxious to get them away from Tehran. There are rumors galore about more Poles descending upon Iran from Russia in numbers varying from 30,000 to 120,000.

Letters intercepted by the British censor provide additional insight. Letter from Tehran dated April 20, 1942:

> There has been a drive for clothes and money and medicines for them. Bread is scarce (truly the staff of life here). Yet we do not hear the Iranians grumbling at this addition to the population. We see whole trucks—loads of white bread go out there. The worst factor is the typhus fever they carry.

Several British employees of the oil company in Abadan comment on the arrival of Polish refugees. Letter dated May 2, 1942: "40,000 to 50,000 Polish refugees have arrived in the north of this country from Russia, internees since the Russians walked into Poland in October 1939. They are in a deplorable state with no clothes or money or shelter." Letter from Tehran dated May 5, 1942: "Quite a number of ladies who have children here are sending for Polish girl refugees to look after their children as nannies, instead of the Iranian women. It is a home and they will be well looked after, as I believe in North Persia it is pitiful, so many destitute refugees."

Cable from Bain in Cairo to Davis in Washington on April 25, 1942 (Telegram 655, 891.48/304):

> Supplies for Poles going forward from Egypt to Tehran satisfactorily. Barber reported by air mail April 20 that of 11,893 refugees in Tehran 961 are sick, 337 being typhus cases and 69 total deaths since March 29. Anticipated influx of several thousand more Polish civilians from Russia rumors varying between 40,000 and 80,000.

A follow up communication states that the actual number of deaths was 90 and not 69.

Dreyfus on June 19, 1942 (Dispatch 289 and enclosure, 840.48 Refugees/2976):

> Supplementing my despatch no. 262 of June 12, 1942, I have the honor to enclose excerpts of a communication dated June 19, 1942, addressed by Mr. B.D. MacDonald to Mr. Maurice Barber, Acting Director of the American Red Cross Middle East at Cairo. This report contains interesting information concerning the handling of the Polish Refugee problem, and it deserves careful reading in connection with the proposed evacuation in the near future from Russia of approximately 10,000 Polish children and their mothers referred to in the Department's telegram no. 153 of June 11, 5 p.m.

MacDonald writes:

> The war is resented by the Persians for the same reasons which make the Turks want no part of it. They feel it has stopped their progress along new lines. But Persia is weaker than Turkey and has bowed to British-Russian occupation. After this F.R.'s (Field Representative's) visit to Smyrna and Ghesme where he had the opportunity to observe Turkish reactions to the influx of Greek refugees from nearby islands, he feels qualified to comment most favorably on the way the Persians are receiving the Poles in their arid midst. There is drought in the south and a growing shortage of food that is ominous. There is a serious shortage of medicines all over the country. It must be said that the Persians accept the Poles because they must. But the fact remains that this inrush, which threatens to grow to tremendous proportions, (50,000 is the latest figure) does the Persians no good. Because of the above mentioned shortages of food and medicines, and because of the hospitality that the Persian government is giving the Poles, this F.R. feels it would be a wise and fair move on the part of the American Red Cross and make a larger gift of medicines and food to this country than is presently planned. This increase is urged, even if it means dipping into the Tehran stocks now allocated solely for the use of the Poles. The Polish Red Cross is already receiving substantial amounts of supplies from New York through lend-lease purchases by the New York consulate general. . . . Poles decided to buy liquid milk in the market and to hang on to the klim. This is an unsound idea, for the local milk supply is limited. What the Poles buy up, the Persian children won't get. . . . The Persians feel they have been left out in the cold by the American Red Cross. A not-too-extravagant gesture at this time seems worthwhile for many reasons. . . .
>
> Another group of 10-12,000 refugees are expected very soon. It seemingly is impossible to get any definite information about their arrival

place or date. Local authorities probably will be better prepared to handle this second lot. There is also a very large plan in the making, to bring out 50,000 Polish children from Russia. News of this large scale evacuation of children spread around the city this afternoon. . . . Without question, however, something serious is in the wind. The State Department has cabled Minister Dreyfus to report on the feasibility of such an undertaking and to find out to what extent the American Red Cross, the Polish Red Cross, the British and the Iranian governments can aid. Washington headquarters of Amcross must therefore be aware of the project. In the carefully considered opinion of this field representative, since it now seems fairly certain that large numbers of new refugees are about to descend on Tehran, the American Red Cross should hold a fairly large reserve of stocks here, instead of letting practically everything go into Russia.

On July 23, 1942, Assistant Secretary Breckinridge Long had written to Davis:

I refer to the Department's letter of July 13, 1942 with which was transmitted excerpts from a communication dated June 19, 1942 addressed by Mr. B.D. MacDonald to Mr. Maurice Barber, Acting Director of the American Red Cross Middle East at Cairo, which had been sent to the Department by the American Legation at Tehran. In view of the existing situation in the Near East the Department believes that it would be most unfortunate if the Iranians were given cause to feel that they were being imposed upon and were receiving unfair treatment. The Department, therefore, is inclined to support Mr. MacDonald's recommendation that the American Red Cross plan to make a larger gift of medicines and food to Iran than is presently contemplated.

Second Wave of Refugees

Dreyfus on July 9, 1942 (Telegram 227, 860C.48/743):

I am informed by American Red Cross representative that following additional Poles are on the point of arriving from Russia: 70,000 soldiers and 20,000 or more civilians mostly wives and families of soldiers. A further project to evacuate 50,000 children to Iran is expected to materialize shortly. Arrival of first contingents expected at Pahlavi where obligatory delousing under British military supervision is arranged. British military unable to provide food for civilians, but Poles

> themselves with Amcross aid can handle situation easily using large stocks food and clothing already in Tehran. Further arrivals also expected at Badjgiran, and a second reception camp being established at Meshed-i-Sar. This large influx refugees will temporarily tie up existing transport making impossible further movement Polish Lend-Lease food to Russian Tashkent region where increased suffering entire population reported. In assessing Iran's needs under procedure of CSC it should be borne in mind that Iranian stores of food, clothing, medicine and other goods will be still further depleted by this influx and prices driven even higher. . . . Amcross representative insisting Poles make immediate use Amcross beans, flour, milk, clothes, medicines. Representative also hopes to make larger gift of medicines to Iran from large Amcross stocks new Middle East Relief Refugee Administration (MERRA) set up Cairo by British to coordinate relief work in regard to food, transport, camps evacuation et cetera. Iran Government not yet advised of these arrangements nor is Iranian assistance expected.

Dreyfus follows up on July 10, 1942 (Dispatch 308 and enclosure, 840C.48/750):

> Referring to the Legation's telegram No. 227 of July 9, 1942, with reference to the evacuation from Russia to Iran of 70,000 Polish soldiers, 20,000 civilian refugees and possibly an additional 50,000 Polish children, I have the honor to enclose for the Department's information a report on this subject prepared by the Field Representative of the American Red Cross.

Excerpts from MacDonald's report of July 9, 1942, to Barber:

> Eight days ago, Mr. Matthews, director of the newly formed Middle East Refugee Relief Administration (MERRA) arrived from Cairo with the information that no more Polish refugees would be allowed until after the present number is evacuated to central Africa. But this decision on the part of the British is evidently by the board. On July 6, instructions came from London to prepare for the immediate reception of 70,000 Polish soldiers and 20,000, plus, civilian refugees. A plan to bring out an additional 50,000 Polish children was also announced. The large scale evacuation of children will probably take some time to arrange, but the soldiers and their civilian relatives are believed to be on their way. A large number are reported at Krasnovodsk, rail head on the Caspian, at this moment. Naturally there is a rush of preparation. Reception camp at Pahlevi and also at Meshed. Delousing and

new clothes issue will be obligatory. The same British officers who handled the first influx at Pahlevi are arranging feeding, temporary shelter, transport to Tehran where an additional 10,000 can be received at the two existing camps. The Meshed camp will be a new one and designed for those who cross the frontier at Badjiran. The Tenth Army will issue rations for the Polish soldiers but is not able to bear the strain of handling and feeding the civilians. Under present conditions in the Middle East this is understandable. Tenth Army headquarters, by the way, are at Baghdad.

The earlier flood of refugees poured into Pahlevi for nine days at the rate of five thousand a day. Just what will happen in the near future no one knows, but details of reception are being worked out to eliminate unnecessary confusion and suffering. This sudden impact of another 100,000 people on the semi-desert Tehran area will place a severe strain on the Persian economy. There has been far too much buying out of the limited market, especially of milk, and there seems to be no one able to control this practice which is causing a rise in prices, a scarcity of milk and vegetables and deterioration in the friendly feeling that once existed between the refugees and the Tehran population. The local government has not been consulted about the new refugees nor is any aid expected from it. . . . As the last sentence of this report was being typed, Mr. Dashnisky, one of the London delegates, rushed in (3:15 p.m.) with the wild information that 20,000 soldiers and civilians were on their way from Krasnovodsk. What this means he can't say. But it is possible that this number may arrive in Pahlevi within two or three days. . . . The incoming 20,000 referred to above represents the first wave. 100,000 can be expected as a minimum—probably more. With the British caring for the soldiers, this leaves about 30,000 for the Poles to worry about themselves, with Amcross aid of course. Adequate stocks of staple foods, clothes and blankets are on hand. . . . Whereabouts of the sixty tons of medical and surgical supplies is not known. They left Cairo June 26 by trucks for Baghdad, presumably. Local R.T.O. does not believe they will come clear thru by truck. Probably will be offloaded by Baghdad and come on by rail via Basra and Ahwaz, not arriving until the end of July. Unfortunate. For the Persian hospitals are out of supplies and are eagerly awaiting their promised portion. Since this medical shipment is so large, F.R. begs that the Persian allotment be doubled or tripled. Such a gift to Iran would fill a desperate need. It would improve Polish-Persian relations. And it can easily be spared. How, for example, are we going to be able to use up to 3000 pairs of rubber gloves, 1000 cases of surgical

> dressings, and some of the drugs and hospital supplies in the amount shipped? F.R. once again stresses that the local need of medicines is urgent. He also points out that the Poles themselves have been buying medicines from the tragically limited Tehran market for shipment to Russia.

Minor on August 18, 1942 (Dispatch 330 and enclosure, 840.48 Refugees/2977): "I have the honor to enclose a copy of a letter addressed by the Tehran representative of the American Red Cross to the Cairo director of that organization, which contains yet another chapter of the fascinating and tragic story of the Polish refugees." MacDonald's letter to Barber is dated August 14, 1942:

> The second mass exodus of Polish soldiers and civilians is finally under way. The first ship with about 3000 persons arrived in Pahlevi harbor at 1:20 a.m., August 12. Col. Drummond, British medical officer in charge of this area, arrived from Pahlevi yesterday, reporting that the physical condition of both troops and civilians was bad, four persons suffering from night blindness, all weak, thin, and clad in filthy clothes. This F.R. plans to leave Tehran August 17 to spend two days at reception camps. . . . The entire 70,000, of which 27,000 will be civilians, are expected to swarm into Pahlevi rapidly. The civilians accompanying the troops are, in the main, relatives. Mr. Stiburski bitterly remarked that the hundreds of thousands of Poles remaining in Russia would surely die unless food was rushed to them. Sympathy was expressed and no mention made of the tragic fact that lack of transport both in Russia and Iran will allow very little relief. . . . From now on, the problem of caring for the Polish refugees in Iran will be largely a transport one. . . . It gives this F.R. no great pleasure to refer back to his final two pages of report No. 1, written in mid-June. He pointed out the folly of rushing more supplies unless transport could be secured. On June 12, he begged Mr. Kollat to stop bringing food and clothing from America and to use the allotted cubic space on ships for trucks and tires. Nothing was done. Nothing is being done. Long strings of camels have made their appearance again on the broad streets of Tehran. The slow, deep clang of their bells is heard everywhere. Until a few years ago the camels and donkeys carried the goods of Persia and the trip to Meshed took a month. . . . The past is coming back.

The flow of Polish refugees had continued. Cable from Foley and MacDonald in Tehran to ARC, received August 25, 1942 (Telegram

270, 891.48/312): "Twenty thousand Polish civilians newly arrived Pahlevi 10,000 more immediately expected."

Dreyfus on August 29, 1942 (Dispatch 336 and enclosure, 860C.48/774):

> I have the honor to enclose a copy of yet another communication addressed by the Tehran representative of the American Red Cross to the Cairo director of that organization, regarding the latest developments in the Polish refugee problem in Iran. This communication is particularly interesting because it reports the arrival of fresh contingents of Polish refugees and the departure of part of those who found temporary refuge in Iran.

MacDonald's report to Barber is dated August 20, 1942. Excerpts follow:

> Despite the military events in Russia and to the surprise and amazement of officials here, above half of the second influx has arrived at Pahlevi: about 15,000 civilians and twice as many soldiers. Almost a thousand have already arrived in camp No. 2 on the outskirts of Tehran. Conditions of this last mentioned is certainly not bad, considering the long, crowded, hot journey by freight train, tankers and trucks. . . . There are four camps: two for military, two for civilians. One of each is called "the dirty one" where incomers are placed before being bathed and deloused and issued clean clothing. "The clean camp" is where the soldiers and civilians remain until buses and lorries bring them south over the mountains. The British are pressed to find enough transport to keep the necessary food and other supplies rolling into Pahlevi. The Transport manager of UKCC remarked tonight that he had been obliged to cut his deliveries to Russia in half to take care of the new Polish rush. The strain, of course, will largely be removed within three weeks or so.

MacDonald also reports that between August 5 and August 19, 1942, six trainloads of refugees containing 3,006 Poles had left Tehran for Ahwaz en route to Africa via India:

> Reports have it that evacuation to Africa will cease when 4000 have been moved and that the remainder plus the new arrivals now swarming into Pahlevi must winter in Iran. Of the original wave of civilians that arrived here in the early spring, less than 5000 remain in Tehran: men 574, women 2722, children 1616. Approximately another thou-

> sand children are in Isfahan and Meshed. These figures do not include the women in uniform who are regarded as auxiliaries attached to the Army, nor the several hundred office workers in the many bureaus and camps, the nurses, doctors, orderlies, nor the estimated four hundred who have found work in the city. Total of this uncounted group will run well over a thousand.

He also adds: "The medicines which were sent by twenty lorries from Cairo June 26, are now arriving in Tehran. . . . Plans of distribution have been explained in earlier reports. Thus far, six cases are missing. Many have been broken and part of contents taken."

Polish refugees in Iran had been well cared for. Dreyfus on April 7, 1943 (Telegram 364, 860C.48/855):

> For Stettinius OLLA from (George) Washington. British officers in close touch with refugee problems have furnished the following information: (drug) needs of Polish refugees in Iran (about 17,000) have recently been supplied by Tehran's Pasteur Institute and British Military. No more biologicals appear to be needed. Complete evacuation by August or sooner is expected. Poles have all been protected against small pox and typhoid. In Kazekestan and Uzbekistan refugee Poles estimated at 70,000.

A follow-up telegram from Washington to Stettinius dated June 11, 1943, reveals that the remaining Poles in Russia were expected in Iran shortly (Telegram 610, 860C.48/892):

> British and Polish relief authorities believe that Russians will send additional refugees perhaps 25,000 to 50,000 from Russia to Iran possibly in the next few weeks. Inquiry raised whether Lend-Lease goods now in Iran will be available to feed incoming refugees. This might prove wisest use of supplies.

More than a year after they were supposed to have left Iran, Polish civilians continued to resist plans to "evacuate" them. Ford on May 22, 1944 (Dispatch 949, 840.48 Refugees/6180):

> I have the honor to inform the Department that roughly 1,000 Polish refugees left Tehran recently by train for Ahwaz and Khorramshahr en route to Kenya in East Africa. . . . The refugees selected to make the move were all volunteers. It is understood that there was some diffi-

culty at first in obtaining a sufficient number of volunteers to make up a group of the size which it had been decided to move. . . . The Legation has heard that some of the refugees, who had volunteered to make the shift, changed their minds at the last minute, and demanded to be allowed to remain here, and that others, after having entrained at Tehran, endeavored to leave the train at way stations between here and Ahwaz. . . . The Legation understands that a further movement of Polish refugees from Iran will take place in the near future with India, this time, as the destination. A group of 1,000 refugees are said to be already in the Ahwaz area, awaiting completion of the necessary arrangements.

Chapter 11

The American Red Cross and Iran

The ARC's response to Iran's request for the typhus vaccine was noted in chapter 8. As noted in chapter 10, ARC had been urged by its Tehran representative to donate to Iran some of the medical supplies destined for the Poles, and the State Department had advised the ARC to avoid giving the impression that they were in Iran solely to assist the Poles. Dreyfus on August 22, 1942 (Dispatch 332 and enclosures, 860C.48/769):

> It has been evident for some time that relief supplies of all kinds for Polish refugees in Iran have been piling up in warehouses faster than they can be transported or consumed. The committee (Central Supplies Committee), which has viewed with concern the large shipments from the United States for Polish refugees without proper control or examination by it, was particularly perturbed to learn from Mr. MacDonald of the American Red Cross that $600,000 worth of additional supplies, amounting to some 6,000 tons, have been allocated for shipment to Iran for this purpose. This would be in addition to the perhaps 10,000 tons of goods stored in Tehran warehouses, and some 1,000 tons a month are coming forward by purchase by the Poles from Lend-Lease funds. It should be mentioned that a serious difference of opinion exists between the American Red Cross and the Polish authorities concerning relief supplies for the Poles. The American Red Cross take the view that no supplies can be sent into Russia for the Poles unless consigned to the Russian Red Cross and Crescent while the Poles have insisted that the Polish Red Cross should handle these supplies. The question, however, at the moment is purely academic since the transport facilities for moving these goods to Russia do not

exist. This is an absolute fact which should not be disregarded in considering this problem. In addition to the difficulties of transport northward from Tehran, it should be observed that Polish supplies are putting a severe strain on the railway transport from the ports in the south to Tehran, and impeding the transport of essential war goods to Russia. Some goods are now on sidings awaiting shipment to Tehran. The Poles, unhappy that the supplies are not going forward to Russia for the relief of their starving compatriots, refuse to use Red Cross supplies in Tehran, holding them in the vain hope that they can eventually find their way into the Soviet Union. The result is that part of the supplies are approaching the point of deterioration, the beans being about ready to sprout. This is, of course, a ridiculous situation considering the sacrifices of shipping space which were made to get the goods here.

Another angle must be taken into consideration. The Poles are well taken care of in Iran and are far from suffering. I see no reason why they should receive treatment superior to that accorded the local population. The diet for Poles, suggested by the Red Cross, which was read out in the Central Supplies Committee meeting, caused much amusement. We are living in a country of near starvation, where the common people have nothing to eat but bread (which they can hardly get now because of the shortage) cheese, rice (almost never) onions (sometimes) and small amounts of fruits in season. The mothers and children are terribly undernourished and if milk is to be given away in large quantities it could find no better outlet. It pains those of us who have affection for Iran to see this condition while the Poles are given such special treatment. This brings us to the question of shipping space. The committee is of the opinion that our precious shipping space is being needlessly wasted and I concur in this finding. The Poles in Iran are well taken care of during their temporary stay here from the produce of the country and with the enormous supplies now in their warehouses. I might mention, too, that the Poles have not acted in a particularly fitting manner. Many are living in luxury, going in for parties, automobiles, fine living, picnics, theaters, etc. Mr. MacDonald had the unfortunate experience, reported by telegram to the Red Cross in Washington, of having almost five thousand bags of Red Cross flour taken from one of his warehouses by the Poles without his consent. There are many angles of this problem. Such as requisitions by the Poles for medical supplies, particularly quinine, with which Mr. MacDonald is displeased.

> It would be wise, in my opinion, to permit no supplies of any kind to be shipped to the Poles in Iran, whether Red Cross or Lend-Lease, unless recommended by the Central Supplies Committee. This committee was set up to control goods destined for Iran in order to see that shipping space is not wasted and unless it can control all shipments the ends for which it was instituted will be defeated. The Central Supplies Committee and the British and American Legations will soon make definite recommendations regarding the shipment of these supplies to Iran. In the meantime, it is strongly recommended that no shipments of any kind or amount be made.

Dreyfus on September 15, 1942 (Dispatch 346 and enclosure, 891.48/314):

> It may be appropriate here to record public reaction to a gift made by the American Red Cross of medicines to Iranian institutions. This generous act on the part of the Red Cross has had a most favorable reaction and comment locally. I have remarked in previous despatches that I felt it unfortunate that Polish refugees should be given treatment far superior to that accorded the local population. Polish refugees have created here serious social and economic problems and have caused considerable resentment among the population. This small gift by the Red Cross to the Iranians will help somewhat to dispel this feeling and cause the Iranians to remember that the Americans have not, in fact forgotten them in their difficulties. Typical of press comment regarding this gift is the following from the *Journal de Tehran* of September 10: "Colonel Neuwirth has recently remitted, on behalf of the American Red Cross, to the Ministry of Public Health 321 cases, representing about three tons of dressings, blankets, clothing, etc., for the poor, destined to hospitals, and about 200,000 ampules for the Pasteur Institute. At a time when we have urgent need of such aid, particularly for pharmaceutical goods, the American Red Cross has been very helpful to us and has demonstrated the friendly American spirit toward our country." The Red Cross has made substantial gifts, in addition to those to the Pasteur Institute and Iranian hospitals, to the Iranian Red Lion and Sun (Iranian Red Cross) and to British and American missionary hospitals. On September 10, the eight American and four British missionary hospitals were given miscellaneous drugs amounting in value to more than $50,000 and containing such scarce valuable items as sulfa derivatives, quinine and surgical dressings. A duplicate was also made to the Iranian Red Lion and Sun on September 11. The Red Cross representative informs me he is holding in reserve 350,000 qui-

nine tablets, which may be delivered to the Iranians if necessary. He further states that approval has been given to make available for Iranian relief part of the large medical stores now en route from the United States. I have suggested to Mr. MacDonald that these gifts be brought discreetly to the attention of the Iranian press to counter persistent reports that the allies are not furnishing Iran with much needed essential goods.

ARC Response to the Fall 1942 Crisis

In the fall of 1942 Iran was faced with a severe bread crisis, described in chapters 13 and 14. The ARC, however, had shown little sympathy and even less desire to help. Telegram from Bailey in Cairo to the ARC headquarters in Washington dated November 16, 1942 (Telegram 2016, 891.48/329):

> Arrived Cairo twelfth. Wiens departed (for) Tehran today replacing MacDonald December 1. Previous stores now completely liquidated with the exception of surgical dressings. Three ships carrying supplies have not yet reached Persian Gulf and due to slow offloading and forwarding may not commence arriving Tehran from one to three months. Consider Iranian wheat and food crisis entirely governmental responsibility and, since white flour cannot be used in native ovens and shipment of tomatoes is equivalent of coals to Newcastle and other foods en route no shortage or particular need, recommend one quarter of distribution Polish transit in Egypt, 5000 refugees Ahwaz, balance Tehran for Poles remaining there for winter months. Typhus outbreak reported among refugees and native population Tehran. British and Iranian officials taking measures to control but will keep you advised.

Dreyfus on November 20, 1942 (Dispatch 387 and enclosures, 860C.48/806):

> I have the honor to report a recent development of importance caused by the presence in Iran of a considerable number of Polish refugees during the present food crisis. The Department has been kept currently informed of the progress of the evacuation of Polish refugees from Russia to South Africa through Iran and will recall that the first group consisting of between 11,000 and 12,000 civilians and about 30,000 Polish soldiers arrived during the latter part of April, 1942. They were all sent to other destinations, the civilians to South Africa and the

soldiers to points West, before the arrival in August, last, of a second group which included about 26,000 civilians and an undisclosed number of soldiers. The civilians in this group are still in Iran. According to both British and Polish authorities who are responsible for this movement, there were at the beginning of November, 1942, about 22,000 Polish civilian refugees in Tehran, between 2,000 and 3,000 in Isfahan and about 1,500 in a camp in Ahwaz. Details regarding the movement of the Polish soldiers have not been given out, but the same authorities assert that that the number still in the vicinity of Tehran is not large and that they are being moved westward steadily and will soon all have gone.

The Department has also been kept informed concerning the growing scarcity of wheat and bread and the rapidly rising prices of all foodstuffs as well as rents and most commodities. It has caused alarm and discontent among Iranians of all classes. The press of Tehran has been very bitter on the subject and blame for these developments has generally been laid on the large number of foreigners who now occupy the country, particularly the British and Russians. The presence of Polish civilians and soldiers has also been pointed to as a factor contributing to the scarcity and high prices of foods, particularly since many of them have been seen daily on the streets and in the food shops buying liberally. The fact that the Polish refugees are given white bread while the Iranian public must be satisfied with whole wheat bread has not helped matters. Charges that excessive purchases were being made daily in Tehran markets for the Polish refugees became the subject of discussion at a meeting of the Iranian Council of Ministers on November 2, instant, when it was decided that some action should be taken to reduce the burden on Tehran markets imposed by the heavy purchases of foodstuffs made for the refugees. To discuss this possibility, a meeting of representatives of the British, Polish and Iranian Governments in Tehran was called on November 3rd by Mr. J.P. Sheridan, American Supply and Food Adviser to the Iranian Government, and this Legation was asked to send a member of the Staff to observe and assist if possible. At this meeting, Mr. Sheridan read a list of purchases of foodstuffs made by a contractor in the open market for the Polish refugees on October 26, 1942, as evidence of the excessive extent and variety of these purchases. It showed that total purchases that day amounted to 62,600 kilograms, or an average of 2½ kilograms per person not including 52,000 eggs, bread, sugar, and several other less important commodities. Bread for these refugees is baked specially for them from white flour furnished by the American Red Cross or other foreign sources, whence come their sugar, beans and some other supplies. . . . The Polish Minister then had read a list prepared by his assistants showing the average daily requirements of the Polish civilian refugees now in Tehran that have been met by purchases in the open market. . . . It was pointed out by the representatives of the Iranian Government that even the Polish list of daily purchases was greatly in excess of similar purchases made by many of the better class Iranians in Tehran; that it includes a large number of items that are completely beyond the reach of the average Iranians and that the total constitutes a heavy burden on Tehran markets and might easily be an important factor in bringing about the recent increases in prices of foodstuffs. . . . The committee thereupon agreed to appoint a sub-committee of medical experts to decide upon the diet and fair rations for (1) Polish adult refugees; (2) Polish children; and (3) Polish sick in hospitals. The American representative on this committee was Dr. A.A. Neuwirth, Lieutenant Colonel, United States Army Medical Corps, who has been acting as adviser to the Iranian Government. It included one British, one Iranian and three Polish representatives. At a subsequent meeting the recommendation of the medical sub-committee was considered and adopted. . . . Mr. MacDonald, Red Cross representative in Tehran, pointed out that . . . the diet recommended by the sub-committee as very satisfactory indeed under the circumstances, since the normal ration contains 2565 calories. The Iranian representative stated that, while his Government wished to extend every possible courtesy and all possible hospitality to the refugees, the welfare of the residents of Tehran required a reduction in the demands on the markets, particularly for eggs, butter, tea, coffee and vegetables. He hoped the rations recommended by the sub-committee would be approved by the committee. The First Secretary of the British Legation pressed for the return of the diet of the fresh vegetables that had been entirely eliminated, and it was finally decided to sanction the purchase of one ton of cabbage per day in lieu of fresh vegetables of all kinds. With this amendment the recommendation of the medical sub-committee was approved for trial for one month. At the end of that time, the refugees are to be examined to determine whether the rations have been detrimental to health. . . . The Polish representatives pointed out that the new rations will effect a reduction in purchases on the open market of a total of 13,000 kilograms and of 23,000 eggs. The most important reductions were in the daily purchases of milk (4,250 kilograms), meat (2,200 kilograms), butter (140 kilograms), potatoes (1,600 kilograms), and fresh fruits (2,800 kilograms).

A report of the decision to reduce the purchases of food stuffs was inserted in the Tehran press following the last meeting of the committee and no adverse criticism or other mention of the Polish refugee question has been observed in the press since this action was taken, although the wheat and bread situation has worsened and the price of foodstuffs and most other commodities have continued to rise. It would seem that the action of the Committee and the publicity which has attended it has gone far to create a better understanding of this situation and to relieve as much as possible the burden on the Iranian economy caused by the presence of the Polish refugees in this country. This burden may be expected to lessen as they are moved out of the country.

ARC Desire to Divert Supplies from Iran

On November 30, 1942, Dreyfus had written to Ralph Bain, Director, ARC, Cairo:

> I have received your letter of November 7th. . . . In reply to your request for observations and suggestions as to how your organization can operate most effectively in this area, I am informed that the Iranian Government is now organizing all of the twenty-five or more charitable organizations into one group under the aegis of the Red Lion and Sun, which in Iran corresponds roughly, in theory at least, to the American Red Cross in the United States. The Prime Minister is the titular head of the Red Lion and Sun but he has designated the Minister of Food to represent him in this capacity. Your representative in Iran may find it convenient, therefore, to work closely with the Minister of Food in the distribution of American relief supplies that may be sent to this country. He has doubtless written you that, while there is always destitution in some parts of Iran, the situation now is probably more acute than usual because of the shortages of shelter, clothing, medical supplies and food.
>
> I understand that Red Cross supplies coming to the Persian Gulf will be diverted to Egypt, with the exception of that part destined for Polish use in Ahwaz. This would, in my opinion, be a great mistake, since it appears not unlikely that famine and general distress may develop in Tehran and throughout the country during the coming winter. I would suggest, therefore, that you keep a representative here, at least for the time being, and that emergency stores be brought to or retained in Iran to meet this threatening crisis. I have heard it stated frequently that white flour cannot be used in Iran. I do not believe that this is the case.

White flour would be most useful for mixture with other flour in any period of shortage and Mr. Sheridan is desirous of obtaining as much of it as possible.

As you know, arrangements are being made by the British and American Governments to supply this country with enough wheat to satisfy its needs over the coming winter. Your representative, at present Mr. Wiens, will doubtless keep you fully advised as to the manner in which your organization can best supplement the flow of supplies into Iran so as to meet the real needs of its population.

I have pleasure in assuring you that Mr. MacDonald, your representative in Tehran up to today, has kept me fully advised of the manner in which he has conducted the work of your organization and that, in my opinion, it could hardly have been done better. I have no doubt that Mr. Wiens will prove equally competent. I shall be glad to assist him with advice and suggestions any time. Mrs. Dreyfus and I hope you will be coming up this way again for a visit and that we can then hear all about your trip home.

On December 4, 1942, Henry W. Wiens, the new ARC Special Representative in Tehran, had written to Charles E. Bailey, Assistant Director, ARC, Cairo:

I have at hand your letters: IRL-1 indicating that a portion of the goods landing in the Persian Gulf are to be transshipped to Cairo for use of the Men's Service Club; IRL-3, ordering the transshipment to East Africa of two cases of goods (surgical and dental supplies) from Agwi Prince; IRL-8, ordering the shipment to East Africa of 10,000 blankets for the use of the Polish refugees; and Telegram No. 35, asking for an inventory of undistributed medicines and other items, so that you can answer a request for drugs for refugees in East Africa. In IRL-1, page 2, you indicate there is a possibility that none of the incoming supplies may be sent to Tehran and that the work here will probably be diminishing. The situation here is deteriorating rapidly. In connection with Bain's request to Dreyfus for recommendations on our local program, the Minister called me into conference and inquired concerning our current program, especially regarding the disposition of the goods shortly to arrive in the Persian Gulf. He was very upset when I informed him of my orders, as indicated above. And he asked me to urge you to reconsider these orders. He also asked me to discuss this matter with army and other appropriate officials.

Dreyfus has called me in several times during the last few days, and today he said: "I am extremely anxious for Cairo to know that the food situation here is extremely grave, but actually dangerous." The situation is so critical that Mr. Dreyfus asked for permission to buy five tons of our flour for Legation purposes, as the lack of it is hampering their work. I told him that the request would have to be referred to you. It is obvious, as you pointed out when I was in Cairo, that the problem of feeding Tehran is too big for the Red Cross, and no one is suggesting this. But if the food were at hand, we might in an emergency prevent food riots and violence. This is no exaggeration. Any day now Tehran might actually be without wheat. The inside news is very discouraging today.

LATER: I was interrupted in writing and called into conference concerning the food situation at this very moment. Tomorrow and for several days to come, Tehran will be entirely without wheat. Mr. Sheridan showed us an announcement to be read over radio tonight, attempting to quiet the population, for already the situation is dangerous. Gendarmes were protecting the Ministry of Food where important conferences have been going on despite today being Friday. Gendarmes are everywhere in evidence. In the last few days, several people have died of exhaustion or suffocation in the crush before bakeries. I have seen these frantic mobs before bakeries, and Mr. Dreyfus says that it is the worst he has ever seen.

The radio will announce tonight that tomorrow the government will sell potatoes and day after beans and peas at bakeries at the same price that bread was formerly sold. Hoarders of wheat are given 72 hours to sell to the government without penalty, after which Timmerman will arrange a house to house search. The government will confiscate all wheat and punish the offenders severely. Informers will be paid in cash 20% of the value of the stocks concerning which they have informed. The immediate crisis should be over in a few days as wheat is being imported from Iraq. But it might well reoccur. The 25,000 tons of wheat ordered from Canada will arrive in lots of about 5,000 tons a month, beginning about the end of January. Sheridan literally begged the Red Cross today not to deliver any supplies from Iran. Our white flour and other foodstuffs, he says, are entirely usable for Iranian relief. White flour would be mixed with six parts dark flour donated by the Iranian government, and the bread distributed free to poor Iranians. The American Red Cross would thus get credit for the six time augmented gift!

Some supplies should come in to be distributed in Tehran, while others should be distributed in the more critical Southwestern and Yezd area, the Iranian government furnishing free transportation. The British Movement Control has also promised to rush our supplies on the railroad. Part of the supplies should be allocated to the Poles, and this would help to relieve the general situation. Describing an American Red Cross contribution as of "inestimable value" to the Iranians, Sheridan said, "I can't state too emphatically how important this would be to the poor people." A growing resentment and a tendency to blame the allies for Iran's woes create a tailor-made situation for the ever active local fifth columnists. Sheridan insists that this constitutes the perfect opportunity for the Red Cross to build goodwill toward the United States. A public announcement in the near future that the American Red Cross would make a contribution to poor Iranians would receive wide publicity and materially bolster the morale of the people.

Even if the situation should not continue to be extremely dangerous, the food could be used to magnificent advantage to the extremely poor, who are really "made destitute by the war." Prices are rising almost hourly, and the poorer classes simply can't afford to eat. The American Red Cross has the opportunity of doing what would be the equivalent of "disaster relief." Although we are interested in doing relief on the basis of need, it should be noted that this is perhaps the best opportunity in the entire battle area for doing relief which will advertise the American Red Cross and build up the American "reservoir of goodwill." It would be tragic to miss this opportunity.

The commanding officer of this area (General Connolly), in my interview with him, was thoroughly aroused, almost indignant over the possible diversion of supplies from this area. He used strong language in characterizing this "waste of shipping space." He pointed out (as the British Control Movement has since confirmed) that it would take at least two months, possibly much more, to ship anything from the Persian Gulf to Cairo, as it would have to be reloaded at Karachi. Both he and later the British thought it would take less time to bring something from America to Cairo than to re-ship it from the Persian Gulf. Any removal of any goods from Iran creates a vacuum which must be filled by the use of the extremely critical shipping space. He added that if the purpose was to supply the SAF men's club in Cairo, we should consider the fact that the SAF should be establishing immediately clubs in Iran, where we would find the problem of supply ten times more difficult. He directed me not to divulge any information concerning

> the size of the operation in this letter, but I am able to say that it will be much larger than all of the rest of our operations in the Middle East or than our operations in India and China combined. You of course realize that this information is strictly confidential. He recommended the immediate consideration of establishing men's Service Clubs at least in Tehran and Ahwaz. And he categorically stated his opinion that nothing in Iran or the Persian Gulf should be shipped out of this area. (I should like to recommend personally that the SAF try very soon to find places in Tehran and Ahwaz for their club purposes, as rents are rising almost daily. I should be most happy to render any possible assistance.)
>
> The Polish situation presents a new problem. For the present no Poles are leaving Iran. How long this will last, no one knows, but Col Drummond estimates that evacuations will possibly not be resumed for three months. Others think they may possibly be resumed in a month or two. At best our medicines and supplies could not reach Africa for a considerable time. Col. Drummond advised keeping all of our stocks of medicines here, and he believes the medical and especially the dental instruments arriving in the Persian Gulf should be kept here. Medicines and surgical instruments are worth their weight in gold here. One British hospital of 1200 beds, for example, lost all of their equipment en route. They could not be operating without our contributions of a sterilizer, surgical instruments, and syringes. The men in charge hardly know how to thank the Red Cross enough for supplying their emergency needs. This situation might well be duplicated for American army hospitals, as ten of them are to be established in Iran shortly. Col. Van Vlack and Capt. Norem have indicated that our recent donations to them have been a god-send. Dental instruments are especially in demand. As for the blankets, we have only 6,150 left. As you know, 20,000 were recently allocated to the Poles here for overcoats and use in camps. Recently we contributed 10,000 blankets to the American military hospitals, who were desperately in need of them. A great shortage of blankets exists here and will become more acute during the approaching winter, while it is summer in East Africa now.
>
> In view of the Minister's and others' requests, I am sending you this information and awaiting your further instructions.

Wiens' letter had elicited a long response from Bailey. In a letter of December 9, 1942, the day after Tehran was shaken by bread riots, Bailey writes:

My dear Mr. Wiens, We have received your letters . . . and have given considerable study to the various remarks and suggestions. I realize that the food problem in Iran is extremely grave, but in my report to Washington regarding the present situation, I have stated that the problems in Iran are those of Governments and not American Red Cross. . . . It is perfectly well known throughout Persia that the more wealthy classes, as well as many of the villagers, are hoarding wheat, sufficient in many cases to take care of the families of the hoarders for periods of from two to four years. Since there is enough hoarded wheat in Iran to take care of all requirements during the next two months, until wheat can be brought in from Canada (or from India which is much nearer) it seems to me that the Iranian Government should immediately take steps to confiscate wheat from the hoarders to relieve the present crisis. When I left Tehran, a very short time ago, I had understood that ration cards were to be issued to every citizen of Tehran who could prove his residence in that city. At that time definite plans had been made to close every bakery in the city and all bread was to be made in a Government bakery which was a converted glass factory. It was stated that such arrangement would immediately stop the food riots in the city of Tehran. What has happened to this plan?

You mentioned the crisis developing in Yezd and Kerman. The Iranian Government has had plenty of time to supply these two areas with wheat since the date of the report submitted to the Minister of Food after my return from an inspection of these areas. The authorities in the city of Isfahan, through which city wheat for Yezd and Kerman had to travel, had been holding up wheat en route to Yezd and Kerman to such an extent that they had built up a sizable surplus for themselves. Had the Iranian Government followed up the recommendations, that Isfahan should be forced to relinquish some of its surplus, Yezd and Kerman would have received a supply of wheat from Isfahan in sufficient amounts to carry them through until additional wheat could be brought in from India or even Canada. The city of Shiraz has more than a three months surplus of wheat. Has the Government taken any of this wheat for distribution to more needy areas? If the Government authorities are not competent to force the hoarders of wheat to relinquish their stores in order to meet the present crisis, I cannot see why the American Red Cross should be expected to give their limited amount of valuable stores which were sent across the ocean for the benefit of war refugees. It is also well to remember that the supplies which were sent to Iran by the American Red Cross were heartily ridiculed around Tehran a few weeks ago as being unwanted, not needed and not adapted to general use in Iran. The Amcross supplies which are arriving at the Persian Gulf are not sufficient in amounts to be of any particular benefit to the poor people of Iran taken as a whole. The city of Tehran could use our entire supplies in one day, but the crisis would continue the next day.

At no time have we stated that all of our supplies would be diverted from Iran to other areas. We have intimated that they might never be sent to the city of Tehran itself. For the war effort it is our duty to save shipping space whenever possible, particularly on the route of war supplies to Russia. If we can help the war effort by using our food supplies at the Polish refugee camp at Ahwaz we will be saving railway cars for war materials and at the same time reducing the amount of food supplies the British would be forced to import in order to feed the Poles at Ahwaz. You stated that the SS Samuel Moody was due to dock on December 3rd at Khorramshahr. According to our records there is no flour on this ship. There are 3,873 cases of canned tomatoes and 7,222 cases of oleomargarine. There is certainly no shortage of tomatoes in Persia. The poor people rely almost entirely on wheat so that this first shipment would in no way relieve the food crisis in the city of Tehran. Since this food was originally sent from Washington for the benefit of the Polish refugees, we wish you to discuss with Col. Drummond and Mr. Hankey the matter of need among the Polish refugees in Ahwaz and obtain their suggestions as to the most intelligent use of the oleomargarine and the tomatoes among the Poles not only at Ahwaz but also in other parts of Iran including Isfahan, Tehran and Meshed.

We are also asking you to discuss with Col. Drummond and Mr. Hankey and obtain from them specific recommendations as to the need among the various Polish refugee camps throughout the country in relationship to the flour, rolled oats, syrup and additional tomatoes that are coming in on later ships. If it is definitely stated by the British authorities that the Poles will not need certain amounts of our supplies during the next five or six months of their stay in Persia, we can then determine the disposition of the balance. We shall appreciate having you send us a letter from Col. Drummond or from Mr. Hankey of the British Legation, who is keyman of MERRA in Iran, giving recommendations, and as soon as we receive such a letter we shall be able to intelligently instruct you as to the allocation of the incoming supplies. Please keep in mind that any distributions of Amcross supplies made in Iran are to be determined in Cairo in collaboration with Washington and with MERRA, and although we desire recommendations from you, the control must remain here where we have an opportunity of examining without bias the needs of the entire Middle East area.

We realize that you have been placed in a very difficult position, a new man unexperienced in Near Eastern operations and unfamiliar with the intrigues of the various factions in Tehran. We are perfectly confident in your ability "to keep your feet on the ground" and as you have an opportunity of remaining longer in Persia you will be in a better position to weigh the problems and give them their proper values. I am sure that you will be able to give excellent advice, and as an intelligent American citizen, to such people as Mr. Sheridan and others who are interested primarily in local Persian problems, but if you are asked to sit in on conferences, relative to the local problem, we ask you to be mindful of the fact that the problems discussed are not necessarily the affairs of the American Red Cross. We have our own little job to do, namely, to assist the British authorities, who have accepted continuing responsibility for the welfare of the Polish refugees and we have no authority nor are we in a position to take any leading part in the management of the refugee camps or in accepting responsibility in Persian affairs. Naturally our activities in Iran will diminish in ratio to the speed with which the Poles are moved to East Africa.

Bailey had followed with another letter on December 9, 1942:

Dear Mr. Wiens, In connection with your discussions with officers of the American Army, Persian Gulf Command, it is well to keep in mind the fact that your responsibility is restricted to civilian war relief and that any matters referred by the Army to you should be immediately forwarded to us in Cairo, to be acted upon by the Field Supervisor. There are three SAF field representatives (about to arrive) in Persia at the present time assigned to their respective units. For the time being, you will have plenty to keep you busy with your own problems and we certainly do not wish you to become involved in matters which should be handled by the SAF staff assigned to the Middle East. We shall be very pleased if you pass along to us any suggestions or requests made by the military so that proper action can be taken by Mr. Bain and Mr. McDermott.

Bailey had followed with yet another letter on December 10, 1942:

In connection with the problems of the Iranian Government it is well to keep in mind that the British are responsible for seeing that sufficient

> supplies are available for the Iranians. This is the affair of the Middle East Supply Council (sic) which collaborates with Lend-Lease. Therefore, any requests to American Red Cross for emergency relief among the Iranians should be routed through Major Hobson, of the MESC who, in turn, will make formal requests to you in Teheran. You in turn will send such requests to this office in Cairo for approval. In insisting that the above channels be followed you will be relieving yourself of all the direct calls upon you for assistance from various local organizations and the Iranian Government officials.

Bailey's attitude was in part at the instigation of the British in Cairo. On December 18, 1942, C.A. Pickard of the Middle East Relief and Refugee Administration (MERRA), Office of the Minister of State, Cairo, had written to Lt. Col. A. Ross of the British Legation in Tehran. It reads:

> Dear Ross: We have been discussing with the American Red Cross the disposal of ARC stores in and en route to Iran. Briefly we have agreed that in present circumstances all ARC stores should be held for Polish refugees and not released to the Persians. ARC are asking their representative to consult with you about the storage of margarine and canned tomatoes due at Basra shortly. We thought that it might be possible to hold it at Ahwaz. I hope to visit Tehran on January 4th with Bailey of the ARC to try to settle all outstanding supply problems.

In forwarding the above correspondence, Dreyfus had commented in his dispatch of December 27, 1942 (Dispatch 414 and enclosures, 891.48/324):

> The questions raised by Mr. Bailey require some clarification. I have no quarrel with the Red Cross if, as Mr. Bailey states in his letter IRL 16 of December 9, they desire to consider Iranian problems as those of the Government and not of the Red Cross. However, I should like to point out that the consequences of this short-sighted policy might well be a serious decline in prestige in Iran not only of the Red Cross but of Americans in general. There is not the slightest doubt that there is at present great suffering on the part of the masses of the Iranian people and that this unfortunate condition will grow as winter progresses. It is of no constructive value to state, as Mr. Bailey does in his letter, that the Iranians have wheat and other goods hoarded which they should bring to light before asking aid from abroad. I have tackled this ques-

tion in frequent despatches and telegrams; even if it be admitted that there is wheat hoarded in Iran and that the Iranians should put their own house in order before turning to us, there are numerous difficulties which should be taken into consideration. I suggest that my despatch No. 409, December 21 on the background, facts and consequences of the Tehran riots of December 8, 1942, be consulted in this regard, since I explained therein some of the reasons why the Iranians have not had the ability, the strength or the courage to do many of the things which seem to us so obvious and which are so easy to suggest.

I am sorry that I find it necessary to criticize Mr. Bailey's letters on several scores; I should like to point out that these criticisms are intended to be constructive and friendly. First, it seems to me he takes a somewhat callous and unfeeling view of the Iranian situation and seems uninclined to look behind the scenes to discover the true reasons why the Iranians are in the present predicament. Secondly, I believe he is unduly harsh on Mr. Wiens, who reported in his letter of December 4th the facts as he saw them and with, in my opinion, a considerable degree of perception and truth. Thirdly, Mr. Bailey's suggestion of subordinating Mr. Wiens to Mr. Hanke of the British Legation and Colonel Drummond of the British Army would seem to me unworkable and unreasonable. It would also prevent the Red Cross taking a truly American line; this may, in fact, be seen by careful reading of enclosure No. 4.

Again I should like to make it quite clear that I have no desire to dictate or even suggest Red Cross policy. I merely feel it is my duty to call these matters to the Department's attention. I explained in my despatch No. 346, September 15, 1942 the bad impression made on the Iranians by the fact that the Polish refugees in Iran have liberal food rations and comparatively are lavishly cared for while so many Iranians are in dire need. I agree with Mr. Bailey that the Red Cross supplies cannot possibly be of sufficient volume to solve Iran's difficulties. I feel however, and in this Mr. Wiens and Mr. MacDonald (formerly Red Cross representative in Tehran, now employed by Mr. Kidd of Lend-Lease) agree, that small and well directed gifts to Iranian hospitals, organizations, etc., would have a very good effect and correct to some extent the feeling prevalent here that the Red Cross has little regard for the Iranians. At least, a more friendly and sympathetic approach to the Iranian problem would be of value. . . . I should explain, in closing, how the enclosed copies of Red Cross correspondence were obtained. The Red Cross having failed to answer my letter of November 30, I inquired of Mr. Wiens whether or not he had received any communications which might throw light on the matter. He replied that he had and delivered to me the originals of the enclosed communications.

State Department–ARC Correspondence

Dreyfus' comments had been communicated to the ARC and on February 27, 1943, Philip E. Ryan, Assistant Director, Insular and Foreign Operations, had replied. The letter and the memorandum of agreement between ARC and the British throw considerable light on ARC's attitude (Letter and enclosure, 891.48/333):

> The American Minister raises a question of basic policy when he expresses his opinion that the American Red Cross should take greater initiative in Iran, and operate on its own responsibilities rather than through the British. We have kept the Department informed of our position with respect to operations throughout the Middle East, and it has been our consistent policy that the basic responsibility for relief operations in that area rests with the British authorities, since the Middle East is under the military control of the British, and since that area is generally considered within the British sphere of influence. American Red Cross operations are considered as supplementary to the work which the British are prepared to do for civilian refugee relief. In pursuing this policy we have experienced satisfactory relationships with the British officials and it appears to us desirable to continue such cooperative operations rather than embark upon independent action in that area.
>
> There is in the American Minister's letter some indication of a possible misunderstanding with respect to the supplies which the American Red Cross has sent into Iran, designated to be used for relief of Polish refugees. In this connection, reference is made to Mr. Mitchell's letter of October 3, 1942, to Mr. George Brandt, which contains a summary of the negotiations with respect to Polish relief in Iran and Russia. You will note that in this letter Mr. Mitchell points out that the dispatch of supplies to the Middle East was made with the definite understanding that such supplies should be available for Polish refugees or "for the Iranian population and other groups in the Middle East as need may arise." It has unfortunately been assumed that the supplies were intended solely for the Polish population and could not be diverted from that purpose. This position and further statements

> with respect to our operations in Iran were concisely stated in our cable ME 179, October 13, 1942, a copy of which is attached. In pursuance of this policy, the American Red Cross representative in Cairo has developed an agreement with the Middle East Refugee Relief Association, a copy of this agreement is also attached.
>
> We have assumed that this policy with respect to American Red Cross operations in the Middle East has had the continued approval of the State Department. If, however, there has been a change in the Department's position, we shall be prepared to discuss the matter with representatives of the Department, with a view to working out any modification which may seem to be necessary.

The accord between the ARC and MERRA is entitled "Memorandum of Agreement between the Middle East Relief & Refugee Administration and the National American Red Cross," dated January 5, 1943, and consists of eleven articles, including the following:

> 1. The ARC recognizes MERRA as the official British agency responsible for certain indigent evacuees, and refugees in the Middle East. 2. The ARC will endeavor to meet all requests made by MERRA for services or supplies within the limits of ARC policies and resources. . . . 6. MERRA will arrange for transportation, warehousing and final distribution, without cost to ARC, for all supplies handed over to MERRA by ARC for distribution. . . . 10. ARC assistance in its present form is primarily of an emergency nature and intended only as temporary. The continuing care of refugees and for the provision of relief supplies in the Middle East is the responsibility of MERRA and other British agencies. Therefore, such ARC assistance as is provided will be of temporary supplementary nature. 11. This Agreement may be amended or modified at a later date by written mutual agreement by MERRA and the ARC. Signed on behalf of the Middle East Relief & Refugee Administration, W.T. Mathews, Director General. Signed on behalf of the American National Red Cross, Egypt, R. Bain, Director Middle East Operations.

Ryan's letter to Secretary Hull had elicited a note from Alling to Murray dated March 15, 1943 (Memorandum, 891.48/340):

> The elements of the American Red Cross position in Iran, as shown by the attached file, would seem to be as follows: 1) Although Red Cross

officials in Washington have taken the position that their supplies in Iran could and should be diverted to Iranian relief if not needed by the Polish refugees in the country, Amcross headquarters in Cairo has, in general, opposed such diversion. However, this is water over the dam, since Cairo now recommends disposal of remaining supplies by distribution first among the Iranian population. 2) Both in Washington and Cairo the Red Cross has followed a policy of merely supplementing British relief work in the Middle East, under the overall planning of the Middle East Relief and Refugee Administration, which is British. This policy has been applied to Iran as well as the other territories of the area. 3) In view of the expected departure of the Polish refugees, Amcross headquarters at Cairo recommends the discontinuance of American relief work in Iran, evidently following the thought that Iran is a British sphere of responsibility and that it is entirely up to the British to take care of any purely Iranian needs.

NE believes that in replying to Mr. Ryan's letter of February 27, 1943, we should call attention to certain factors which differentiate Iran from the rest of the Middle East. Because of its function as a supply line to the Soviet Union and because of its petroleum production, Iran is vitally important to the United Nations. It is also the most difficult of all the small nations of the Middle East to keep in line and is precisely the territory where British influence is least effective and American influence is greatest. Consequently, the Department's policy is to take an active part in Iranian affairs, cashing in for the benefit of the United Nations as a whole the high standing of the United States in that country. We most definitely do not regard Iran as a purely British sphere of political responsibility. This has been recognized and welcomed by the British Government.

It follows, therefore, that activities tending to increase American popularity and convince the Iranians of our interest in their welfare are directly in line with our foreign policy and are helpful in attaining the objectives of that policy, and it is obvious that judicious relief work by the Red Cross would fall in this category. Conversely, a withdrawal by the Red Cross from Iran would be taken as evidence that we are interested in that country only to the extent that it can be used to assist our non-Iranian friends, such as the Poles, and would weaken our position. From Red Cross and other reports it is clear that there is need for relief in Iran. It would be foolish to suggest that the Red Cross try to feed the population; as Mr. Bailey pointed out, that is a job for governments, and we are doing our best to provide wheat. But the

> presence of one Amcross representative in Tehran to make small gifts of medical supplies, special foods, clothing for the destitute, and to assist the Iranian authorities in meeting sudden emergencies, would have a great moral effect.
>
> This Division feels that the Red Cross officials here should be requested to reconsider their policy with respect to Iran, looking at it not as simply one of a number of Middle Eastern territories but rather as a country of special interest and importance to the United States, with a view to undertaking at least a small program of specialized assistance to the Iranian people themselves. It should also be pointed out that such a program would be most appreciated by the Iranians, and hence most effective from our point of view, if it were entirely independent of any British relief operations.

The ARC-MERRA agreement had also elicited some caustic comments by American officials. A telegram from the American Legation in Tehran dated June 21, 1943, reads:

> For Norman Davis Amcross from Sulzberger. Passing through Tehran enroute to Moscow I have learned of Amcross MERRA agreement of January 5, 1943, and would appreciate advice care of Amembassy, Moscow as to whether modifications are now contemplated. From a business viewpoint it would seem unwise that Amcross funds be distributed by British. You, of course, sense strong Russian British rivalry in Iran. Furthermore, despite instructions or possible facts themselves impression prevails assistance largely Polish not Iranian. Therefore we have American funds used by British on behalf of Poles who are unliked by the Russians just when we are doing utmost to cultivate Russian relations. I appreciate this is a British sphere but we are here sufficiently heavily to be independent. I am returning via Tehran in two or three weeks so I can check further if you will advise. Regards.

On April 7, 1943, Assistant Secretary Long had written to Davis incorporating verbatim the contents of the above Alling to Murray memorandum. The letter concludes (891.48/333): "The Department would appreciate receiving the views of the American Red Cross in this matter before any action is taken by it upon the joint recommendation of Messrs. Bailey and Bain that all Red Cross representations be withdrawn from Iran."

Long's letter had received the following initial response dated April 14, 1943, from Davis (Letter, 891.48/335):

> Since receiving your letter of April 7th . . . I have dispatched a cable to Mr. Bain in Cairo, asking him to wire Mr. Bailey, who is now in Tehran, to take no action which would be construed as indicating a prospective complete removal of the American Red Cross from Iran. Your suggestion is being given further consideration here, and we shall communicate with you on the subject shortly.

Davis followed up on May 8, 1943 (Letter, 891.48/336):

> American Red Cross representatives were assigned to the direction of relief operations in Iran because of the movement of Polish refugees into that country from Russia. In response to the pressing needs for supplementary assistance to such refugees, and to Polish nationals concentrated in south Russia, the American Red Cross provided supplies from stores then available in Egypt and Syria, and later by direct shipment to Iran, to a total estimated value of some $2,000,000. These supplies have now been practically exhausted, although a small reserve remains in our control in Iran. During the course of these operations, certain drugs and surgical supplies have been turned over to the Iranian Red Lion and Sun Society for distribution through institutions in Iran, for the benefit of the native population. In addition, some five hundred bags of flour have been distributed to the Iranian population as a gift of the American Red Cross, and more recently, additional flour has been provided on a loan basis to meet emergencies.
>
> It appears that the principal cause for relief needs among the Iranians is the present failure of normal processes of distribution within the country and the lack of transportation facilities for imports normally brought into Iran. It has been reported that because of the work projects engaged upon by the British and American armies, there are certain unusual opportunities for employment in Iran. Presumably, therefore, if normal imports and distribution facilities within the country could be maintained, there would be little necessity for free distribution of relief supplies. Any attempt on the part of a relief agency to deal with the problem just described will require the procurement and shipment of substantial supplies, particularly food; but if these problems can be solved, there apparently would be no need for a relief operation. It seems to us, therefore, that the situation is largely one which should be

met with the resources and through the collaboration of the Iranian, British and American Governments. The American Red Cross will, as heretofore, give sympathetic consideration to any supplementary effort which may assist in the solution of the problem.

With the prospective removal of the Polish refugees in Iran by the first of July, and unless a program of relief for the Iranian population is approved, there would not seem to be justification of the presence there of an American Red Cross representative for the sole purpose of giving relief. During this time, however, as our program of services to the American armed forces has developed in Iran as well as in other points throughout the Middle East, we now have several representatives there, and we will be adding to that staff as transport facilities permit. Thus, the possible removal of one representative who has been stationed in Iran for civilian relief operations probably need not be interpreted as the withdrawal of the American Red Cross from Iran. Nevertheless, if the State Department wishes us to do so, we can maintain our representative now engaged chiefly in relief operations in Iran until it is clearly apparent that there is no longer a need for his services. . . .

In all the relief operations undertaken by the Red Cross in territory in the Middle East under British control, we have taken the position that the primary responsibility for the organization of relief and the assembly of supplies for that purpose rests with the British authorities. The American Red cross has undertaken to supplement British resources and, as you know, has done so, both in the direction of relief operations and by the shipment of relief supplies purchased in the United States. Largely as a result of the efforts and advice of Mr. Kirk and our representative, Mr. Bain, the Middle East Relief and Refugee Administration (MERRA) was established. So far as I have been informed this organization has functioned satisfactorily. If the American Red Cross is to undertake independent relief operations in the Middle East, certain agreements with the British and our own agreement which will permit the necessary freedom of action on the part of the Red Cross must be established to succeed the agreement under which our operations have been maintained to date. If the Department believes that such steps should be taken at this time we will be happy to give further consideration to the matter.

Long's reply of June 16, 1943 (Letter, 891.48/336):

> I acknowledge the receipt of your letter of May 8, 1943 in further regard to the possible modification in the American Red Cross program in Iran. The Department appreciates the Red Cross' position, and agrees that the American Red Cross could hardly be expected to undertake a broad program which would involve the feeding and clothing of millions of Iranians whose incomes are at present insufficient to meet their minimum needs. The American Minister at Tehran . . . has suggested that the American Red Cross might interest itself in meeting special cases, such as emergency needs for certain medical supplies. The Department is of the opinion that it is highly desirable, from a political standpoint, that the American Red Cross continue the assignment of a civilian representative at Tehran until such time as it is clearly apparent that he can serve no useful purpose there.

ARC had relented. Assistant Secretary Howland Shaw's letter to Davis dated July 14, 1943 (Letter, 891.48/336):

> In Mr. Long's absence, I have received Mr. Allen's letter of June 24, 1943, in regard to the American Red Cross program in Iran. The Department is pleased to hear that the Red Cross has decided to continue the assignment of a civilian relief representative in Tehran, and is in complete agreement with the action and policy expressed in the last paragraph of Mr. Allen's letter under reference.

Chapter 12

Deepening Crisis and Weakening of Soheily Government

An OSS report of February 11, 1943, entitled "Food in Iran," gives a background on food and economic conditions in the spring of 1942 (Research and Analysis, 891.5018/22):

> Although Iran is normally self-sufficient in food, except for tea and sugar, the stress of war has brought a serious dislocation of its economy. The occupation of the country in August 1941 by Russian and British troops, with subsequent augmentation of these forces using the roads and railroads for forwarding supplies to Russia, had several consequences: (a) more mouths to feed, (b) serious curtailment of transport facilities available to customary domestic trade, (c) transfer of considerable labor to these projects from production of food, and (d) preemption of shipping so that foreign trade was curtailed. Moreover, the government lost control of exports to Russia, the amount of which no one knows. Soon considerable numbers of Polish refugees entered the country, and, although tens of thousands were sent on to other countries by the British, continued to be a heavy drain upon supplies. Hoarding, holding for higher prices, and increase of the paper money issues to meet Allied need inevitably followed, stimulating inflation. Prices soon sky-rocketed. The cost of living index, based on the year 1936-37 as 100, had risen to 163 by November 1940, and a year later was 260. The predominant item in this index is food, something over 75%. Yet this was only the beginning of the Allied occupation: much worse was to come. In January 1942 the Government was compelled to ration sugar, one of the chief imports, and issued books to the heads of families for that purpose. As the year progressed the same method

should have been applied to other staple foods, but the Government lacked the courage to deal resolutely with the developing crisis. So serious had become the problem that governments rose and fell on the issue. February 28, 1942, the government of Foroughi fell because of its failure to cope with the problem successfully. Foroughi was succeeded by Soheily, his Minister of Foreign Affairs, (on March 9, 1942). He pressed for a devaluation of the pound sterling in relation to the Iranian currency, but the British resisted vigorously because of the precedent and effect elsewhere in the Middle East. The Majlis authorized the Ministry of Finance to exempt essential food-stuffs from the regular customs: all cereals, flour, dates, live animals, butter and potatoes. A steep rise in prices occurred in the first quarter of 1942 so that some prices in April were three to four times those of the previous April; whereas wages of unskilled labor for the same period had only doubled. From the beginning of this soaring prices, hoarding was evident, but the amount of it was in dispute between the Iranians and the British. March 18, 1942 the Majlis passed a strong law against it, but the Government was slow in publishing a list of articles affected, and never, according to the British, vigorously enforced it. Apparently this hoarding has been as prevalent among the masses, in their small way, as among the big dealers and landlords. Certainly speculation has been rife on the part of these rich landlords and large dealers. In June the Majlis passed a law establishing close control over food and clothing, preparatory to creating a Ministry of Supplies and Transport, in an effort to implement the law against hoarding. Food prices receded somewhat in the spring and with the coming of the food harvest. But, even so, widespread hardships and increasing resentment were the inevitable result. Soheily's greatest achievement was the announcement of Lend-Lease to Iran, but it made little immediate difference on the food situation. By September 1942, the cost of living index stood at 418.

By the spring of 1942, Iran was on the verge of famine. Minor on April 1, 1942 (Dispatch 238 and enclosure, 891.50/48):

I have the honor to enclose a translation of a law on hoarding and profiteering voted by the Majlis on March 18, 1942. . . . The general question of providing food, particularly wheat and sugar, for the population, preventing profiteering and controlling hoarding has become the most urgent problem facing the Iranian people.

Dreyfus on April 23, 1942 (Telegram 121, 691.003/62):

> With a view to alleviating the food scarcity in Iran the Majlis on April 20, 1942 enacted an urgent law authorizing the Ministry of Finance to exempt from all customs charges wheat, rice, barley and other cereals, flour, dates, live animals, butter, clarified butter and potatoes imported from abroad. It is stated that the law will go into operation immediately.

Dreyfus on June 15, 1942 (Dispatch 284, 891.50/49):

> I have the honor to enclose a translation of the Regulations on the Enforcing of the Hoarding Law, which were approved by the Majlis on May 25, 1942. A translation of the Law on Hoarding and Profiteering, voted by the Majlis on March 18, 1942, and intended as a basic law to cover these and any other regulations issued, was enclosed with the Legation's despatch No. 238 of April 1, 1942. The law and regulations on hoarding and profiteering, it would appear, give the Government authority to deal with these important problems. More important, though, than the text of the regulations will be the manner of enforcement. The Government has delayed and procrastinated for almost three months in the passing of the regulations on hoarding, permitting in the meantime speculation, hoarding and graft to run rampant. This dilatory action, or lack of action, on the Government's part has been extremely harmful, having permitted large stocks of medicines and foods, particularly wheat, to find their way into the pockets of speculators who are reaping a rich harvest. It is commonly stated that high officials including members of the Majlis are engaged in these unpatriotic and reprehensible activities. Therefore, if the Government's action in enforcing the regulations be in the same weak vein, there is little hope that they will be properly enforced. The Government, it should be remarked, is asking the Majlis for plenary powers in the two fields of food and transport which, if given as they doubtless will be, would greatly enforce its ability to enforce the regulations. An interesting angle of this matter is the possibility that an American may be, as the Department is already aware, appointed as food and relief administrator. This step would be welcomed by both the Iranian public and Government, the former in the hope that soaring prices may be controlled and the latter in the hopes that the regulations may be properly enforced.
>
> The situation in Iran with regard to hoarding, speculation and prices has, indeed, become serious. Stories are current, some perhaps untrue

but most bearing some kernel of fact, of speculation and hoarding by high Government officials. The Prime Minister, rumor has it, is part of a ring of officials who have made large sums in speculation in medicines. It is said that the Government itself refused to buy a stock of medicines offered to it, valued at something like 2,000,000 rials, in order that certain officials, including the Prime Minister, might buy them personally and sell them at exorbitant prices. The medicines are said to have found their way eventually into the hands of a pharmacist named Dr. Namdar. It is reported that two deputies who were sent to Khuzistan to investigate into the wheat situation ended up buying quantities of wheat themselves, holding it for a double price. Tales of this kind are legion, including graft of all kinds, selling of Government offices and other forms of dishonesty. It is said that the Prime Minister has retained the three portfolios of President of the Cabinet, Minister of Interior and Minister of Foreign Affairs in order to be able to sell the minor positions in these Ministries. Whatever truth there is in any of these individual stories, there is not the slightest doubt in my mind that the Iranians are sinking ever lower in a morass of graft and dishonesty. Iranian morale, I might say, has been shattered by the events of last August and the subsequent virtual occupation of the country by the dreaded Russians and unpopular British. The Iranians, confronted with this face-destroying situation and the loss of their great leader who acted and thought for them for twenty years, have not yet been able to get a grip on themselves. I have called to the Prime Minister's attention on several occasions to the necessity of reducing graft, putting a brake on personal ambition and preventing exploitation, but so far without visible effect. I told him in the presence of the Turkish Ambassador, in order to let him know that the diplomatic corps were aware of abuses, a story now circulating to the effect that Dr. Etebar, a deputy and close friend of the Prime Minister's, had told the Minister of Education that unless he appointed a certain individual to lead a division in his Ministry the Minister would be removed from the Cabinet.

Something must be done to remedy this situation. The poor people, who have suffered much and complained little in these years, are now reduced to near starvation. Prices of foods are outrageous; medicines sell for several times the equivalent American price, completely beyond the reach of the average person. The press and government offer sympathy, weep crocodile tears, promise remedy, but nothing is done. Prince Firouz, now Governor General of Fars, told me the other day that natives in his area are existing on Iranian bread (when they can get it), tea with a tiny bit of sugar, sometimes a little cheese and grass.

What is the remedy? The answer, easy to give but difficult to realize, is a strong and honest Government which will distribute food, deal harshly with hoarders and control prices. An American who would come here and take over food and relief administration would be a God-send. It is possible, also, that a member of the proposed American financial mission to Iran could take over these duties. I am of the opinion that an American could succeed in this important task where an Iranian would fail. For example, the local manager of General Motors told me yesterday that he doubted if tire distribution could be properly carried out by the present set-up in the Ministry of Finance. No Iranian, he said, would dare refuse tire to a high official. However, he was sure that with an American at the head of the organization it would function reasonably well for the Iranian employee would be able to "pass the buck along" to the American, relieving himself of the impossible situation of having to deal with a high official.

The British seem to feel that the Iranians are hopeless, that they are incapable of running the country well or of meeting and remedying situations such as those of hoarding and prices. Many Iranians, themselves, feel the same way, particularly a certain honest minority, some of them educated abroad. This feeling of despair and impotence, as I suggested above, comes from the shock of the invasion, the consequence loss of face, the disruption of life due to violent change from dictatorship to democracy, and the disheartening situation caused by virtual loss of independence. I, for one, perhaps naively, do not admit the thesis of Iranian inability to govern. What the Iranians need at this point is help and sympathy, friendly but firm, and this they can get only from us. They are clamoring for American advisers, as indicated in my despatch No. 279, June 11. Here is an anomaly which I believe has gone heretofore unnoted and which contains a suggestion as to the eventual solution of the Iranian problem. The very politicians who are lining their pockets with money at present are clamoring for American advisers of all kinds. They must know, for this was well impressed upon them by the Shuster and Millspaugh missions, that the Americans would not stand for widespread graft on the present variety and that the goose that lays the golden egg will, with the arrival of a large number of American experts, die a natural death. The fact that this does not deter them for asking for Americans to come and break up their comfortable rackets, shows there is something of patriotism and decency in their makeup. They are, to a great extent, victims of a vicious system. There is much good in them which they themselves scarcely recognize. They ask for our leadership; they will follow it if

> given. I cannot emphasize too often the necessity of sending to Iran the highest type of American adviser, men of tested integrity and character. The sending of one dishonest or unscrupulous American would be disastrous for Iran; it would be like employing a rascal as a teacher in a primary school.

Dreyfus on June 16, 1942 (Dispatch 286 and enclosure, 891.5018/3):

> I have the honor to enclose the text of a law passed by the Majlis on June 14, 1942, which gives the Government plenary powers to deal with food control and transportation in cases not covered by the laws and regulations on hoarding and profiteering. . . . It is useless to conjecture on the possible effects of this new law. The machinery for combating hoarding, profiteering and soaring prices is now in the hands of the Government. It remains to be seen whether the Government's dilatory handling of these matters during the last three months will now be converted into positive action.

Meanwhile, an OSS report expresses pessimism (891.00/1912):

> From an entirely reliable source, the Agency has received a report from Teheran dated July 4, 1942, covering . . . (s)teps taken by the Persian Government for regulating the hoarding and profiteering in foodstuffs, particularly wheat: "The impression which one has here now is that the government has finally set up the machinery for dealing with hoarding and profiteering in foodstuffs. This has been done with great public flourish of resentment against malefactors. The regulations are one thing, but whether, considering the number of minor administrators involved and their probable venality, the rules will be enforced, is another. In the case of wheat, the government is offering a premium to those growers who turn over their crops promptly. But in practice, the price the government pays is still less than the growers can obtain from private illegal sales. The wheat harvest in Azerbaijan and Khorasan, the two great wheat producing provinces, has been very good—better than last year. These two provinces lie in the Russian occupied area. It is alleged, though so far not proven, that the Russians are making indirect purchases in these regions. Even if that is true, a shortage of wheat for the native population in those areas would probably be due to ineffective collection and distribution of wheat by the government."

The government had also tried to prevent hoarding of medical and pharmaceutical goods. Minor on August 18, 1942 (Dispatch 331, 891.50/50):

> I have the honor to enclose a translation of anti-hoarding regulations with respect of medicines, which came into force by publication in the Ministry of Justice Gazette on August 16, 1942. These regulations are based on the Law on Hoarding and Profiteering voted by the Majlis, March 18, 1942 (quoted in despatch No. 238 of April 1, 1942) and on the regulations based thereon, passed by the Majlis on May 25, 1942.

In a classic dispatch of May 13, 1942, Dreyfus discusses the rising anti-British sentiments in the context of deteriorating conditions (Dispatch 264, 741.9111/69):

> I have the honor to enclose a translation of a notice in all Tehran newspapers by the Imperial Police calling the attention of the public to the fact that Iran is in treaty relations with the British and Russians and that propaganda in favor of Axis countries or concealing of Axis nationals are inconsistent with the interests of the country and the terms of the pact. This notice was directly inspired by the British Legation in an endeavor to check pro-axis propaganda, which has been on the increase throughout Iran, and in a belated effort to improve their Iranian relations which, particularly since the events of August last, have been none too cordial. The British wished, at the same time, to call to the attention of the Iranians the fact that their treaty with the British and Russians involves obligations as well as advantages, a condition they are wont to forget. . . . Relations between these unnatural allies have been marred since August by a number of knotty and aggravating problems. First of these was the treaty of alliance, which had literally to be forced on Iran; the long and complicated negotiations from September to January put a severe strain on British-Iranian relations. . . . A second cause of friction was the matter of the expulsion of the Japanese Legation which, up to the denouement of April 23, 1942, caused considerable hard feeling. . . . A third irritating factor has been the negotiations with regard to financial matters, particularly the questions of supply of rials for allied war work, which is inevitably tied up with the exchange rate and the conversion of sterling holdings into dollars or gold. These negotiations are now approaching, it is hoped, a settlement which will be satisfactory to both Iran and the British. . . . A fourth disturbing element has been the arrest at British demand of a

number of Iranians for pro-axis activities. . . . There have been other irritating problems, principally involving the supply of wheat, sugar and other essential goods to Iran by the British. The Iranians have, on the whole, failed to appreciate the magnitude and difficulty of these problems of supply. They have preferred to adopt an attitude of complaint that supplies were inadequate rather than one of appreciation for what has been furnished. This shortsighted and opportunistic policy, abetted by German propaganda, has led the average Iranian to believe that the British, far from supplying the country with needed goods, have actually taken them out of the country. Iranians complain widely of the lack of wheat, which they attribute to the British, although the British have brought into the country since August more than 50,000 tons of this essential commodity. To counteract this mistaken belief, the British have begun to use newspaper media to explain to the Iranians the extensive supplies they have been bringing into the country.

This viewpoint on the part of the Iranians which has amounted to a policy of non-cooperation, is based on inherent dislike for and resentment of the British. The British have been forced, therefore, on numerous occasions to exert strong pressure on the Iranians to obtain their ends. There is enclosed, as an example of this kind of pressure so frequently put on the Iranians, a copy of a British Legation Note dated April 4, 1942, which virtually threatens Iran with stoppage of supplies if the Japanese Legation were not expelled from the country. This note, I might add, was quite unnecessary for it seemed likely at the time it was delivered that the Iranians would accede to the British-American representations without the necessity of resorting to strong and formal pressure. These strained relations between Iran and Great Britain have not been helped, to say the least, by German propaganda. The Germans, through agents in Iran, and by their effective daily propaganda broadcasts in Persian from Berlin, playing on the credulity of the anti-British masses, have been most successful in discrediting the British in Iran. This feeling of comradeship for the Germans and repugnance for the British is, as I have frequently pointed out, based more on general anti-British sentiment than any affection for the Germans. In any event, the masses are impressed. The people talk openly of the arrival of the Germans. One of our missionaries heard a porter saying to another that they would have much better pay and treatment when the Germans arrive. The same missionary reported that the audience at a cinema in the poor section of the city cheered wildly for Hitler at decidedly the wrong places when a British war film was shown. With regard to the German broadcasts in Persian, which have had more effect on the Iranians than any other single propaganda item, I am happy to report that these broadcasts have been effectively jammed by the Russians. An amusing sidelight on this radio campaign was the British inspired action on the part of the Iranian police removing all radios from public places. They were quickly restored, again at British request, when it was found, quite strangely, that one could not tune in to *British* broadcasts without a radio.

One cannot blame the Iranians too severely for their short-sighted and unrealistic policy of refusing to cooperate voluntarily with a nation at whose hands they have suffered so much; on the other hand, one is reluctant to criticize the British, for their action in Iran is essential to the prosecution of the war. This whole affair serves as an excellent lesson in practical international relations. Relations based on force and exploitation rather than on mutual help and goodwill do not pay dividends when the day of reckoning arrives. This is brought more forcefully home by contrasting these strained relations with the cordial ones between Iran and the United States. We have had in many of these Iranian-British disputes, notably the expulsion of the Japanese Legation, supply of wheat, and the financial negotiations, to intervene to assist in effecting settlements. The attitude of the Department in these matters has been helpful and constructive. By refusing to join the British in putting pressure on the Iranians in matters not essential to the war effort, we are maintaining our prestige in Iran and following our traditional policy of disinterested help to this country; on the other hand, by supporting the British where essential to the war effort and by refusing to be placed in the position of backing the Iranians against the British, we are playing fair with our allies and contributing to the prosecution of the war. This intelligent, middle of the road, policy has so far worked admirably as regards both the British and the Iranians. British-Iranian relations are at the moment, I am happy to report, better than they have been at any time since the events of last August. All of the more aggravating problems have been disposed of and the financial dispute seems well on the way to a settlement satisfactory to both parties. The British Minister informs me that, with these irritating problems out of the way, there is a noticeable tendency on the part of the Iranians to offer more cooperation and less tendency to resort to the delaying and obstructing tactics of recent months. There will undoubtedly be other disputes in the future, as for example the incipient one in regard to tires mentioned in my telegram No. 147, May 10, but on the whole relations between these two nations have shown improvement.

The "improvement" was short-lived.

Dreyfus on May 30, 1942 (Telegram 181, 740.0011 EW 1939/21860):

> British civil and military authorities here are now taking more seriously than they have in the past year possibility of German thrust into Iran. This borne out by statements to me of prominent British officials, by construction of air raid trench in British Legation compound and by recent visit here of General Quinan, GOC Iraq, who came examine Iran defenses against invasion via Caucasia. Reports he has available three British divisions for defense Caucasia not taken too seriously because of fact that British have no such forces available unless they are withdrawn from theaters farther west. British officials consider German arrival here in July, August definite possibility. Few seem to take seriously threat which I feel should not be overlooked of invasion via Syria when Libyan campaign reaches its peak. British here aware of danger of disorder, famine, sabotage and vengeance against their citizens should Germans approach nearer to Iran. This is definite possibility which I will bear in mind in considering welfare of our citizens. Iranians becoming increasingly nervous as German threat grows. They fear particularly that famine will develop if Germans penetrate into Caucasia. Rumors are being spread present Government would in such case flee taking the gold and crown jewels. I consider it not unlikely pro-German elements which predominate in the country particularly in army will get out of hand if Germans penetrate deep into Caucasia. I hazard prediction that German ultimatum to Iran delivered when they arrive at or near Baku would not be effectively resisted by Iranian people.

Dreyfus on June 3, 1942 (Telegram 186, 891.00/1882):

> The relative calm which has prevailed since advent of Soheily Government has given way to atmosphere of political intrigue and uncertainty. Rumors are current of Cabinet changes, for example, that Ahy (perhaps the best man in Cabinet) will become Ambassador to Russia while Saed Ambassador there will become Minister of Foreign Affairs. This political unrest is caused to considerable extent by growth of graft and unbridled personal ambition. Stories are widespread of graft in high position, sale of high offices, speculation in essential commodities and other reprehensible acts. The Prime Minister is widely accused of keeping three portfolios in order to sell positions, of having taken money from his Minister in Washington for privilege of staying there and of being a ring speculating in medical supplies. While I do

not believe all of the stories, I am convinced there is much truth in them. I consider situation as unsatisfactory and have told Prime Minister frankly that I have heard some of the stories and believe he should do all possible to eliminate graft. While I have been satisfied with Soheily's cooperation with Allies, I must express disappointment with his lethargy in putting essential reforms such as hoarding bill into effect, with his inability to control politicians and with the scandalous graft situation he has permitted to arise and contributed to. A group of officials is working for appointment as Prime Minister of Qavam-es-Saltaneh. Qavam is said to have Russian support but British have been no more than lukewarm to him. British Minister told me recently he would like to back Taqizadeh now Minister in London for Prime Minister if Soheily fails. . . . I do not recommend any immediate action since our war activities in Iran are going forward satisfactorily but we should bear the situation in mind in our future dealings with the Iranians.

Dreyfus on June 26, 1942 (Telegram 316, 891.01A/176):

Reference my telegram 191, June 9 and despatch 279, June 11. Prime Minister called me today to express his deep concern over failure of American Government to respond to his many requests for advisers, particularly Food Administrator and financial mission. He said he had promised the Majlis on occasion of expulsion of Japanese Legation and when other action favorable to the Allies was taken that effective aid from the United States would soon be forthcoming. He added in evident agitation that he is "getting near the end of his rope" and that his position may soon become untenable unless American help is extended.

Dreyfus on June 30, 1942 (Dispatch 298, 891.00/1896):

I have described in other despatches and telegrams the pro-German, or rather anti-British and Russian attitude of the Iranian masses, a turn of mind especially noticeable among the army. The feeling has grown apace until at present the Iranians have in their hearts only bitterness and hatred for the invaders of their soil. Some Iranians talk openly of revenge when the day of deliverance arrives. It is reported that radical elements among the masses intend to take revenge on Christians and there are even reports that our missionaries are in danger because they have had a leading part in encouraging and developing Christian minorities. . . . I am distinctly apprehensive of civil disorder of a wide-

> spread and violent nature if, as seems at least possible, the Germans enter Iran or even approach its borders.

Dreyfus on July 2, 1942 (Telegram 221, 740.0011 EW 1939/22613):

> Prime Minister and other high officials especially those closely connected with Allies express deep concern over German victories in Egypt which are being interpreted here as prelude to conquest of entire Middle East. The Iranian masses are almost jubilant over British reverses and voice hope that Egyptian campaign will lead to their liberation from Anglo-Soviet domination. Few if any stop to consider consequences of German occupation their only immediate thought being that of getting rid of the invaders of their soil. There seems little doubt that the Germans would be welcomed here as liberators. Resentment over allied occupation, near starvation in certain areas, extremely high prices, scarcity of goods, disruption of normal life and recrudescence of tribal disturbances have put the masses in an ugly mood. There is in my opinion danger of civil disturbances and acts of revenge against foreigners should the Germans enter or approach Iran. The danger is particularly great for Christian communities in the north.

Weakening of Soheily Cabinet

The wheat and food situation had continued to deteriorate, the harvest notwithstanding. Dreyfus on July 6, 1942 (Telegram 224, 891.24/214):

> Reference the Department's memorandum instruction of May 12 regarding food supplies. Shortage is reported of wheat, ghee, sugar and imported food products. Disruption of transport facilities makes distribution difficult and hoarding aggravates situation. Shortage of wheat is particularly acute and is causing considerable suffering especially in south. It is impossible as yet to estimate wheat crop now being harvested. Iranian Department of Agriculture states crop this year will be 1,400,000 metric tons as compared to normal of 1,700,000. British Legation believe normal is much lower and that this year's crop will be between 80 and 100% of normal. British have several wheat specialists attached to Consulates throughout Iran to study the situation. Meanwhile Iranians complain that because wheat crop will be below normal they will need to import 100,000 tons during next twelve months. During the year ended March 20, 1942, 73,509 metric tons wheat were imported from India and Canada. Iranians estimate 350,000 tons will be needed this year to supply urban needs.

The latter figure turned out to be accurate.

Dreyfus on July 7, 1942 (Telegram 225, 891.00/1894):

> Reference my numbers 186, June 3 and 210, June 22. The internal political situation has become more tense. The Government is being widely attacked in the press and Majlis for its failure to insure the essential food and transport needs of the country, for the closing of three newspapers, and for unfulfilled promises. The Prime Minister went to the Majlis Sunday to present new Minister of Interior but found the atmosphere so hostile that he left without doing so. The Russian Ambassador considers the present Government too weak to meet the present emergency. He informs me that he favors the entry of Qavam-es-Sultaneh as Prime Minister and the formation of a strong Government. The Turkish Ambassador favors the holding of new elections in order to bring in a truly constitutional Majlis but the Soviet Ambassador feels the time for this is not opportune. While I have been satisfied with Soheily's cooperation, there is no doubt that his Government has failed to deal effectively with internal problems and that a stronger Government is needed (see my number 186). I see no reason why we should oppose a Qavam Cabinet particularly since he has signified his intention of cooperating fully with the United States. There is, of course, potential danger in the Soviet intention to take a more active part in internal politics of Iran. The Russian Ambassador told me frankly that "if the situation deteriorates, it will take two Soviet divisions here to keep order unless a stronger government is put in power." I agree with him fully in the need for more forceful action in internal matters, particularly food distribution, transport problems, prices, hoarding and internal security.

Dreyfus on July 17, 1942 (Telegram 237, 891.24/218):

> Wheat situation has become more critical with resultant acute shortage of bread. Since stocks on hand in Tehran are adequate for only few days Government is urgently endeavoring to uncover stocks in provinces to tide country over until new crops harvested. This situation as suggested in my no. 225, July 7, is one of the main causes of present political crisis. British Legation Tehran has maintained up to present a rather intransigent attitude taking view that the 60,000 tons imported are sufficient, that no wheat should be furnished Iran after the harvest and that Government should requisition stocks alleged to be in hands of hoarders before requesting imports. Iranians have taken view that arrivals have been inadequate, that 100,000 tons will have to be im-

> ported before 1943 harvest and that relatively small stocks are in hands of hoarders. Iranian view as to hoarding has been proved substantially correct by recent investigations which failed to reveal large stocks in hands of persons designated by British. British Legation in staff memorandum takes stand that Iranians are largely responsible for present situation for failing to bring true facts to its attention. This explanation in my opinion is weak since Iranians have frequently pointed out to Allied representatives the urgency and seriousness of the matter. British now recognizing seriousness of situation, are lending Iran 5600 tons of wheat from military stores to be repaid by wheat purchased by Saleh and now en route. They are also trying to obtain five thousand tons of barley to be mixed with wheat for bread. Soviets have promised to return 3000 tons of wheat that they borrowed. These measures will assist tiding country over until new crop is harvested during July and August. The transport problem is grave; Iranian transport is so depleted that crops cannot be moved until UKCC furnishes tires. British Minister has proposed to me and Soviet Ambassador formation of an Anglo-American-Soviet-Iranian committee to handle matters of this kind and has suggested that an Iranian Ministry of Food be established. Soviet Ambassador does not favor the committee but has consulted his government. For my part I feel such a committee would be useful but that it might better be formed as a subcommittee to CSC. A definite step forward would be afforded by designation and early arrival of an American food adviser the Department is seeking for Iranian Government. As to future wheat needs of Iran, I recommend an open mind until the harvest is finished. If crop is normal it may be possible under guidance of competent food adviser to squeeze through next year without imports. We must however carefully watch 1943 crop indications since a crop failure then might result in wide-spread famine.

The British desired the establishment of a "food board." Winant on July 21, 1942 (telegram 4050, 891.5018/5):

> We have received a communication from the Foreign Office which in substance reads as follows: "The Foreign Office has been giving much thought to the supply situation in Iran with particular reference to the need for insuring more efficient collection and distribution of foodstuffs if famine conditions such as arose in the last war are to be avoided. The allies have been obliged during the last nine months to import into Iran over fifty thousand tons of wheat from all sources including the United States. This was necessary as emergency measure to prevent

famine conditions during the winter. But the shipment of such bulky commodities as wheat to Iran by sea besides placing an additional strain on allied shipping resources can only be effected at the expense of supplies for the Soviet Union to which the largest possible share of Iranian port and transport capacity must be devoted. At the same time it is clearly desirable on grounds both of humanity and interest to see Iran does not go short of supplies and that order is preserved within an area so vital to allied communications. The problem therefore is to find means of insuring that Iran is adequately provisioned without the need for large imports. Normally Iran is self-sufficient in all staple foodstuffs except sugar. Recently shortages have been mainly local and are due partly to the breakdown of administration following the Anglo-Soviet occupation last autumn and partly to transport difficulties resulting from war conditions. Given suitable administrative action the Foreign Office feels that these difficulties should not prove insuperable but the Iranian Government 'who have many awkward tasks on their hands have not yet shown themselves able to deal adequately with the food problem.' The British Legation at Tehran has done everything possible to impress the Iranian Government with the gravity of the present position but fears that more positive steps are necessary to prevent famine. If famine occurs, the Allies would be faced with the alternatives of allocating more shipping, which can ill be spared, for the transport of supplies to Iran or allowing disorder and distress to continue unchecked.

The British Government have already appointed additional officers to service in certain Iranian provincial towns whose main duty is to assist the authorities in the collection of this year's harvest. But the British Chargé d'Affaires believes some more effective central control is necessary to effect any substantial improvement in the food situation. He has accordingly suggested that a food board should be constituted, with American, British, Soviet and Iranian members; and that this board should have executive power and direct the food policy of the country in all its aspects. The British Chargé has not yet sounded the Iranian authorities whose agreement would clearly be necessary, 'but he has reason to believe that the scheme would not be unwelcome to them.' He states that the American Minister has expressed himself as personally in favor of some such scheme provided the Iranian Government agrees, and feels that one of the United States relief experts 'for whose services the Persian Government are understood to have applied, might usefully represent the United States on such a board.' The Foreign Office concludes that the proposal is at present 'a tentative

> one only' but that it is anxious to have the views of the United States Government and the Soviet Government before any steps are taken to put it to the Iranian Government. If the American and Soviet Governments agree in principle that some such measures are desirable, it is the Foreign Office idea that the details be worked out 'by our representatives in Tehran in collaboration with the Persian Government.' "

The State Department replied to Winant on July 25, 1942, with copy to Dreyfus (Telegrams 191 and 3460, 891.24/218):

> Your 4050, July 21. British suggestion that an Anglo-Soviet-American-Iranian food committee be formed was reported by Minister Dreyfus in his cable no. 237, July 17 to Department, to which following rely has been sent as Department's 191 of July 25, 1 pm. "Department agrees with your view that it would be preferable to handle food matters through a sub-committee of CSC rather than an independent body. Soviet representatives might be invited to sit on subcommittee in advisory capacity if it should be found necessary. With respect to British Minister's suggestion that Iranian Ministry of Food be established, Department would authorize you to support this proposal, provided a) you think idea would be acceptable to Iranians and b) you are convinced such a Ministry would increase efficiency in food supply matters within a reasonable time. However, in view of inevitable delays in organization and resulting confusion, we are inclined to think it would be well to postpone any such undertaking at least pending the arrival of an American food and supply adviser." You may convey the substance of the above to the Foreign Office, adding that we hope to be able to despatch a food and supply expert to Iran within next few weeks.

Chapter 13

Appointment of Qavam and Rising Friction with the British

Dreyfus on July 30, 1942 (Telegram 244, 891.00/1897):

> Refer my Nos. 186, June 3 and 225, July 7. Political crisis has become more acute and reconstitution of present cabinet or formation of a new government may be expected soon. Situation has been aggravated by bread riots which have taken place in various parts of country despite fact wheat harvest is being reaped. Soheily is endeavoring reform his cabinet to include opposition politicians and thus satisfy dissident elements. However, British and Russian envoys are of opinion that Soheily has failed to deal efficiently with internal situation and feel he has played politics at time when energetic action was required. British Minister will see Shah today to suggest that Qavam es Sultaneh be called to form new government. I see no reason to oppose entry of Qavam who as stated in my 225 also has strong Soviet backing. We should, I feel be prepared for entry of Tadayyon into cabinet but I pointed out to the British Minister the undesirability of having him in education post especially now that arrival of Monroe mission is imminent.

On July 30, 1942 (Telegram 246, 891.00/1898): "Reference to my no. 244, July 30. The Soheily Cabinet has resigned."

OSS telegram of August 7, 1942, from Richard Lowe in Tehran (Telegram 252, 103.91802/720):

> Soheily cabinet fell largely due failure solve food problem new cabinet being formed Ahmad Qavam experienced politician retired twenty years.

> Popular tension and minor rioting on increase due following: poor quality and scarcity of bread; high cost foodstuffs often prohibitive; fear government will not execute 17 former officials including General Mokhtari on trial for revolting political murders they performed under former regime; popular disgust practice ministers deputies officials placing personal gain over national and popular needs; distrust governments failure stop hoarding and profiting; growing resentment against allied troops and Polish refugees popularly blamed for food shortage and high prices. Noticeable increase police and military patrol activity Tehran. Allies cannot count on support Iranian army. . . . British now expect Germans in Iran in September.

An OSS report of February 11, 1943, entitled "Food in Iran," gives additional background (Research and Analysis, 891.5018/22):

> The situation deteriorated so that by early August (1942) there were minor food disturbances in Tehran at the time Soheily resigned and Qavam was called from long retirement to form a new government. He immediately formed a department of food-stuffs with its director general, Mehdi Farrokh, directly responsible to the premier. September 22, 1942, this department was upped to a ministry and the economic sections of the Ministry of Finance transferred to it. The Qavam government has struggled vigorously with the food problem. These efforts of the Government failed because it was unwilling to take strong measures against hoarders and speculators. Moreover, considerable difficulty arose in the provinces, which refused cooperation with the central government, an increasing phenomena since the exile of the former Shah. An important contributing cause of their failure was the serious shortage of transport, especially tires and spare parts, since even in normal times food must be brought some distance to Tehran, carried from the north to the south of the country. Most of the trucks in the country had been commandeered by the Allies upon their occupation; and imports were beyond Iranian control. Early in 1942 the Iranian government approached the USA in regard to furnishing advisers in various departments. Among those was to be one on Food Supply. By August 8th Joseph P. Sheridan was appointed to the post; he arrived in Iran about October 1st. His presence and work have done considerable to stabilize the situation and prevent its further deterioration, although not to improve it. The latter was impossible because of the complex nature of the problem, linked as it is with international politics and especially financing of the allied military efforts in the country.

Dreyfus on August 2, 1942 (Telegram 248, 891.00/1899): "Reference my no. 246, July 30. The Majlis yesterday expressed approval of Ahmad Qavam (formerly Qavam-es-Sultaneh) for post of Prime Minister by vote of 51 out of 87 deputies present. The Shah has requested Qavam to form a cabinet which should be presented to Majlis within a few days." Dreyfus on August 5, 1942 (Telegram 250, 891.00/1900):

> My 248, August 2. Qavam has assumed duties as Prime Minister and is actively engaged in forming cabinet which he expects to present to Majlis next Sunday. United Press and Associated Press representatives in interview with Qavam yesterday were much impressed with evident warmth of his statements that he desires strengthen relations with the United States and to obtain American advisers. He spoke of things American to exclusion other topics. When asked what his program would be Qavam picked up a piece of bread from his desk and replied "this is my program. If I can put bread of good quality in hands of all Iranians other problems will be easy to solve." There are indications Qavam will form relatively strong cabinet and he intends to deal with Iran's pressing food, transport security and other internal problems with dispatch and energy. I see no reason to believe he will fail to cooperate with allies. Perhaps to test him on this point British Minister is seeing him today to insist on arrest of a number of persons suspected of pro-German activities.

Friction with the British had come at the outset. Dreyfus on August 9, 1942 (Telegram 253, 891.00/1901):

> Reference last two sentences my 250 August 5. A rather serious divergence of opinion has arisen between British Minister and Prime Minister over arrest of persons considered by British to be engaged in pro-German activities. This may adversely affect British relations and future of Qavam Government which is being presented to Majlis today. Qavam consented readily to the arrest of the 40 persons listed by British but now asks that written evidence against them be presented within 24 hours in accordance with Iranian law. British expect arrested persons to be turned over to them without hearing or trial by Iranians. I have frequently called Department's attention to danger to British Iran relations of such arbitrary treatment. British disregard of Iranian susceptibilities is causing Iran public to become increasingly bitter against them. This additional aggravation of British Iran relations seems unnecessary since Iranian Government will assent to arrest and intern-

ment of persons against whom proper evidence is submitted. British Minister takes view "I can't work with a Government like this" an attitude which may cause another political crisis at time when Qavam has succeeded in forming a relatively strong Cabinet. If Qavam Cabinet falls or resigns I see little hope for constitutional Government here in the near future and the only alternative would seem to be direct allied interference internal affairs of this country.

Dreyfus again on August 5, 1942 (Telegram 251, 891.24/224):

Reference my 237, July 17 and Department's 191, July 25. Wheat situation continues serious. British Legation view is that "unless wheat situation is taken seriously in hand, famine with all its accompanying difficulties may soon become a reality." I agree with this view. Minor food riots in provincial towns continue and cavalry has been parading in Tehran to forestall riots here. I met with British and Soviet envoys today to discuss situation. It was decided for each of us to approach Qavam, the new Prime Minister, (my 250, August 5 as to Qavam's status and attitude) to urge that transport board, mentioned in my 242, July 7, be set up without delay and that most energetic steps be taken by Iran Government to obtain control of wheat now being harvested. Qavam, it is reported, intends to set up Ministry of Food and Supply in his Cabinet.

Dreyfus on August 9, 1942 (Telegram 254, 891.00/1902):

Refer to my 250, August 5. Qavam presented his Cabinet to Majlis today. . . . Vote of confidence will be taken late in week after usual study and discussion of Government program. . . . I consider the Cabinet to be strong and above average of recent Cabinets in ability, integrity, and prestige. This coalition Cabinet of elder statesmen and young career officials containing few politicians should be able to deal with Iran's pressing problems with energy and confidence.

On August 13, 1942 (Telegram 258, 891.00/1905): "Medjliss today gave Qavam Government vote of confidence by vote of 109 out of 116 deputies present with seven abstentions."

American Advisers and Establishment of Food Ministry

Qavam had wasted no time in hiring American advisers. Cable to Dreyfus on August 8, 1942 (Telegram 205, 891.24/232A):

> Your 250 and 251, August 6. The Iranian Minister has reached an agreement with Joseph P. Sheridan for the latter's appointment as Food and Supply Adviser to the Iranian Government. Minister has cabled Tehran for approval of the terms agreed upon. . . . (H)e will be able to depart for Tehran immediately after September 7. In your discretion you may inform the Prime Minister that the Department considers Sheridan a very able man and believes that if given full cooperation by the Iranian Government he will be of great assistance in solving the pressing supply problems confronting Iran.

Sheridan arrived in Tehran on September 26, 1942. It turned out that, unfortunately, he was unsuited to the task.

Dreyfus on August 11, 1942 (Telegram 257, 891.24/233):

> Department's 205-6 and 7, August 8. I have discussed question of American advisers with Prime Minister along lines suggested by Department. Qavam assured me he strongly favors employment of American advisers who will be given wholehearted support by his government. . . . Qavam was delighted with suggested appointment of Millspaugh but stressed he would have less broad powers than on previous mission due to present democratic form of government. I personally am of opinion that the Department has executed a grand coup in the Millspaugh appointment which will have most favorable repercussions here. Qavam was also pleased with appointment of Sheridan.

Murray on August 13, 1942, in a memorandum to Assistant Secretary Berle and Under Secretary Welles (891.24/238):

> It is of course gratifying to note that Mr. Dreyfus feels that "the Department has executed a grand coup in the Millspaugh appointment, which will have favorable repercussions here." . . . The point is, to my mind, that the name Millspaugh, like that of Shuster, has become almost legendary in Iran and his return at this time, regardless almost of what service he renders, will act as a powerful stimulant to Iranian morale. It will at the same time enormously enhance American pres-

> tige in that country. It is interesting to note that, whereas the British laid down all sorts of conditions to their support of Dr. Millspaugh during his earlier tour of duty in Iran, they are apparently only too anxious now to see an American financial mission, however composed, operating in Iran at the earliest possible moment.

Qavam had also taken steps to establish a Ministry of Food. Dreyfus on August 25, 1942 (Dispatch 234, 891.24/252):

> I have the honor to report that pending the creation of a regular Ministry of Food, a temporary Bureau for the procurement and distribution of foodstuffs has been set up in Tehran under Amanollah Ardalan, a man of wide experience who will probably be named Minister of Food if legislative authorization for the creation of the new ministry is given by the Majlis. All other agencies dealing with provisioning will be bound by the instructions of this new office. These include the offices of grains, of grain storage, army purchases, sugar and tea, transportation, and textiles. The agencies now engaged in enforcing the anti-hoarding and rationing laws will also be subject to the orders of the new bureau. A special budget for the office has already been created by the Ministry of Finance.

Contrary to expectation, Ardalan was not appointed. Dreyfus on September 25, 1942 (Telegram 299, 891.00/1920): "Prime Minister yesterday presented Mehdi Farrokh to Majlis as Minister of Food simultaneously with presentation of bill for creation of Food Ministry. Qavam also presented himself to Majlis as Minister of War."

Dreyfus on October 31, 1942 (Dispatch 367, 891.24/307):

> I have the honor to enclose herewith a copy of the French text of the Law for the Creation of a Ministry of Food. The Minister of Food, Mr. Mehdi Farrokh, a man of some experience but not particularly high reputation, is not well regarded in certain circles and may not continue very long. His most recent post was that of Minister of the Interior for a few weeks shortly before the fall of the Soheily Cabinet. Mr. Ardalan who was head of the preliminary Office of provisioning and who was expected to become Minister of Food, was instead appointed Undersecretary of Finance. It is fortunate that the arrival of Mr. Joseph Sheridan as Food and Supply Adviser coincided with the actual creation of the Ministry in order that his recommendations may be put in force before the Ministry is too thoroughly organized. Mr.

Sheridan has already announced that he plans to suggest a reorganization of the Ministry as it now exists.

Discussion of Recent Developments

Dreyfus on August 24, 1942 (Dispatch 333, 891.00/1918):

The Soheily Government has passed into the great beyond with scarcely a sigh to mark the passing and the Qavam Government has taken its place to face the vagaries and uncertainties of Iranian politics. This despatch will endeavor to suggest the reasons for the premature demise of the Soheily Government, to describe the agitated conditions under which the new Government takes over. . . . The present situation may be described as political opportunism run rampant. Let us consider the reasons for this situation. First of all, it must be sought in a serious defect in the Iranian character—an almost total lack or sense of social responsibility, a condition which makes the operation of democratic government extremely difficult. Add to this a series of soul-shattering and face-destroying events: the invasion of this country in August, 1941, by the dreaded Russians and hated British and the feeling of shame occasioned by the poor record of resistance by the Iranian army; the imposition of an unwanted treaty with the British and Russians; lack of security throughout the country, especially in the tribal areas; political interference by the allies in the affairs of the country, such as arrest and detention without trial of persons suspected of pro-German activities; general belief that the allies have not lived up to their pledges to do their utmost to supply Iran with much needed food and other supplies; deterioration in Iranian economy; virtual loss of control over the richest producing areas in the north; and lately near famine because of wheat shortage and breakdown of the road transport system. These facts must then be viewed in the light of the confusion, helplessness and inefficiency which resulted from the sudden switch-over from a dictatorial to a democratic regime after the departure of Shah Reza. Take the above ingredients, add a dash of the bitterness which Iranians feel because of the unfortunate events of last year, shake well by a vindictive and irresponsible press, and you have a distinctly unpalatable cocktail.

On the fall of the Soheily cabinet:

It became apparent some weeks ago, as indicated in the Legation's telegrams 186 of June 3, 210 of June 22 and 225 of July 7, that popular feeling against the Soheily cabinet was growing to such an extent that its position was untenable and its existence circumscribed. Primary causes of this were unfavorable reaction to arrests of pro-Axis persons at British instigation, dissatisfaction with cabinet's lack of action in vital food and transport problems, which had resulted in acute food shortage, a general feeling that the cabinet had not lived up to its promises, displeasure with the extensive graft which had grown up in government circles and considerable dose of plain vindictiveness on the part of disgruntled elements in the Majlis and press. The cabinet position became so weak and its position in the Majlis so unsatisfactory that it resigned on July 30. Here are some of the things the press were saying about the Soheily Government: *Tajaddod-e-Iran*, July 8: "The most important thing achieved by the Cabinet of Soheily is the devastation of Rezayieh, the famine in Fars, the suppression of newspapers and the massacre of prisoners. The newspaper *Azad* was suppressed for Shirvani, *Omid* for Ahy and *Setareh* for Haji Bibi Khanum (woman attached to the court)." *Tajaddod-e-Iran*, July 28: "There were riots in Borujerd on July 26 for bread. The municipality and the granary were raided, damage done, many wounded and two killed. This is an example of the sagacity and efficiency of the Government." *Payam*, June 27, printed a cartoon which showed a dead man being brought to a store where textiles are sold, the pall-bearers having to fight to get two meters of goods. The influential *Ettelaat* of July 5 printed an article questioning the government on its food supply policy and demanding an immediate reply. It also questioned the government on the suppression of newspapers and asked for a reply within 24 hours.

On Qavam's appointment:

Immediately upon the resignation of the Soheily cabinet, a Majlis delegation was sent to Hossein Pirnia. . . . Upon the refusal of Pirnia and after the Majlis had expressed its informal approval on August 1 by a vote of 51 out of 87 deputies present, the Shah invited Ahmad Qavam to form a cabinet. Qavam immediately assumed his duties while engaged in forming his cabinet, which was presented to the Majlis August 9. The Majlis gave the Qavam cabinet a vote of confidence on August 13 of 109 out of 116 deputies present. . . . The cabinet formed by Qavam is perhaps the most adequate in both ability and prestige of any formed since the fall of Shah Reza ushered in a pseudo-democratic system. . . . Qavam, now 70 years of age and considered a leading elder statesman, has had a colorful career. His return to power after two decades on the shelf is welcomed by the people generally, since he

> represents a complete break with the unpopular Shah Reza regime. Qavam . . . was Governor of Khorrasan in 1918, was arrested in 1921 by persons responsible for the coup d'état but shortly after released, became Prime Minister in 1921, and headed the cabinet in which Reza Khan was Minister of War. Arrested in 1923 for an alleged plot against the life of Reza Khan, his estates were sequestered and he was exiled to Europe (apparently Reza Khan had not learned at that early stage of his career to dispose as quietly and efficiently of opponents as in later days when his technique became highly perfected). Having been granted amnesty, he returned several years later to Tehran, built a beautiful house (with what funds it is not clear since his estates had been taken) and lived in retirement, the while keeping his political eye peeled but his hands clean. Qavam is considered to be able and strong in spite of his age, but ambitious and somewhat unscrupulous. It is even said that he aspires to greater position than that which he holds at present. Of a religious turn of mind, he may be expected to play in somewhat with the mollas but it seems probable that he will be able to control them. It is interesting to note that he was Prime Minister when Millspaugh arrived; he states, in fact, that it was through him that American advisers were brought to Iran and an oil concession was granted to an American oil company. His policy at present seems to be pro-American and cooperation with the United States and bringing of American advisers in all lines a cornerstone of his policy. He is popular with the Russians but the British appear no more than lukewarm to him and he in turn could hardly be described as pro-British. . . . The Prime Minister very wisely refrained from drawing up a long, impressive program. . . . Instead he faced the problem with realism, limiting his program to three essential points on which he must succeed or fall. These are: 1. Full observance of the interests of the country in foreign policy; application of the Treaty of Alliance and other treaties in vigor, notably intimate collaboration with nations whose interests are closely allied with those of Iran. 2. Amelioration and maintenance of security in the entire country. 3. Insuring the food and pharmaceutical supply for the entire population. . . . The Qavam Government is of more than average strength, capability and integrity but it faces a gigantic task. It is most unfortunate, and not at all its fault, that it should have to face the present violent public criticism in the matter of the arrests mentioned above. This might conceivably result in the fall of the Qavam Government, which would be most unfortunate at the present critical time.

Qavam also faced violent criticism over the trial of former police officials who, thanks to Foroughi, were to be spared the gallows. Dreyfus on August 11, 1942 (Dispatch 322, 891.00/1914):

> The current trial of the ex-police chief General Mokhtari and 16 other subordinate police officials, I have the honor to inform the Department, is deeply stirring the Iranian public and contributing to the general feeling of unrest in the country. I had occasion in despatch 209 of February 12, 1942, to call the Department's attention to the fact that General Mokhtari and other police officials had been arrested and held for trial and I indicated that popular feeling was running high against all persons responsible for atrocities and injustices committed during the regime of Shah Reza. Feeling against Mokhtari and the other accused is being whipped up by a vindictive and irresponsible press until the public is literally crying for blood. Particular indignation is being expressed that the trials are being conducted by a special court set up about 1928 to deal with cases of embezzlement and bribery by government officials, a court which cannot by law hand down death sentences. The press is demanding that the cases be transferred to the criminal courts, which are permitted to give death sentences, and a petition to this effect has been introduced into the Majlis by a number of deputies.

The penultimate part of the dispatch reads:

> This surging and seething of the spirit is a sign of the times in Iran; it springs from the chain of events following on the invasion of Iran in August, 1941. Humiliated by the invasion of the country by the dreaded Russians and the hated British, overcome by a feeling of impotence at his inability to cope successfully with pressing problems, dissatisfied by the treatment meted out by the occupying powers, unable to grasp the meaning or method of the democratic processes into which he has willy-nilly been plunged, surrounded by grafting and inefficient politicians, observing the lack of security and disruption of internal life and now faced with severe food shortage, the average Iranian has perhaps sought solace and compensation in vindictive outcry against those connected with the former regime. Iran has, in short, not taken well to democratic processes. The Majlis has played politics to the detriment of the interests of the country in the many political crises which it has itself helped to aggravate; bribery and graft among government officials has reached a high, or rather a low, point; the press has degenerated into an instrument for personal gain with little regard for the welfare of the people and without thought of social responsibility; and the people have drunk deep of disillusionment and despair.

The final part reads:

> We should, I feel, bear in mind this surly state of Iranian temper in considering our plans for the coming difficult months. As the Germans move ever nearer Iran's borders, the tendency is clearly for pro-German elements to become more active and articulate and for smoldering hatreds to burst into flame. Already there have been isolated incidents, such as attacks on British soldiers, events relatively unimportant in themselves but foreshadowing things to come. I have ventured to predict in recent cables and despatches that rioting, acts of personal vengeance, and perhaps a coup d'état will take place if and when the Germans arrive at or near Baku. I see no reason to change that view at present.

In a memorandum to Assistant Secretary Berle and Under Secretary Welles, dated September 4, 1942, Alling wrote:

> The attached despatch no. 322, August 11, 1942, from Tehran is interesting, primarily because of the Minister's statement that the Iranian people are in a surly mood which might lead to serious repercussions as the Germans approach the borders of Iran. . . . I think you will agree that this points out very clearly the urgent advisability of placing Americans in strategic positions in the Iranian Government, and, in particular, shows the necessity of sending a military mission to observe and, if possible, check any internal plots in the Iranian Army which might lead to the coup d'état that Mr. Dreyfus fears. I am calling this to the attention of the appropriate officer in the Operations Division of the War Department, Colonel J.E. Upton, Chief of the Africa-Middle East Section.

On August 31, 1942, Dreyfus comments on the deteriorating security as Germans advanced in the Caucasus and North Africa (Dispatch 337, 891.00/1919):

> The internal security situation in Iran remains unsatisfactory. It might be supposed, in the absence of sensational developments such as those reported in previous despatches, as for example Kurdish depredations in Rezaieh area, organized banditry in Khorassan, and large-scale fighting in southern Kurdistan, that there has been a general improvement in the situation. I do not believe that this is the case. On the contrary, there seems to be a strong and increasing undercurrent of unrest among

> the tribes and the masses. Rebellion against Government authority, inherent in the tribal spirit, was chased underground by Shah Reza but not killed. Tribal defiance has grown as the central Government has shown itself incapable of reestablishing its authority. The tribes have steadily strengthened their control over isolated regions until it is now almost secure, particularly in the Kashkai area south of Shiraz, Kurdistan north of Baneh and Saqiz and the more inaccessible parts of the Bakhtiari country, Luristan and Kerman. Government inability to assert authority in these remote regions derives from several factors—the breakdown in army morale as a result of the events of last year, lack of adequate leadership, immobility of the army forces due to lack of transport, general weakness of the central Government, the serious food situation which has made the masses more unruly and Government forces less loyal and hatred of the British and Russians which has grown in the twelve months of occupation and rankled in the Iranian spirit. The masses have been favorably impressed with German victories and adversely affected not only by allied defeats but also by the weakness of British policy in Iran. Latent dissatisfaction and hatred come ever nearer the surface as German victories continue and as the Germans approach Iranian soil. This crescendo of dissatisfaction and hatred may be expected to grow to fortissimo proportions in the coming weeks as the German threat to Iran becomes more real. It seems to me not unlikely that it will manifest itself in riots, general disorder, rebellion and acts of violence against foreigners and Christians. The position of the Christian communities as indicated in my despatch No. 298, dated June 30, 1942, is especially dangerous.

Bullard-Qavam Exchange on Wheat

In addition to resisting British demands for the arrest of Iranians suspected of pro-Axis activities, Qavam was involved in a not-so-friendly exchange with the British Minister over the supply of wheat. Soon after, there was another currency dispute, as well as friction over the matter of housing in Tehran. Dreyfus' report entitled "Wheat Situation in Iran," is dated September 18, 1942 (Dispatch 350, 891.5018/9):

> I have the honor to enclose copies of (1) a letter of August 24 addressed by the British Minister to the Prime Minister, (2) the Prime Minister's reply of August 26, (3) the British Minister's latest communication to the Prime Minister dated September 3 and (4) a memorandum prepared by the British Legation official in charge of wheat matters. These letters, read together with the Legations telegrams . . .

> will, it is hoped give the Department a clear picture of the background and present status of this important and difficult wheat problem. The Department has approved of a course of action requiring the Iranians to put their domestic house in order by enforcing the hoarding laws and making every human endeavor to get possession of stocks of wheat in the country before turning to us for additional supplies. There are signs that the new Prime Minister and Mr. Ardelan, the Minister of Food, are taking a much more positive and energetic line in this regard than did the Soheily cabinet. The task, however, particularly in a country like Iran, is a gigantic one and it is scarcely to be hoped that all of the hoarded wheat will come to light. I remarked in my telegram No. 271 that it was unlikely that any substantial part of the surplus wheat in Azerbaijan would find its way to Tehran. However, an effort in this direction is being made by the Allied Consular representatives in Tabriz, which gives some hope of success since the Soviet Consul General is taking part in the démarches. I have asked Consul Kuniholm to do all he can in this regard.

The latter part of the dispatch reads:

> There seems little doubt to me that the Iranians should have been able, given a fair crop and the fact that the country is normally self-sufficient in wheat, to get along until the next crop year without outside help. However, there have been many impediments in the way—disturbed conditions in the rural areas, a weak policy on the part of the government, occupation of the north by the Soviets, disrupted transport system and a mania for hoarding which the peasants and landowners learned by a dint of bitter experience. It is no good telling the Iranians what they should have been able to do; one must face realities. It seems clear beyond question to me that war goods cannot be carried through a starving countryside. An excellent example of this was provided a few days ago when Colonel Shingler and other officers of the American Persian Gulf Command came to Tehran urgently to endeavor to arrange for the delivery of wheat to workmen employed by us in the south of Iran. Without bread in this country, work stops. I have high hopes that Mr. Sheridan, who should arrive in Tehran late in this month, will be able to render effective assistance in this matter.

In his letter of August 19, 1942 to Qavam, Bullard blames the Iranians for the wheat and transport shortage and tries to wiggle out of any obligation to assist in solving these problems, the Tri-Partite Treaty of Alliance notwithstanding:

In order that there may be no room for misunderstanding on the subject of wheat supplies and transport in Iran, I think it desirable to explain to Your Excellency the views of His Majesty's Legation in this matter. 2. In the Majlis recently, and in your conversation of the 15th August with Mr. Squire, Your Excellency mentioned the figure of 120,000 tons as the quantity of wheat which the Allies had undertaken to bring into the country. This figure, as was admitted to Your Excellency by Dr. Amini in Mr. Squire's presence, was only an estimate of what the Imperial Government considered its last year's requirements to be, but in the absence of reliable statistics of the country's production and consumption, it was not accepted by the Allies as necessarily correct. In actual fact the amount imported from all sources, as Dr. Amini's figures showed, was 90,000 tons and this assistance has enabled the Imperial Government to tide over the difficult period until the ripening of this year's harvest. 3. The situation for the present year is that the obligations of the Allies as defined by Article VII of the Treaty of Alliance which states that the Allies "will use their best endeavors to safeguard the economic existence of the Iranian people against the privations and difficulties arising out of the present regime." This claim involves the right and indeed a duty for the Allies first to ascertain what exactly are the economic means of the country and then to see how best they can be supplied. It does not necessarily mean that the Allies should use valuable shipping space for the importation of wheat supplies unless it is established beyond all controversy that these are really necessary.

4. It is true that the harvest in some parts of the country has not been good, but against this there must be set the following facts: (i) In many areas such as Azerbaijan and Isfahan the crops have been well above the average, while in Khorassan they have never been better, and a rough estimate by our Consul-General in Meshed gives the surplus as over 40,000 tons. (ii) In other areas, notably Gurgan and in some parts of the Hamadan district, the areas sown with wheat are more extensive than they have been for many years. (iii) Last year's crops were excellent, and would, under ordinary circumstances have easily sufficed for the country's needs. There should, therefore, have been in the country at the present moment a surplus from last year of at least 80,000 tons, the equivalent of Allied imports, and in spite of the extensive smuggling over the Western frontiers, for which the Iranian Government cannot escape all responsibility, a great part of this surplus must still exist. 5. In the absence of reliable statistics, therefore, it is reasonable to assume that the country will have sufficient surplus for the greater part, if not the whole, of the present year, and Your Excellency will

doubtless agree that, before calling on the Allies for assistance from abroad, it is the duty of the Imperial Government to do all in its power to obtain these vital supplies by the strict application of the Hoarding Regulations, by energetic action to collect the proprietor's share of the harvest, by offering sufficient inducement to cultivators to sell any stocks they may hold to the Government and by the institution of rationing in order to conserve the country's supplies. . . .

6. The problem of transport needs to be tackled on the same lines. The UKCC have only hired about one-quarter of the total number of lorries in the country, but there is as yet little sign that any effort has been made by the Imperial Government to organize or in any way regulate the use of the remaining three quarters. Surely it is unreasonable to ask that the UKCC should come to the help of the Imperial Government until this has been done. In actual fact the UKCC have already given a great deal of assistance to the Imperial Government and I am happy to hear that the organization of all Iranian civil transport is now being taken seriously in hand. An Allied Transport Board has also been proposed which will, I hope, be able to solve this most difficult problem. In this connection may I also draw Your Excellency's attention to the necessity of dealing with the question of touring cars as well as with that of heavier lorries. Reports are constantly reaching me that the work of provincial administrations is seriously hampered by the inability of the Central Government to supply tires for the essential tours of many of its officials. Particularly is this the case in the Kermanshah Ustan, where not only the officials of the Finance and Amlak Departments in Shahabad are unable to do their work for lack of transport, but the Farmandars and even the Ustandar himself are immobilized for the same reason. 7. May I also invite Your Excellency's attention to my letter No. 1159 of the 27th Khordad (17th June) to Monsieur Soheily, on the subject of the maximum use of animal transport, and urge that all possible steps should be taken to supplement the available motor transport by the greatest possible employment of whatever animals are available in the country or can be obtained from the neighbouring territories.

8. If these problems are tackled with energy and good will, I am confident that it will be possible to overcome all difficulties. May I add that His Majesty's Legation are at all times ready to do anything in their power to assist the Imperial Government in order that the Allied Powers may achieve victory in the present struggle at the earliest possible moment. Yours sincerely (sgd) R. W. Bullard.

In Qavam's reply of August 26, 1942, it is made clear that despite the recent harvest Iran was on the verge of a very grave wheat and transport crisis:

> I thank you for your letter No. 1232 of the 28th Mordad (19th August) giving explanations in respect to the wheat needed by Iran and I have the honor to set forth the following points. The figure of 120,000 tons which was given as quantity needed by Iran in the course of the conversations with Mr. Squire was fixed as the result of studies into the 1321 situation made by the Department concerned: as Mr. Squire himself will be aware, in the course of the numerous conversations between himself and the Ministry of Finance and in the course of the explanations which were given about the Government's policy in the matter of wheat collection, the situation in respect of the present wheat crop of Iran was clearly explained; but although a repetition may be a source of trouble to Your Excellency, I think it necessary, in order to remove any possibility of misunderstanding, to give Your Excellency a brief summary of the facts of the situation.
>
> The practice of the Government in the wheat question since the wheat monopoly was introduced has been to obtain undertakings for the handing over of their surpluses from landowners all over the country and to allot the surpluses of areas which supply more than they need to assure the needs of areas which produce less than their consumption requirements. Accordingly, since both in buying and selling the Government takes the surpluses of the landowners only and does not touch the peasant's share, it has to do in reality with only part of the country's output and consumption. In order to achieve the object in view the Department-General of Cereals prepares in the month of Khordad (22 May – 21 June) before the harvest is lifted a forecast of the wheat crop; this forecast is prepared in accordance with the information which is collected from the provinces about the condition of the crops; and a programme for the transport of wheat from surplus to deficiency areas is then drawn up on the basis of this forecast. Last year the country's output was, as Your Excellency has pointed out in your letter, not bad on the whole, but in most of the wheat producing areas in which the lifting of harvest begins in the month of Shahrivar (22 Aug – 22 Sept) the crops on the threshing floors were seriously damaged owing to the events of Shahrivar (August '41), and a great part of them disappeared; subsequently Government officials were unable despite of strenuous efforts to move even the quantity which it was possible to collect owing to lack of transport; thus a part of the difficulties of supplying

Tehran, Isfahan and other towns with bread last year and at the beginning of this year arose out of the events of Shahrivar.

At that time the Iranian Government requested HBM's Government to provide assistance from abroad to make up the deficit to the extent of at least 150,000 tons of wheat to make up the deficit but unfortunately they were not successful in delivering more than 80,000 tons, including the quantity delivered to the Russians, owing to shipping difficulties. As has been repeatedly explained to Mr. Squire, one of the essential conditions of success in collecting wheat and preventing hoarding is to have a sufficient quantity of wheat in Government depots and this was the Government's object in insisting on the provision of sufficient quantity of wheat last year. But unfortunately the bread situation in Tehran, as Your Excellency will have observed, shows with what difficulties we are faced even now at the beginning of the harvest and the difficulties of the situation is itself a powerful factor causing anxiety in the population and encouraging hoarders and opens the door to every sort of abuse; whereas if the Government had a reserve of not less than 20,000 tons in the Tehran depot it would be able, without causing an uncalled for rise in the price of wheat, to collect easily all the surpluses and to proceed with the outmost severity against hoarders.

2. In your letter Your Excellency referred to the balance of last year's crop and assessed the surplus of Khorassan at 40,000 tons, but you will recall that similar arguments were adduced from the British Consular officials at Isfahan and Hamadan and that finally, in order to establish the facts of the case and to make clear that the Government had made the necessary efforts to collect surpluses, permission was given to Colonel French to buy such quantities as he could in Hamadan and Isfahan through his own officials acting with the official approval of the Iranian Government; if you will ask Mr. Squire you will find that the quantities purchased by these officials were negligible compared to the figures estimated by the British Consular officers; so much so that Mr. Squire himself agreed that these estimates were baseless. Your Excellency may therefore rest assured that the figure of 40,000 tons given for the surplus over consumption needs in Khorassan is based on no foundation.

Your Excellency will naturally be aware that at least 10,000 tons of Azerbaijan wheat used to be allotted every year for the consumption of Tehran, whereas last year, owing to the lack of security in that region and to the opening of the Iranian frontier on the Turkish and Iraqi sectors, the bread supply of Tabriz was assured only with the greatest difficulty and the situation in that city is still very difficult. I am sure that Your Excellency will agree that the Iranian Government could not have done more to check smuggling than it was able to do with the means at its disposal.

3. With regard to the collection of this year's crop the estimates made in the month of Khordad of the current year forecast the total to be collected at about 194,000 tons and the total consumption at 342,000 tons, leaving a deficiency of 148,000 tons to be supplied from abroad. Of course the estimate of the quantity to be collected is a maximum figure, and since reports from the provinces indicate that owing to the dryness of the year a part of the harvest has totally failed, the amount which is left is so small that we may only with difficulty reach the estimated figure; nevertheless extraordinary efforts will be made to collect the crop by every possible means and in order that the peasant's surplus, with which the Government ordinarily has nothing to do, shall not fall into the hands of hoarders and hucksters, orders have been given that it shall be purchased by means of exchanges against monopoly goods and through merchants offering free market price; however, owing to the dryness of the year and unsatisfactory weather conditions, a deficit of the quantity indicated above is certain and energetic steps should now be taken to send this quantity to Iran; I therefore trust that Your Excellency, in order to assist the Government in its measures designed to collect the entire cereal crop, will take urgent steps to have a quantity of the wheat required shipped as soon as possible; Your Excellency may rest assured that the extension of this assistance will not merely not cause the Government to diminish its strenuous efforts to collect the harvest and to combat hoarding, but will fortify it in its resolve.

4. With regard to transport, as you are aware, the Government has instituted energetic measures and it is hoped that with the formation of the Transport Committee this difficult problem which has a fundamental effect on the whole economic life of the country will be solved in a satisfactory manner, but it must not be forgotten that the regulation of the transport problem and the satisfaction of the country's fundamental needs depends on the delivery of a sufficient quantity of lorries and tires. Since most of the lorries already in the country are laid up for lack of tires and a number were destroyed during the events of Shahrivar and a number are at the disposal of the UKCC, the transport needs of the country cannot be met without sufficient help from abroad. Accordingly I have the honor to request Your Excellency to extend your

full assistance in this matter also, in order that no crisis may arise in the provision of the country's food supplies and in the satisfaction of the country's other needs. Yours sincerely, (Sgd.) Ahmad Qavam.

Bullard's follow up memorandum of September 3, 1942:

Thank you for your letter No. 11082 of 4th Shahrivar (26th August). There is one point in Your Excellency's letter to which I must reply; that is the reference in para. 2 to Brigadier French's experiment in Hamadan and Isfahan. It is true that this did not meet with the success it was hoped for, but reports that have since been received show that this was not due to any lack of wheat in the areas concerned, but to other causes. In Isfahan the holders of stocks were unwilling to sell at the Government price to which Brigadier French was limited, and I have still to hear that any action is being taken against them under the Anti-Hoarding Regulations. But the main cause of failure was obstruction in the Finance Department itself in spite of Mr. Bader's personal orders that all possible assistance was to be given. Holders of stocks in Hamadan and Kermanshah districts were willing and eager to sell their grain, but in many cases were prevented by Finance Department officials from doing so, and those few who, in order to comply with Monsieur Bader's instructions, were allowed to sell to Brigadier French, had first to bribe Finance Department officials in order to obtain this permission. All these reports agree that large amounts of last year's wheat existed and still exist in these districts. 2. I am very glad to know that strenuous efforts are now being made to collect the greatest possible quantity of wheat and to hear from Mr. Squire of the energy being displayed by Mr. Ardalan in his difficult task. I hope that these efforts, backed by Your Excellency's firm attitude towards hoarders will meet with complete success.

Rising Anxiety over Wheat and British Propaganda

Sheridan arrived in Tehran on September 26, 1942. Dreyfus on October 30, 1942 (Dispatch 365, 891.24/309):

I have the honor to enclose a copy of a letter addressed to me by Mr. Joseph P. Sheridan, adviser to the Iranian Ministry of Supply, concerning the efforts to insure Iran's wheat supply. . . . Mr. Sheridan has taken hold of his job with energy. He has surrounded himself with a group of young Iranians, who seem to have become imbued with his

> restless energy and drive. It is interesting to note that Mr. Sheridan's impressions, admittedly based on very short experience and observation, are that many young Iranians are intelligent and capable, responding to forceful leadership with loyalty and action. Even the Minister of Supply, Mehdi Farrokh, has been working from 10 to 14 hours a day and Mr. Sheridan reports that he has had his Minister's full support as well as the backing of Qavam. It will be most interesting to observe, and I shall report in due course, whether Mr. Sheridan retains these favorable impressions, which are contrary to those obtained by so many foreigners on arrival here.

Dreyfus next discusses the wheat and transport situation:

> Iran's primary food problem is wheat, for the staple and almost exclusive diet of the people is bread. The main phase of this problem is the uncovering and transportation to urban centers of surplus wheat, much of which has found its way into the hands of hoarders and speculators. By surplus wheat is meant not wheat in surplus of the needs of the country but that part in excess of the needs of the peasants and land owners for their own needs and for seed for the coming season. This phase is aggravated by the lack of motor transport but I hope this problem is on the way to being solved. An Iranian-American-British transport board has been organized and is now engaged in drawing up a basic decree on transport, which will give the committee broad powers to organize and control transport and will place all truck transport directly in their hands. Already the Iranian transport organization set up in the Ministry of Supply under this committee is functioning with some 130 trucks and it is hoped that this number can be increased considerably if the decree is published and trucks are no longer permitted to do unessential work. All trucking, in fact, will be done either by the Iranian Government or by one of the allied bodies, such as UKCC or Iransovtrans. If, therefore, tires and trucks are forthcoming from the United States as promised, there is reason to hope that wheat can be moved. It will, however, be difficult to accomplish this if the allies, notably UKCC and Iransovtrans continue to "gobble up" Iran's tiny resources of civilian trucks. For example, the UKCC now controls 1200 trucks, Iransovtrans 400 and the Iranian Government only 130.
>
> An important angle of this question concerns the willingness and ability of the Government to obtain control of wheat. This includes, first, finding the wheat; secondly, requiring provincial officials to permit its

transport to Tehran since they often feel that their own food for the winter is being taken away from them; and, thirdly, making hoarders and speculators disgorge. The Qavam Government has shown considerable energy in this direction but it is probable that more drastic action will be necessary. Mr. Sheridan a few days ago found 800 tons of wheat in the hands of four important persons in the Tehran area and at once obtained possession of it. One of these hoarders, General Khodayar, a very large land owner and possessor of some 15 villages, was relieved of 200 tons, and was, in Mr. Sheridan's words "pilloried in the press." It is hoped that the wide publicity given his hoarding activities will deter others and make them voluntarily disgorge. An amusing sidelight of this hoarding angle was that of getting the Queen-mother to give up her wheat, a case which Mr. Sheridan and the Minister of Food handled very astutely. Rather than denounce the Royal family as hoarders, the Minister of Food called on the Shah, explained the critical food situation and allowed the Shah the "out" of offering his mother's 200 tons of wheat as a gift for public welfare. Newspapers next day played up the gift of the Royal family as a highly patriotic and unselfish act.

At this point international politics enters into the picture. As I indicated in my telegram No. 339, October 23, it is reasonably established that the British, Russians and Poles have been buying up Iranian food on a scale which has been detrimental to the Iranian food situation. As I stated in this telegram, the Russians are now asking for 5,000 tons of wheat, 15,000 tons of barley and 30,000 tons of rice. It is not at all certain that this will be a final demand, as the Russians pretend, for already they have asked Mr. Sheridan for 15,000 tons of wheat. . . .

I have taken the view in recent months that a wheat shortage would probably develop this winter and I see no reason to alter this view. It may be that there is sufficient wheat in the country to meet Iran's needs but I see little hope of getting it into the urban centers in time and sufficient quantities to prevent a serious shortage. There were many adverse factors this year—the harvest last year was harmed by the invasion of the country, sowing was limited last fall by the unstable and insecure conditions, spring rains were poor, crops in the south were very bad, transport has been lacking, peasants and landowners have hoarded in honest fear of shortage, speculators and others have hoarded to obtain higher prices, and the allies have bought to some extent. The British and Mr. Sheridan are now swinging around to this view, especially in view of the open Russian purchases of grain. I am, therefore, of the studied opinion that we should begin wheat shipments to Iran as soon as possible, particularly in view of the months which must necessarily expire between the time of shipment and receipt in Tehran.

Another interesting phase of the food problem is that of distribution after the wheat is found and milled into flour, a phase which Mr. Sheridan discusses in his letter. Mr. Sheridan found a most unsatisfactory condition in this regard upon his arrival, flour being mixed with all sorts of extraneous materials. Bread was poorly baked, loaves were underweight and sold in bakeries to mobs of undisciplined and riotous customers. He found that the public usually paid two or more times the legal rate of one rial per kilo. His plan is to fix the price at two rials a kilo, give honest weight and good quality, and to mix wheat flour up to 30 per cent of barley flour when the latter can be obtained. To prevent the psychologically bad bread lines and riots, he plans to bake the bread at night so that customers will not have to wait, as is now the case, while the bread is being baked. The bread would then be taken out of the bakeries and sold by the police to customers who would be required to form queues (this would perhaps be the first queue ever formed in Iran). I am constrained to observe that in spite of Mr. Sheridan's efforts, bread is still of poor quality and queues are still seen in front of bread shops. Yesterday, in fact, there was a bread riot in which a group of soldiers almost destroyed a bakery. It remains, therefore, to be seen whether his measures will produce positive results.

The press and public are much perturbed over the wheat situation and generally take the line that the allies are responsible for this and other Iranian woes. *Nabard* of October 24 wailed that truckloads of bread are taken away by the allies in the very face of hungry Iranians, who devour the very dust of such bread trucks. *Nabard* was suppressed by the Government the following day for a series of violent articles of this kind, but particularly for an open letter to the Minister of State Casey, who was visiting Tehran, in which the allies were taken severely to task. *Javan* of October 26 printed a leading editorial called "On to Chaos," criticizing the Government for the bread situation and stating that people are saying that famine is imminent. Deputy Safavi in the Majlis on October 16 called attention to Mr. Sheridan's statement that the wheat supply of the country is assured until the next harvest and stated that within one week of this statement a most serious shortage had developed. *Kushesh* on October 19 stated: "We will never ask why the allies are providing Greece with wheat. Never, for we admire

> this action to save the Greeks from starvation. But we say sell us a sufficient quantity of wheat to save us from this crisis." *Setareh* on October 19 referred to allied promises to furnish necessary supplies to Iran and added "there is a Persian proverb which says 'the patient bitten by a snake will die before they bring the antidote from Iraq.'" . . . *Ettelaat*, always more dignified and restrained than the other papers, in a leading article on October 17 stated that Tehran had been almost without bread for several days and a famine was imminent. The editor called on the allies to furnish Iran 100,000 tons of wheat, particularly since they are giving Turkey 200,000 tons.

As noted, on October 21, 1942, the Soviet Government had formally requested to purchase 5,000 tons of wheat, 15,000 tons of barley and 30,000 tons of rice. Additional information on this and other matters is found in Sheridan's letter to Dreyfus dated October 24, 1942. Excerpts follow:

> From all figures given to me by British Consular representatives, our own field workers and private sources, it appears that the maximum wheat surplus possible of export from the various provinces to Teheran is as follows: Azerbaijan East & West, 35,000 tons; Khorassan, 15,000 tons; Kordestan, 3,000 tons; Kermanshah, 3,000 tons; Teheran area, 2,000 tons; Arak, 1,000 tons. We will note that I make no reference to any of the Southern Provinces. Quite frankly, I cannot organize during this present Autumn crisis any collection of surplus wheat from any Southern Areas for Teheran. All of the Southern Provinces are bordering on a famine stage more particularly Khuzistan, Fars, Kerman and Southern Baluchestan. Northern Baluchestan I am assured by the Governor will probably be taken care of from Zabol Area. From a political point of view the Teheran situation is the most pressing problem today; from the humanitarian point of view all of Southern Iran is equally serious.
>
> I have been in the country exactly 4 weeks. Immediately upon my arrival I was . . . confronted, as we were, with the pressing problem of Teheran (and) we have been compelled to put practically 100 percent of our time in feeding the 700,000 people of Teheran. . . . If we are permitted by the authorities occupying the northern half of the country to purchase wheat and without competition from their own purchasing agents and also granted the back loading facility of both railways and lorries I am convinced that we can carry through the winter in Tehe-

> ran. In view, however, of the demands made upon this Ministry on Wednesday the 21st instant for arrangements to supply the Russian Army with food-stuffs including wheat, barley and rice I now feel that the Allied nations must seriously consider their responsibility to Iran in so far as the import into the country of wheat and barley. . . . In conclusion I wish to assure Your Excellency that I am taking the necessary steps to open soup kitchens probably in the bakery shops themselves throughout the city at a fortnight's notice. I am planning on a diet in a form of soup or vegetable stew consisting principally of potatoes, lentils and beans. At the present moment the crops of all these commodities are reasonably abundant but I am informed that the British Army has been steadily purchasing these items for export to Iraq and I have written to the Commercial Secretary of the British Legation regarding this matter on the 20th instant. Finally there is still one other possibility of relieving the situation. The rice crop in the two Northern Provinces has been excellent. If no obstacles are placed in our way either as to quantity permissible of purchase, and its transport to Teheran, the use of the rice flour which can be steadily milled in our own mill will relieve the situation considerably. However during the last week the price of all vegetable commodities including rice have risen tremendously. Rice is a monopoly of the Government and I am giving instruction at once that the entire rice crop must be purchased and forwarded to Teheran less the requirements of the northern provinces and of the necessary needs of the Russian Army.

The British had embarked on a propaganda campaign. Excerpt from the British Legation's "News Bulletin" of September 9, 1942, and entitled, "Iran has plentiful food and yet many people believe that there is a critical shortage." It reads:

> Great Britain has imported over 64,900,000 kilos of foodstuffs into Iran, and the harvests this year have produced an adequate supply. German propaganda asserts that there is a food shortage, owing to British consumption here, and this story is spread by a number of people in Iran. Is there any truth in this? None. On the contrary, apart from the imports mentioned above, all staple foodstuffs for the British and the Poles are also imported from abroad. Why is this story supported by certain people in the country? For this reason: that there is a large class of men cornering, hoarding and speculating in wheat. If people knew that these men were deliberately starving their compatriots they would be torn to pieces. So, to conceal their crimes, they support German scare rumours that the shortage is caused by the Brit-

> ish. But their day of retribution is coming fast. Mr. Churchill and Mr. Wilkie were both disgusted to find such practices in a distressed country.

The "News Bulletin" of November 11, 1942, has a piece entitled, "The Food Situation in Iran":

> Before the negotiations between Iran and her Allies are concluded one point should be made clear. The solution of the food problem in Iran, as for almost any problem, should rest on a basis of simplicity: simplicity in deed and thought. The landlord-speculators, who are largely responsible, have helped to bring about this situation by trying to be too clever and complicated. Instead of being satisfied with a normal profit they try to become millionaires. They become millionaires only by selling at a fantastic price. Having obtained these fantastic prices on the Black Market they complain that they are afraid of inflation: the invariable result of extravagant speculation. Complicated action such as this always tends to be inconsistent, and the complicated explanations of these evildoers are equally inconsistent. The British import 70,000,000 kilos of grain. The landlord-speculators use it, not to feed their country, but to speculate with. To avert suspicion they produce the most complicated explanations: that the British having imported this grain have now exported it! Why they should do this is explained by further wild contortions of the truth, incomprehensible to all but their inventors. Then comes a new situation. The landlord-speculators, terrified at the situation they have created, appeal to Britain for more grain. So, at the moment, the great speculators, declaring that Britain the importer has exported all the grain, ask Britain to import some more. Something wrong there. With one hand they scrawl a swastika on the wall, and hold out the other for more grain from Britain. Is it not time that these people were dropped by parachute over Germany, their spiritual home?

These were forwarded by Dreyfus with a report dated November 19, 1942, and entitled "British Propaganda in Tehran on Food Problem" (Dispatch 386 and enclosure, 891.48/322):

> I have the honor to enclose excerpts from two propaganda bulletins of the British Legation Public Relations Bureau in Tehran touching on the food situation. These propaganda items are most interesting in showing the distortion of facts to which the British in Tehran have resorted in order to present themselves in a more favorable light and to overcome to some extent the strong feeling against them which has devel-

oped in Iranian minds. Their endeavors in this regard, however, have been almost useless for the Iranian is not a particularly gullible individual and a preconceived prejudice once developed in his stubborn mind is difficult to eradicate. The British Legation publicity department consisting of some 80 persons has, at least so it appears to me, done more harm than good to the British cause in Tehran.

Gold for Wheat Proposal

On November 5, 1942, Assistant Secretary E.V. Rostow had addressed a memorandum on the wheat situation in Iran to various divisions in the State Department (Memorandum, 891.24/328):

> The attached excerpt from a personal letter from Mr. Kidd, representative of lend-lease affairs in Iran, states his proposal that we use gold to get wheat out of hoarding. I should appreciate your views on these questions: Should we sell gold to the Iranians for rials, on their undertaking to use it for the purchase of wheat? Should we have the USCC buy the wheat for gold? . . . Should we get the Russians in their purchasing, to buy wheat for gold?

Philip Kidd's letter to Oscar Cox is dated American Legation, Tehran, October 19, 1942, and reads in part:

> Food conditions in Iran are very bad—not because actual shortage of wheat but because of hoarding. The people still remember that about one quarter of the population died of starvation twenty five years ago. There is also wheat hoarding by speculators that the government isn't strong enough to go after. There are some signs of famine already in Ahwaz and Shiraz. If we had gold we might be able to get a lot of wheat out of the hands of speculators but not out of the hands of people who are afraid of starving. A lot of people are going to starve in this country before the buds come out next spring. As far as I can find out there is only one thing people would rather hoard than wheat—gold. I have talked to Sir Arthur Rucker about it; also to Walter, the Head of the Imperial Bank; also to Dreyfus—none of us know how much wheat we would get by offering gold but we all agree that we would get some, possibly a lot, and that it would save lives and shipping space. I have been told that it is silly for me to think of getting our Government to provide the gold because of the ramifications involved. If gold will save shipping or save lives (and it will out here) I don't know why we should be so God Damn dumb or so God Damn stupid to insist on

> saving it to put in our teeth. If it is to be done it must be done soon because the winter will soon be on us and we won't be able to move wheat. If you don't think I am crazy on this idea take a crack at it and shoot me a cable. It would be a simple operation to handle. Maybe we could get the gold from Russia or South Africa.

General opinion was opposed. Cable from Cairo on December 14, 1942 (Telegram 2190, 891.24/323):

> Department's 1571, December 7, 6 p.m. Following from Fred Winant. "Use of gold to extract hoarded wheat has been much discussed subject in the Near East. . . . British opinion here divided on use of gold in Iran for that purpose. London opinion I understand questions advisability of proposal. . . . In our opinion approach should be directed against hoarding of wheat, applying greatly stiffened penalties against hoarding and seeing that those penalties are actually put into effect. So far as the terms of purchasing wheat are concerned we believe that the existing monetary system be used with appropriate grading in prices to encourage wheat coming out and to discourage wheat in hiding. General opinion would seem to be that gold cannot be restricted to dealings in wheat alone, that all commodities will tend to gold transactions and that such a situation existing in Iran would likely be duplicated in other nearby territories. Volume of gold on such a scale it is pointed out would be difficult in handling and transportation for quick operation."

Dreyfus on December 16, 1942 (Telegram 445, 891.24/324):

> Department's 362, December 7. All informed persons with whom I have discussed possible purchase of wheat with gold with exception of Kidd are of opinion it would be inadvisable. British Legation considered procedure but advised London against it. Main difficulties in way of scheme are: (1) It may render difficult collection of wheat in subsequent years except by payment in gold. (2) It might become necessary to extend gold purchase scheme to other articles in Iran and perhaps to other nearby countries. (3) It might have bad effect on rial. (4) It would be difficult to fix a gold price it is true that Iranians much prefer gold to paper but the seller can at present convert rial proceeds of his wheat sales into gold by purchase in open market. The extra inducement to the seller, therefore, would be amount of gold he is offered for wheat. Same thing could be achieved by raising rial price of wheat so that seller could purchase more gold sovereigns. British Legation feels that if gold is to be brought to Iran at all it would be preferable to sell

> in open market with idea of bringing gold price here down to nearer world level which might have effect of forcing down price level. A proposal along this line has been made to London. Kidd is still of opinion that plan is workable. He believes it involves psychological factors that have not been taken into consideration and that its disadvantages are far outweighed by good effects it would have. I have suggested that he prepare and forward a memorandum setting forth his views.

Matthews in London on January 22, 1943 (Telegram 605, 891.24/352):

> We called today on Waley at the Treasury to get Treasury's views on suggestion to buy Iranian grown wheat for gold. . . . It seems at first sight to be an attractive idea to conserve shipping space by transporting a ton of gold rather than some 26,000 tons of wheat if, as a result, an individual who otherwise would hoard wheat would, instead, hold gold. This idea which has been advanced not only in connection with the Middle East but in connection with North Africa and China as well has been given a great deal of consideration by Treasury. . . . Current British expenditures in India and the Middle East amount to as much as two billion dollars annually, financed by increasing the paper sterling holdings of these countries. . . . Treasury feels that much as it dislikes to increase British overseas liabilities to the extent of over two billion dollars annually it should be very chary about starting in these countries a demand to be paid in gold on the ground that at present neither dollars nor pounds are of any use because goods are unobtainable due to supply and shipping difficulties. Anything which is at all likely to undermine confidence in the local currencies would be, in the view of Treasury, very dangerous. . . . Treasury has learned of the suggestion that the United States might purchase wheat that is hoarded in Iran. As Treasury sees it, this would not be the right procedure for, if gold is once used to pay for commodities, the risk is at once increased of people declining to offer commodities for sale except for gold and the use of the local currency as a purchasing medium might increasingly decline and become discredited.

A subsequent proposal to import gold bars to be exchanged for Iranian gold coins, however, had caused great opposition because, apparently, the Iranians did not trust the purity of British bars. Schnare on February 12, 1943 (Telegram 165, 891.24/379):

> My 445, December 16. British Legation has obtained approval of British Treasury to a plan by which gold would be made available for circulation in Iran in hopes bringing down price of gold and hence of commodities and of countering inflation. Plan contemplates importation into Iran of British gold bars to be exchanged for gold coins held by Bank Mellie and forming part of cover for rial. Coins would be placed in circulation leaving Iran gold cover unchanged. Iranian press Majlis and people are protesting violently against the plan alleging British have ulterior motives harmful to Iran. As result of these protests bill was introduced yesterday which would prevent plan being carried out. British are indignant at this Iranian reaction to what they had intended a helpful gesture. Millspaugh is studying desirability and possible effects on Iranian finance and economy of any such scheme of circulating gold coins or small bars. Meantime, Department is requested to indicate whether American Government would be willing to make gold coins or very small bars available for this purpose.

Housing Shortage in Tehran

At about the same time as the gold controversy, the British desire to requisition housing in Tehran had further strained relations. Dreyfus on December 22, 1942 (Dispatch 412 and enclosures, 891.502/6):

> I have the honor to enclose copies of notes written to the Iranian Government by this and the British Legations suggesting that a commission be appointed to examine into the question of high rentals in Tehran with a view to preparing corrective legislation. The bidding of American and British military authorities for all available houses in Tehran has become so keen that rentals have been forced up to several times their former level. Fantastic rentals sometimes as high as $1500 a month, are asked for large premises suitable for housing military or civilian personnel or for use as offices, and prices continue to soar. It was considered necessary, in the interests of both the allied Governments and of Iran, to suggest to the Iranians that corrective measures be taken. I cannot but draw attention to the haughty and sarcastic overtone of the British note, which is a fair sample of the manner in which the British are accustomed to approach the Iranian Government. The second sentence contains a rebuke for the long delay in the Iranian answer to an earlier note. Paragraph two begins by venturing to believe the Iranian Ministry of Foreign Affairs was mistaken. This is followed by a most sarcastic statement to the effect that the Prime Minister is well aware of the fact that the enthusiasm of the deputies

for the allied cause is very great, a statement deliberately concocted to convey the opposite meaning.

Dreyfus' note of December 22, 1942, to Foreign Minister Saed points out the acute housing shortage and rising rents and adds:

> I venture to suggest to Your Excellency, in order to effect a remedy to this unsatisfactory situation, that a commission be named without delay to examine urgently into the matter with a view to drawing up corrective legislation. In making this suggestion, I am thinking mainly of aiding (the) Iranian economy and trust Your Excellency will take my recommendation in the light in which it is intended.

In contrast, Bullard's note to Qavam (No. 1345) of November 29, 1942, reads:

> In a memorandum No. 487 dated 22nd August, His Majesty's Legation suggested to the Minister for Foreign Affairs that the Imperial Iranian Government should make arrangements whereby property required urgently by the British Military Authorities should be requisitioned for them by the Iranian authorities, as is done in Iraq. After some two-and-a-half months the Minister for Foreign Affairs replied, in a memorandum No. 15917/1909, dated 9th November, that the laws of the country do not permit of such an arrangement and that to pass a new law might meet with difficulty in the Majlis. I venture to believe that the Ministry of Foreign Affairs are mistaken in supposing that a bill in the required sense would meet with difficulty in the Majlis. As Your Excellency is well aware the enthusiasm of the deputies for the cause of the United Nations is very great, and it is my opinion that they would welcome the opportunity to pass such a Bill into law, with a view to assisting the war effort of the United Nations and at the same time helping to keep the general level of rents from rising. I should therefore be glad if the question could be reconsidered and a speedy decision taken in the sense suggested in the original letter.

Dreyfus on January 9, 1943 (Telegram 31, 891.044/145):

> British military supported by British Legation are pressing Iranian Government to enact an emergency law giving the Iranian civil authorities power to requisition buildings and lands for use of Allied military authorities. British contend law is essential because Allied armies are

finding it almost impossible to obtain suitable quarters or offices and because inflation and competition have driven rents to fantastic levels. Law would give the Allied military authorities priority in renting (one) buildings completed after date of act (two) existing buildings not inhabited by owners and (three) buildings inhabited by owners if other suitable quarters can be found for them. Tenants would be evicted by Iranian authorities where necessary. Disputes over rental amounts would be settled by president of court of first instance. First British-Iranian meeting to discuss question was attended by two members of American military and by Kidd. I have neither taken part in discussions, nor delegated anyone to attend meetings. I am of opinion that Iranian Government will refuse to sponsor this law and that in any event the Majlis will almost certainly refuse to enact it. If the Allies insist on the law Qavam's position may be weakened and another political crisis precipitated. The matter if pressed may also have harmful effects on American-Iranian relations. I shall discuss question with General Connolly, Prime Minister and British Minister after which I shall report fully to Department.

Dreyfus on January 18, 1943 (Telegram 59, 891.044/146):

My 31, January 9. General Connolly informs me that although he is faced with serious housing shortage he is unalterably opposed to any show of force in obtaining properties or to putting pressure on Iranians to enact proposed requisitioning law. I am in full accord with his views. Prime Minister strongly opposed to project and states neither his government nor Majlis will support it. I do not believe British, in view of strong Iranian opposition and lack of active American support, will insist on enactment of this law. However British Minister has made it clear to me that British cannot accept continuance of present unsatisfactory housing situation and will be forced to take action on own initiative. This he said will probably consist of arbitrarily taking possession of properties for which they are negotiating and discussing fair rental with landlords at later date.

Chapter 14

Renewed Financial Dispute and Tripartite Food Declaration

Barely four months after the financial agreement of May 26, 1942, there was another currency crisis. Taking advantage of the acute wheat shortage, the British forced the Iranian government and Majlis to cede control of the note issue to a currency board. Having obtained an unlimited supply of rials, the Allies failed to deliver the promised wheat. With the ensuing hyperinflation, the burden of Allied military activities fell entirely on the Iranian people. The OSS report of February 11, 1943, entitled "Food in Iran," gives a useful introduction (Research and Analysis, 891.5018/22):

> By late October (1942) the bread shortage in Tehran was becoming acute since the Russians from their occupied area did not send to Tehran any of their excess wheat, 35,000 tons in Azerbaijan, and 15,000 tons in Khorassan. In addition the Russians wanted to buy in the open market. By mid-November things were critical, Sheridan had only a half day's supply of wheat in storage in Tehran. Deliveries to the capital from the provinces were slow, so deficient were transport facilities under Iranian control, and so poor their provincial management. The situation was aggravated by an influx of people from the provinces, convinced that at least Tehran would be supplied with sufficient bread. Sheridan prepared to set up soup kitchens in case of emergency, while the US put on unavailing pressure to have wheat moved from India.
>
> The problem of food supply and especially the cost of living have been greatly complicated by the financial dislocations attendant on the Al-

lied needs for rials within the country. As the legal limit for the issuance of notes was soon passed each government had to ask the Majlis to authorize extensions. By November 1942 Allied war expenditures had become 400,000,000 rials per month. Between August 1941 and October 1942 the note issue had increased from 1,600,000,000 to 3,000,000,000 rials, with the proposal then made that it be increased 2,000,000,000 more. Without adequate controls this naturally meant inflation. It also meant that the Majlis had a whip in hand for a certain amount of political jockeying. The British refused to move resolutely to alleviate the food situation until the government would give them unlimited rials for use in the country. Finally (on November 19, 1942) the Majlis conceded their control over the note issue, and the British agreed to the issuance of a Joint Food Declaration on the part of the Iranian, United Kingdom and United States governments. Control over the issuance of notes was delegated to a Note Reserve Control Committee, still dominated by a majority of Iranian representatives from the cabinet. Their decisions, however, need not be made public as were those of the Majlis, thus minimizing their inflationary effect. The British seemed satisfied and London pressed for the forwarding of grain to Iran from Iraq. But, for some reason, this did not arrive although later 5,000 tons were produced by the British from Ahwaz!

The Food Declaration was signed by the three parties on December 4, 1942. This declaration asserted that responsibility for feeding Iran lay with the government, but because of war's distress the US and UK agree to take measures guaranteeing sufficient bread until the 1943 harvest, provided Iran undertakes to carry out the recommendations of the American food adviser, including those pertaining to hoarding and rationing, as well as the recommendations of the Road Transport Committee! Cereals will be imported to the degree of proved need, but distribution rests with the Iranian government.

Dreyfus on September 11, 1942 (Telegram 228, 891.5151/239):

Another currency shortage has developed with Banque Mellie holding only 100 million rials which it wishes to hold as reserve. Iranians are reluctant to fulfill their promise to supply British with rials because they fear inflation. British insist Iranians live up to letter and spirit of signed agreement. Majlis last evening in secret session approved issue of 300,000,000 rials of new currency and it is thought open session tomorrow will give formal approval. This amount should suffice for allied needs for two or three months but solution is at best temporary.

> What Iranians need is long range financial policy providing for adequate note issue, price control and measures to prevent inflation.

The 300 million had lasted a month. Dreyfus on October 12, 1942 (Telegram 319, 891.5151/240):

> Reference my 288, September 11. Another of recurrent financial crisis has developed, the 300,000,000 rials issued in mid-September having become exhausted. Prime Minister has promised to introduce double urgent bill in Majlis at once for issue of 700,000,000 rials additional currency. British Minister and Soviet Ambassador and I have called separately on Prime Minister to impress on him absolute necessity of adequate supply of rials for allied war work in Iran. Iranians are reluctant to issue new currency because of their great fear of inflation. The threat of inflation in Iran is indeed real and little thought to checking it has been given. The arrival of the American financial mission would be most helpful in this respect. Allied monthly rial needs for war purposes are roughly as follows: American about 15,000,000 rials and steadily increasing; British about 300,000,000 rials; Soviets about 100,000,000 rials.

Proposal for Anglo-American Food Declaration

By mid-October 1942, there was a full blown crisis. Dreyfus on October 17, 1942 (Telegram 327, 891.00/1922):

> The political situation in Iran has suddenly deteriorated and position of Qavam Cabinet is precarious. The situation derives from strong calling for issue of two billion additional rials coupled with widespread dissatisfaction at British refusal to furnish wheat and general discontent at treatment accorded Iran (by) Allies. These matters were brought to the fore by statement made to press by Sheridan, pertinent passages of which follow: "I would like to emphasize that before leaving my country I was assured that the United Nations will not permit Iran to suffer through no fault of her own. Unfortunately Iran occupies a geographical position which makes it necessary for United Nations to use roads and railroads for transport of war supplies to Russia. This has caused a complete disruption of your transport services and this as I said above is all due to no fault of the Iranian people. Every freedom loving individual in the world, yourselves included, must do everything they can to aid the destruction of the German menace. Rest assured therefore that both the United States and Great Britain have a

sincere desire to help you in every way possible but you must help yourselves up to the maximum limit of your own resources. As the months progress if we find that your own resources are insufficient then I assure you that you will have a sympathetic and helping hand from both Britain and America." British took exception to Sheridan's statement since they felt he had no right to bind them to furnish wheat to Iran. Sheridan has assured me he will make no further statements of political nature without consulting me. Situation was further aggravated by Casey who, on a short visit to Tehran, offered to trade Iranians 5,000 tons of wheat (half for Iranian Government and half for British troops in Iran) in exchange for 25,000 rifles. Iranians refused on grounds that British have not yet paid for 100,000 rifles and 1,000 machine guns bought several months ago. Casey, because of this refusal and urged by the British Minister who takes stand that no wheat should be supplied Iran, then told Iranians British did not intend to furnish them any wheat and that "I know about the shipping situation more than Mr. Sheridan."

Prime Minister was then in throes of facing a rebellious Majlis over question of issue of two billion additional rials in currency (see my No. 319, October 12. The amount was changed to two billion to allow one billion for Allied war needs and one billion for internal needs principally wheat program which calls for huge subsidy in wheat price to endeavor to bring wheat out of hoarding). The Government and Majlis feel it is useless to make sacrifices for the Allies when the latter refused to furnish wheat or other commodities and when Allies take their potatoes, vegetables and cattle out of Iran. Qavam is discouraged and wishes to resign. Majlis in fear of inflation and starvation do not wish to pass monetary bill. Prime Minister has telegraphed Churchill and Shah telegraphed King asking for benevolent British cooperation in present acute situation.

Crux of the situation is wheat. British maintain there is sufficient wheat in hoarding to take care of Iran's needs. I have consistently (see my No. 271, August 26 and Department's 277 August 29) advised an open mind on wheat shipments until we can determine whether measures taken will bring sufficient wheat to light. I recommend we await Sheridan's judgment after he has had more time to study food situation. Iranians are at present one jump ahead of bread shortage which here is tantamount to starvation. Sheridan has been able to keep no more than two days supply of wheat on hand in Tehran and is working desperately to bring in stocks from provinces; he is confident he can obtain 35,000 tons in Azerbaijan and 15,000 tons in Khorassan if only he can obtain cooperation of Soviet railway and military authorities. My opinion is there will be wheat shortage within a few months and we should keep in mind possible necessity of shipping some 50,000 tons. Iranians seek promise from Allies their essential needs especially in wheat will be met before they commit themselves to further cooperation or issue of currency. If Qavam Cabinet resigns bill for additional currency must necessarily be tabled in which event Allies will be placed in difficult position of suspending war work or taking matters in own hands. I would recommend we give Iran Government guarantee we will undertake, on Sheridan's statement that he is unable to uncover enough wheat to last till next harvest, to furnish deficit or at least much as we are able. This would I realize run counter to British policy in Iran. I have impression that British Legation is playing again game of divide and rule and may be endeavoring to force out Qavam and obtain a more suitable Quisling. At any rate British policy here seems to me to lack comprehension and vision.

Cable to London on October 19, 1942 (Telegram 5155, 891.00/1922):

Tehran's telegram no. 327, October 17 reports crisis has arisen as result of severe wheat shortage and British Government's refusal to furnish wheat. Situation is complicated by need for issuance of large additional supply of currency (Bill has been presented to Iranian Legislature calling for issuance of two billion additional rials). Iranian Government contends its recent harvest will fall far short of meeting domestic requirements for wheat and insists that Allies make up deficit. J.P. Sheridan, newly arrived American food and supply adviser to Iranian Government, has made public statement that Iran must help itself to maximum extent of its resources but that if those resources prove insufficient, Britain and America will extend "a sympathetic and helping hand." British authorities Middle East have taken exception to Sheridan's statement. Minister of State Casey offered Iranians five thousand tons of wheat in exchange for twenty-five thousand rifles. Iranians refused and Casey informed them Britain would furnish them no (repeat no) wheat, adding "I know more about the shipping situation than Mr. Sheridan."

Iranian Cabinet and Legislature unwilling to make sacrifices for Allies in view of refusal to furnish wheat and other urgently needed articles, and Prime Minister Qavam threatens to resign. Legislature does not wish to authorize proposed currency increase. Shah and Prime Minister has cabled King and Churchill requesting benevolent cooperation in present acute situation. Wheat supply appears to be crux of situation and present shortage appears largely due to hoarding by growers, shortage of transportation material, and inefficient organization for internal distribution. Both British and American Governments have urged Iranian Government to take strong measures to deal with hoarders before requesting supplies of foreign wheat. It is hoped that Sheridan will be able to deal with this situation and to improve transportation and distribution. It is further expected that he will be able to provide exact information regarding available domestic supplies of wheat and whether or not imports will be necessary. Accordingly, our Minister recommends, and Department agrees, that no final decision regarding imports should be taken until Sheridan has had time to survey the situation and make a report. He is fully occupied at present in maintaining the day to day supply of wheat in Tehran. Minister Dreyfus believes, however, that there will be a real shortage within a few months and that Iranians must be given some assurance from the Allies with regard to meeting their future needs before further cooperation can be expected of them. He points out that if present Cabinet resigns, currency increase bill will be tabled and Allied military forces will find themselves unable to obtain Iranian currency to carry on operations. In addition, Department feels that frequent Cabinet changes are undesirable from point of view of United Nations, since they tend to increase existing Iranian confusion and to foster discontent with regime sponsored by Allies.

Please inform Foreign Office urgently that this Government believes it advisable to give Iranian Government immediate assurance with respect to future wheat supplies if and when it is determined such supplies are necessary. Therefore, we propose that the British and American Ministers at Tehran be instructed to advise Iranian Prime Minister that if Sheridan in due course reports domestic wheat supplies are insufficient to meet minimum requirements for current year, Britain and United States will see to it that within the full limit of their ability wheat from other sources is furnished to make up deficit. In support of this proposal you may inform Foreign Office that this Government feels it is essential to the proper functioning of the supply route to Russia through Iran that the Iranian people should be adequately fed. A starving and rebellious population would, we feel, be an extremely serious obstacle. The United States Government is especially concerned on this account because of the recent arrangement whereby the American Army is to take entire charge of the transportation supplies to

> Russia through Iran. As an instance of the difficulties created by the food shortage, you may mention that Colonel Shingler, present head of the American military mission in Iran and Iraq was recently forced to make a special trip to Tehran to urge that bread be provided for the Iranian workers in Persian Gulf ports in order that work on the transshipment of Russian supplies should not be interrupted.

The above telegram was repeated to Fred Winant in Cairo with the following addition: "Following telegram has been sent to London as Department's 5155, October 19, 10 pm. In your discretion you may discuss this matter with British authorities and endeavor to obtain their agreement with Department's viewpoint. Please report immediately any action you may take." The State Department on October 19, 1942, had also given Dreyfus a tentative go ahead (Telegram 279, 891.00/1922):

> Your 327, October 17. Department concurs in your recommendation regarding assurance to be given Iranian Government if Sheridan determines wheat supply will be insufficient to last until next harvest. However, you should give no (repeat no) guarantee to Iranians pending further instructions. We are sending summary of your telegram to London and instructing London Embassy to endeavor to obtain British agreement to joint assurance. Winant at Cairo is also being informed and authorized in his discretion to take question up with British Middle East authorities.

Dreyfus on October 20, 1942 (Telegram 333, 891.00/1923):

> Reference my 327, October 17, 10 p.m. After protracted discussions between Prime Minister, Soviet Ambassador, British Minister and myself the Prime Minister has been persuaded to present and defend the currency bill in the Majlis provided American and British Governments agreed to provide any cereal deficiency which may occur up to end of war or at least until next harvest. Prime Minister informs me he will go to Majlis today to seek legislative authority for immediate issue of 500 million rials of currency for purchase of wheat, of which he will then earmark 150 millions for Allied war use. This amount should last about a fortnight. If the Allied assurance as to cereals is given he would then press for authority to issue remainder of 2 billion rials. Because of urgency of currency question we have been seeking a formula which will solve this problem and at the same time save the Qavam Government and quiet Iranian fears of starvation. A joint Anglo-

> American declaration that Iran's cereal deficiency will be met if such deficiency is clearly established and if Iran takes certain steps to help herself has been suggested by the British Legation and the Prime Minister as a way out of the present impasse. A draft declaration is now being worked on and will be cabled to Department as soon as completed. Such a joint declaration would have decided advantage over unilateral declaration recommended in my No. 327 in that it would also bind the British and would prevent British from gaining impression that we are backing the Iranians against their interests. British Legation is recommending to London approval of this declaration. . . .
>
> An important factor in Iran's wheat problem is Azerbaijan surplus of about 35,000 tons. While Soviet officials have expressed willingness to assist in transport of this wheat to Tehran little actual cooperation has been given. I have impressed upon them the fact every ton of wheat shipped into Iran means one ton less of vital raw materials for Russia and I hope this argument will have some effect. There are strong indications however that the Soviet military intends buying up this wheat for their own use. Department may wish to call to attention of Soviet Government the harmful effects to Iranian economy of their purchase of large quantities of wheat, cattle and other goods in Iran. . . .
>
> British Legation is dissatisfied at these recurring financial crises and favors solution along following lines: (1) legal limit on currency issue be removed; (2) setting up of a currency board consisting of an Iranian, Russian, American and British members; (3) elimination on issue of further currency except by sales of foreign exchange in order to prevent continuance of Government's present policy of avoiding taxation by expediency of long term borrowing. It is doubtful if Iranians would voluntarily approve setting up of currency board suggested. It might be advisable to await Millspaugh's arrival before making any commitment in this regard.

Deepening October Crisis

Qavam had delivered on his promise. Dreyfus on October 22, 1942 (Telegram 335, 891.00/1924): "Reference my telegram No. 333, October 20, 5 p.m. Medjliss has passed bill authorizing issue of 500,000,000 rials currency." But there was no respite. Dreyfus again on October 24, 1942 (Telegram 340, 891.00/1928):

> Refer to my telegrams of past week on wheat and finance. Developments disturbing effect on public opinion and have brought about a state of political confusion and uncertainty. Majlis is in state of near rebellion criticizing government and the Allies openly and bitterly. Bill for additional issue of five hundred million rials had literally to be jammed though Majlis. Not at all certain if Qavam will be able to force through bill for issue of remainder of two billion rials even if he obtains promises of wheat shipments from Allies. Deputies fail to understand Iran's basic monetary questions or to comprehend the urgent and overriding nature of Allied problems in Iran. They are so obsessed with dangers of inflation and starvation they cannot see conditions in realistic or practical light. Qavam on the other hand while personally distrustful of British shows every indication of basic comprehension of problems and of desire to cooperate in practical sense. Present situation in Majlis is unsatisfactory and if it continues must inevitably end in one of two alternatives – either Qavam will fall or Qavam will be compelled dissolve Majlis on grounds it does not represent will of people because improperly elected during former regime. Press and public also deeply stirred, taking generally view Allies are pushing Iran into inflation and starvation. While American prestige still high there is growing tendency to group Americans with British and Russians and to hold us to a certain extent responsible for present conditions. Prices are soaring and poor classes can hardly afford to buy bread, their only staple food. Profiteering is scandalous and Government has not taken corrective measures such as taxation or price control. Financial situation is so unsatisfactory and chaotic that every effort should be made to hasten departure of Millspaugh.

Reaching agreement was no easy task. Dreyfus on October 21, 1942 (Telegram 334, 891.00/1925) provides the text of the proposed Anglo-American declaration on food, adding,

> Iranians have introduced new clause which British had stricken from an earlier draft as objectionable. Clause states British and American Governments are at once importing into Tehran twenty-five thousand tons of wheat to be stored in silos as reserve to be supervised by Ministry of Food and Sheridan and disposed of only case necessity and then only on consent of a majority of following: Minister of Food, Sheridan, American and British Legations. . . . British state that Iranian allocation on railway is only 200 tons a day so that it would take 125 days to move 25,000 tons of wheat to Tehran from the port to the exclusion of other goods. This argument is hollow for if Iran's press-

ing needs for essential goods is established it is the duty of the Allies to lend their assistance. In view of length of time involved in shipping wheat and transporting it to Tehran and considering great possibility of a wheat deficiency I am of the opinion that we should approve the Iranian Government's demand for a reserve of 25,000 tons.

Taking advantage of Iran's vulnerability, the British had piled on the pressure. Winant on October 22, 1942 (Telegram 5908, 891.24/266):

> We discussed the situation in Iran as outlined in Department's 5155, October 19, 10 p.m. with the Foreign Office and stressed the advisability of giving the Government of Iran an assurance as to future wheat supplies. Foreign Office, however, had just received a message from the British Minister at Tehran transmitting the text of a statement which the Government of Iran desires to publish. In it the public would be told that the British and American Governments have assured the Iranian Government that under certain conditions supplies of wheat, if needed, would be furnished. Foreign Office stated in this connection that it understood that a copy of this proposed statement had been telegraphed to the Department by Minister Dreyfus. Foreign Office feels that it would be well if the Government of Iran were to issue some form of public statement but the Foreign Office does not approve of the proposed statement of the Government of Iran as presented through the British Minister at Tehran. When a decision has been reached as to the kind of statement the Foreign Office feels might well be issued, Foreign Office will inform us of the proposed text. In discussing the question further with the Foreign Office of giving the Government of Iran joint assurances as to future wheat supplies, it would be very helpful for us to have the Department's views on the advisability of the issuance by the Government of Iran some form of public statement.

As reported in chapter 13, in the midst of this crisis the Russians had demanded to purchase a large quantity of grain. Dreyfus on October 23, 1942 (Telegram 339, 891.00/1926):

> Soviet authorities in Iran have presented Iran Government formal request for purchase of 5,000 tons of wheat, 15,000 tons of barley and 30,000 tons of rice. British Minister is trying to exact from Soviets promise that if this request is met they will make no further demands until next harvest, that they will lend every assistance to Iran Government in collection of wheat in Azerbaijan and Khorassan and in its

> transport by rail or road to Tehran even to extent of providing military trucks to railhead and that they will help Iranians to build up wheat reserve in Tehran to give Allies time to meet new situation caused by their purchases. In my opinion there is no assurance Soviets will refrain from making additional demands. For example Sheridan says they informed him that they wish to take 15,000 tons of wheat. British Minister telegraphed his Government requesting 20,000 tons wheat be sent to Iran as soon as possible to meet situation caused by Soviet purchases. In note to Soviet Embassy British Minister stated success of this operation will depend on extent of Soviet cooperation and if the Soviets intend to request additional grain later this be made clear at once to the British and American Legations. Note calls attention to fact that political situation of Allies is weakened by Soviet purchases and argument heretofore used that since Iran sorely needed its own wheat for its internal use Allies were not buying Iranian wheat is no longer valid.

The telegram concludes:

> This Soviet demand brings out into the open what has been known for some time—that Russians, British and Poles are buying up large quantities of Iran food products to detriment of local food situation. . . . It is becoming obvious that frantic Iranian appeals for wheat in recent months have been based on more than avarice or caprice. British are slowly swinging to view this Legation has held for several months, that a wheat shortage would probably develop and that we should be prepared to meet. There are strong indications Iran's food situation will become acute during winter and that it would be well in my opinion to begin wheat shipments to Iran without delay.

The State Department quickly approved the Russian purchase of Iranian grain (Telegram 299, 891.00/1926, October 29, 1942):

> Your 339, October 23. For your confidential information, the Soviets are asking America and Britain to supply a large quantity of wheat to Russia. Consequently, Department considers it unwise to raise any blanket objection to Russian purchases of Iranian wheat. It would seem advisable to allow reasonable quantity of Iranian wheat to go to Russia, making up any Iranian deficit with Anglo-American wheat. However, we regard it as most important that Russian purchases should be carefully calculated to avoid stripping any part of Iran of the grain needed for local consumption. . . . Department feels it would be ex-

tremely unfortunate if exports to Russia, or consumption by local Russian forces, should cause a critical shortage in the interim period before replacement supplies could arrive.

The MESC's request that Iran make an "inventory" of drugs, described in chapter 9, was a pretext to delay imports. The same ploy was used in the case of wheat. Winant from Cairo on October 24, 1942 (Telegram 1872, 891.00/1827):

> On the subject of Persian wheat the British authorities here feel strongly that there is needed a realistic substantiation of the true situation regarding supply. They cannot reconcile an acute shortage of wheat in Tehran, based on any lack of wheat in the country, with the fact that the current harvest has just been gathered. They believe that the difficulty is the direct result of unsatisfactory mechanics of Iranian distribution; that is, inability of the Iranian civil authorities to prevent large scale hoarding, inadequacy of the motor transport system and ineffective administrative organization of internal distribution. The British authorities therefore insist receiving more accurate information on the present supply and adequate control for the handling of wheat supplies in the future. To this end there is proposed the establishment of a joint Anglo-American-Russian-Persian food board. . . . The British are fully aware of the importance of avoiding unrest and disorders in a country used as a supply route to Russia. It is in the interest of maintaining supplies to the Russian front that the British authorities are loath to import for delivery to Tehran a commodity such as wheat which will necessarily displace the hauling of an equal amount of war munitions. It is hoped by closer cooperation with the Russians there may result a better system for handling the Persian cereal situation. For instance instead of importing wheat to Basra for hauling over the railroad to Tehran it might prove better for the war effort to draw on some of the wheat stocks in the Russian zone.

The reply to Winant in Cairo, October 26, 1942 (Telegram 1305, 891.00/1927):

> Department and Foreign Office London are now considering suggested Anglo-American-Iranian announcement whereby British and American Governments would undertake, under certain conditions, to make good any deficit in Iranian cereal supplies which may be determined by Food Adviser Sheridan. Foreign Office and Department approve announcement in principle but are studying possible modifications of

draft prepared at Tehran. British understood to object to Iranian request for clause binding Allies to provide immediately 25,000 tons wheat as reserve at Tehran in order to restore public confidence in ability of Iranian Government to maintain food supply. You may wish to consult MESC on this point and may say Department favors Iranian request, which is supported by our Minister Tehran. Dreyfus indicates food situation will become acute during winter and feels steps should be taken now to meet anticipated situation. Soviets are asking Iranians for 5,000 tons wheat, 15,000 tons barley and 30,000 tons rice. If made, these purchases will aggravate situation and increase responsibility of Allies for ensuring Iranian supplies.

Cable to London on October 26, 1942 (telegram 5300, 891.24/266):

Your 5908, October 22. Department is studying draft announcement prepared by British Legation Tehran and alternative draft drawn up by Iranian Government. It is understood both drafts have been submitted to Foreign Office. Principal divergences appear to be (a) that Iranians place responsibility for road transport organization on Food Adviser Sheridan, whereas British leave this authority in Anglo-American-Iranian Transport Committee; and (b) Iranians request undertaking by British and American Governments to transport 25,000 tons wheat to Tehran immediately in order to constitute a reserve which would improve public confidence in Iranian Government's ability to maintain food supply. British Minister Tehran objects to this request. Department approves proposed announcement in principle and favors Iranian request for early supply of 25,000 tons wheat. However, pending clarification of certain points on which we are consulting Tehran, we are not prepared to make a decision on the exact terms or wording. In this context we should be glad to have any text agreed upon by Foreign Office and we shall submit our own as soon as sufficient information is received. From reports which we have received, we believe food situation in Iran is becoming steadily more serious and that it may become disastrous if preparations are not made now to meet later contingencies. Minister Dreyfus reports that Soviets are seeking to buy substantial quantities of Iranian wheat, barley and rice. Such purchases will, of course, aggravate shortage in Iran and will also place a greater and more direct responsibility upon the United Nations for maintaining Iranian food supply. Cairo now informs us British authorities there contemplate establishment of British-Russian-American-Iranian food board to deal with all phases of grain supply distribution. We should be glad to have Foreign Office reaction to this proposal.

On October 28, 1942, Winant had sent from London the text of the proposed announcement (Telegram 6015, 891.24/271):

> The text of the announcement has been telegraphed to the British Minister at Tehran with instructions to hold it until informed by Minister Dreyfus that the Department's concurrence has been given. The Foreign Office is of course prepared to consider any changes in this proposed announcement that the Department might wish to make. It is also prepared to consider carefully any draft the Department prepares. With reference to making some wheat available as soon as possible Foreign Office states that it has advised the Ministry of War Transport here that it approves supplying 20,000 tons. Foreign Office adds in this connection that it would not object to having 25,000 tons supplied, the figure mentioned by the Department. In order to meet the serious currency situation Foreign Office states that in agreement with the Iranian authorities arrangements have been made within the framework of the Anglo-Iranian Agreement of May 26, 1942 for issuing rial currency in the amount estimated to be sufficient to meet the needs at least until November 2 of this year. Foreign Office is very much concerned over the currency situation and feels strongly that an early solution of this problem must be found. With a view to facilitating this Foreign Office inquires whether the Department would not consider instructing Minister Dreyfus to tell the Iranian authorities that the Department regards the carrying out of the terms of the Anglo-Iranian Financial Agreement to our interests as well. As to the proposed British-Russian-American-Iranian Food Board mentioned in the Department's telegram 5300 of October 26 Foreign Office states that it feels that before new steps are taken in this respect the Soviet Ambassador in Tehran ought to recommend the establishment of such board to his Government. The British Minister in Tehran has been asked to suggest to the Soviet Ambassador that he may care to submit such a recommendation to his Government. Foreign Office like Department views situation prevailing in Iran as serious. It appreciates having been kept so fully informed of Department's attitude and it wants to cooperate closely with the Department in meeting the situation there.

New British Demands

Following El Alamain, the British had been emboldened to seek additional concessions, and as noted in the previous telegram, they now desired to link the wheat and currency issues. The request for the fulfillment of the May 26, 1942 accord was changed to a new set of demands.

Dreyfus on October 30, 1942 (Telegram 350, 891.00/1933):

British Legation has received authorization from Foreign Office to proceed with negotiations for a tripartite declaration on the bases of amended version of draft given in my 334, October 21. However British Legation is now of opinion this declaration does not meet situation fully for while British and Americans would be bound to supply wheat until next harvest the Iranians could again resort to what British term "blackmail" when the two billion rials are exhausted within a few months. The Minister has therefore proposed to London the abandonment of present basis of negotiation and proceeding along following lines (1) British and American Governments undertake to insure Iran's wheat supply until war's end and to ship 25,000 tons as soon as possible, (2) Iran to remove legal limit (on note) issue, to take out of hands of Majlis right to restrict note issue, and to set up currency board outlined in my 333 October 20. Draft declaration given in my 334 had weakness from American viewpoint that while we were bound to supply Iran with wheat the Iranians were not bound . . . to supply us with rials.

Dreyfus on November 4, 1942 (Telegram 359, 891.00/1936):

A reply to my no. 350, October 30, is urgently requested as local conditions continue to deteriorate and is rapidly reaching critical stage. Prime Minister informs me allied delay in this matter is very embarrassing to him and is causing local situation to become hourly more critical. There have been a number of bread riots and suicides in the last few days. Prime Minister has placed another 100 million rials of that 500 million recently voted by Majlis at disposal of Allies. This should last a maximum of 10 days which time currency crisis will become acute. Allied food declaration should no longer be delayed. Its publication should not only relieve political situation somewhat but would also strengthen hands of Government in obtaining Majlis approval of pending currency bill.

Confidential. It is quite possible that British are deliberately delaying solution of food and currency problems by making additional demands and suggestions, such as those outlined in my no. 350. I should not be surprised if they intend to occupy Tehran on pretext that Iranians have not lived up to agreement to furnish rials. This would be done with large forces which are now in Qum, having arrived there ostensibly for winter quarters and to make room in Kermanshah area for Polish troops.

State Department replied on November 5, 1942 (Telegram 306, 891.00/1933):

> Your 350, October 30. Department is advising London that we agree to Foreign Office draft announcement, with two minor changes of phraseology. Principal change is substitution of words "Iran" and "Iranian" for "Persia" and "Persian" throughout. Provided British believe necessary shipping will be available we are proposing that announcement be accompanied by simultaneous public statement that American and British Governments will transport to Iran as soon as possible 25,000 tons of wheat to be stored under supervision of Iranian Ministry of Food in whatever parts of country may seem most desirable, this reserve stock to be used only in an emergency and with approval of majority of Iranian Food Minister, American Minister, and British Minister. We are suggesting to Foreign Office that future currency needs would seem to be adequately assured if terms of Anglo-Iranian Financial Agreement of May 26 were strictly fulfilled by Iranian Government. To guarantee this fulfillment, we are suggesting that agreement be formally approved by Majlis, thus binding that body to take whatever legislative action may be necessary to carry out its terms, and we have offered to support British in requesting such approval as condition to our agreement to wheat undertaking. Department feels this procedure would be less offensive to Iranians than suggested four-power currency board and would also present fewer administrative difficulties. We are not (repeat not) inclined to favor British Minister's proposal that we guarantee Iranian wheat needs for duration of war, as this would commit us too far in future and would also remove some of incentive for Iranians to put own house in order. Department is somewhat puzzled at recurrent need for ever-larger Iranian note issues. Unless United Nations expenditures and general price level have risen to a point far higher than we have understood, it is understood that cause must be failure of currency to complete normal cycle and return to banks for reissue. . . . Department feels that urgent consideration should be given to some means of ensuring supply of rials to United Nations without continuous increases in currency circulation, which will soon be more than double June 1941 volume, and we are expressing this view to London.

Dreyfus commented on the Allied expenditures in Iran on November 18, 1942 (Telegram 378, 891.00/1944):

> Reference that part Department's 306, November 5 dealing with finance. Causes of Iran's currency crisis are: (1) Large allied war expenditures of about 400,000,000 rials monthly. Iranian note issue increased from 1550 million rials in August 1941 to three billion in October 1942. It is now proposed to issue some two billion additional for allied war needs and Iranian wheat purchasing program, (2) Rise in price level. Banque Mellie price index rose from base of 100 in 1937 to 193 in August 1941 and 331 in September 1942. Cost of living index for the same period was 100, 209 and 418. This is perhaps main cause of need for ever larger note issue and also an effect of increased circulation. (3) Failure of notes to complete normal cycle and return to banks for reissue.

Dreyfus again on December 14, 1942 (Telegram 438, 891.00/1967):

> My 378, November 18. American military in Iran inform me their rial needs during 1943 will be approximately 300,000,000 rials monthly as compared with former figure of 15,000,000. This will bring total Allied rial needs to the colossal figure of about 750,000,000 monthly, which is half of the total Iranian pre-war note circulation and one fourth of the present total. This amount should decrease of course as British turn over communications to Americans. Rials for Allied war needs should be readily forthcoming from currency committee (see my no. 386, November 20 reporting enactment of law by which Majlis surrendered currency powers to committee) however, it is difficult to see how inflation which already a fact in Iran, is to be prevented from assuming disastrous proportions unless some system is devised by which Allied war needs are to be met without recourse to ever larger note issue. I have impressed on General Connolly necessity of keeping personal expenditures of highly paid American technical forces to minimum to relieve rial situation.

Cable to London on November 5, 1942 (Telegram 5534, 891.24/271):

> Your 6015, October 28. Department agrees to text of announcement prepared by Foreign Office, with following minor changes: One. Wherever the words "Persia" and "Persian" are used, we would very much prefer to substitute "Iran" and "Iranian." We suggest this amendment not only because it accords with our own practice but because of the definite preference of the Iranian Government, which would be a party to the declaration. Two. For clarity, we suggest changing first part of

second paragraph to read as follows: "Considering that the responsibility of feeding the people of Iran rests primarily on the Imperial Iranian Government, but that it is desirable, in as much as war conditions may bring economic distress to the people of Iran, and in as much as it is the general policy etc."

Provided British are confident that necessary shipping will be available, Department suggests that simultaneous announcement be made that British and American Governments will transport to Iran as soon as possible 25,000 tons of wheat, which will be stored under supervision of the Iranian Ministry of Food in whatever parts of the country may seem most desirable, this reserve stock to be used only in the event of an emergency and with the approval of a majority of Iranian Food Minister, American Minister, and British Minister. Department understands there is some apprehension lest proposed joint undertaking with respect to wheat leave Iranians free at some later date to raise new difficulties with respect to currency issue. We assume, however, that provisions of Anglo-Iranian Financial Agreement of May 26 would be adequate, from British point of view, to cover any situation which might arise, provided this agreement were strictly fulfilled by Iranian Government. As we see it, the difficulty is that the agreement was never approved by the Majlis, which consequently does not consider itself legally bound to take the legislative action required to implement it. Accordingly, you may inform Foreign Office that this Government would be willing to support British in requesting that financial agreement be given Majlis sanction as a condition to our agreement to undertaking with respect to wheat.

We believe, however, that continuous expansion of Iranian currency circulation cannot be considered satisfactory solution to the problem. It is pertinent to note that in June, 1941, authorized circulation was less than two billion rials, while it is now three billion five hundred million and it is proposed to increase it to five billion. In view of Iranian fears of inflation, further expansion of note issue at this rate would seem likely to encounter increasing official and popular opposition and might provide the basis for inflationary developments which would be difficult if not impossible to control. Consequently, we feel that urgent consideration should be given to some method of making rials available for the United Nations without repeated new issues. We should be glad to have views of Foreign Office on this matter, together with any information available to British which would shed further light on basic causes of existing situation.

Cable to London on November 6, 1942 (Telegram 5581, 891.24/271):

> Department's 5534, November 5. Following telegram has been received from Tehran: "359, November 4, 6 p.m. A reply to my no. 350, October 30 is urgently requested as local situation continues to deteriorate and is rapidly approaching critical stage. Prime Minister informs me allied delay in this matter is very embarrassing to him and is causing local situation to become hourly more critical. There have been a number of bread riots and suicides in the last few days. Prime Minister has placed another 100 million rials of the 500 millions recently voted by Majlis at disposal of Allies. This should last a maximum of 10 days which time currency crisis will become acute. Allied food declaration should no longer be delayed. Its publication would not only relieve political situation somewhat but would also strengthen hands of Government in obtaining Majlis' approval of pending currency bill." Please convey substance of above to Foreign Office and state that Department hopes action on wheat declaration and announcement regarding shipment 25,000 tons may be taken immediately. Please advise us urgently of British decision.
>
> Confidential. For your information and comments there is quoted below Section two of Tehran's telegram under reference: "It is quite possible that the British are deliberately delaying solution of food and currency problems by making additional demands and suggestions, such as those outlined in my no. 350. I should not be surprised if they intend to occupy Tehran on pretext that Iranians have not lived up to agreement to furnish rials. This would be done with large forces which are now at Qum, having arrived there ostensibly for winter quarters and to make room in Kermanshah for Polish troops." Additional demands and suggestions mentioned included removal of currency control from Majlis and establishment of four-power currency board.

Foreign Office was clearly playing for time. Winant on November 7, 1942 (Telegram 6257, 891.24/280):

> Substance of Department's 5534, November 5, 8 p.m., and the first three paragraphs of Department's 5581, November 6, 10 p.m. conveyed to Foreign Office. Replies and comments to date of Foreign Office on points dealt with in Department's telegram are: One. Foreign Office agreeable to the minor changes in the proposed announcement on Iran which are suggested by the Department . . . on its 5534

of November 5. Foreign Office asks that Department inform American Minister at Tehran accordingly and give him the necessary instructions to enable immediate publication of announcement. Two. Foreign Office also requests that Department seriously consider instructing our Minister at Tehran actively to support British Minister at Tehran in his discussions with the Iranian authorities on proposals to find a long-term solution of the currency situation, the first step towards such a solution being a proposal to divest the Majlis of control over currency matters and to vest this control in a currency commission. Three. With reference to the immediate shipment of a supply of wheat to Iran Foreign Office states that it is trying to arrange for the shipment of 20,000 tons, this figure having been taken because that is the amount of wheat and barley which it is understood the Soviets have purchased in Iran and the 20,000 tons serve, therefore, as a replacement for Soviet purchases. If after arrangements have been completed for shipping these 20,000 tons, Department still desires that an additional 5,000 tons be shipped the British authorities Foreign Office states, would probably not object. Foreign Office adds that it prefers to have the 20,000 tons of wheat looked upon as a replacement for that which the Soviets have purchased rather than as a reserve. Foreign Office prefers this because it believes because it believes that if the Iranian authorities look upon this supply of wheat as a "reserve" rather than a replacement, they will be less inclined to cooperate in meeting the situation that has arisen in Iran.

With further reference to the shipment of wheat Foreign Office states that it has been told by the British shipping authorities that it will be very difficult to find the tonnage necessary for transporting immediately 20,000 tons to Iran. Moreover, it is felt that the arrival of this whole amount at once would increase the delay of clearing other goods through the ports of Iran. It has consequently been decided to ship 5,000 tons of the wheat this month, another 5,000 tons in December and the remaining 10,000 tons as soon thereafter as possible. Mr. Casey at Cairo has been asked to advise the Middle East Supply Center to make the necessary local adjustments, Mr. Eden in the meantime has told the Soviet Ambassador here, Mr. Maisky, of these arrangements pointing out at the same time that the shipment of this amount of wheat to Iran would necessarily entail a reduction proportionately in the transportation of supplies to Russia over the Iranian route. Foreign Office adds further that the Ministry of War Transport is very anxious that those authorities of the United States Government having charge of shipments to the Iranian Gulf should understand the situation fully

> so that arrangements will be made for shipments to Russia to be reduced in proportion to the quantity of wheat sent to Iran. Such arrangements must be made in time, it is stressed, to avoid serious congestion at the Iranian gulf ports.
>
> Four. Foreign Office also states that when Mr. Eden informed Mr. Maisky of the proposed announcement on Iran Mr. Maisky replied that he thought his Government would like to become a party to the announcement and also to participate on the Road Transport Committee mentioned in the announcement. Mr. Eden told Mr. Maisky that he saw no objection to that so long as the Soviet Government assumed the obligations accompanying such participation. Mr. Maisky then said he would consult his Government which he has done, but he has not yet received a reply. When informing us of the foregoing the Foreign Office made it very plain that it felt that the effort that are being made to find a solution to the critical problems that have arisen in Iran should not be slacked in any way pending further word from Mr. Maisky nor, specifically, should the issuance of the announcement on Iran be delayed.
>
> Five. With reference to Section Two of Tehran's telegram referred to in the Department's 5581, of November 6, we can say emphatically that at no time during the discussions which we have had during the past weeks with British officials on Iran have we felt that the British were trying to delay the finding of a solution to the food and currency problems. On the contrary these officials have throughout shown great concern and full appreciation of the seriousness of the situation prevailing in Iran and of the necessity of finding a solution as quickly as possible.

To further complicate matters, the British had announced the discovery of a plot. The "Franz Mayer Documents" which was used as a basis to arrest numerous Iranians, is described in chapter 17. Dreyfus on November 6, 1942 (Telegram 361, 891.00/1938):

> British Minister informs me British intelligence officers have uncovered widespread plot by German agents to seize power and commit sabotage in case Germans near Iran. Plot is alleged to have been discovered as result of seizure of documents belonging to a German named Meyer (sic). British commanding officer Iran said to have asked London for permission to take action at his discretion. Situation here is already so critical that should attempt be made by British to arrest

> large number of prominent Iranians said to be involved in this plot Qavam Government would probably fall and conditions become so chaotic military occupation of Tehran would be inevitable. It is not beyond realm possibility that British have exaggerated or manufactured this plot as excuse for military occupation of Tehran (see last paragraph of my 359, November 4).

This telegram was forwarded to Winant in London on November 7, 1942, adding (Telegram 5604, 891.00/1938):

> Please urgently advise Foreign Office that we hope British authorities will proceed with utmost caution and regard for Iranian sensibilities in any action which they may take with respect to alleged conspirators. We consider it especially desirable that no action of any kind be taken against Iranian nationals until tension caused by wheat and currency problems has relaxed.

Winant's reply on November 10, 1942, must have further convinced officials in Washington of his ineffectiveness (Telegram 6327, 891.00/1939):

> Triple priority. Secret for the Secretary and the Under Secretary. Immediately on receiving the Department's 5604, November 7, 7 p.m., the last paragraph was called to the attention of the Foreign Office. I felt, however, because of the confidential insert in paragraph two that I should take this subject up at length with Mr. Eden himself. I did so this morning. I read to him the entire message excepting the confidential section. He confirmed the statement of a German plot and told me he was in agreement with the message. I then went on to say that there has again arisen some question as to British policy in Tehran. We went into this in great detail and, I am certain, with complete frankness on his part. I saw both the secret minutes of the cabinet meeting on this situation and the file of his exchanged messages with his Minister in Tehran. Eden does not (repeat not) want to occupy that country and in this he has the support of the War Cabinet. The plot was not manufactured for political reasons but was a seriously organized conspiracy by the enemy. It was discovered by General Wilson, a general I know, who has a great deal of common sense and is not at all interested in politics. In a recent message to his Minister, Eden explained that no occupational program could be undertaken without first consulting both the United States and Russia. It is true, in my opinion, that the British would take action if military necessity required it but after notifying

us. The strategic value of this area has, I believe, taken on added value since the British victory in Egypt and our African operations. I am certain that Eden is set against any intrigue to take over this country for selfish British interests.

Additional British Demands

The British were not about to relent. Dreyfus on November 7, 1942 (Telegram 362, 891.00/1937):

> Urgent. My 359, November 4. British Legation has again altered attitude toward food declaration and now takes view that in view of serious deterioration of situation in Iran, the declaration should be made only against greater concessions and assurances on part Iranians. They believe it is useless to obtain satisfaction on currency matter alone only to be presented later with new problems and demands which will require concessions and negotiations. They consider now time set stage for complete Iranian cooperation. British Minister is therefore telegraphing London recommending British and American (if United States agreement can be obtained) are prepared to support Qavam or any other Iranian Government only in following circumstances: One. Iran Government must be prepared to support war effort and to give assurances that hoarding laws will be enforced, rials guaranteed, price control instituted, press controlled and security maintained. Two. To enable government carry out these engagements government should seek full powers from Majlis for six months or full year. Three. Allies may call on Prime Minister to modify Cabinet as they see fit. Four. Food declaration will be given only against Iranian acceptance above conditions. British Minister in his cable admits this course of action may lead to fall of government and even necessity of use of force but states that alternative is political and economic chaos. He also states he is now considering composition of alternative governments. Seems to me certain that Majlis will not grant these full powers nor even those outlined in my 350, October 30. Result of attempts to obtain their compliance will be fall of Qavam either through resignation or no confidence vote. In this event British must be prepared (one) to install alternative government which will close Majlis, throttle press and generally do Allied bidding or (two) occupy Tehran and set up Quisling Government.
>
> It would appear that British have determined on a policy of presenting Iranians with demands that could not possibly be accepted with ultimate intention of occupying Tehran and setting up puppet govern-

ment. Their reasons for this are not clear but may include (one) honest belief that present confused and unsatisfactory situation can only thus be remedied or (two) intention of getting Iranian situation under control (see my 361, November 6 as to Fifth Column plot) in view of possibility of German threat toward Iran this winter. I am in agreement with British that government should seek full powers from Majlis and have gone so far as to suggest this course informally to Prime Minister. This is necessary to eliminate destructive influence of Majlis, to be able to control irresponsible press and to accomplish anything substantial. However, I am not convinced that the British have chosen the proper method of accomplishing this aim and I cannot conscientiously recommend that we support these new British demands. I am hopeful that the same thing can be accomplished by the use of informal and friendly, but firm, pressure on government. I am anxiously awaiting Department's reply to my 350 in order to inform Qavam who has been summoned to Majlis session Sunday for Interpellation on food situation. I fear the new British move reported above will so confuse the situation that Qavam's position will become untenable.

Dreyfus on November 9, 1942 (telegram 365, 891.00/1940):

Department's 306, November 5. Iran Government has suggested following changes in food declaration: (1) they ask assurance that declaration in no way changes British obligations under British Soviet Iran treaty; (2) they wish to alter article one of declaration to provide that we will "undertake to arrange for importation of cereals" rather than merely to take all steps within the full limit of our powers; and (3) they desire that in article two we undertake to move cereals from an area with a surplus to a necessitous area in case they are for reasons beyond their control unable to do so. In making last two suggestions Iranians have in mind both heavy Allied purchases of their food and constant Soviet obstruction to shipment of wheat from Azerbaijan. British agree to comply with one but firmly refuse to agree to two and three. Both British Minister and I have informed Prime Minister that Anglo-Iranian financial agreement of May 26 must be ratified by Majlis as condition to our making food declaration. Prime Minister is taking British refusal to accede to his suggestion under consideration and promises early reply. An expression of the Department's attitude toward these proposed changes will be appreciated in case Prime Minister persists.

Iranians base their requests enumerated above on sincere belief that Allies, far from having lived up to their pledges to Iran, have pillaged the country to such an extent that a firm and inescapable rather than a vague promise must be obtained. There is much to be said for Iranian viewpoint for the country has indeed been pillaged of food and transport by Allies. Allies have taken over Iran railways; UKCC has taken 1700 Iranian trucks and Soviets 400 while newly formed Iranian transport organization has only 180. UKCC has created major passenger crisis by taking about 200 of Tehran's 300 buses. British appear to be bent on obtaining a puppet government. British Minister hinted to me that if necessary he is prepared to seize bank notes in Banque Mellie by force. In my 362, November 7, I suggested two possible reasons for this British attitude. A third reason might be that British wish to entrench themselves solidly in Iran for fear that ever increasing American influence and activity here may have adverse effects on their long range interests. British Legation is cold and harsh in dealing with Iranians. For example, aide mémoire presented to Iranians today began: "Irrespective of any other consideration His Majesty's Government intends to secure the fulfillment of the financial agreement and the necessary supply of rials."

Cable to London on November 10, 1942 (Telegram 5640, 891.24/280):

Your 6257, November 7. 1. We are instructing our Minister Tehran to propose immediate publication of wheat announcement as amended. We assume Foreign Office has sent similar instructions to British Minister Tehran. 2. By telegram dated November 7, 1 a.m., Minister Dreyfus reports British Minister is now recommending that wheat announcement be made conditional upon following Iranian undertakings: (a) Iran must support war effort, and give assurance that hoarding laws will be enforced, guarantee supply of Iranian currency to United Nations, institute price control, institute control of press, and maintain internal security; (b) Iranian cabinet must seek full powers from Majlis for six months or year; (c) Allies to have right to call upon Prime Minister to modify cabinet as they see fit. 3. Dreyfus believes these demands would be unacceptable to Iranians and would result in fall of cabinet. Ensuing situation would probably compel Allies to set up alternative puppet government, undertake military occupation of Tehran, or both. 4. Department maintains its previously expressed view that any action leading to the fall of the cabinet would be unfortunate. Please so advise Foreign Office and explain our conviction that advantages of Allied Military occupation of Tehran or establishment of puppet government would be more than offset by adverse reaction of Iranian people and other Moslem peoples. Even if another cabinet could be formed without undue Allied interference, we fear that repeated changes cannot fail to increase general disorder and undermine confidence in government. 5. Accordingly, we are instructing Dreyfus that wheat announcement may be made, in his discretion, without attaching any condition precedent. It is our understanding that this is the desire of the Foreign Office. If Dreyfus considers it desirable, however, we are authorizing him to suggest that Prime Minister seek full powers from Majlis, and we are likewise giving him discretion to urge strict fulfillment of Anglo-Iranian financial agreement. 6. Please inform Foreign Office that we are much disturbed by apparent tendency on part of British authorities Tehran to make repeated changes in bases of negotiation during a period of crisis such as the present. It is our view, and we gather from your telegram under reference that Foreign Office takes same position, that the wheat situation should be cleared up without further delay, leaving other problems to be worked out in the more favorable atmosphere which would be created by the announcement agreed upon. We feel the more strongly about this matter because of the added responsibilities being assumed by United States in Iran through operation by our Army of supply routes to Russia and furnishing of numerous American advisory missions, notably the financial group to be headed by Dr. Millspaugh, which will need the willing cooperation of a stable Iranian Government with popular support. 7. We would not object to Russian participation in announcement and in Road Transport Committee, provided Soviets assume corresponding obligations and provided such participation does not in any way delay issuance of wheat announcement. 8. We would appreciate explanation of reasons causing British Government to favor four-power currency board. As stated in our 5534, November 5, we feel that the Anglo-Iranian agreement of May 26 should be adequate to cover British needs if it is fulfilled by Iranians. 9. We shall advise appropriate authorities regarding contemplated shipment 20,000 tons wheat, and we should appreciate being kept currently posted on developments in this connection. We understand, however, that Middle East shipping programs are primarily decided in London and assume Foreign Office is taking necessary steps at that end.

Also on November 10, 1942, the State Department had sent a long cable to Dreyfus (Telegram 314, 891.00/1937):

Your 362, November 7 and Department's 306, November 5. One. London telegram dated November 7, 6 p.m. states Foreign Office agrees to our suggested changes in draft announcement and "asks that Department inform American Minister at Tehran accordingly and give him the necessary instructions to enable immediate publication of announcement." Complete text of draft is being sent to you separately. Please present this to the Iranian Government and British Minister and request their agreement to its immediate publication. We assume Foreign Office has sent corresponding instructions to British Minister. Two. London is trying to make arrangements for shipment of 20,000 tons wheat as replacement for equal quantity said to have been purchased by Russians. It is proposed to ship this as follows: 5,000 tons in November, 5,000 tons December and remainder as soon as possible thereafter. Foreign Office considers earlier shipment impracticable because of shipping situation and probable congestion at Persian Gulf ports. Additional 5,000 tons may be sent if United States considers it essential. Three. Foreign Office prefers to consider this shipment as replacement, rather than as emergency reserve, since otherwise Iranians "might be less willing to cooperate in meeting situation which has arisen." Four. Department is not (repeat not) informed regarding conditions which Foreign Office may wish to attach to use of this "replacement" shipment, but we consider it desirable that they should not (repeat not) exceed those originally proposed for suggested 25,000 tons reserve, namely, approval by majority vote of Iranian Food Minister, American Minister and British Minister. Five. Department approves your attitude toward additional demands proposed by British Minister. We are opposed to repeated changes in the bases of negotiation in a period of crisis such as the present. We believe any action which would bring about fall of cabinet is to be avoided if possible, since we fail to see how repeated cabinet changes may be expected to bring about greater order to enhance public confidence in Government. We are even more strongly opposed to forced suppression of Majlis and constitutional procedures or military occupation of Tehran. In our view, such advantages as might be gained would be more than offset by adverse reaction of Iranian people and probable repercussions among other Moslem peoples. We feel the more strongly on this matter because of the added responsibilities being assumed by United States in Iran through operation of supply routes to Russia and furnishing of numerous American advisory missions, notably the financial group to be headed by Dr. Millspaugh, which will need the willing cooperation of a stable Iranian Government with popular support. Department is expressing above views to London and, if you see fit, you may convey their substance to British Minister as representing Department's attitude. Six. In your discretion, you may formally urge

> upon Prime Minister advisability of seeking full powers from Majlis. You may also urge fulfillment of terms of Anglo-Iranian financial agreement and, if it seems advisable, approval of that agreement by Majlis. However, neither these nor any other measures need be considered as essential conditions precedent to issuance of wheat announcement. Department leaves to your discretion whether any assurances should be obtained from Iranians prior to publication of announcement. We gather that Foreign Office is prepared to go ahead at once on wheat and work out other questions later, and we agree with your opinion that our objectives should be sought by informal and friendly pressure rather than by ultimatum. Seven. Foreign Office now appears to favor four-power board as long-term solution of currency problems. We are not (repeat not) convinced that this is the best procedure and are again stating our view that strict fulfillment of Anglo-Iranian agreement should be sufficient. However, in making any recommendations in this connection, you may wish to take into consideration probability that American expenditures in Iran will soon increase greatly and fact that we are not (repeat not) covered by Anglo-Iranian agreement.

The Millspaugh appointment mentioned in the latter cable is reported by Dreyfus on November 12, 1942 (Telegram 372, 891.24/285): "My number 364, November 9, 2 p.m. Majlis today passed law for employment of Millspaugh. Prime Minister urges that he come forward as soon as possible since important financial legislation will be suspended pending his arrival."

On November 12, 1942, the State Department had followed with another instruction to Dreyfus (Telegram 317, 891.00/1940):

> Your 365, November 9. Regarding undertaking to import wheat, Department feels unable to give stronger guarantee than that contained in text of agreement cabled to you, nor do we see how Iranians can expect us to do more than "take all steps within the full limit of our powers." With respect to internal distribution, we assume Iranians fear that Soviets will interpose physical obstacles to movement of wheat from Russian-occupied zone, even if adequate transport is available. We cannot undertake to control action by Soviets, nor could we well use British or American trucks to bring wheat out of Azerbaijan and Khorassan in the face of Russian opposition. However, in your discretion, you may assure the Prime Minister that this Government will, if occasion arises, endeavor to use its influence with Soviet Government

> to ensure that Iranians are permitted to move surplus grain from Soviet zone to other parts of Iran. Russian Ambassador London has stated his Government may wish to become a party to wheat declaration and also participate in transport Committee. Department and Foreign Office seem to agree that there would be no objection to this, provided that Russians assume corresponding obligations and provided conclusion and publication of wheat agreement is not, thereby, delayed.

Currency Commission

Foreign Office strategy consisted of making demands that the Iranians could not possibly meet, and then abandon them in favor of more realistic ones. Winant on November 13, 1942 (Telegram 6340, 891.24/284):

> The substance of Department's 5640, November 10, 8 p.m. concerning Iran has been given to the Foreign Office and the various points raised by the Department have been discussed with the Foreign Office. One. Foreign Office confirms report that British Minister at Tehran has recommended that the announcement on wheat be made conditional on undertakings by Iran as outlined by the Department. Foreign Office has already advised British Minister that it does not (repeat not) view the proposed undertaking favorably. Foreign Office however, now states definitely that it wishes the announcement on wheat to be "bound up" with a long term solution of the currency problem. It feels as pointed out in the Embassy's 6257 of November 7, 6 p.m. that the establishment of a currency commission with full control over currency matters would be an effective approach to such a solution. Two. Foreign Office agrees with Department that Anglo-Iranian agreement of May 26 would be adequate to meet British needs if fulfilled by the Iranians. Difficulties as frequently created by the Majlis, however, make fulfillment questionable. The Foreign Office believes therefore that the creation of a purely Iranian Currency Commission, the only kind of a commission which it feels there is possibility of getting authority to set up, would not only result in more expeditious meeting of currency and related problems but it would at the same time remove the danger of the Majlis obstructing solutions in the hope of getting further concessions. Foreign Office feels that unless the establishment of a commission is insisted on now before the announcement on wheat is issued a good opportunity for finding a long term solution of the currency problem will be lost. British authorities, the Foreign Office stresses, do not want to be left in the position where whenever a solution to some pressing phase of the currency situation is to be found,

the Majlis has to be approached. Three. Foreign Office states that the proposed wheat announcement, as amended has been presented to the Iranian authorities for their information and that the Iranian reaction to it is favorable. British Minister has, however, been instructed not to agree to its publication until, as indicated above, the establishment of a Currency Commission has been authorized. Four. Foreign Office today referred to the view which was expressed in the Department's 5534, November 5, 8 p.m. that a continuous expansion of the Iranian currency could not be considered a satisfactory solution. It stated in this connection that it is in entire agreement with the Department's view and that it had, consequently, placed all pertinent facts before British Treasury officials with the request for suggestions on how the currency problem in Iran might be met without resorting to repeated expansion of the currency. Five. With respect to the final paragraph of the Department's 5640, Foreign Office states that it will be glad to keep us informed of developments in connection with the shipment of wheat. It stated further that the Department's understanding that Middle East shipping programs are decided here is correct and added that it is taking all the necessary steps here.

The State Department on November 13, 1942, had consented to the establishment of a currency commission (Telegram 5687, 891.24/284):

Your 6340, November 11. Provided Iranian consent can be obtained without objectionable pressure, Department has no fundamental objection to creation of purely Iranian currency commission as condition precedent to wheat agreement. Our previous opposition to commission was based upon understanding it was to be composed of British, Russian, American and Iranian members, which we felt would have been unacceptable to Iranians. We assume Foreign Office contemplates action by Majlis to vest full control of currency in proposed commission. Please confirm this and indicate what would be relation of commission to Iranian Cabinet. As Foreign Office is aware, Iranian Government is engaging a financial mission, under leadership of Dr. Millspaugh, in this country. It is also seeking an American to act as technical director of Banque Mellie Iran. Under terms of Millspaugh's proposed contract, which Iranians are reported to have accepted, he will have extensive responsibility for, and control over, Iranian national finances, and he will necessarily be vitally interested in the currency question. The technical director of the Banque Mellie will, of course, be directly concerned with currency matters. Consequently, we feel that if the proposed commission is formed, there should be a definite understanding

> that upon the arrival of Dr. Millspaugh and the Banque Mellie adviser they will become members. If you deem it advisable, you may point out to Foreign Office that inclusion of these two men would not repeat not change the essentially Iranian character of the commission, since they will be employees of the Iranian Government and will not repeat not in any way represent the American Government or any American business or financial interest. We are repeating this to Tehran.

On November 13, 1942, Dreyfus received additional instructions (Telegram 320, 891.24/284):

> Department's 314, November 10. London cable of November 10 reports Foreign Office has advised Bullard it does not repeat not favor proposed demands for Iranian concessions. However, Foreign Office wishes wheat announcement to be linked with Iranian undertaking to create purely Iranian currency commission as long-term solution of currency problem. It has instructed British Minister Tehran to withhold agreement on wheat until establishment of such a commission has been authorized.

The British, meanwhile, had resorted to threats. Winant from Cairo on November 14, 1942 (Telegram 2000, 891.00/1942):

> Middle East authorities have just advised me that they have been informed that crisis in Tehran has become more acute due to near exhaustion in supply of rials. If a stoppage of rials occurs it is believed British will resort to measures of coercion. British military taking precautionary measures and will in case of stoppage take over national bank where note forms are lodged.

Dreyfus on November 14, 1942 (Telegram 375, 891.00/1941):

> Department's 317, November 12. Wheat situation in Tehran has taken even more critical turn. Sheridan has only a half day supply in silo and wheat is coming in from provinces very slowly. Famine may come at any time and Sheridan is preparing to open soup kitchens if necessary. In view of this dangerous situation I feel we should take positive and immediate steps, with British consent or without it. I recommend that Department arrange urgently for shipment of wheat to Iran from India at rate of about 5,000 tons a month and further that 5,000 additional tons referred to in paragraph two of Department's 314 come forward

> without delay. Wheat from India could (one) be considered to represent the 20,000 tons. . . . Shipment from India is recommended because wheat from more distant sources might not arrive in time to meet the crisis should it arise. While Sheridan may possibly be able to obtain sufficient wheat to tide country over for several months, my opinion is that we cannot afford to gamble while the lives of several thousand people are at stake. In line with the views expressed in paragraph six of Department's 314, November 9, with which I am in full accord, I have urged British Minister to agree to immediate publication of wheat declaration but he prefers first to obtain definite assurance of Iranian concessions, particularly as to unlimited supply of rials. Prime Minister informs me he is presenting declaration to Majlis tomorrow. My suspicions that British are carrying on machinations to obtain puppet government or even occupy Tehran (see my no. 362, November 4) have been confirmed by two documents which originated in British Legation, copies of which have fallen into my hands. One of these outlines an entirely new cabinet with Mohammad Sadiq Tabatabai as Prime Minister and containing many persons known to be pro-British or British tools. The other gives a proposed government program which would reduce powers of Shah, increase number and powers of American advisers, control press, set up war council with American military adviser as one member, require more Iranian cooperation with allies and make government more subservient to British. Copies of these documents are being sent Department by next airmail.

The documents mentioned by Dreyfus are discussed in chapter 16. Dreyfus' telegram 375 of November 14, 1942, had prompted the State Department to seek Indian wheat for Iran. Given famine in India, it came to nothing. It also elicited a sharp response from Murray. In a memorandum dated November 16, 1942, addressed to Assistant Secretary Berle and Under Secretary Welles, Murray writes (Memorandum, 891.00/1969-1/2):

> I am of the opinion that the situation described by Mr. Dreyfus in the attached telegram makes it all the more desirable that Mr. Welles seek an early moment to impress upon the British Ambassador the serious concern which we feel over the steadily deteriorating situation in Iran. I am not at all surprised at Mr. Dreyfus' suspicion "that the British are carrying on machinations to obtain a puppet government or even occupy Tehran, which have been confirmed by two documents originating in the British Legation," copies of which have fallen into Mr.

Dreyfus' hands. Indeed, judging from my own personal experience in Iran and my observation of British methods there, I should have been surprised if such was not the case.

Referring to the conversation which took place, at our instructions, between Ambassador Winant and Mr. Eden on this subject, when our Ambassador felt that Mr. Eden "was entirely frank" in placing all his cards on the table, it may be observed that this episode is in no way surprising. The fact is that the British Legation in Tehran has always been, and still is, staffed by officials of Indian Civil Service background, who traditionally conduct their own foreign policy with regard to Iran, almost independently of the British Foreign Office. The presence of American advisers in Iran and the successful accomplishment of their duties has always been looked upon with a jaundiced eye by the British Legation staff in Tehran, and it is safe to say that such still is the case despite recent radical changes in the situation in Iran which render it practically impossible for British subjects to function there in any civil capacity.

You will recall our earlier interest in encouraging younger patriotic Iranians to assume important posts in the Iranian Government at this time and our earnest endeavor to gain British collaboration to this end. You will also recall that, in reply to such suggestions from us, the British Foreign Office pointed out rather unctuously, the undesirability of such a policy, on the grounds that such young and competent Iranian officials as either the American Legation or the British Legation might sponsor in Tehran would be handicapped by the very act of such sponsorship. The catch in this was, of course, that British sponsorship is in fact a deadly handicap to any Iranian, whereas American encouragement, and, if you will, even sponsorship, is the greatest possible asset, as has been exemplified by the rise of Mr. Allah Yar Saleh, who is now in this country and whom both of you have, I believe, met.

With the British admonishment to us on this subject fresh in our minds that we should under no circumstances concern ourselves with the advancement of young patriotic Iranian officials, we are now confronted with the sordid design of the British Legation to install stooges of its own in the Iranian Government to be hired and fired at will by that Legation. Such being the case, it seems to me that Mr. Eden's assurances are not adequate to meet the actual situation prevailing in Tehran, and I am of the opinion that the situation calls for frank words with Lord Halifax, without of course mentioning the source of the information conveyed in the strictly confidential section three of Mr. Dreyfus' attached telegram of November 14, 5 p.m.

As described in chapter 17, Lord Halifax subsequently received a stern lecture from Welles. On November 17, 1942, two First Secretaries at the British Embassy had called at the State Department (Memorandum, 891.24/301):

> Mr. Hayter and Mr. Thorold called, under instructions from the Foreign Office, to explain the British point of view with regard to the existing critical situation in Iran. Mr. Jernegan set forth the Department's understanding of the developments of the past several weeks, explaining that we had agreed to the Foreign Office suggestion that the establishment of a purely Iranian currency commission should be made a condition precedent to the issuance of the Anglo-American-Iranian wheat declaration. We had not agreed to attaching any other conditions. We assumed that the British Minister at Tehran would proceed with the signature of that declaration, in conjunction with our Minister and the Iranian Government, as soon as agreement had been reached on the currency commission question. Mr. Hayter said that this was substantially his understanding, except that he gathered that the Foreign Office wanted a very definite assurance at this time that a long-term supply of rials would be made available to the Allied forces. He was not clear as to the exact form this assurance would take, and he agreed that if the proposed currency commission were given, by the Majlis, full powers over note issue, this would probably meet the desire of the Foreign Office. Mr. Hayter emphasized that the supply of rials was vital to the maintenance of the supply route to Russia and that the British Government did not wish again to be faced with the prospect of a complete stoppage of rial sales. In this connection, he said that the British need for Iranian currency was largely caused by the necessity of operating and protecting the Russian supply route and that, therefore, Britain was really acting on behalf of the United Nations in dealing with this knotty problem.
>
> Mr. Murray, Mr. Alling and Mr. Jernegan stressed very strongly the view of the Department that every other alternative should be employed before resorting to force, or the overthrow of the Iranian Government, to ensure the supply of rials. We agreed that it was vitally important to obtain currency and that it was conceivable that a situation might arise in which the Allies would be compelled to use force. However, we did not feel that things had come to such a pass as yet.

Even failing Iranian agreement to the proposed currency commission, Great Britain and United states could still go ahead with the wheat agreement, on the understanding that the Iranian Prime Minister would then, as he had assured our Minister some weeks ago, obtain from the Majlis authority to issue an additional 1,500,000,000 rials in bank notes. This amount would take care of our needs for a few months, at least, and in the meantime Dr. Millspaugh's financial mission would have arrived and conditions in general might have improved. In our opinion, the Allied policy should be to play for time, carrying on such expedients as might prove practicable, and avoid forcing the issue to a showdown which might compel us to undertake military occupation of the entire country. In this connection, Mr. Murray recalled the views expressed by Mr. Berle at the time of the previous financial crisis last spring, to the effect that more could be obtained from the Persians by kindness than by bludgeoning. Mr. Murray also said that Mr. Welles has been much concerned over the present crisis situation in Iran and planned to speak to Lord Halifax about it. Mr. Hayter said that the Foreign Office entirely agreed that the use of force should be avoided if at all possible, and he pointed out that although the British had been in occupation of Iran for more than a year, they had not yet resorted to force on a single occasion, despite the fact that they had no other means of pressure open to them. However, he appeared to feel that the Iranians should be made to understand that as a last resort force would be used.

With reference to the wheat shortage, Mr. Hayter and Mr. Thorold were informed of the latest report, dated November 14 from Minister Dreyfus, in which he stated that Tehran stocks were sufficient for only half a day and urged that immediate shipments be made from India. Mr. Thorold said that the Embassy had received a cable from Tehran dated November 13 reporting that the Soviets had agreed to release 7,500 tons of wheat from Russian-occupied Azerbaijan for the Tehran population. It appeared that 3,500 tons of this was being sent forward at once. The total amount would take care of the city's consumption for a little less than a month. According to Mr. Thorold the British Minister at Tehran had taken a very strong line with the Russian authorities in order to obtain release of this wheat, as he felt that the city ought to have a reserve good for at least four months. It was agreed that if the 7,500 tons should reach Tehran in the near future it would relieve the situation to some extent, but Mr. Alling and Mr. Nielsen pointed out that this amount would be used up before the 20,000 tons being sent by the British could possibly arrive. Accordingly, it was asked that Mr. Thorold consult his Government on the possibility of making immediate shipment from India or from the "wheat pool" of the Middle East Supply Center. Such advances could be replaced later by the contemplated shipments from North America. The suggestion was also made that a total of 25,000 tons, instead of 20,000, should be programmed. . . . In passing, Mr. Thorold mentioned that the Soviet Government was very much interested in maintaining in power the present Iranian Cabinet, headed by Ahmad Qavam.

On November 27, 1942, Thorold had written to Jernegan (Letter, 891.24/298-½):

> You will recall that at the recent meeting which we had regarding Persian matters, we discussed the possibility of some immediate supplies of cereals being made available to Persia from either the MESC pool or from India; such supplies to be replaced from the United States or Canada at a later stage. We have now been informed by the Foreign Office that in order to meet the present shortage in Tehran 3,500 tons of Iraq barley is being sent from Ahwaz, partly at the expense of supplies to Russia. We are also informed that in order to assist building a small reserve in Tehran the Minister of State in Cairo is being advised that it is hoped that he would be able to arrange for 3,000 out of 5,000 tons wheat programmed for shipment in November to be advanced, either from military stocks in Iraq or from India against subsequent replacement. I hope these quantities together with the supplies which we understand are being provided by the Russians, will serve to tide over the immediate crisis.

As reported later, of the 7,500 tons of wheat "promised" by the Russians, "not one ton" had reached Tehran, and barley from Iraq failed to arrive on time.

Cable to Dreyfus on November 18, 1942 (Telegram 327, 891.00/1944):

> Your 375, November 14. We are asking Foreign Office London and Indian Government New Delhi to give urgent consideration to immediate shipment wheat from India or Middle East rather than more distant loading areas. Could you not arrange through Frederick Winant for temporary loan of wheat from so-called "MESC wheat pool"? Department considers it unwise, from standpoint of general policy, to attempt shipment without British concurrence. Furthermore, such ac-

> tion would seem impracticable, since all possible sources in Middle East and India are under direct or indirect British control and British authorities, as we understand it, control priorities in handling of cargo in Iranian ports and within Iran.
>
> Reference Department's 320, November 13, Foreign Office has expressed its agreement with Department's views on currency commission and approves inclusion of Millspaugh and Banque Mellies adviser. It feels, however, that exact composition of commission should be worked out with Iranian authorities by you and British Minister. . . . Please advise present status of negotiations with respect to currency issue and wheat declaration. What is exact nature of assurance British Minister is seeking with respect to rials? Is he still asking concessions with respect to other matters as well? In conversation with British Embassy here November 17, Department strongly expressed views that force should be used to secure currency supplies only repeat only as last resort. Rather than use force, we would prefer to issue wheat declaration without any conditions whatever, if by so doing there were a reasonable prospect of obtaining even a temporary supply of rials and improving general internal situation.

Iranian Consent to Currency Commission

Dreyfus on November 19, 1942 (Telegram 382, 891.00/1948):

> Prime Minister called Russian Ambassador, British Minister and me tonight to inform us he will dissolve Majlis unless they pass currency bill tonight. He would issue order himself in order not to embarrass Shah. He has been opposed and blocked at every turn by Majlis which has held up for three days passage of vital currency law. He would exercise emergency powers subject to ratification by next Majlis.

The next day, Majlis had surrendered. Dreyfus on November 20, 1942 (Telegram 386, 891.00/1951):

> My 382, November 19. Majlis last night enacted bill surrendering its currency powers to the existing currency committee. Prime Minister promises delivery of rials to the Allies from Banque Mellie tomorrow and immediate meeting of currency board to consider additional issue. British feel they have now received satisfaction on currency question and we are proceeding at once with wheat declaration. Majlis was

> badly frightened by threat of dissolution and promised Shah to cooperate with Government. While I am not hopeful that Majlis intends permanently to alter its obstructive tactics there is no doubt that its action last night has considerably eased the political situation. Much, however, will depend on its reaction to a new bill presented last night in which Government asks for additional powers. Noteworthy in negotiations of last few days was helpful attitude of Russian Ambassador based on new instructions from his Government to take more active part in joint Allied dealings with Iranians. I must express opinion that internal situation will go into another crisis if British carry out intention of arresting four very prominent Iranians including a deputy and two Generals on grounds of implication in plot (see my 361, November 6). I have pointed out to British Minister bad effect of these arrests would have unless the evidence of guilt is conclusive but he seems determined to proceed on grounds of security.

Instruction to London on November 24, 1942 (Telegram 5924, 891.00/1938):

> In telegram dated November 20 Tehran reports Iranian action vesting control of currency in existing Iranian Note Reserve Control Committee. British Minister reported satisfied with this action and proceeding at once with wheat declaration. Dreyfus feels this has relieved political situation but fears another crisis if British authorities in Iran carry out expressed intention of arresting four prominent Iranians, including a deputy and two generals, on grounds of implication in plot mentioned in Department's 5604 November 7. Dreyfus has pointed out to the British Minister effect such arrests would have unless evidence of guilt is conclusive but Bullard appears determined to proceed on grounds of security. Please reiterate to Foreign Office views expressed in 5604. You may say this Government is no repeat no less anxious than British to preserve security of Allied position in Iran, but that we are most anxious to avoid another crisis, especially since the wheat-currency difficulties are still in process of settlement. If action against alleged conspirators is considered absolutely necessary, we hope British authorities Tehran will be instructed to proceed with all possible observance of Iranian laws and procedures. It would be preferable to allow Iranian themselves to make arrests and conduct proceedings.

London replied on November 25, 1942 (Telegram 6651, 891.00/1953):

> Views expressed in Department's 5604, November 7, 7 p.m., repeated to Foreign Office and substance of Department's 5924, November 24, 10 p.m., conveyed to it. Foreign Office states that it, too, feels that caution should be exercised, particularly as wheat and currency problems are not definitely settled, and that it has telegraphed British Minister at Tehran to this effect. In the same telegram it has asked for fuller information regarding the charges against the four prominent Iranians who the British authorities in Iran wish to arrest. Foreign Office adds that the possible arrest of these individuals will be considered by it in the light of the additional information that has been requested but that it hopes, in any event, that it will not be necessary to take any action against the wishes of the Iranian Government.

Dreyfus on December 3, 1942 (Telegram 412, 891.00/1956): "Political situation continues to drift hopelessly. . . . Political intrigue against Qavam is increasing. . . . It seems likely the rapidly developing food shortage will bring about new crisis which will result in Qavam's fall or dissolution of Majlis." Dreyfus again on December 3, 1942 (Telegram 413, 891.00/1957):

> Department's 327, November 18. Food situation in Tehran is deteriorating and it is not unlikely a major crisis is at hand. Sheridan has only one day's wheat supply in silo and is ready if necessary to open soup kitchens. He reports wheat from Azerbaijan is not coming as hoped but he attributes this more to Iranian inability to gather wheat than any lack of Russian cooperation. I am informed British Army can at present promise to furnish only 1500 tons of flour and MESC reports it has no reserve stocks which could be made available. In my opinion British here do not take a sufficiently serious view of this situation. Could not Department urge British to arrange for a loan of wheat from some nearby country against replacement from the 25,000 tons being shipped.

On December 3, 1942, Thorold had telephoned Jernegan (Memorandum, 891.24/329-½):

> Mr. Thorold called in reply to my inquiry regarding what, if any, progress had been made in shipping wheat to Iran. He stated that up to November 27,145 tons had been dispatched from United States ports. It had been planned to ship the balance of the scheduled 5000 tons before the end of November, but Mr. Thorold did not yet have definite information as to whether this had been done. He promised to let me

know within a few days. Mr. Thorold said he understood it had now been decided to ship a total of 25,000 tons, instead of 20,000, and that some statement to this effect should be included in the Anglo-American-Iranian wheat declaration.

Signature of Tripartite Food Declaration

The declaration was finally signed on December 4, 1942 (Dreyfus, Telegram 419, 891.24/312):

> Food declaration was signed this afternoon by Foreign Minister, British Minister and myself. Text is substantially same as that given in Department's 315, November 10. British Minister and I simultaneously presented two notes to Foreign Office. First informed Iranian Government that British and American Governments are jointly arranging to bring into Iran 25,000 tons wheat. Second stated that if Soviet Government wishes to participate in declaration a revised text will be signed to replace the present one. British Minister also presented note declaring that declaration in no way diminishes British obligations under Tripartite Pact of January 29, 1942. Original of declaration and copies of notes being forwarded by airmail. Declaration will be published at once in Tehran and London.

In forwarding copies of the agreement and the various notes on December 4, 1942, Dreyfus provides the following observations (Dispatch 399 and enclosures, 891.24/329):

> The signing of this agreement brings to a close negotiations which grew out of a suggestion made in my telegram No, 327 of October 17 that a unilateral American pledge be given the Iranians that we would undertake, under certain specified conditions, to endeavor to make up Iran's wheat deficit. After discussions with the British Minister and Prime Minister, as reported in my telegram No. 333 of October 20, it was decided to recommend a joint Anglo-American declaration in this regard. There has been considerable delay in signing the agreement, caused principally by British-Iranian quibbling over unimportant questions or phraseology. . . . I feel that the signing of this declaration and the shipment of 25,000 tons of wheat were necessary and constructive steps. My consistent viewpoint that there would be wheat shortage in Iran has been vindicated earlier than I had expected. A serious food crisis has already come about, as indicated in my telegram 413, December 3, and I fear that the situation this winter in Tehran will be

desperate. It may well be that shipments of wheat in addition to the 25,000 tons agreed on will have to be made during the next few months to avert famine.

Annex: Text of the Tripartite Food Declaration

The approved text was given to Dreyfus in a cable of November 9, 1942 (Telegram 315, 891.24/271):

> The Governments of the United States of America, the United Kingdom of Great Britain and Northern Ireland, and the Imperial Iranian Government; Considering that the responsibility of feeding the people of Iran rests primarily on the Imperial Iranian Government, but that it is desirable, in as much as war conditions may bring economic distress on the people of Iran and in as much as it is the general policy of the Governments of the United States and the United Kingdom to safeguard the economic existence of the peoples of the Middle East against such distress, to take all possible steps to ensure the supply of bread for the people of Iran until the gathering of the harvest in 1943;
>
> Having regard to the undertaking given by the Imperial Iranian Government to carry out (a) all measures recommended by the United States adviser to the Ministry of Food, including measures to prevent hoarding and the introduction of the rationing of foodstuffs, and (b) all recommendations of the Road Transport Committee which are certified to be essential for the regulation of the means of road transport in Iran by the majority votes of the following three members of that committee, namely the Chairman appointed by the Imperial Iranian Government and the members designated by the British and United States Ministers at Tehran respectively; Have agreed as follows:
>
> (1) If the Iranian Minister of Food, with the concurrence of the United States adviser, and the United States and British Ministers at Tehran decide, by a majority vote, that they are satisfied that all practical steps have been taken by the Imperial Iranian Government under their undertakings referred to above, and that nevertheless the supply of cereals (wheat and barley) within Iran is insufficient to cover the minimum needs of the population of Iran for the current year ending with the gathering of the 1943 harvest, the Governments of the United States of America and of the United Kingdom will take all steps, within the full limit of their powers, to ensure that supplies of cereals will be brought to Iran from other sources sufficient to make up the deficiency.

(2) The Imperial Government of Iran are responsible for the distribution of cereals within Iran and for ensuring that a deficiency in one area is met by supplies from another area in Iran when the total supply of cereals within Iran is sufficient for the needs of the population of the country as a whole. The Imperial Iranian Government are also responsible for the distribution to necessitous areas of any supplies brought into Iran from other sources in fulfillment of the undertaking of the other two Governments in Article 1 above. The Governments of the United States of America and of the United kingdom will take all steps, within the full limit of their powers, to ensure that the means of transport at the disposal of the Imperial Iranian Government shall be sufficient, if put to the best possible use, for the proper distribution of these cereals. In witness whereof the undersigned, being duly authorized to this effect by their respective Governments, have signed the present agreement and have affixed their seals. Done at Tehran this – day of – in triplicate.

Chapter 15

Tehran Bread Riots

The Declaration, too little, too late, had no impact on the crisis. Dreyfus on December 8, 1942 (Telegram 424, 891.00/1958):

> My 412 and 413, December 3. Political situation continues to deteriorate with relations between Majlis and Government at breaking point. Situation aggravated by bread shortage, Tehran living today on reduced rations and with less than a day's wheat supply in silo. Several thousand people including women and children have been demonstrating all day in front of Majlis crying "You may kill us but we must have bread!" Crowd is growing but so far has not got out of hand. Situation was further aggravated by arrest today by British Army and internment at Sultanabad of General Zahidi, Governor General of Isfahan. . . . Why British deliberately chose this delicate moment to arrest Zahidi is not at all evident.

Dreyfus again on December 8, 1942 (Telegram 425, 891.00/1959): "My 424. Crowd is now out of hand and rioting has developed on widespread and severe scale. Shopping area is being looted by uncontrolled mobs. Police and army coming belatedly into action. Damage is heavy and there have been casualties."

Dreyfus on December 9, 1942 (Telegram 426, 891.00/1961):

> My 424, December 8. Situation quieter today though nervous tension is high and shooting is still to be heard in the city. Tehran commerce tightly closed and potentially dangerous crowds throng streets. Shah

placed Field Marshal Ahmadi in charge to restore order. Police and army patrolling city today in force. Riots started with demonstration in front of Majlis by school children demanding bread. Accumulating crowds grew increasingly restive as it became clear police were not taking action. Afternoon mobs marched to business section breaking windows and looting food stores first and later any shops into which they could gain access. It was not until situation was desperate that police received orders to take action. Police and army went into action with a few tanks and machine guns clearing main mobs although isolated acts of looting, personal violence, robbery and attacks on cars continue. Responsibility for early shameful lack of police action not yet established who was responsible for allowing school children led by teachers to demonstrate. Tehran's business section is badly damaged, numerous stores being gutted and little exposed glass left intact. House of Prime Minister was sacked. Majlis was entered and some damage done. Several persons were killed and many injured. No Americans reported to have suffered injury or damage to property. Drastic action will be necessary to prevent recurrence. It is reported British will bring into Tehran some of their forces now stationed at Qum. Political aspects will be covered in separate telegrams.

Dreyfus again on December 9, 1942 (Telegram 427, 891.00/1962):

My 426. British Minister informs me a battalion of British troops now at Qum will arrive in Tehran this afternoon marching through the city and taking up quarters at race track. He states this action necessary to protect British property and military installations in Tehran. It is not known whether Russians will also bring troops to Tehran. The exact cause of the Tehran riots are obscure. British Legation is spreading story that it was part of a German plot and Russian Ambassador in conversation with me supported this view. I am not at all convinced it is true. Iranians believe that riots were inspired by the British or Russians. It seems probable to me riots grew spontaneously as uncontrolled crowds increased, crowds desperate (on) account of food shortage and made bitter by belief their woes are due to British and Russian invaders. However, in long range it seems to me British have much responsibility. I should not like to state categorically that British have incited disturbances or connived at deterioration of situation in order to bring troops into Tehran with ultimate objective of gaining political control. There are, however, numerous indications that this is true. (See my Nos. 359, 361, 362, 365, and 375 of November four, six, seven, nine and fourteen). I know that British have failed for some

> reason to bring to Tehran 3500 tons barley and 1500 tons flour earmarked for Iran and held at Basra at a time when they were desperately needed. Sheridan informs me Prime Minister told him today that when he urged British Minister to hasten arrival of these cereals latter replied to effect he did not see why he should help Iranians when British are being abused and slandered in streets of Tehran. Counselor of British Legation told me today British Minister will tell the Shah today he cannot favor bringing cereals to Iran when the country is so hostile to Allies. I still urge Department to expedite shipment of 25,000 tons wheat and so arrange, if possible, for wheat loan for Iran from a nearby country.

Dreyfus again on December 9, 1942 (Telegram 428, 891.00/1963):

> My 426. Riots have plunged Iranian political situation into a stage of even greater confusion. Shah asked Qavam to resign yesterday. He refused. Qavam was encouraged to take this stand by promises of British support. Shah wished to form a military government under his own domination but was prevented from doing so by British support of Qavam. British Minister talked to Shah today frankly and severely making following suggestions amounting almost to an ultimatum: (1) military governor and police chief to be removed, (2) Qavam to be asked to form a new government and given full support, (3) Prime Minister and others to be compensated for damage to their properties, (4) corrupt and pro-Axis officials to be eliminated from army, (5) inquiry to be held into causes of riots, (6) British will not look with favor on importation of wheat into Iran unless government is favorable to Allies, (7) government must severely enforce hoarding laws and control (prices) and Majlis. Shah accepted proposals in principle and promised to adjust his differences with Qavam and ask him to form a new government. . . . Press has been suspended and curfew imposed at 8:30.

Cable to Dreyfus on December 9, 1942 (Telegram 363, 891.00/1959):

> Your 412 and 413, December 3 and 424 and 425, December 8. As we have previously indicated, Department favors maintenance of Qavam cabinet and its strengthening in any way feasible. From your reports we gather you concur in the view no (repeat no) gain is to be expected from a change in Prime Ministers. Of the steps being considered by the Shah, our thought is that a reform of the Qavam cabinet would be

preferable to a change of government. We should like at the same time to have your views on the possible effect of a dissolution of the Majlis upon popular feeling. Do you believe new elections could or should be held? We have already urged British Government to arrange for a loan of wheat from nearby territories. British Embassy here advises 3500 tons Iraq barley being sent. Foreign Office has also instructed Minister of State Casey to attempt shipment of 3000 tons of wheat from military stocks in Iraq or India. British say they can do no (repeat no) more at present, but we are repeating our representations.

Cable to London on December 9, 1942 (Telegram 6232, 891.00/1959):

Tehran reports political situation has grown worse largely due to obstruction by Majlis. Worsening food shortage has brought on new crisis which threatens to cause fall of Qavam cabinet or dissolution of Majlis. Widespread rioting occurred in Tehran December 8. As we have repeatedly stated, Department strongly favors continuance in power of present cabinet, even though it may be unsatisfactory in certain respects, rather than change to another group which might prove even more unsatisfactory and which would command even less popular support. Please communicate substance of above to Foreign Office and let us have any comments British Government may care to offer in this regard. Please also advise Foreign Office our reports indicate food situation in Iran still deteriorating and we hope British authorities will press their efforts not only with respect to shipment of wheat from North American ports but also in connection with possible advances of grain from near-by territories in Middle East.

Another cable to London on December 10, 1942 (Telegram 6255, 891.00/1938):

Department's 5604, November 7 and 5924, November 24. Tehran reports British Army arrested and interned at Sultanabad on December 8 General Zahidi, Governor-General of Isfahan. Both Shah and Prime Minister reported greatly upset and taking line that action was unfair because Iranian Government was not consulted and arbitrary because had no right to make arrest. Shah has sent personal representative to register protest with our Minister. Dreyfus states arrest has aggravated already critical situation which is evidenced by widespread and serious rioting in Tehran. Please express to Foreign Office our concern over this development. We are particularly surprised that such drastic ac-

> tion should have been taken in the light of Foreign Office attitude reported in your 6651, November 25, from which we had understood that British Government shared our views regarding the advisability of proceeding cautiously and of taking no repeat no action without the concurrence of the Iranian authorities.

A copy of the telegram was communicated to Dreyfus on December 10, 1942 (Telegram 364, 891.00/1959).

Winant on December 10, 1942 (Telegram 6999, 891.00/1969):

> Substance of Department's 6232, December 9, 8 p.m. concerning situation in Iran has been communicated to Foreign Office. Foreign Office states that it was informed of rioting in Tehran by British Minister. With reference to present cabinet, Foreign Office says that it also feels that while this group is in some respects unsatisfactory, a change at this time would be most inopportune. Unfortunately, Foreign Office adds, the Shah himself apparently wishes to dismiss Qavam. As Foreign Office, however, feels so strongly about the advisability of retaining the present Cabinet in power, it instructed the British Minister at Tehran on December 9 to see the Shah and to emphasize how disruptive a change of Cabinet would be at this time. Foreign Office also states that it fully realizes that extreme shortage of wheat, particularly in Tehran, is primary cause of unrest and disorder. According to its information, which is confirmed by the Soviet Ambassador at Tehran, some 35,000 tons of wheat are available in the northern provinces of Iran, which are under Soviet occupation. On two occasions recently the Soviet Ambassador at Tehran reassured the British Minister there that the Soviet authorities would in no way impede the transportation of wheat from this area to Tehran. As the food shortage may become much more acute within the last few days, and as there is this supply of wheat in the northern provinces immediately available, Foreign Office also instructed the British Minister on December 9 to see the Soviet Ambassador and urge him to do everything he can to enlist the support of the Soviet authorities in those provinces in actually transporting this wheat to Tehran. At the same time, the British Minister at Tehran was instructed to report whether it has been possible to obtain wheat in Iraq for Iran and, if so, whether any of this has been shipped, and also to report how much, if any, barley has been shipped to Iran from Iraq. In connection with the possibility of obtaining some wheat and barley in Iraq for immediate shipment to Iran (see my Embassy's 6518, of November 19, 7 p.m.).

Winant on December 12, 1942 (Telegram 7035, 891.00/1965):

> Foreign Office, on being informed of substance of Department's 6255, December 10, 9 p.m., concerning arrest of General Zahidi, stated that, in the view of the British military authorities and of the British Minister in Iran, Zahidi was so deeply and dangerously implicated in the plot organized by German agents that his arrest was considered urgently necessary. Careful consideration was given by these British officials and by the Foreign Office to the advisability of informing the Iranian authorities in advance of their intention to arrest Zahidi but, Foreign Office stated, it was decided that to do so would only embarrass the Iranian authorities. According to its reports, Foreign Office added, the arrest passed off quite unnoticed by the public.

Dreyfus on December 12, 1942 (Telegram 433, 891.00/1964):

> My 427, December 9. As result of urgent representations made by Sheridan and me to British Minister the British military have not only agreed to expedite shipments to Tehran of the 3,500 tons of barley and 1,500 tons of flour but have telegraphed instructions for the immediate advance of 253 tons flour from British army stocks in Tehran and Kazvin. Sheridan read the British telegram, which stresses that publicity value of this so called generous action should not be lost and that trucks of flour should be labeled "British aid to Iran." British now admit these 5,000 tons cereals were being held not in Basra but in Ahwaz where they could have been brought to Tehran without delay. Sheridan also reports that UKCC has procrastinated for two weeks in bringing to Tehran 5,000 tons of rice now in Mazanderan. After this strong representations by British Minister the UKCC now promises to bring the rice at once. It would seem to me that British have deliberately delayed bringing cereals to Tehran in order to exert pressure to require the Iranian Government to pursue a more pro-British policy. Sheridan informs me he is gradually and reluctantly becoming convinced that this is the case.

Cable to Dreyfus on December 14, 1942 (Telegram 372, 891.00/1964):

> Your 433, December 12 and 427 and 428, December 9. For your confidential information, Department has expressed to British Government its surprise and disappointment at recent course of events in

> Iran, which appears to have been contrary not only to the desires of the American Government but also to the policy of the Foreign Office as indicated to Department on various occasions. We drew attention to obstacles placed by British authorities in path of wheat agreement, to arbitrary action of British in matter of General Zahidi, and to entry of British troops into Tehran. We particularly emphasized statements made by British Minister to Shah and Prime Minister regarding wheat supply for Iran and failure of British to move available flour and barley to Tehran, contrasting this attitude with repeated assurances given us by Foreign Office that orders had been issued to ship cereals from Iraq and other nearby source at earliest possible moment. In conclusion, Department expressed hope that Foreign Office would take steps to see that policies laid down in London should be more accurately reflected in actions of British authorities in Iran.

The above-mentioned telegram is given in chapter 17.

Dreyfus on December 19, 1942 (Telegram 451, 891.00/1973):

> Department's 372, December 14. General Ridley has had interesting conversation with British Minister in which he called attention of Minister to fact that arrest of Zahidi by British had completed breakdown of the already low morale in Iranian army. Minister expressed great interest in this view and agreed that in future British should refrain from arrests of army officers but should permit Iranians themselves to handle such cases. It may well be that this was result of Department's representations to London. I am now informed that Zahidi was taken out of country by British by plane. I had feared that my relations with British Legation might be impaired by Department's message referred to. I am happy to report that I do not now believe this will be the case.

Dreyfus on December 19, 1942 (Telegram 450, 891.00/1972):

> Prime Minister has decided to permit Majlis to reopen. He feels his position is now stronger and he will have a comfortable majority. I agree fully with Department that dissolution of Majlis would be most undesirable in its long range effects and should be avoided if possible. While Qavam's position is stronger as result of riots this is mainly because of allied backing. People at large have turned against him and now consider him as an allied tool. British again blundered in bringing troops to Tehran, their position vis-à-vis the Iranians having deteriorated if possible. Russians on the other hand again gained in reputation by not bringing in troops. While Russians cannot be said to be liked by

Iranians there is no doubt that their restraint and good conduct are turning many Iranians increasingly in their favor.

Report on the Riots

On December 21, 1942, Dreyfus had written a long report on the Tehran riots of December 8, 1942 (Dispatch 409, 891.00/1981):

> I have the honor to submit the following discussion of facts, background and consequences of the Tehran riots of December eighth. Before relating the actual facts concerning the riots, it will be useful to glance very briefly at the Iranian political scene of the past year to find therein some explanation of the reason why totalitarian Iran of the last two decades has degenerated to the point where such disturbances are possible. Let us turn the calendar, therefore, back to August 25, 1941, the day when Iran was invaded by the British and Russians. . . . A series of events which have shaken Iran profoundly began with the invasion of the country by the British and Russians on the morning of August 25, 1941, an invasion which had for its stated purpose the removal of the German fifth column menace. The most immediate and important result of the invasion was the abdication on September 16, 1941, of Shah Reza who had ruled Iran for two decades with a hand of iron. . . . With the abdication of Shah Reza, who had acted and thought for Iranians for twenty years, Iran's house of cards came tumbling down. Dormant democracy awakened and the people arose to strike off the chains which had bound them for so long. They plunged boldly into democratic processes which they neither understood nor appreciated and the result was bewilderment, confusion, inefficiency and a fight for power by unscrupulous and self-seeking elements. A people always lacking in civic spirit and sense of social responsibility, the Iranians played the political game for all its worth, seeking only advantage for themselves and their friends with no regard for the welfare of the people at large. This game of political opportunism was accompanied by a widespread feeling of humiliation at the invasion of the country by two hated powers, a feeling which developed into an attitude of despair and impotency. This feeling of demoralization was in turn accompanied by a wave of pro-German feeling on the part of all classes, an attitude of mind which was and is basically more anti-British and Russian than consciously pro-German. Superimpose on this canvas of bitterness and despair the economic stagnation caused by the occupation of the country and add the breakdown in internal security, so carefully built up by Shah Reza, and you do not have a

pretty picture. The bitter feelings just described caused the Iranians to regard the British and Russians with even more suspicion and distrust than was their traditional wont. A period of Iranian non-cooperation and thinly veiled obstruction vis-à-vis the British and Russians ensued. The Soviet-British-Iranian pact of alliance of January 29, 1942, had literally to be forced on the Iranians; the expulsion of the Japanese Legation from Tehran was refused until the American Government intervened; other things desired by the Russians and British were accomplished only after long and difficult negotiations. In this period of trial, the Iranians turned more and more toward the United States for help and guidance, both because they sincerely needed a friend and to a considerable degree to be able to play us off against the British.

The Iranians have by this time developed a complex that their woes are due entirely to the British and Russians, pointing out in particular the lack of security, economic stagnation, the utilization of the Iranian railways almost exclusively for allied benefit, the taking over by UKCC of almost all of Iran's motor trucks, and finally the serious food shortage. They feel that the food shortage is caused by British and Russian purchases in Iran, by the invasion which prevented normal sowings and by the lack of means of transport. They feel that the allies have exploited them in every way. This feeling of bitterness toward the Russians and British has contributed toward the general political instability of a people already grasping blindly at democratic processes. Cabinets have come and gone in rapid successions; they have fallen not only because of the nefarious activities of self-seeking politicians and an irresponsible press but also because the people would not support the Government in actions benefiting the allies, even though it should have been clear that the Government was acting practically under duress. For example, the decline of the prestige of the Qavam Government was due to a great extent to popular dissatisfaction with its financial measures, calculated to make rials available for allied use by colossal note issues. The public have taken the view that the allies are driving the country into bankruptcy and inflation. The most immediate and grievous Iranian complaint at the time the riots developed was that the people were being starved by the allies, who were taking food out of the country and bringing about a condition bordering on famine. There is no doubt that the food situation was serious at the time of the riots, the city being on reduced rations and there being no reserve of wheat in the silo. It should be explained that bread is the staple and almost exclusive diet of the Iranian masses, both because they are accustomed to it and because they are unable with their less than subsistence wage scale to buy any other food. Against this backdrop of threatened famine, political confusion, bitterness, despair and demoralization, the riots took place.

Dreyfus next describes the riots:

The riots began on the morning of December 8 with a demonstration in front of the Majlis by middle school pupils and university students demanding bread. The accumulating crowds, joined by vagabonds and irresponsible elements, became increasingly bold and restive as it became clear that the police had no intention of taking any severe action. By mid-afternoon the mob, now having grown to several thousands, began marching into the main streets of the town, breaking glass, stoning cars, and committing depredations of all kinds. As the police still continued to take no effective action, the more bold began to loot food stores; looting spread into any stores into which access could be gained as the uncontrolled mobs saw what fun it was and what advantage in loot was to be had. Hooligans and small children joined in the fun of smashing windows. Lalezar, Ferdousi, Stambul and Nadiri streets suffered most, little exposed glass being left unbroken and numerous stores being gutted. There is no evidence that the mob had any premeditated intention in the beginning of looting premises of Jews and Armenians but it is a fact that these were much harder hit than those of Moslems. A Jewish radio dealer, for example, lost his entire stock valued at two million rials; a Jewish hotel, the Nadiri, was badly damaged; an Armenian food shop was looted; the Café Continental was completely destroyed; and many other shops suffered the same fate. I can verify as a result of personal inspection that the sacking of the house of the Prime Minister was a remarkably efficient piece of work. Rugs were burned, mirrors smashed, bathroom fixtures demolished, furniture destroyed, clothing torn apart, window and door frames damaged and generally everything of value was stolen or rendered useless. In the late afternoon, the police and army under the direction of Field Marshal Ahmadi who had been placed in charge by the Shah, came belatedly into action, using small tanks, machine guns and cavalry which they had been holding in reserve all day but had not yet used. The main streets were soon cleared of mobs but isolated acts of brigandage, looting and violence continued into the night. The next day the crowds assembled again but were kept under control by the police under the direction of Mr. Timmerman the American police adviser, using among other measures fire hoses. A strong show of force by the police and army, using small tanks and cavalry, prevented continuance of riots. Commerce was gradually opened in Tehran and the likelihood of any recurrence at this moment seems remote. The Prime Minister promised in a broadcast that compensation would be paid for damages suffered, but no official estimate of the losses has as yet been made. Nor has any official statement of casualties been made, but it is generally estimated there were about ten deaths, including three British soldiers, and a few scores of casualties. No American was harmed and the only American property loss was a broken window at the American Presbyterian Mission. Several Americans, however, had their cars stoned, including the Military Attaché, Mr. Timmerman and General Ridley. Mr. Timmerman estimates that 150 shops were looted but that stolen goods valued at six million rials have been recovered. It is understood that 156 persons have been arrested.

On the responsibility for the riots:

The responsibility for the riots is variously fixed, as it suits the fancy of the story teller, on the Shah and his military clique, a civilian group of politicians, Qavam himself for the purpose of discrediting the Majlis, the Majlis in an endeavor to get rid of Qavam, the Germans, in the imagination of the allies, and on the British and Russians by a large part of the Iranian masses. The Americans seem to be the only possible group which has escaped blame in some quarter or other. While the responsibilities are indeed obscure, some reliable facts are beginning to emerge from the welter of wild rumor. This much seems to me crystal clear—that while the ostensible cause of the riots was the food shortage, the deeper and underlying causes were political. Intriguers encouraged the students to assemble in order to further their political ends, using the food shortage as a sentimental issue. It seems further clear that the disorders developed spontaneously as the crowds grew and were joined by riotous elements and as it became clear the police were not taking effective counter measures. If we had the answer to two questions we would perhaps have the key to the puzzle. These are—first, who permitted or encouraged the students to assemble and demonstrate on a school day and, second, who was responsible for the orders which prevented police action until the mob was out of hand. No evidence I have been able to obtain points towards direct connivance by the British, Russians, or axis agents. It would appear unlikely to me that Qavam, as many allege, encouraged the students to demonstrate with a view of preventing the Majlis from voting him out of power, an act which the parliament is said to have contemplated. It is not clear how the demonstration would have prevented or discouraged the vote nor is it explained why, if Qavam had in fact planned the affair, the fury of the crowd was turned on him and his property.

It seems to me fairly established that two groups, one military and one civilian, were working with the common aim of getting rid of the Qavam Government, but perhaps with distinct ultimate objectives. Whether or not they were working in liaison is not clear nor is it likely that this point will be clarified. The military clique consisted of the Shah himself; aided by Radsar, Chief of Police; Yazdan Panah, Chief of Staff of the Army, through whom the Shah has been maneuvering to control the Iranian army; and a group of young and, to a considerable extent, dissolute army officers who surrounded the Shah at the court. The objective of this group was beyond doubt to replace the Qavam Government by a military one; just how the Shah thought this might be accomplished without the consent or blessing of the allied governments is not evident. The second group was large and included the following: Ali Soheily, former Prime Minister; Akbar Massoud, formerly Sarem-ed-Dowleh, now retired but onetime politician and Minister of Finance; various members of the Peikar Party (a youth organization); deputies Bayat (Vice President of the Majlis) Massoudi (editor of *Ettelaat*) and Yamin Esfandiary; Nikpur (head of Chamber of Commerce); Rahnema (editor of *Iran*), Azad (editor of *Azad*), and Safavi (editor of newspaper *Kushesh*); Tadayyon, several times cabinet minister and recently Minister of Education, who may have incited the students through his connection with the university as a language teacher; and the brothers Hassan and Karim Akbar of Gilan. These names were given me by the Prime Minister himself as being the ringleaders of a movement against him and various informed persons have verified to me the participation of one or all of them. I do not mean to infer that either this or the military group actually intended to instigate riots. It is more likely that, separately or in accord, they desired to create further difficulties for Qavam, whose position at the moment was so weak that it appeared he might be forced to resign. As to responsibility for failure to take police action, which would have prevented the riots, it is generally conceded that the onus for this must rest on the shoulders of the Shah. It is reported by Mr. Timmerman that an army officer, thought to have been General Ebrahim Arfa, spoke to assure the crowds that the police had orders to take no action to harm them. Furthermore, the Prime Minister informed me personally, and this is confirmed by various sources, that the Shah telephoned to him many times on Tuesday to insist that he resign. This Qavam refused to do, after having received the assurances of the allied envoys in Tehran that he would have their support. In summary, it seems to me probable that the Shah and his military clique, possibly aided by a civilian group, encouraged the demonstrations for the purpose of discrediting Qavam and they subsequently prevented police action being taken. The onus of this action is great, since Mr. Timmerman's opinion is "this demonstration could have been broken and beaten within a period of half an hour if proper police methods had been applied."

While there is no evidence that the British and Russians had any part in organizing or developing the demonstration or the riots, I have long believed that they must bear a full share of responsibility for the sorry plight of this country today. Consequently, in the long-range sense, some responsibility for the riots must rest on their shoulders. Far from having lived up to their pledges to assist the country economically, they have exploited it by making use of its means of communication, utilizing almost all of its good trucks for the carrying of war materials, permitting confusion to reign, failing to give the army the moral or material support so sorely needed in reestablishing order and in failing to do a thousand and one things which would have assisted the country in getting back on its feet after a humiliating and demoralizing experience. Had the allies assisted the Iranians immediately after the invasion in re-establishing security throughout the country, had they given the Government the support and strength to carry them through this period of adjustment, had they not exploited the communications of the country for their own benefit, had they adopted a policy of friendly guidance instead of one of destructive criticism, it is doubtful if the present unsatisfactory situation would have developed. The food shortage, in my opinion, could easily have been prevented if the Government had had the strength and the transport at its command to take the wheat from the threshing floors in July and August instead of letting it get into the hands of landlords, peasants, hoarders and speculators. The Iranians, it seems to me, had the right to expect from the allies, as occupying powers certainly not invited into the country, considerably more guidance and assistance than they received.

On the consequences of the riots:

Some of the consequences of the riots are becoming evident; not all are bad. The Iranians have had a salutary lesson in democracy. Many have seen the harmful effect of selfishness run rampant, of the political intrigue, of self-seeking without regard for the common good and of political obstructionism. It is hoped that the Majlis and Government will, as a result of the lesson, work together more effectively for the good of the country. The press, too, has had a dose of bitter medicine, all of the newspapers in Tehran having been suspended. Tehran had, since the abdication of Shah Reza, been flooded with small newspapers, some with a circulation of only a few hundred, most of them serving some questionable political or personal end. The influence of public opinion of these sheets, which preached the most utter nonsense, indulged in personal diatribes and dealt in distorted news, was extremely harmful. It may be that the press, also had a lesson in democratic procedure. The Government's position has beyond question been strengthened. Qavam feels so confident of his present position that he is preparing to re-open the Majlis within a few days, with the assurance that he will have a comfortable majority. It seems probable that he will now have sufficient strength to put through some of the reforms, such as enforcement of the hoarding laws, control of prices and rents, etc., which his weak position in the Majlis and his poor support in the press have made almost impossible. The British Minister informs me that Qavam has within the last few days taken favorable action on two important matters which have been pending for many weeks. I have agreed with the Department that the closing of the Majlis should be avoided if at all possible. It may be that the riots have brought Iranian politicians to their senses sufficiently to make this unnecessary. This, however, remains to be seen. The Iranian masses gained nothing; but they had nothing at all to lose for their status was as miserable as it is possible to be. One cannot help but remark (and even take a certain surreptitious and vindictive delight in the fact) that at least they made themselves heard. That they had no other means of expressing themselves is unfortunate. Can it be that this is the beginning of a new era in which the masses in Iran will claim the right to a standard of living by which they may at least obtain food and shelter?

If anyone gained as a result of these riots, it was the British, who have long sought for a government which would do their bidding with less delay and obstruction. It seems likely that the Qavam Government, since it was kept in power largely at British insistence, will fulfill this desideratum. It should be mentioned, however, that the British gain in power was not accompanied by a gain in prestige. Their action in bringing troops into Tehran from Qum was a psychological blunder and resulted only in further reducing the low esteem in which they are held by the Iranians. It might be mentioned here that the British, perhaps in order to make sure they were not blamed for the riots, have spread the story that the disturbances were part of an axis plot. As stated above, no satisfactory evidence that this is true has come to light.

The Shah, it seems to me, has overplayed his hand. I have always wondered whether his protestations of deep attachment to democracy were sincere and whether he would not one day kick over the traces and endeavor to emulate his father. Whatever his part in the Tehran riots, there is no doubt that he interfered in the political affairs of the State and that he played a losing hand. Having come to the throne as the much hated and distrusted son of Shah Reza, he was able gradually to build up a certain prestige as a kindly, constitutional monarch. The events of the last two weeks have done much to destroy that prestige. It appears to me altogether likely that the Shah will one day lose his throne, if not in the near future perhaps when the allies withdraw from the country and the Iranians again become free agents.

The OSS take on the riots given in a report of February 11, 1943, entitled "Food in Iran" (Research and Analysis, 891.5018/22):

The Joint Food Declaration of December 4 did little to stabilize the situation since wheat stocks were barely enough for a day ahead despite restrictions on amounts. Then came the riots of December 8th. By this time it was impossible to alleviate conditions sufficiently to prevent trouble, and there are those who suggest that the British were not sorry since it gave them a chance to put a stronger military hold on Tehran.

Reports of these riots are conflicting as to cause and events. Apparently begun by student demonstrations against the Majlis, toward evening they spread to include a wider populace and area. Neither the police nor the military interfered at first. The original demonstrators at the Majlis beat up (Abbas) Massoudi (editor of *Etela'at*) when he denounced Qavam, the Premier. Later mobs, however, pillaged Qavam's house, as well as the city shops. There was considerable shooting during the night, with twenty Iranian casualties, and three British. British troops took over the race track outside the city, paraded through it during the day, but did not patrol it. They were brought from Qum, ninety miles south of Tehran, wither they had previously been moved from Kermanshah in exchange for Polish troops. Curfew was moved up from midnight to 8:30 p.m. and the capital put under martial law, administered by an Iranian military commander.

> To complete the picture it is necessary to mark the possibility that the British themselves were playing politics. They had consistently refused to admit the seriousness of the situation when it was developing. Then, when it was real, they used it to get firmer control of the government, particularly finances. For their justification it might be said that something like this had proved necessary, while the means they employed to gain their end may be questioned. In any case, they had troops on hand to take over Tehran should it be necessary, and they found 5,000 tons of wheat in Ahwaz which they brought up when they had gained their ends. Moreover, in the midst of the crisis it seems they tried to replace Qavam with Taddayon, a reactionary, but were opposed by the Russians. In the end they backed Qavam against the Shah and the military clique—the Allies agreeing that the situation needed stability in government more than change. Whether their maneuvering also involved discrediting or embarrassing Mr. Sheridan is a matter only for conjecture, but in the light of their past performance in Iran such a conclusion is not impossible. As already intimated, Iran is in the center of long-standing British imperialism and politics. Because of this, even though directives from London may seem quite clear and sincere, there are persons and forces in the Middle East who are capable of deflecting this declared policy in its actual implementation towards ends inimical to the integrity and well-being of Iran. American best interest require the maintenance of this integrity and well-being. Iranians at present have faith in our friendship and sincerity. We should make sure that the policy of the United Nations bears toward that end. This food crisis is at the center of a larger problem, which may well become the testing ground of Anglo-American relations and cooperation in building the better world we have mutually declared to be our goal.

The British had tried to undo some of the damage. Dreyfus on December 22, 1942 (Dispatch 411 and enclosures, 891.48/325):

> I have the honor to enclose a copy of a propaganda item released by the Public relations Bureau of the British Legation in Tehran on December 9, 1942. The information given in this news release is, to put it bluntly, untrue. It is yet another example of the efforts of the British Public Relations Bureau to fix the entire blame for Iran's ills on the Iranians themselves. This devious policy seems to have had surprisingly little effect in deluding the Iranians. Reference is made to similar British propaganda items enclosed with my despatch No. 386 dated November 19, 1942. There is also enclosed, by way of refutation of

the information given in this propaganda item, a copy of a letter addressed by Mr. Sheridan to the British Minister in which the situation is placed in its true perspective. Mr. Sheridan points out in the antepenultimate paragraph, for example, that had the British expedited the shipment of certain cereals lives and property would have been saved. Mr. Sheridan also took the opportunity to call to the Minister's attention the harmful effects caused by the delay of the UKCC in bringing rice from Resht. I might mention here that the reason the Iranian Government must turn to the UKCC and British army movements control for transportation of cereals is that the British have taken over almost all of Iran's serviceable trucks, leaving almost none for Iranian civil use. It should be pointed out that Mr. Sheridan did not send this letter to the British Minister, since he thought that the information could be conveyed in a more telling manner and with better chances of success if done in a personal interview. This, he informs me, he did.

The British "Points from the News" contains the following:

> Bread situation was just going to improve as a result of Allied imports. Speculators, hoarders, political enemies of the Government, and German sympathizers realized that the position would soon get better. So they seized the last chance offered by the temporary shortage, and organized bands of brigands to make trouble. They even sent schoolboys to shout at the Majlis, although they knew that the boys would be in danger if any shooting started.

Sheridan's statement dated December 10, 1942, reads in part:

> In view of the distressing events of last 2 days I feel it necessary to emphasize that all this trouble could have been avoided if I had sufficient wheat to feed the people of this city. . . . I must point out that . . . in order to maintain public order, feed the people the barest essential of life, 800 grams a day, foreign wheat will have to be made available as a reserve against situations such as have occurred the last 2 days. . . . I wish to point out that had the original contract for supply of 3500 tons of barley plus the offer of the British Army of 1500 of Atta flour been properly executed we would have been able to pass over this period of unrest with its unfortunate results in loss of lives and destruction of property. Finally I wish to call your attention to another delay which if avoided, could have helped us during the last few days. On November 26 I requested the Movement Control to arrange with the UKCC to backload 5000 tons rice from Resht. Colonel Donaldson as

usual did his utmost on our behalf but I now learn today from his office that UKCC paid no attention to this request until December 4th and the final instructions were not given by them until December 6th. As a matter of fact nothing has been shipped from Resht up to yesterday.

British Complaint against Dreyfus

On December 22, 1942, General H.M. Wilson, commander, Persia and Iraq Command (PAIC), had complained about Dreyfus to Lieutenant General F.M. Andrews, Headquarters of the United States Army, Middle East, Cairo (Letter, 891.00/1978). Wilson complains about Dreyfus' response to the arrest of Iranians by the British army, adding:

> The US Minister has also submitted to Washington an accusation that the British Army deliberately delayed sending up barley, etc. to Tehran when it was agreed that this should be provided for the Persian Government. This consignment was dispatched from Shuaiba the day my staff received the order, which entailed loading and train conveying to the Basra docks, off loading into barges and conveyance to Ahwaz, (owing to an unforeseen drop in the river a delay of three days was imposed), and finally conveyance by train to Tehran. My stall could have arranged a quicker route by ordering the off loading of the barges at Khurramshahr, but only at the cost of delaying the off loading of ships bringing aid to Russia, which having no indication of urgency was not justifiable. The attitude of the US Minister in Tehran is making things very difficult for me as well as creating a farcical situation. . . . I have brought this to your attention in case you could see your way to communicating with Washington on the subject, as the last thing I want is that harmonious relations between our two armies should be upset by outside interference.

Dreyfus replied on January 4, 1943 (Telegram 4, 891.00/1978):

> I am confidentially informed by both Admiral Standley and Colonel Ens that General Wilson in letter to General Andrews accuses me of being anti-British and of pursuing a line detrimental to British interests, mentioning particularly my attitude towards arrests of pro-Axis suspects. The accusation that I am anti-British is untrue. My personal and official relations with British officials have been cordial and Legation staff has been scrupulously correct and friendly in dealings with British. It is true that American and British views, actions and objectives in Iran from time to time have been divergent (see Department's

364, December 10 and 372, December 14 which may well have caused this attitude on part of General Wilson) but in such cases my action has been dispassionate, frank and open. I have never sensed on part of British Legation any feeling that my actions have been based on bias or obstruction. My objectives have been first to keep Department fully and accurately informed, second to maintain and strengthen cordial relations existing between Iran and United States, third to maintain the most friendly relations with Iranian, British, Soviet and other officials, always with the primary and overriding objective of the war effort in mind. I shall firmly endeavor to continue along this line.

The following incident will show that General Wilson shares callous attitude toward Iran of many British officials. On the occasion of General Hurley's visit to Iran en route to Russia General Wilson remarked to Hurley in my presence, in reply to Hurley's statement that Iran seemed on point of starvation "Then that should make it easier for us to deal with them."[1]

Note

1. In 1915, the British had also accused the American Minister to Persia during World War I, John Lawrence Caldwell, of being anti-British. Majd, Mohammad Gholi. *Persia in World War I and Its Conquest by Great Britain*. Lanham: University Press of America, 2003. 47-48.

Chapter 16

Fall of Qavam and Re-Appointment of Soheily

Distrustful of Qavam, the British sought his removal. In telegram 375, Dreyfus had mentioned the two documents "that had fallen in his hands." He forwarded them on November 18, 1942 (Dispatch 384 and enclosures, 891.00/1970):

> I have the honor to enclose copies of the two documents referred to in my telegram No. 375, November 14th. These two documents were obtained by the Legation's Military Attaché from secret sources within the British Legation. They are highly confidential and the Military Attaché promised that he would not let their contents be made known to anyone except me. One of the documents outlines a suggested Iranian "shadow" cabinet; the other gives the proposed cabinet's program. I have no reason to doubt the authenticity of these papers. I do not, however, over-estimate their importance, since they do not represent a definitive British plan but rather merely the views of one or several British Legation officials. It is not unlikely that they originated with Mr. Trott, the British Legation's Oriental Secretary. The British Minister has informed me, and in fact he has not concealed from his Government, that he is engaged in considering the composition of alternative Iranian Governments. The documents show, at any rate, the extent to which the British are interfering in Iranian internal affairs. The proposed cabinet is headed by a Prime Minister who has a record of being pro-British, who in fact was a firm friend of Herman C. Norman, one-time British Minister here. It contains a number of persons who are more than pro-British and might be described as British tools, notably the Fateh brothers. It would not appear to me to be a

> particularly strong Government, the various members have been chosen apparently because the British believe their compliance would be readily forthcoming.

The proposed "shadow" cabinet included the following: Mohamad Sadiq Tabatabai, 65, Prime Minister; Mostafa Fateh, 47, Deputy Prime Minister; Nasrullah Entezam, 40, Minister of Interior; Mohamad Saed, about 55, Foreign Minister; Zand, 53, Minister of War; Ali Gholi Ardelan, 43, Minister of Food; Abdul Hossein Hajir, about 40, Minister of Propaganda; Ataollah Ittihadieh, 38, Minister of Communications; and Mahmud Fateh, 45, Under Secretary of Agriculture.

It was stated in the OSS report that during the bread riots the British had tried to get rid of Qavam and had only swung to his support after the Russians had prevented his dismissal, thereby strengthening Qavam's position. Dreyfus on January 10, 1943 (Telegram 70, 891.00/1983):

> Prime Minister informed me yesterday he will very shortly reform his government. . . . Prime Minister told me with evident satisfaction that he has adjusted his differences with Shah and I have verified this from other sources. This is a happy development since the disagreeable and harmful relationship which has existed between Qavam and Shah (see my no. 422, December 9) has prevented formation of a unified and strong government. Since the settlement is probably more surface than real it will be interesting to watch the struggles for power between the political fox Qavam and the ambitious young Shah. There are indications that the Shah has won something of a victory; for example, new cabinet contains three of his candidates and it is reliably reported he is obtaining the dismissal of Qavam's two sons-in-law, Amini his Chef de Cabinet, and Azodi who will go to Brazil as Minister. It is expected that Majlis will as result of this rapprochement be forced to cooperate more readily with Government. Ala informs me that the Shah is ready to dissolve Majlis in case it shows signs of obstruction. It is hoped this new turn of events will permit the formation of a Government capable of solving Iran's many problems. Prime Minister informs me in justification of his recent lack of positive action that he must necessarily in most matters await the arrival of Millspaugh.

On January 21, 1943, Qavam presented his newly reconstituted cabinet. Lester L. Schnare, Chargé d'Affaires in the absence of Dreyfus, on January 29, 1943 (Dispatch 451, 891.00/1990):

The reconstituted Qavam cabinet may be rated well above the Iranian average in ability and integrity. It is essentially a young man's Government, eight of the ministers being under 50 years of age. Two elder statesmen have been retained to furnish "window dressing" and prestige. As the British Minister put it "It would seem difficult to obtain a better Government considering the present circumstances." As indicated in my telegram No. 70 of January 20, the new cabinet is something of a victory, be it ever so fleeting, of ambitious young Shah over the wise old politician Qavam. There is little doubt that the Shah insisted on the appointment of at least three of the new ministers—Rais, Motemedi and Entezam. It may be mentioned, too, that two of Qavam's young relatives by marriage were removed from the Government at the Shah's suggestion—the competent Azodi leaving the Ministry of Roads to become Minister to Brazil, and the equally able Dr. Amini leaving the post of Under Secretary to the Prime Minister to head the Iranian Trade Delegation to the United States. I have reported to the Department on several occasions, as for example in telegram No. 428 of December 9, the political rift between the Prime Minister and the Shah and how this animosity was preventing the formation of a strong unified Government. The present rapprochement, which made possible the formation of this new coalition cabinet, is a happy augury and may bear good results if it lasts. It may well be that the Majlis will fall more readily into line and cease some of its obstruction as a result of the new understanding between the Shah and the Prime Minister. For example, the Prime Minister was able to railroad through the Press Bill which the Majlis had previously resolutely refused to pass. It seems likely, however, that this unruly body will slowly gain courage and begin again to assert itself.

The strength of the cabinet, its young men of intelligence and ability, is also its weakness, for there is a cocksure attitude on the part of most young Iranian politicians which often lands them in difficulties. It was reported in a recent despatch how young, competent, Ebtehaj on being appointed head of the Banque Mellie remarked to an officer of this Legation "No one can tell me anything about banking." The instrument of expression of this political kindergarten is "Iran Javan" (Young Iran), three of whose leading lights are Siassi, Fateh and Mosharraf Naficy. Fateh, it may be mentioned, is in the anomalous and inconsistent position of belonging to the Iran Javan party, which is encouraged by the Shah and includes many of Iran's young aristocrats, while at the same time he is the founder of a new socialistic party called "Hamrahan" (persons who travel the same direction). This group's mouthpiece has been the newspaper *Keihan*, which is widely believed to be supported by the Shah. However, it is understood they will soon publish their own organ, to be called *Iran Javan* and edited by Abdul Hamid Zanganeh. While the cabinet is well regarded by the British, the Russians are clearly dissatisfied. As to American interests, the cabinet seems not unfavorable. The appointment of Saleh is particularly welcome. Our advisers might well be forewarned, however, that they are probably in for a series of headaches in dealing with some of these young officials, especially Naficy and Ebtehaj. While skeptics will continue to wag their heads and say Iran cannot survive except under a despotic ruler, the general trend seems to me to be satisfactory. The new cabinet is composed of intelligent, young men who give at least lip service to democracy; the Majlis, its feathers somewhat rumpled, is still in existence; and the press, considerably chastened, is beginning to reappear. There are those, and the number seems to be increasing, who are in rebellion against the Iranian political and economic system by which the masses are strangled by a government composed of, or subservient to, the landed aristocracy and the dishonest merchant classes. These dissatisfied elements can hardly view with satisfaction the formation of another such Government. But the forces of democracy are growing, slowly but perceptibly, and a day of reckoning will surely come.

The Shah had another reason to feel reassured. On January 7, 1943, Mohammad Hassan Mirza, brother of Ahmad Shah and his designated successor, died unexpectedly in Maidenhead, England, at the age of 43. Politically active since the downfall of Reza Shah, and in apparent good health, he had gone for his daily stroll and was found dead in the street.[1] His death came at a most opportune time for the British and the embattled Pahlavi regime, and was also reminiscent of the death of Ahmad Shah at the age of 32 in 1930 in Paris during the tribal rebellions against Reza Shah. Clearly, the dossier on the death of the two brothers needs to be reopened.

Following the death of the Qajar claimant, and taking advantage of Dreyfus' absence, the British wasted no time in getting rid of Qavam. Schnare on February 8, 1943 (Telegram 146, 891.00/1987):

Qavam Government is in throes of another of Iran's recurrent crises. All ministers except Finance, War, Interior have complied with Prime Minister's request for resignation of entire Cabinet. This crisis referred by the press as "artificial" was caused by protocol dispute following an unauthorized visit the Minister of Interior made on Shah. However, matter is deeper than mere protocol and is in fact another manifestation of the struggle for power between Shah and Qavam mentioned in my 70, January 20. British Minister informs me that Shah indicated to him and Soviet Ambassador in separate interviews his intention of supporting Qavam in present crisis and of prevailing on Minister of Interior to resign or apologize to Prime Minister. British Minister, however, is of opinion that Qavam's position is too weak to permit him to continue to end of war and that consequently alternative Prime Minister should be considered. He believes that most suitable candidate is Taqizadeh providing he can be persuaded to alter his consistent refusal to accept. Qavam having received vote of confidence 65 votes to 42 in Majlis secret session yesterday is now reforming his government.

Schnare on February 13, 1943 (Telegram 170, 891.00/1989): "Prime Minister Qavam resigned today."

Second Soheily Government

Schnare on February 14, 1943 (Telegram 173, 891.00/1992):

My 170. I am reliably informed Shah is considering appointment of Ex-Foreign Minister, Mohammed Saed, as Prime Minister. Majlis is pressing for appointment of Ali Soheily but a group of deputies which called on Shah to request this appointment received no encouragement. British Minister is of opinion Saed is weak, and may become involuntary tool of Shah and army. However, in view of lack of suitable candidate and because Saed is well regarded personally British will make no objection to appointment. British Minister says Russian Ambassador takes similar view. While Saed is certainly not of outstanding caliber he has been friendly and frank in dealing with this Legation. Reference Department's 76 February 11. British Minister informs me he has no (repeat no) intention of encouraging return of Tabatabai to Iran. He also states that Taqizadeh refuses to accept post of Prime Minister and in any event should not be encouraged because of his age and poor health.

On February 15, 1943 (Telegram 176, 891.00/1993): "My 173, February 14. Medjliss yesterday in secret session declared in favor of Soheily for post of Prime Minister by vote of 72 out of 110 present. As a result of this vote, Shah last night directed Soheily to form new Government. It is widely reported Soheily will retain several Ministers of Qavam Government including Saleh."

Dreyfus on February 17, 1943 (Telegram 187, 891.002/379):

> Soheily presented to Majlis the Cabinet listed below. Cabinet's program centers on insuring food supply, lowering cost of living, effecting reforms in Agriculture, Education and Justice, safeguarding interests of farmers and laborers, and strengthening relations with Allies. Vote of confidence in program and Cabinet will be considered at next Sunday's session. Cabinet composed of Ministers already known to Department and Legation appears to be adequate . . . and key appointees in War Finance and Interior fit in well with our program of American advisers. Soheily as he has done on past occasions has left open two portfolios (Agriculture and Food) perhaps to use as bait to obtain support at least temporarily of Cabinet aspirants who have been passed over. Prime Minister informed Majlis he will shortly present to them certain special views he holds regarding Ministry of Food.

Dreyfus on February 22, 1943 (Telegram 198, 891.00/1995):

> My 187. Majlis yesterday gave Soheily Government vote of confidence of 89 out 99 Deputies present. Were 8 abstentions and 2 blank ballots but no contrary votes. Two Deputies demanded government explain why American troops have come to Iran without formal agreement having been reached. Prime Minister replied that Deputies need have no fears in this regard as negotiations for an agreement are under way. Deputy Teymour attacked Sheridan in bitter terms stating food situation had deteriorated since Sheridan's arrival, charging Sheridan with incompetence and demanding his removal. This Deputy also attacked transport regulations and organization set up by Iranian Allied Transport Board. Prime Minister in his speech promised investigation and report on these matters and spoke in a very favorable terms of Iran's relations with United States. While Soheily is at present receiving support of press and Majlis almost all observers predict his government will not last for more than two months. I am not sure this will prove the case. If he can weather storm for a few weeks until wheat begins to arrive from United States and until certain economic and financial plans come to fruition he may be able to take personal credit for achievements of substantial benefits to country.

Dreyfus in a report of March 2, 1943, entitled, "The New Soheily Government; Discussion of Iranian Political Situation," (Dispatch 468, 891.00/2000):

> I have the honor, with reference to my telegrams 187 of February 17 and 198 of February 22, to offer the following appraisal of the new Soheily cabinet and general discussion of the Iranian political scene. . . . In my despatch No. 333 of August 24, 1942, I observed, "The Soheily Government has passed into the great beyond with scarcely a sigh to mark the passing and the Qavam Government has taken its place to face the vagaries and uncertainties of Iranian politics." The shoe is now on the other foot and Qavam, completely discredited, gives way to the man he replaced only six months ago. Herein lies a lesson in practical Iranian politics. No matter how discredited and unpopular a politician may be he will rise again if he has sufficient tenacity and political acumen. To prove this, one need only to refer to some of the bitter and damaging remarks which were being made about Soheily when he surrendered power in August. He was accused of selling Government positions; the press stated freely that his accomplishments were confined to the devastation of Rezaieh, the spreading of famine, and the closing of newspapers. One of the more amusing bits was a cartoon showing Soheily driving a cart containing construction materials from the Ministry of Foreign Affairs building to his new home. Some of these press reports were quoted on page four of my despatch No. 333 of August 24. Majlis and press guns are now similarly trained on poor old Qavam. . . . The immediate and obvious causes of Qavam's fall were three. First, his suggestion that the Iranian Constitution be revised was much resented in the press and Majlis. Second, his action in introducing into the Majlis a bill permitting deputies to assume cabinet position was regarded by most members of that body as a trap to obtain parliamentary support. Third, and most important, his political jockeying in the matter of the bill providing for the appointment of the Banque Mellie Director by the Majlis caused suspicion in all circles of his motives and methods. This last question was dealt with in my telegram No. 155 dated February 10 and my airgram No. A-5 dated February 15. The deeper and truer reasons for his departure are two—first, popular dissatisfaction because of Iran's critical problems, particularly the food situation and high prices, continue unsolved; and second, the Majlis and press are still playing politics to such an extent that it is difficult for the best of Governments to survive. In Qavam's behalf, it must be said that he carried on courageously in the face of almost insurmountable difficulties. He is accused of failure to take

steps to correct Iran's ills and of indulging in political maneuvering. In answer to the first accusation, it may be said that he was in fact actively engaged in ground-work which may eventually pay high dividends to Iran. He was responsible for the engaging of the many American advisers and was purposely delaying action on many important financial matters pending the arrival of Dr. Millspaugh. He was giving full support to Mr. Sheridan in the impossible task of feeding the population of Tehran when the supply of wheat was inadequate. He introduced into the Majlis several constructive bills, as yet unpassed, such as one for compulsory education, one providing for women's insurance, and one amending the conscription law. He was able to force through the press law, which, although a constructive measure did not then or now meet with the approval of the Majlis or the press. He was responsible from the Iranian side for the signing of the wheat agreement with the United States and Great Britain, a measure which will bring great benefit to Iran when American wheat begins to arrive in the near future. In short, he did the donkey-work which paid him no personal dividends but which should be of ultimate benefit to the country. In answer to the accusation that he played politics, one cannot help but ask how he could otherwise proceed in dealing with a political-minded and selfish Majlis and an irresponsible press. It is, in fact, a tribute to his political sagacity that he was able to hang on as Prime Minister for six months.

One must strive to keep a sense of balance in the midst of these constant changes of cabinet in order not to come to the conclusion that all is chaos. He must remember that Iranians, at best, are not noted for political constancy. He should not, however, forget that there is basic common sense and hard-headed intelligence in the Iranian makeup. For example, it was interesting and pleasing to note the resounding and unanimous "no" Qavam received from the press and Majlis when he suggested tampering with the Iranian constitution. Yes, the people, the press and the Majlis are dissatisfied with promises which bring no improvement, with allied intervention in their internal affairs, with soaring prices, with shortage of bread, and with dozens of other woes. They turn to the new Government for solution of these problems. They turn also, and this should be carefully noted, to the American advisers for concrete results. Soheily has an unprecedented opportunity to make good. Wheat from the United States is beginning to arrive and in a few weeks should reach Tehran and the southern famine areas for the rest of this crop year even if no grain is obtainable from internal sources. Also, some of the other problems, particularly the financial ones, are

> being energetically tackled by Dr. Millspaugh. If these food and financial projects come to fruition, Soheily may well "cash in" on them and give the lie to those who predict his government cannot last more than two months. . . . The struggle for power between the Shah and Qavam, which I have reported in frequent telegrams and despatches, has ended in a victory for the Shah. The victory was not a complete one, however, for the Majlis succeeded in imposing its own candidate for Prime Minister in preference to the Shah's choice, Foreign Minister Saed. The bid for power by the Shah will undoubtedly continue, both through the career army and by political machinations in the Majlis, but it will probably eventually end, when Iranians are again free agents, in the loss of his throne.
>
> As compared with previous governments and in capacity to meet the present emergency, the new Soheily Government measures up well. However, as I indicated at the end of my despatch No. 451 of January 29, 1943, more advanced and social minded people consider this merely another government of the entrenched classes, robber barons, landowners and merchant princes. They know that this Government, like its predecessors, will play about on the brink of social reform without having the courage to take the plunge so necessary if the lot of the lower classes is to be improved. Many competent observers, including the very well informed Turkish Ambassador, are of the opinion that Iran is on the verge of a great social upheaval. While it is true that the masses are accustomed to being downtrodden and abuses, it must be remembered that in the former days they had Shah Reza to see that they were given abundant bread at low cost. Conditions have changed, too, in that the people now have the Russian example in the north of the country. They also enjoy tacit, if not actual, Soviet protection in the spreading of socialistic doctrine, whereas under Shah Reza this was heresy punishable by imprisonment and even death. The socialist press is whipping up popular feeling to encourage the cowed and inarticulate masses to open revolt. . . . This interesting and important question will be made the subject of a separate despatch.

The fall of Qavam and the re-appointment of Soheily was a great victory for the Shah. In March 1943, shortly after the advent of second Soheily government, the Shah had felt confident enough to begin to transfer his money from Iran to the United States. As described and documented in another study, in March 1943, the Shah had opened a personal bank account at the Guaranty Trust Company of New York with an initial deposit of $1 million, courtesy of the American diplomatic pouch.[2] At a time when Iran was in the midst of a famine and a raging typhus epidemic, the Shah was transferring his money out of the country.

Upcoming Majlis Elections

The elections to the 14th Majlis are considered the most free, democratic, and meaningful elections held in modern Iran. Dreyfus on March 20, 1943 (Airgram-9, 891.00/2007):

> One of the most important and controversial political topics today in Iran concerns the Majlis elections which are due to be held in August. Most high Iranian officials in their growing fear of communism (see my despatch No. 478 dated March 6, 1943) are apprehensive that as result of elections almost all of the 55 deputies from Soviet occupied zone and many from other areas will be socialists or communists. There is therefore, widespread desire on part of politicians, merchants and representatives of entrenched classes to postpone elections. The British Minister told me frankly that he favors postponement; his stand is undoubtedly dictated by fear of increase in Soviet influence in Iran in detriment to long range British interests. Prime Minister confidentially informed me that Soviet Ambassador has urged him to have elections held as scheduled. Prime Minister expressed opinion to me that, while it may become necessary to postpone elections or even dissolve the Majlis, it is too early yet to consider such matters. . . . I have expressed no views on subject because I feel it is unwise and dangerous to meddle in internal affairs of this kind. Personally I feel that democratic processes should continue in spite of the fact that interests of privileged Iranian classes or foreign powers may suffer.

The elections and the political situation are further discussed by Dreyfus in a report of July 2, 1943 (Dispatch 598 and enclosure, 891.00/2030):

> I have the honor to enclose a translation of a Royal Firman ordering the Minister of the Interior to prepare for the election of the Fourteenth National Consultative Assembly, known in short as the Assembly or Majlis, and to offer a brief discussion of the political aspects of the approaching elections. The elections called for by this Firman are routine and in conformity with the existing law which requires the election of a new National Consultative Assembly biennially. The present law provides for 136 deputies from specified sections of the country. This number will be elected unless, as is being considered, the Majlis amends the law to provide for a greater number, perhaps

200, candidates for election to the Majlis must be 30 years of age, of Moslem religion, well known in their communities and without criminal record. The election law requires that the Shah issue a firman calling for elections five months before the end of the existing legislative term and that elections be held two months before the end of the term. In conformity with this law, the decree was issue on Khordad 31 (June 23) since the Majlis term is completed at the end of Aban (November 22). There is also some talk of the institution of a Senate, which is provided for by the fundamental law but has never been brought into being. The Senate, if instituted, which seems very unlikely, would consist of 60 members, 30 elected from various sections of the country and 30 to be appointed by the Shah. The Russians would hardly look with favor on the formation of a Senate in view of the fact that half of the members would be appointees of the Shah.

These, if they materialize, will be Iran's first free elections in more than fifteen years. I use the word "free" advisedly to mean that one is now free to make himself a candidate, to nominate and back a person of his choice, to organize or develop a party or group, to conduct an open campaign without fear of persecution, to play politics to his heart's content, and, above all, to criticize opponents to the point of slander without bringing down retribution on his own head. That is not to say, however, that the elections themselves will be free and honest. There will undoubtedly be a great deal of political maneuvering and in the end a substantial amount of vote buying for cash or promise of some privilege to come. The approaching elections have stirred a veritable hornet's nest of political activity and intrigue in Iranian circles. The principal internal pressure groups are four: the political "ins" represented by the Majlis members, the Shah and his military clique, the leftists, and the mollas. The deputies, working feverishly to insure their own reelection, have offered Soheily their support of his government in exchange for assurance that they will be kept in office. This assurance, as I indicated in my telegram No. 619 of June 14th, Soheily is unwilling or unable to give. The existing Majlis, a rubber stamp creature of Shah Reza, can hardly be said to represent the free choice of the people. It represents much of the worst in Iranian life—corruption, egoism, power of the entrenched classes, political obstructionism, and unbridled greed. There is no doubt that these politicians would welcome suspension of the elections and prolongation of the thirteenth Majlis.

The Shah and his military group are apparently playing a waiting game, standing by for the proper moment to establish a military dictatorship.

The Shah confided in me in a personal conversation that he considers the Soheily Government too weak to cope with the present situation, that he favors Ali Mansur for the post of Prime Minister, and that he is prepared to dissolve the present Majlis if such a step becomes necessary. The Majlis, bad as it is, represents a democratic bulwark and is in addition what the Department recently referred to as a safety valve. Its dissolution, given the weakness and corruption of the Government, might offer a golden opportunity for the Shah, working through his career military clique especially his Chief of Staff Yazdan Panah, to insinuate the group gradually but surely into power. I have a feeling that nothing like a military coup or sudden movement would be attempted but rather a slower and surer penetration. The Shah has nothing to gain and much to lose by holding elections this year since any change in the political complexion of the Majlis would be toward the left, a movement obviously opposed to his interests.

The left wing is offered perhaps the best opportunity in Iranian history of entering the Government in strength and curbing the vicious rule of the favored classes. The moment is even more favorable than that presented by the constitutional movement of 1906 because of the present occupation of part of the country by sympathetic Soviet forces. There are those who predict that left wingers of varying degree will obtain half of the seats of the fourteenth Majlis. While this may be an exaggerated view, it is quite possible that there will be a movement toward the left, especially in elections in the Soviet occupied zones. The Department's attention is invited to despatch No. 478 dated March 8, 1943 entitled, "Increase in Socialistic Proselytism in Iran," for a discussion of the general subject of the socialist trend in Iran. The mollas are using the elections in support of their bid for return to power, a trend I have indicated in despatches since the departure of Shah Reza. Many mollas in Tehran are actively engaged in electioneering. A leading molla of Tehran assured the Legation's interpreter that he is in a position to insure the election or defeat of any candidate. While this is an obvious exaggeration, it shows that at any rate the mollas are not unmindful of the opportunity now presented them to improve their position. It is reliably reported that a delegation of mollas met the Shah on the occasion of his recent visit to Qum and presented a number of demands, among them the right of women to wear whatever costume they desire (which would remove the present legal prohibition against the veil and make it possible for the mollas to exert pressure to require women to veil), and increased influence of mollas in the Government. Religious leaders would beyond question like to put into active operation the existing but unobserved provision of the constitution which calls for five mollas to sit in the Majlis to pass on all legislation. Something like the eternal triangle is taking place. The Shah courts the mollas while the Majlis woos the Shah!

Foreign powers are not uninterested or inactive in these elections. The Russians, naturally, desire that they proceed in accordance with the law, since the election of a number of socialist deputies seems likely. The Soviet Ambassador has told the Prime Minister pointedly on several occasions that dissolution of the Majlis or postponement of the elections would not be favorably received by the Embassy. The Ambassador has expressed to me and to Sir Reader Bullard less pointedly this same view. It is difficult, in view of this Soviet stand, to see how Soheily can do otherwise than proceed with plans for the elections. He may find, of course, at a later date some method or formula for postponing or delaying which would not meet with too violent Soviet disapproval. The British would much prefer to have the elections postponed indefinitely. They would, as I have often informed the Department, even prefer to see Majlis dissolved. Their action with regard to postponement of elections or dissolution of the Majlis has, however, been restrained and, while they have left the Prime Minister in no doubt of their views, they have not demanded any positive action along these lines. While dissolution of the Majlis might improve allied position in Iran somewhat at the present moment and make it infinitely easier to control the Iranian Government, I am not sure that the long range effects of such an action would be favorable. It would destroy the fiction of democratic government in Iran, a fiction on which a more real and effective democracy must be built in the future. It would perhaps play into the hands of the Iranian military clique by presenting them with a reasonably valid pretext for stepping into the breach at some future date with a military dictatorship. It might, furthermore, strengthen rather than weaken the Soviet position by causing the socialists to redouble their efforts. It might serve, also, to make the Soviets even more suspicious of the activities and designs of their allies in Iran. With regard to British-Iranian relations, it is important to record that the British Minister has expressed to me his great dissatisfaction at the interference and intrigues of the Shah in political matters. To say that the British look with general disfavor on the Shah and his Minister of Court (Ala) would not be indulging in exaggeration.

As far as this Legation is concerned, I have refrained from taking sides or expressing an opinion in this internal and controversial matter of

> elections. Personally, it would seem to me that the elections should go forward and let the chips fall where they may. This is the democratic way and perhaps, all things considered, the best course from our own point of view. Certainly, no Majlis could be more corrupt, inefficient and selfish than the present one. The election of a number of socialist deputies might in the long run be all to the good in bringing about a gradual improvement in the intolerable system of government by the privileged classes. Unless such a change is brought about gradually and in a democratic way, it eventually will have to be achieved suddenly and drastically. The publication of the firman calling for the elections does not necessarily mean that they will take place. There are, as I have shown above, numerous internal and external forces being brought to bear, so that almost anything may happen between now and election time. It is not unlikely that even if elections are fully agreed upon they will be postponed, dragged out, confused and disputed to such an extent that there may be a hiatus between the thirteenth and fourteenth legislatures which will serve the interests of those who desire the demise of the Majlis as adequately as would out and out dissolution. There are many who predict that there will be riots if elections are held. This view has been confidentially expressed by General Ansari, who is generally well informed. The British Legation support this view, possibly to support their contention that the elections should be postponed. The possibility of riots developing must not be overlooked, however, in view of the bitterness and heat with which the elections will be disputed. A newspaper states that Dr. Jordan once remarked that if there were political parties in Iran they would number 15,000,000 since no two Iranians could agree, while another newspaper declares that there are only fifteen million candidates for the 136 seats in the Majlis. There are said to be, seriously, as many as 150 candidates for Tehran's 12 seats as the horses go to the post. The race should not be without excitement.

Additional comments on the forthcoming elections are contained in an OSS report of July 22, 1943 (Communication No. 37, 891.00/2037):

> The life of the Iranian Parliament is two years. Elections for the current XIIIth Parliament were held in August, 1941 and the first return were just coming in at the time of the joint British and Russian occupation of Iran on August 25, 1941. Thus the present deputies were men who had been handpicked by the dictator, Reza Shah and who were suddenly confronted with the real responsibility for government instead of merely voting in favor of policies drawn up by Reza Shah.

> The XIIIth Parliament opened on November 13, 1941 and its term expires in November of this year. An Imperial Firman stating that elections for the XIVth Parliament are to take place has already been issued and voting is to begin soon after Shahrivar 1st (August 24th). For the period of the voting, it is a long drawn out process, and probably for some time in advance martial law will be abrogated to permit public meetings and other activities connected with the campaign to take place. In spite of many rumors, chief of which is that the present Shah will attempt to intervene in the elections, these elections will undoubtedly be the first free ones for many years: since the early days of Reza Shah and before he had established a machine to assure the election of mere puppets. Nearly all of the present deputies will strive to keep their seats; the chances of using devious methods towards this end are greater in the provinces than in Teheran. Many new people will be elected. At least one elderly and highly respected opponent of Reza Shah has declared his intention to run for a Teheran seat and other men will be supported by reviving political parties or by the host of new ones coming into being. . . . An interesting summary of the situation in Teheran is condensed from an editorial of July 18th in the non-partisan paper "Iran." "Teheran elects 12 deputies to Parliament and there are now about 1000 candidates for these seats. Teheran has now some 40 newspapers and is said to have some 20 political parties. At this moment we in Teheran are speaking about our regained national rights, about the crooked leaders of the old regime and the men without honor who were prominent during the past 20 years. It is good to be able to speak once more of freedom and righteousness. But not so easy to do anything about it: for if you ask anyone you know to name 10 really good men from among these 1000 candidates, they are at a complete loss to do so."

On the forthcoming elections in Azerbaijan, Consul Richard Ford from Tabriz on August 11, 1943 (Dispatch 3, 891.00/2047):

> I have the honor to present herewith a discussion of current political developments in the province of Azerbaijan. The usual public announcement has been made by the Governor General to the effect that the coming election of deputies to the (14th) national parliament must be kept clean, that free balloting must be observed, and that any coercion of voters will be appropriately punished. It is reported of course that practically with the same breath the Governor General gave verbal orders to his private henchmen to make sure that the appropriate appointments and transfers of the right gendarmerie and ballot-takers are

made forthwith in order to insure that voting not get out of hand and not too heavy for the wrong candidates. At two different political rallies in Tabriz during the past week, one by liberal elements on the anniversary of Iran's constitutional regime and the other couple of days later by the Anti-Fascist Society of Tabriz, the deplorable condition of election practices in Azerbaijan was the subject of much comment, particular emphasis being given to the charge that the present deputies in the parliament are puppets of the ex-Shah and that the workers of the province have neither appropriate representation in the government nor any likelihood of getting it under present conditions. The meetings are reported to have adjourned amidst cries of "Death to Pahlavi" and "Annihilation of Fascism," respectively. . . . At the anti-fascist rally mentioned above, at which 2000 workers are reported to have been present, the first speaker devoted considerable time and energy to an impassioned eulogy of the Russian soldiers, and of how these splendid troops had saved the workers of the world including Azerbaijan from slavery and worse under the axis. . . . That this speaker was followed immediately on the program by the above-mentioned denouncer of election frauds in Azerbaijan was probably a coincidence. Nevertheless, one cannot help remarking the number of cases which continue to arise in this province in which appreciation of Russian soldiers is linked to the sorry state of the workers of Azerbaijan. . . . Under the auspices of the Governor General and the Armenian Archbishop, the Moslems and Armenians of Tabriz are taking up a collection for the purpose of participating in the reconstruction of the city of Stalingrad.

Notes

1. Majd, Mohammad Gholi. *August 1941: The Anglo-Russian Occupation of Iran & Change of Shahs*. Lanham: University Press of America, 2012. 364-370.

2. Majd, Mohammad Gholi. *Great Britain & Reza Shah: The Plunder of Iran, 1921-1941*. Gainesville: University Press of Florida, 2011 Reprint Edition. 324-330.

Chapter 17

Anglo-American Exchanges and American Views on British Policy in Iran

On December 11, 1942, Lord Halifax had called on Under Secretary Welles (Memorandum, 891.00/1985):

> The British Ambassador called to see me this morning at his request. I read to the Ambassador appropriate portions of London's 6999, December 10, 10 p.m., and Tehran's 426, December 9, 10 a.m., and 427, December 9, 4 p.m. I emphasized in the strongest terms the very grave concern of this Government at the way in which British authorities in Iran seem to be undertaking to pursue a policy not only at complete variance with the policy which this Government believed to be wise, but also with the policy which the British Foreign Office was informing this Government the British Government itself was pursuing. I said it seemed to me utterly incredible that at the very moment that the British Foreign Office was informing us that it was instructing its representative in Iran to move heaven and earth to get wheat and barley to Tehran and our own Minister in that capital was informing us that 3,500 tons of barley and 1,500 tons of flour were at Basra and earmarked for Tehran, the British Minister in Tehran should be telling the Iran Government that the British Government did not see any reason why cereal should be sent to Tehran so long as British subjects were abused in the streets of that city. I stressed again the importance of Iran as the one sure means of furnishing supplies to the Soviet Union, and emphasized the fact that in our judgment if the British authorities in Iran continue their present policy, the nation would be in

such a state of foment as to make it altogether impossible to control the situation, even with a military strength far greater than that which the British Government had available in that area. I concluded by saying that our considered views in this matter were being cabled to Ambassador Winant for communication to Mr. Eden. The Ambassador said that he fully agreed with the policy of this Government with regard to Iran. He said he thought it was criminally stupid for the British authorities in Iran to pursue the policy they were following when there was nothing to be gained by it and only trouble to be anticipated. He said he would cable Eden himself, indicating in the clearest terms our concern in the matter and expressing the belief that appropriate action should be promptly taken by the British Government.

American-British Exchange of Notes

As indicated by Welles, on December 11, 1942, a long instruction was sent to Winant in London (Telegram 6280, 891.00/1964A):

Please urgently transmit to the Foreign Office substance of the following:

During the past year the Government of the United States has felt itself to have an increasingly direct interest in conditions in Iran. We have been led to adopt this position primarily because of the importance of Iran in the war effort of the United Nations, an importance which is of course fully recognized by the British Government. In addition to our general interest, in common with all the United Nations, in the successful prosecution of the war in all theaters, we have felt special responsibility in connection with Iran for the following reasons. A. American prestige in that country places this Government, we believe, in a position to exert powerful influence on behalf of the United Nations, and it is felt that this is an important asset which should be conserved and utilized. B. The Iranian Government has requested a large number of American advisers to strengthen the internal administration of the country, and we feel obligation to see that the work of these advisers is begun and carried out under conditions favorable to their success. We understand that the British Government has been heartily in favor of the dispatch of these advisory missions; on several occasions the British Government has, in fact, taken the initiative in suggesting their formation. It is, of course, obvious that such advisers can exert a most effective influence on behalf of our common cause. C. The American Government has made heavy commitments in connection with the furnishing of supplies to the Soviet Union and is therefore directly concerned in the maintenance of the route by which a large part of these supplies must necessarily be transported. In addition, the United States military authorities have recently agreed to undertake the physical operation of the Iranian ports, railroads, and highways by which supplies for Russia are moved through Iran.

We have been given to understand on various occasions that the British Government welcomed the interest of the United States in Iranian affairs and that our active cooperation in settling the problems which arise from time to time was desired. We feel sure that the British Government understands our policy is in no way motivated by considerations of self-interest but is directed solely toward the furtherance of the common war effort and the preparation of foundations for satisfactory and lasting peacetime conditions in Iran, as in the rest of the world. With this in mind the Government of the United States has, as the British Government is aware, taken an active part in the exchanges of views and negotiations which have taken place since the middle of October 1942 in connection with the acute political and economic situation in Iran. It has been the consistent view of the Department of State that a satisfactory solution of the problem could only be achieved through adequate provision, in one way or another, for the minimum economic needs of the Iranian people and through the maintenance to the maximum possible extent of Iranian authority and responsibility in the internal affairs of the country. Quite apart from the obvious moral principles involved, principles to which the United Nations are pledged and to which we know the British Government subscribes without reservation, it has been the opinion of the Department that purely practical considerations would in any case dictate that the military forces and civil responsibilities of the United Nations Governments concerned should be kept to a minimum in Iran, in order to permit the employment of those military forces and of the civilian personnel in other areas where they would be of more immediate value in the prosecution of the war.

Accordingly, in its communications to the British Government and to the American Minister at Tehran in connection with the crisis which began in October, the Department has repeatedly expressed its desire that early and adequate arrangements be made for the transportation to Iran of supplies of wheat which would prevent famine in areas deficient in grain stocks. In taking this position, the Department has recognized that the Iranian Government might be in part at fault in not taking proper steps to ensure the best use of available food supplies within the country. However, we have felt that the urgency of the matter precluded prolonged discussions or reorganization of the Iranian agencies concerned and we have further felt that the use of coercion upon the Iranian authorities would not only have undesirable repercussions but would also fail to achieve the objective sought. From the exchange of communications which has taken place between Washington and London, we have gathered that the Foreign Office was in substantial agreement with this point of view. With particular reference to the question of coercion, the Foreign Office will recall that the Department has more than once expressed its feeling that a military occupation of Tehran or the establishment of a puppet government would be undesirable, and in the light of views expressed by the Foreign Office to our Embassy in London and by the British Embassy in Washington to the Department, we have believed that the British Government was in agreement. The Department has likewise on three occasions expressed its fear that action taken by British authorities against Iranian subjects alleged to be engaged in activities inimical to the United Nations would have serious and unfortunate repercussions unless handled with great care. In particular we urged that the Iranian authorities themselves be allowed to handle such matters. On November 28 the Foreign Office advised our Embassy that it, too, felt that caution should be exercised and that it had telegraphed the British Minister to this effect. Foreign Office stated that it hoped it would not be necessary to take action against the wishes of the Iranian Government.

In view of the apparent agreement, as above indicated, of the Foreign Office and the Department with respect to the principal questions involved, the Department has noted with surprise and regret that events in Iran during recent weeks do not seem to have been in accord with the policies of our two Governments. These events, as they have been reported to the Department, may be summarized as follows:

A. Despite the clear recognition by all three governments of the urgency of the matter, signature and publication of the Anglo-American-Iranian agreement for the supply of wheat to Iran was delayed for several weeks, apparently in large measure because of the desire of the British authorities in Iran to impose successively more difficult conditions upon the Iranian Government before proceeding to signature. Whatever the reason, however, the agreement was concluded only on December 4, when popular dissatisfaction in Iran had become so great that it failed to have the reassuring effect anticipated. B. Despite the assurances given to the American Embassy at London on November

> 25 with regard to the contemplated arrests of prominent Iranians, the British authorities in Iran on December 8 proceeded to intern the Governor General of Isfahan. We are informed that this action was taken without prior consultation with the Iranian Government and that it produced a most unfortunate effect. C. The British Minister at Tehran informed the American Minister on December 9 that a battalion of British troops would enter the city that same afternoon. D. The American Minister at Tehran reported on December 9 that the British authorities in Iran had for some reason failed to bring to Tehran the 3500 tons of barley and 1500 tons of flour earmarked for Iran and held at Basra. Likewise on December 9 the British Minister advised the Shah that the British Government would not look with favor on the importation of wheat into Iran unless the Iranian Government were favorable to the Allies. It is understood that the British Minister made a similar statement to the Iranian Prime Minister. It is superfluous to point out that this attitude is in direct conflict with the previous action of the Foreign Office in instructing the Minister of State at Cairo and the British Minister at Tehran to arrange immediate shipment of barley and wheat to Iran from Iraq and from other near-by sources. It is likewise in striking contrast to the statement made by the Foreign Office on December 10 to the American Embassy at London to the effect that the Foreign Office fully realized that the extreme shortage of wheat, particularly in Tehran, is the primary cause of unrest and disorder in Iran.
>
> In the light of the foregoing, which is submitted solely with a view to a closer coordination of British and American action, the Department ventures to express the hope that the British Government will take such steps as it deems desirable to bring about a more accurate reflection in Iran of the policies laid down by the British Government in London.

Eden's response was conveyed by Winant on January 7, 1943 (Telegram 282, 891.00/1979):

> Foreign Office's comments and questions affecting Iran, mentioned in Embassy's 7114, December 15, 8 p.m. have just been received in memorandum form with a covering letter dated January 6 signed by Mr. Eden. Mr. Eden's letter reads as follows: "I hope that this memorandum clears up any minor misunderstandings which may have arisen between our two governments on Persian problems. I believe that on the main issues we are both in substantial agreement. There is one

further point, not dealt with in the memorandum, which I should like to bring to your personal attention. It is implied in the State Department comments that, although our two governments see more or less eye to eye, nevertheless Sir Reader Bullard is carrying out a policy of his own, which is not in accordance with our views, but creates unnecessary difficulties with the Persians. I hope that the State Department will dismiss this possibility completely from their minds. I am convinced that Bullard is loyally carrying out the policy of His Majesty's Government to the best of his ability, and I have the fullest confidence in him. It is true that he has sometimes had to take action of a nature displeasing to the Persians, who thereupon are apt to run around to Mr. Dreyfus to complain. But on these occasions he has acted with the full approval of His Majesty's Government and as I believe in the interest of the United Nations. If, as I hope, the United States representative in Persia is able to cooperate more actively in future in maintaining the interests of the United Nations, I think we shall encounter far less difficulty than hitherto in our dealings with the Persian authorities."

The Foreign Office memorandum of January 4, 1943, had papered over the differences:

> The United States Embassy's memorandum of the fourteenth December, communicating the observations of the State Department on recent developments in Persia, has been considered in the Foreign Office with the greatest care and sympathy. It is believed that the policy of His Majesty's Government towards Persia corresponds very closely with that of the United States Government. At the same time it is felt that a full and frank exchange of views on this subject will be of great value, lest misunderstanding should arise on points such as those enumerated in the latter part of the memorandum under reply.
>
> Two. In the first place, the Foreign Office wish to confirm their entire agreement with the views expressed in the Embassy's memorandum as regards the increasing importance of the United States Government's interests in Persia. Indeed, the growing interest which the United States Government have shown in Persian affairs has been very welcome to His Majesty's Government, who, as the State Department point out, took the lead in suggesting that United States advisers should be sent out to Persia to strengthen the internal administration of the country. His Majesty's Government therefore fully understand and share the anxiety of the United States Government that these advisers should be

enabled to carry out their work under favorable conditions, and are confident that their work will prove of the greatest value in reorganizing the finances of Persia and in putting the administration on a sound and efficient basis. His Majesty's Government also recognize that the arrangement whereby the military authorities of the United States are to take over the operation of Persian ports, railways and roads greatly increases the interest of the United States Government in the maintenance of law and order throughout the country.

Three. His Majesty's Government also confirm that it has for long been their desire that the United States Government and the United States authorities in Persia should cooperate more actively in settling the questions arising from time to time. Until recently the task of maintaining the interests of the United Nations at Tehran has fallen almost exclusively on the British Legation. It is hoped that it may henceforth be possible for the United States representative at Tehran to take an equally active part in helping to solve the important problems of common concern to the Allied Governments, and it is believed that the task of the two Legations may be greatly eased by the steadying influence which will be exercised on the Persian authorities through the United States advisers.

Four. As the State Department are aware, it has been the policy of His Majesty's Government not to occupy Tehran by military forces, but to allow the Persian Government to continue to administer the country with as little interference as possible. In order to encourage a spirit of collaboration in the Persian authorities, His Majesty's Government took the initiative in the negotiations which culminated last January in the signature of the Anglo-Soviet-Persian treaty of alliance. By this treaty Persia acquired the status of a non-belligerent. This policy has on the whole been successful hitherto, the degree of collaboration afforded by the Persian authorities has in general proved sufficient, but on three problems of major importance it has been necessary, in the interest of the United Nations war effort, to bring strong pressure to bear upon the Persian Government and to contemplate measures which have, as it appears, led the Persian Government to put forward complaints to the Government of the United States. These three problems are: (one) The provision of local currency for the United Nations forces in Persia; (two) The wheat problem, and (three) security measures against Axis agents in Persia.

Six. In the United States Embassy's memorandum under reply, it is stated that considerations of self-interest in no way motivate the policy of the United States, but that this policy is concerned only with the furtherance of the war effort of which the United Nations and with the laying of a basis for satisfactory and lasting peace time conditions in Persia, as well as in the rest of the world. His Majesty's Government readily accept this assurance, and they must request the United States Government in return to accept a corresponding assurance on their behalf. In dealing with the three problems mentioned above, and in all their dealings with the Persian authorities, His Majesty's Government have not been moved in any way by consideration of self-interest but have been concerned with the furtherance of the war effort of the United Nations.

Seven. The difficulties raised by the Persian Government in connection with the supply of rials to the British forces in Persia were, in fact, difficulties which had to be surmounted by some means or other in the interests of the war effort. Without rials it would have been impossible for the Allied forces in Persia to pay for local purchases and local labor. It was absolutely essential that rials should be forthcoming. Otherwise, the trans-Persian lines of communication for supplies of war material to the Soviet Union would have broken down. After difficult negotiations, a solution appeared to have been reached through the conclusion of the Anglo-Persian financial agreement on the 26th of May, and it was therefore all the more deplorable that the Persian authorities, despite the clear terms of the agreement, should again have sought only a few months later to withhold the necessary currency from the Allied forces. The State Department are aware how, mainly as the result of the common front displayed on this occasion by the Allied representatives at Tehran, it proved possible to solve these difficulties without having recourse to forcible measures, and it may be hoped that, with the forthcoming arrival at Tehran of the United States Financial Mission, a further Persian threat to withhold the currency essential to the United Nations need no longer be apprehended.

Eight. Again, as regards the wheat problem, the policy of His Majesty's Government has been directed solely towards furthering the essential war interests of the United Nations, with due regard to the minimum requirements of the Persian people. It has been based upon two governing considerations. The first is that, quite apart from the shortage of shipping, the clearance capacity of Persian ports and transport routes is strictly limited, so that every ton of wheat imported into Persia for Persian consumption involves a reduction in the quantity of vital war supplies sent to the Soviet Union by the trans-Persian routes. The second point is that Persia in normal times grows sufficient cereals for her own use, and the 1942 harvest is believed to have fallen very little short of a normal harvest, so that there must exist in the country sufficient stocks of cereals to last nearly until the harvest of 1943. It will be recalled that, during the period between military operations of August 1941 and the summer of 1942, some 50,000 tons of wheat were imported from British and United States sources to satisfy in the exceptional circumstances then existing the needs of the Persian civil population. But the Persian Government, almost immediately after the harvest of 1942, complained that there was already a serious shortage and requested that further wheat should be imported for their use. It was evident that they were reluctant to take drastic and unpopular measures against hoarders, speculators and profiteers, and thought it easier to appeal to the Allies to solve their difficulties for them by arranging further imports. This attitude was clearly inadmissible. It would have meant a reduction in the supplies sent across Persia to the Soviet Union, for reasons which could not have been justified to the Soviet Government. His Majesty's Government agree that it is in itself desirable that steps should be taken to save the Persian people from want, but it is clearly necessary to insist upon the Persian authorities making the best use of the food supplies available within Persia, and the only wheat imports to which His Majesty's Government have hitherto agreed during the present season are the 25,000 tons of wheat which are being imported to replace the Persian-grown cereals required by the occupying Soviet forces.

Nine. Security measures against Axis agents have also been the cause of serious difficulties with the Persian Government. For many years past German influence in Persia has been extensive, and it was largely owing to the presence of Germans and German agents in key positions throughout the country that it became necessary for British and Soviet forces to undertake the military occupation of certain areas in August 1941. At the present moment, there are still some Germans in hiding in the unoccupied districts of Persia, there are still German agents who are active throughout the country, and there is still a considerable amount of pro-German sympathy in influential Persian circles. His Majesty's Government regard it as absolutely essential to take such steps against German agents as may be required to safeguard the Allied troops and communications in Persia. Some Germans and some German agents have already been arrested, others have been allowed to escape by the Persian police or are said to be untraceable. But proof has been obtained of a widespread conspiracy organized by the Germans with the help of a number of influential Persians, involving definite plans for sabotage against Allied communications, and risings against the Allies in the event of a German invasion of Persia. It is clear that drastic action is justifiable and necessary against those implicated in such matters though such action has hitherto been confined to a minimum.

Ten. The foregoing general observations are intended to cover the main aspects of British and United States policy in Persia, and although emphasis has naturally been laid upon these points which have caused most difficulty and on which differences of outlook are most likely to arise, the Foreign Office believe that on the whole the views of the two governments are very closely in agreement as regards the major issues. There remain the four questions referred to at the end of the United States Embassy's memorandum under reply.

(one) It is true that the signature of the Anglo-United States-Persian agreement for wheat was delayed because it was desired to ensure, in connection with the wheat agreement, a satisfactory long term agreement of the currency dispute. As stated above, rials are absolutely essential for the United Nations forces in Persia. His Majesty's Government felt therefore that it was essential to insist on some new currency arrangement, whereby the Majlis would no longer created difficulties on every occasion when they were asked to provide the necessary rials. As soon as a satisfactory solution on these lines was reached, there was, so far as His Majesty's Government are aware, no further question of delaying the signature of the wheat agreement in order to impose on the Persian Government more difficult conditions. And, as distinct from the agreement, His Majesty's Government have at all times and irrespective of their disputes with the Persian Government, sought to accelerate the despatch of the wheat which was urgently needed owing, primarily, to the Soviet requisitions in Northern Persia. (two) General Zahidi, the Governor General of Isfahan, was arrested because he was implicated in the serious conspiracy referred to above. Careful consideration was given to the question whether the Persian Government should be consulted in advance, but it was decided that to adopt this course would involve the risk of leakage, and would in addition be most embarrassing to the Persian Government themselves. The information at the disposal of His Majesty's Government indicates that the effect locally of General Zahidi's arrest has been very salutary. (three) The sole reason for the despatch of a battalion of British troops to Tehran during the recent rioting was to protect Allied property and military stores.

(four) The Foreign Office were surprised by these reports from the United States Minister at Tehran, which implied that the despatch of certain consignments of foodstuffs to Tehran was being delayed by the British authorities for political reasons. This, as in the case of wheat shipments, would certainly have been opposed to the views and intentions of His Majesty's Government. They therefore telegraphed to Sir Reader Bullard, who has explained that there is of course no foundation whatever for any suggestion that the despatch of this flour and barley to Persia had been deliberately delayed in order to put pressure on the Persian Government. On the contrary, the British Legation had done everything possible to hasten its despatch. (Such delay as occurred seems in fact to have been due partly to an unexpected fall in the level of the Karun River while the barges conveying the grain were on their way to Ahwaz, but mainly to the physical difficulty of moving it from Cshaiba to Margil, thence by water to Ahwaz, and thence by rail to Tehran). Nor did Sir Reader Bullard speak to the Shah or the Persian Prime Minister on the lines mentioned, or threaten them in any way with the possibility that supplies already arranged might be withheld. It is hoped that it may be made clear to the United States Minister at Tehran that he has been misinformed on these lines.

Dialogue with Casey

On January 7, 1943, Casey had met with Welles (Memorandum, 891.00/2095-1/2):

Mr. Richard Casey, former Minister of Australia in Washington and at present British Minister of State in the Middle East, called to see me today. I spoke to Mr. Casey of my very great concern with regard to the policy being pursued by the British Government in Iran. I said I felt that, in the first place, from the standpoint of achievement of satisfactory results, the British policy of the withholding of food supplies and the constant recurrence to military force was not conducive towards the creation of a situation of relative tranquility in Iran which alone could give us the assurance that this vital means of access to southern Russia would remain open to the United Nations. Furthermore, I said, the attitude taken by so many of the British officials in Iran towards United States officials, and particularly towards the American Minister in Tehran, was anything but helpful. I said I did not have to tell Mr. Casey that the United States had no selfish interest of any kind or description in Iran, but that this Government did feel that during the war period it was just as vitally concerned in the maintenance

> of satisfactory conditions in that country as Great Britain. I said I consequently felt that close and friendly cooperation between the officials of the two Governments in that area was indispensable for the sake of our common military objectives, and I also felt that our views with regard to the policy to be pursued towards the Government and officials of Iran should be taken into consideration by the British Government before it embarks upon any undertakings of any serious character in the region. Mr. Casey told me that he had arranged to see Mr. Murray this afternoon, and I told him that Mr. Murray would undoubtedly give him chapter and verse for the statements and suggestions I had just made to him.

In the meeting with Murray, Alling, Merriam, Allen and Jernegan were also present (Memorandum, 891.5018/ 31-1/2):

> Mr. Casey said that he and his staff at Cairo had long ago come to the conclusion that ultimately it would be necessary to ship wheat to Iran in order to tide the country over until the 1943 harvest. However, his economic advisers had strongly urged him to make no announcement to this effect until the last possible moment, since otherwise the Iranians would make no effort to bring out the large stores of hoarded wheat in the country. This policy had, accordingly, been followed until recently. It was, of course, abandoned with the signing of the American-British-Iranian food agreement of December 4.
>
> Mr. Murray said that the Department had felt that there was complete agreement between Washington and London on the subject of policy in Iran, but that there appeared to be a lack of coordination between London and Tehran, as policies laid down in London did not seem to be followed by British officials in Iran. Mr. Casey said that Mr. Welles had raised the same point with him during the conversation earlier in the day. Mr. Welles had also indicated his feeling that the British authorities had been using wheat as a weapon to force Iranian compliance with British wishes. Mr. Casey had assured him that the British in the Middle East had not used wheat in any way as a political weapon and that the sole purpose in withholding an undertaking with regard to wheat had been to induce the Iranians to take steps to bring into the market their own supplies of domestic wheat before recourse was had to imports. As regards the apparently unfavorable impression which the Department had received of British policy in Iran, Mr. Casey was inclined to attribute it to the fact that the British and American Ministers in Iran "did not see eye-to-eye." In expressing this opinion, how-

ever, he was not attempting to apportion blame or praise, since he was not sufficiently familiar with the local situation to do so.

Mr. Murray said that the Department had been very disturbed at the reported remarks of certain British officials in Iran to the effect that they would not favor supplying wheat to Iran so long as Iranian sentiment remained hostile to Great Britain. He remarked that it seemed hardly possible to win the love of the Iranians by starving them, and he went on to emphasize the fear of starvation engendered in the Iranians by their unhappy experience at the end of the last war. Mr. Casey did not reply directly, except by saying that anti-British feeling was not, in fact, manifest in Tehran during the recent riots and by saying that the Iranians did have reason to hoard wheat, both because of their fear of starvation and because of attraction as an investment under present circumstances.

Mr. Casey spoke of the difficulties the Allied Governments had had in connection with obtaining supplies of local currency in Iran. He said that the British Government had been faced with a most difficult situation during the crisis which began in October, 1942. At one point they had only sufficient rials to continue operations for two or three days, and the Majlis was refusing to issue additional currency. Since the British were engaged in work vital to the transport of supplies to Russia, it was impossible for them to suspend operations; yet it was almost unthinkable to resort to the use of force in order to obtain the necessary currency. His own instructions had been to use force only as the very last resort. He had gone himself to Tehran, had talked to Iranian officials and had asked for suggestions from every possible quarter but no one had seemed to have any constructive ideas on the subject. The Prime Minister, Qavam, had done nothing but wring his hands and express the forlorn hope that some way might be found whereby the Iranian Government could live up to its obligation under the Anglo-Iranian Financial Agreement of May 26, 1942. The American Minister, Mr. Dreyfus, had likewise been unable to suggest anything.

Mr. Murray referred to the previous financial crisis, in the spring of 1942, which had been resolved by the conclusion of the agreement of May 26. He pointed out that the British Government had appealed to the Department at that time and had found it necessary to change its previously uncompromising attitude toward the Iranians and to make concessions in connection with the conversion of sterling exchange

> into gold and the provision of dollar exchange to meet Iranian needs. It was also pointed out that the later crisis in the fall of 1942 had been settled ultimately through a concession with respect to supplies of wheat, in return for which the Iranian Government had transferred control of currency issue to a committee, in accordance with British desires. These developments were cited as evidence that it was, in fact, possible to deal with the Iranian Government on a basis other than the use of force, to which the Department was firmly opposed.
>
> Mr. Casey was asked whether he believed that the Iranian Government had the administrative organization and capacity to enforce anti-hoarding laws and bring out of hiding the wheat known to exist in the country, provided it set itself to the task. He indicated that he thought it possible, if all branches of the Government cooperated whole-heartedly. He mentioned in particular the gendarmerie, saying that the cooperation of Colonel Schwarzkopf would be necessary. In passing, Mr. Casey spoke highly of Colonel Schwarzkopf and also of Mr. Sheridan, the Food and Supply Adviser.

On January 8, 1943, there was another meeting between Casey and Murray at which Alling and Jernegan were also present. In a note of January 12, 1943, addressed to Under Secretary Welles and Assistant Secretary Berle, Murray writes (Memorandum, 891.00/2004):

> I had two long conversations with Mr. Richard Casey, British Minister of State in the Middle East, while he was in Washington last week. I think you may be interested in the attached strictly confidential memorandum regarding British and American policy in Iran. As you will note, on page 4 I made a strong appeal to Mr. Casey to join with us in bringing about the introduction into public life of younger British and American-trained men, such as Allah Yar Saleh, the new Iranian Minister of Finance, and the elimination of old-time corrupt politicians. I also strongly urged Mr. Casey to support us in endeavoring to handle the Iranians by conciliatory, rather than by "crack down" methods. In reply to Mr. Casey's rather critical attitude toward Mr. Dreyfus, I pointed out that Mr. Dreyfus had at all times been acting under close instructions of the Department, which were formulated in consultation with the British Foreign Office.

The memorandum of January 8, 1943, follows:

Mr. Murray opened the conversation by reverting to the previous day's discussion on Iran and reading to Mr. Casey the Department's long telegram of December 11 to London setting forth our general attitude toward Iranian affairs, vis-à-vis the British Government, and our surprise and regret at the apparent lack of coordination between the policies of the Foreign Office at London and the actions of the British authorities in Iran. Mr. Casey expressed his entire agreement with the first part of that telegram, in which the Department explained the reasons for its special interest in Iran in connection with the furtherance of the common cause of the United Nations and its understanding that the British Government welcomed this interest and was in substantial accord with the American Government with respect to the policy to be followed. He appeared to feel that we might have been misinformed or have misinterpreted British actions, with respect to the various incidents cited in the final portion of that cable. Specifically, he said that the delay in conclusion of the Anglo-American-Iranian Food Agreement of December 4 was not due to any desire of the British to cause such a delay. It was, rather, because of the necessity for carrying on three-cornered telegraphic correspondence between Tehran, London and Cairo with regard to phraseology and various details as well as questions of policy which had to be decided. At later stage in the conversation, Mr. Casey said that he himself had been responsible for one change in the bases of negotiations, which doubtless contributed to the delay, since he had suggested that the food agreement not be concluded unless a satisfactory long-term solution of the currency question were reached at the same time. He pointed out that we had been proposing to bind ourselves for a period of some twelve months in connection with wheat supplies, whereas no arrangement had been made which would assure us of a supply of rials for more than a month or two.

Mr. Murray then went on to read excerpts from certain telegrams received by the Department: 1) Tehran's 362, November 7, in which Mr. Dreyfus reported new conditions proposed by the British Minister as essential requirements to signature of the food agreement, the most notable being that the Iranian Government must support the war effort, must seek full powers from the Majlis, and must agree to modify the cabinet in accordance with the wishes of the Allies. Mr. Casey expressed surprise at this and indicated that he had not hitherto been aware of these proposals. He seemed particularly struck by the suggestion that Iran support the war effort, indicating that he did not think such an undertaking could mean very much. Mr. Murray stated very emphatically that the British Minister's proposals had astonished the Department, which had been unable to comprehend the reasoning behind them and regarded them as most unwise and as indicating an unfortunate point of view on the part of the British Minister at Tehran. 2) Mr. Murray then read a part of London's telegram 6340, November 11, confirming Mr. Dreyfus' report regarding conditions proposed by the British Minister and saying that the Foreign Office had already advised the Minister at Tehran that it did not regard them favorably. 3) With further reference to the attitude of the British Minister, Mr. Murray next read the statement in telegram no. 427 of December 9 to the effect that the Counselor of the British Legation had told Mr. Dreyfus of the intention of the British Minister to tell the Shah that he could not favor bringing cereals to Iran while the country was so hostile to the Allies. Mr. Murray again remarked that the Iranians could not be expected to become more friendly in the face of such attitude. 4) Finally, with reference to the British policy in arresting Iranians suspected of pro-Axis activities, Mr. Murray read the first sentences of Tehran's telegram No. 451, of December 19, reporting General Ridley's conversation with the British Minister. He pointed out that Sir Reader Bullard had agreed, after the damage had been done, that the British authorities should refrain from arrests of Iranian army officers but to permit the Iranians themselves to handle such cases. Mr. Murray went on to say that this was the policy the British themselves had always followed in Egypt, and he felt that it was surprising that it had not been adopted in Iran.

Mr. Casey said he would like to explain that all the British authorities in the Middle East had been greatly worried by the Iranian situation. He himself had gone to Tehran and spent three or four days there seeking light on the matter. He had found an impression on the part of the British Legation that the American Minister was not taking an active interest in the problem and was not cooperating in the effort to find a solution. Mr. Casey appeared to believe that there might be some basis for this impression, although he himself was not in a very good position to judge. So far as he could gather, the entire weight of the crisis had fallen on the British, since the Russians, as usual, were unhelpful and would not even provide information regarding their own activities in northern Iran. Consequently, the British had felt that they must go ahead and do the best they could on their own.

Mr. Murray said that any apparent holding-back on the part of the American Minister might be attributable in part to a feeling that the

British were, after all, in occupation of Iran and, therefore, should properly take the initiative. A further consideration might be a belief that general British policy in the area was too much influenced by a "crack down" spirit, a spirit which had long-since gone out of favor in the United States. The Department was strongly of the opinion that the Iranians could be better handled through conciliatory methods than through the application of pressure. Mr. Murray emphasized that Mr. Dreyfus had acted throughout under the instructions of the Department and in entire accord with the policies of the Department. In this connection, Mr. Murray read an excerpt from Tehran's telegram no. 4 of January 4. He omitted any reference to the letter written by General Wilson to General Andrews, but mentioned that Mr. Casey might have heard that Mr. Dreyfus had been accused of being anti-British. He then went on to read Mr. Dreyfus' remarks regarding his personal and official relations with British officials and his general attitude toward the British, Russians and Iranians. He also read the final sentence of the telegram, as a further illustration of what he considered an unfortunate attitude of certain British officials toward the Iranian situation. Mr. Casey said that he expected to revisit Iran in the near future and at that time would do his best to straighten out any differences of viewpoint which might exist between Mr. Dreyfus and Sir Reader Bullard. Mr. Murray expressed his hearty approval.

Mr. Casey then referred to the generally weak moral fiber of the Iranian people. He said that the Shah had spoken of this to him and had expressed the wish to do something about it. Mr. Casey had suggested that the Shah gather together a group of the better type of younger men and use them as an influence on the rest of the population. In particular, he had mentioned a young man, whose name he had forgotten, the head of the mortgage bank, who had impressed him with his character and understanding of Iranian problems. The Shah had agreed that this man was a fine type, but had expressed doubt as to the possibility of finding others.

Mr. Murray said that he welcomed Mr. Casey's attitude on this question, since it coincided exactly with our own. He emphasized our belief that the only hope for improving conditions in Iran lay in introducing into public life the younger British and American-trained men, such as Allah Yar Saleh, new Iranian Minister of Finance, and eliminating the old-time corrupt politicians who had taken turns for so long in holding all the important posts in the Government. We had, some months ago, suggested this to the British Foreign Office but the reply had not been encouraging. The Foreign Office had taken the position that any attempt by Great Britain or the United States to push forward any individuals would result in the branding of those persons as foreign "tools" and would destroy their usefulness. Mr. Murray pointed out that this Foreign Office view was hardly in accord with the drastic measures which had been proposed by Sir Reader Bullard in connection with the alteration of the Iranians Cabinet at the will of the Allies. He went on to say that he hoped very much that Mr. Casey would join with us in supporting the entrance into public life of young men of the right type, and he emphasized that the important thing for the future was to have good men in office with minds of their own, not someone who would take orders from any foreign power which supported him. Mr. Casey said that he entirely agreed. Mr. Murray then spoke of certain suggestions which had been made that the Majlis should be dissolved. He said that we had been inclined to consider this proposal, but that we had now come very much to the conviction that it would be unwise, since the Majlis, with all its faults, served as a safety valve and was regarded by the Iranian people as the safeguard of their liberties. Mr. Casey agreed with this view and said that dissolution of the Majlis had been considered only when it seemed that it might be the only way to solve the currency impasse.

Finally, Mr. Murray said that he would like to throw out a thought with regard to the Russian position in Iran. Our reports indicated that the Russians, by following a conciliatory policy and by engaging in elaborate propaganda, have established themselves very strongly in northern Iran. One of our reports had even gone so far as to say that a Soviet could be set up in Azerbaijan overnight, if the Russians gave the word. This trend seemed very reminiscent of the policy followed by Russia twenty years ago in the early days of the communist regime. All that time, the USSR had made a grand gesture of taking Iran under its protection and had given back to Iran all of the Russian rights and concessions, such as the railroad, the bank, et cetera. The purpose of this policy had been, of course, to put Great Britain on the defensive in Iran, weaken her influence there, and it had succeeded. A parallel might well be drawn with the present situation. As a specific instance, the Russians had not followed the British example in moving troops into Tehran last month, and in consequence Russian standing had improved and British had declined. Mr. Murray felt, therefore, that the British Government should keep this in mind. It was worth considering *why* the Russians were taking such pains to establish themselves in northern Iran. In any case, it would be advisable for the British and

American Governments to coordinate their policies and stand together in Iran.

Dreyfus on British Policy in Iran

On January 15, 1943, all the memoranda of conversations with Richard Casey had been sent to Dreyfus (Instruction 180 and enclosures, 891.00/1964A). On February 24, 1943, Dreyfus had submitted a long report on British policies in Iran (Dispatch 462, 891.00/1999):

> I have the honor to offer the following comments on the matters discussed in the enclosures to the Department's instruction No. 180 of January 15, 1943. Before turning to relations between this Legation and the British Legation in Tehran or considering the various points raised in the Department's instruction or discussing general problems of common interest to Great Britain, the United States and Iran, it will be well to make certain that our policies and objectives in Iran are clearly understood and stated. I am in full agreement with the statement of American policy and aims in Iran contained in the Department's telegram No. 6280 of December 11, 1942, addressed to the Embassy in London. Proof of the fundamental soundness of the Department's policy with regard to Iran and of its appreciation of the country's difficult problems have been given on many occasions. . . . I quote, as evidence of my agreement with the Department's statement of our aims and objectives in Iran, the following excerpts from my telegram No. 66 of March 13, 1942: "(4) American Position. American prestige in Iran is very high. Our aims should be, first, a short range objective of using Iran's strategic position for prosecution of the war, which aim nothing should be permitted to thwart, and second, maintenance of our high prestige for constructive use in post-war period. . . . Iranians cannot be expected to cooperate fully and voluntarily with two powers regarded with suspicion and distrust and if they are to be converted from passive appendage to willing partner it will be only through American sympathy and assistance. (5) Conclusion. I recommend that we give Iran our sympathetic support in this hour of need and furnish where possible the goods and advisers requested. I advise that any action suggesting force or open interference in internal affairs be avoided unless necessary for the war effort. I recommend that we avoid if possible joining British representations for fear we thereby lower our own prestige and share to some extent the historic onus which is certain to attach to British action in Iran. We must of course

continue close collaboration and friendly relations with British officials in Iran in matters connected with the war effort."

He next discusses British policy in Iran:

It is difficult to define or appraise British policy in Iran. For general background on British-Iranian relations, the Department is referred to "A Review of the Joint British-Soviet Action against Iran" enclosed with despatch No. 144 of November 1, 1941, and for a resumé of more recent British-Iranian relations to despatch No. 409 of December 21, 1942, which dealt with the Tehran riots of December 8. The latter despatch reviews British-Iranian relations since the invasion of the country, developed the theme of ever-increasing Iranian hatred and distrust of the British, and described the impotence, confusion, breakdown in morale, inefficiency in Government and growth of political opportunism which attended the change over from dictatorial to democratic Government. It revealed how the Iranian complex of attributing all of the country's ills to the British and Russians has prevented the building up of a spirit of cooperation on the part of the Iranians in dealing with the British. This intransigent attitude of the Iranians explains to some extent why the British have felt that nothing can be accomplished except by show of force.

It is impossible to determine how much British policy in Iran is accidental and how much calculated, to what extent the British were merely endeavoring to make the best of an admittedly bad situation and to what degree they have kept the country in insecurity and hunger for the purpose of being able to retain control. There seems no doubt whatsoever to me that the British missed their great opportunity in Iran by not encouraging the reestablishment of security immediately after their invasion of the country. This could quite easily have been done at that time and would have prevented a chain of events which robbed the country of its internal security, its communications, its morale and finally its food. With internal security maintained, which means also that communications would have been preserved, I have no doubt that wheat could have been collected in sufficient quantity to tide the country over until the next harvest.

I, personally, should describe the British policy as shortsighted than evil-intentioned. Mr. Joseph Upton, American representative of the Metropolitan Museum and a keen observer of Iranian affairs, attributes to the Indian Civil Service the muddle into which the British have permitted themselves to fall in Iran. The Indian Civil Service, which still has a great deal of influence in British affairs in Iran, is, according to Mr. Upton, reactionary and given to dealing harshly with what the British consider as "inferior races." Many other informed and unbiased observers are of the same opinion. There is, of course, something to be said for the British view, for the Iranians have been stubborn and uncooperative, a fact which has often required the British to take strong measures to insure steps essential to the war effort, such as insuring the supply of rials for allied operations. The British error would seem to be not that there is no merit in their individual complaints or actions but rather that they have adopted an unfortunate and overbearing manner in dealing with the Iranians. They might well have taken lessons from the Russians, who, as the Department pointed out on page 5 of the memorandum of January 8, 1943, are slowly gaining the confidence of the Iranians by pursuing a conciliatory policy and by treating the people as friends and equals. This the Russians are accomplishing in spite of the fact that at the time of the British-Soviet invasion of Iran they were equally hated with the British and infinitely more feared. The British, I might add, are somewhat touchy on this point. For example, the British Minister, at a recent meeting in reply to Mr. Sheridan's statement that the Iranians are saying that the Russians have fed the Iranians in their zone while the British are starving the people in theirs, replied warmly that such an allegation is unfair because the Russians have the wheat-bearing zones while the British have only the starvation areas. It would be an unfair over-statement of the case to say that the British have deliberately and as a matter of policy prevented the reestablishment of internal security or permitted famine to develop. However, there is ample evidence that they have used these situations as a lever to obtain their desires and improve their position.

Dreyfus next discusses his relations with the British:

Turning now to the impact of our policy on that of the British and specifically to the relations of this Legation with the British Legation in Tehran, I should like to emphasize that I have scrupulously endeavored to be fair to the British in reporting to the Department. Let me quote, in substantiation of this claim, from two of my telegrams. In reporting on the matter of the arrest of Iranian nationals, the Legation stated in telegram No. 111 of April 18, 1942: "While I believe the arrests will not have the desired salutary effect but will only to further serve to alienate Iranians, I should be reluctant to criticize British actions. Iranians while giving lip service to allied cause have frequently obstructed the British and have offered little of the cooperation which their treaty obligations and official statements have given the Allies the right to expect." In No. 271 of August 26, I telegraphed: "Summary. Saleh's statement that Iran faces a critical situation is true but his inference that the blame therefore lies entirely with the allies is unfair. It has been very difficult to get Iranian cooperation and there has been great delay, confusion and inefficiency on the part of Iranian Government. Both British Minister and I have had to press Prime Minister repeatedly in above matters and our efforts are just beginning to bear fruit."

This brings me to the important point of the relations existing between this and the British Legations. Believing that I have always been fair to the British and having thought that our relations in Tehran were cordial, I was pained to read Mr. Casey's statement that "the British and American Ministers do not see eye to eye." This I believe to be a harmful and exaggerated statement of the case. Relations between the two Legations and between the British Minister and myself have, in fact, been cordial. We visit each other several times a week, consult each other on all matters, and maintain a great deal of social exchange. The British Minister, who has a staff some ten times that of mine, is most kind in furnishing this Legation copies of documents, translations of laws and bits of information which come his way. His staff is also on the best of social and official relations with mine. It is quite true that we do not always agree, but I have made it a policy to place my cards on the table in all frankness where there is a divergence of opinion. I have never, in any of my reports, made comments personally unfavorable to Sir Reader Bullard, for whom I have the highest regard. That there is close cooperation between the two Legations is shown by the fact that Mr. Schnare attends the British weekly press meetings, Mr. Minor attends the British weekly staff meetings, and the delegates of this Legation work in close harmony with the British in committees dealing with supplies, transport, the proclaimed list, et cetera.

It is true, as remarked by the British Foreign Office on page 1 of the Embassy's telegram No. 282 of January 7, 1943, that the Iranians if displeased at British action, may come running to me to complain. I have called the Department's attention on several occasions the danger which must constantly be guarded against of permitting the Iranians to play us off against our allies. When they come to me, therefore, an honest endeavor is made to examine into the merits of the particular matter in dispute and to take dispassionate action. There is always latent friction in this respect, since by and large British regard the Iranians coldly and harshly in contrast to the sympathetic attitude of this Legation and almost all Americans in Iran. I hope, in any event, that my action is such cases is based on good judgment and not on any anti-British bias. The British statement contained in paragraph 3 of the London Embassy's telegram No. 282 to the effect that this Legation has not cooperated fully in allied affairs in Iran is an exaggeration hardly worthy of consideration. What the Foreign Office really meant was that this Legation has not cooperated fully in purely British actions, such as the matter of the arrest of pro-Axis suspects, questions connected with the tripartite agreement and disputes in which the American Government was not primarily concerned. I will consider in the following paragraphs, in support of this statement, some of the important Allied-Iranian questions and will at the same time make reply to certain statements contained in the enclosures to the instruction under acknowledgment.

(a) Political Problems. In matters of Iranian politics, there has been close cooperation between the two Legations and I have never felt, knowing my Government's attitude, that I could accompany Sir Reader in questions involving interference in internal affairs or pressure on the Iranian Government. As an example of the use of pressure by the British Legation, especially as an instance of the use of wheat as a political instrument, I enclose a copy of a British Legation office memorandum dated November 6, 1942, and a copy of a British Legation telegram addressed to the Foreign Office on the subject of the wheat agreement. Incidentally, this telegram is the one which seemed to surprise Mr. Casey according to the memorandum of conversation of January 8. I honestly feel that this Legation has been a restraining and stabilizing influence in the relations of the British with the Iranians. For example, it is likely that a word from the Legation, based on instructions from the Department, would have resulted in the dissolution of the Majlis. I am convinced, upon mature reflection, of the basic soundness of the Department's belief that the Majlis is a valuable safety valve and, in spite of its faults, should be retained or at the worst, suspended pending new elections. This matter was commented upon on page 4 of the memorandum of January 8. In the matter of the expulsion of the Japanese Legation from Tehran, this Legation played a dominant role and demonstrated its ability to act in positive support of the British when the matter is one in which we are vitally concerned. . . . In the matter of British propaganda, too, I have been unable to accompany the British. British effort in this respect is so labored and obvious that it defeats its own ends. The Department is referred, for an example of this kind of propaganda, to the enclosure of my despatch No. 386 of November 18, 1942.

(b) Wheat. This Legation has taken the view that, although there may have been some hoarded wheat in Iran, it would not be possible to make it available to the people because of conditions of insecurity, lack of transportation, and breakdown in government machinery and morale. The result, the Legation has contended, would be famine in the winter. The British view has been that there is plenty of hoarded wheat in the country and famine would not develop if the Iranians only took steps to help themselves. I supported the British view that the Iranians should be required to help themselves, as shown most clearly in telegram No. 271 of August 26, 1942. When it became apparent to me that despite all Iranian efforts, or as the British put it lack thereof, a shortage would develop, I recommended to the Department that wheat be shipped without delay. I must point out in all modesty that my stand in this matter was completely vindicated by the riots of December and the present severe bread shortage. British Legation policy in the matter of wheat is directed largely by Counselor Squire, an Indian civil servant. Mr. Squire has clung stubbornly to his view that there is sufficient wheat in hoarding to feed Iran, a belief to which he is obstinately committed. In endeavoring to justify his contention, he has often overreached himself in making estimates of hoarded wheat and judging the quantity available in various areas.

To turn now to some of the statements in the Department's instruction, the Foreign Office is misinformed in remarking on page 6 of the London Embassy's telegram No. 282 that Sir Reader Bullard did not, when speaking to the Shah and Prime Minister, threaten to withhold supplies previously arranged for. My telegram No. 427 of December 9, 1942, was based on a memorandum which Counselor Holman of the British Legation delivered to me at my house. This memorandum, on a small piece of paper, enumerated the points which the British Minister proposed to make to the Shah in his conversation the same afternoon. My No. 428 later in the same day was based on a talk with the British Minister in which he stated he had in fact made this point in his conversation with the Shah. Sir Reader told me a few days ago that he had been misunderstood in this question since he had intended merely to give friendly counsel decidedly not in the form of ultimatum. It is also true that Sir Reader, in Mr. Sheridan's presence, remarked to the Prime

Minister that the Iranians could hardly expect to receive wheat from the British when British subjects were being insulted in the streets of Tehran. It is also true that Mr. Casey, on the occasion of his visit to Tehran, told the Prime Minister the Allies would not furnish one grain of wheat for this country. Notwithstanding this pronouncement, Mr. Casey proposed a trade of 5,000 tons of British wheat for 30,000 Iranian rifles. But, Mr. Casey now explains that the obdurate stand of the British on wheat was based on a desire to make Iranian hoarders disgorge. How were the Americans, much less the Iranians, to know what was in the back of Mr. Casey's mind!

While there is cause to believe the British purposely delayed the shipment of cereals to Tehran, it should be noted in all fairness that in my No. 427 of December 9 I did not state the delay was calculated but merely reported "I know that British have failed for some reason." I regret that there are at the present moment similar delays in bringing Iraq barley to Tehran. If this condition does not improve in the next few weeks I shall report fully to the Department. In closing this section, I should like to point out that the tripartite food agreement originated with my telegram No. 327 of October 17, 1942, which proposed a unilateral American declaration. The idea of changing this to a tripartite agreement was given in my 333 of October 20.

(c) Transport. This Legation has played a leading part in solving Iran's transportation difficulties. . . . The Department will recall the Legation's struggle with the UKCC, which was endeavoring to monopolize Iranian transport. As a result of a joint approach by the British and American Legations, as reported in my No. 242 of July 27, 1942, an Iranian-American-British-Soviet transport board was set up. This board, on which the Legation is represented by Mr. Kidd and Mr. Minor, is doing a constructive job of organizing and operating Iranian road transport. A large part of the success of this important venture is due to this Legation.

(d) Finance. In this field, the Legation has cooperated closely in full harmony with the British Legation. The Department's advice has been helpful; see for example instruction no. 96 of May 11, 1942, enclosing seven memoranda on the subject of Iranian finance. The Legation followed closely the British negotiations for a financial agreement with Iran and reported general Iranian financial matters. . . . There is inconsistency in the statements contained in the memoranda enclosed with the Department's instruction under reference regarding this

Legation's part in financial negotiations. Mr. Casey is said on page 3 of memorandum of conversation of January 7, to have stated, "The American Minister, Mr. Dreyfus, had likewise been unable to suggest anything," while the Foreign Office is reported in paragraph 7 of London Embassy's telegram No. 282 to have said, "Largely as a result of the common front displayed on the occasion by the allied representatives at Tehran, the State Department are aware of how it proved possible to solve these difficulties without having recourse to force." . . .

(e) Middle East Supply Center. This Legation also cooperated with the British and played an equal role in establishing the Combined Supplies Committee in Tehran, the local branch of the Middle East Supply Center. The Legation was largely responsible, through its high prestige with the Iranians, in persuading the reluctant Iranians to submit to MESC routine. The Legation's action in this regard was reported to the Department in 1942 telegrams 119, 192, 204, 214 and 271. The Combined Supplies Committee now includes strong American representation.

Arrests. In the matter of the arrest of pro-Axis suspects, the Legation has indeed not seen "eye to eye" with the British Legation. . . . However, I can lay claim to having been extremely frank in informing the British Minister on several occasions that I was of the opinion that the harm done by the arrests, especially if carried out by the British themselves, would be far greater than the advantage to be gained. In addition, I feel that I have not been blind to the British viewpoint but have dealt fairly with the British in reporting to the Department. For example, I stated in my No. 256 of August 10: "British are to a certain extent justified in their present attitude (see last paragraph No. 111 April 18) because of Iranian lack of cooperation." As a result of our restraining influence the British are proceeding in this matter of arrests with far more care and regard for Iranian susceptibilities than was formerly the case.

Conclusion. The above discussion is not intended as a polemic against the British nor yet as a vindication of the viewpoint of this Legation. It is aimed rather at proving that this Legation has cooperated with the British in matters of mutual concern and at disproving that there has been any basic friction between Sir Reader Bullard and me or between our Legations. I fully appreciate the difficulties of the British in dealing with a stubborn race which offers little voluntary cooperation and in addition suspects British motives even in cases where only good is

> intended. The following story illustrates the difficulties under which the British labor in Iran. Mr. Minor inquired of Mr. Khonsari, a director of the Agricultural Bank, as to why the Iranians responded so rudely and negatively to a British offer to bring gold bars into Iran to place in the Banque Mellie in exchange for Iranian gold coins, which would then be placed in circulation as an experiment (see my telegram No. 165 of February 12, 1943). In reply to this question, Mr. Khonsari answered, "There is an Iranian proverb which says 'When one has been bitten by a snake he is ever after afraid of a black cord.'"
>
> I should like, in closing, to express agreement with the Foreign Office statement made in paragraph ten of London Embassy's No.282 to the effect that on the major aspects the views of our governments are in close agreement. This Legation will, for its part, redouble its efforts to maintain the most cordial relations with the British and to contribute its full share in matters of mutual interest. When there is difference of opinion, I shall continue to make it a point to express my disagreement to the British Minister in frank, constructive and friendly terms. I am hopeful that, as a result of the very frank discussion which has taken place concerning American and British policy in Iran, our relations with the British here will retain their cordial character, a fact which should contribute not only to the war effort but also to laying the foundation for a constructive post-war era in this unfortunate country.

Bullard's urgent telegram of November 6, 1942, to the Foreign Office, mentioned by Dreyfus above, which was based on a memorandum of November 6, 1942, by Iliff, Childs, and Squire to Bullard was repeated to the British Embassies in Moscow and Washington as well as to the Minister of State in Cairo and to India. Thus, Casey's display of "surprise" at its contents when meeting with State Department officials was feigned:

> Your telegram No. 1440. 1- I am grateful for your helpful guidance. 2- General situation, however, has seriously deteriorated during the past few days and continues to do so. Any satisfaction from the Persian Government on currency issue alone is insufficient, if other important issues are left completely at the mercy of the Government's dependence on the Majlis. Concession on wheat in return for currency will only mean that later we shall find ourselves compelled to make further concessions when other issues arise, as inevitably they will.

3- In these circumstances I consider that now that we have something substantial to offer the present is the time to set the stage for a role of complete co-operation on the part of the Persian Government. I recommend therefore that we should inform the Prime Minister forthwith that the Government of the US (if they agree) and we ourselves are prepared to support his Government (or any other Government) only in the following circumstances: (a) If we have an assurance that the government is prepared unequivocally to operate a policy of co-operation with the Allied War effort in not only the letter but the spirit of the Treaty and Financial Agreement, and in particular gives us immediate satisfaction on the following points. A guaranteed supply of currency, rigorous enforcement of anti-hoarding legislation, an effective system of price fixing, control of the press, and security. (b) To enable the government to honour its engagement under (a) we shall expect the government to obtain emergency powers from the Majlis for a year or six months on the lines of our Emergency Powers Act, and, if thought necessary and desirable, leaving the Majlis in being for debate but without the power to reject any measures introduced by Decree of the Council under its emergency powers. (c) We may call upon the Prime Minister at any time to modify the composition of his cabinet so as to rid it of uncooperative elements, and to include ministers (military officers if necessary) recommended by us.

4- Only if the Prime Minister is prepared to accept the conditions in para. 3 above should he be given the concession contained in the proposed food declaration. 5- I fully realize that this line of action may lead to the fall of the Government but I feel that the situation has now deteriorated to a point where if measures of this kind are not taken, we may be faced with economic and political chaos. I am of course considering the composition of alternative governments, and I have not overlooked the possibility that it may be necessary to use force either to maintain the supply of currency or as a result of action by the C.-in-C. out of purely military considerations. (Ref. his tel to Troopers). 6- US Minister is reporting my above-mentioned recommendations to Washington and asking for instructions. He states he is in personal agreement with my proposals, but is reluctant to put them to Washington as being his own. In the meantime, however, he is prepared to press Government "informally" to obtain emergency powers on the lines suggested in (b) above.

On March 29, 1943, W. Strang, the British Deputy Under Secretary for Foreign Affairs, had a meeting with Murray, Alling and Jernegan.

The Russian policy and attitude referred to is discussed in chapter 19 (Memorandum, 891.00/2015):

> Mr. Murray spoke of the interest of the United States in Iranian affairs, in consequence of that country's importance to the war effort, and referred to the American program of assistance to Iran in the form of advisers and technical experts. He asked whether the British Government did not agree that some form of outside assistance would be needed to put Iran back on her feet and whether it did not seem desirable that this aid be provided by the United States in order to avoid the difficulties which had arisen in the past when Great Britain and Russia have judged it necessary to intervene in Iran. Mr. Murray recalled that the British Government itself had taken the initiative some time ago in suggesting that the United States furnish a military mission and other advisers. The United States, in fact, had responded to a number of Iranian requests for advisers and believed that it would be advantageous to the common cause to continue to expand this program, since otherwise there might be a collapse of the Iranian Government with a resulting serious drain upon the resources of the Allies in maintaining order and keeping the Russian supply route open.
>
> Mr. Murray then went on to speak of disquieting reports which had recently been received regarding the attitude of the Soviet authorities in Iran. It appeared that the Soviets were increasing their influence in northern Iran and at the same time looking with suspicion upon the efforts of the American advisers to assist the Iranian people. They had complained against the American Consul at Tabriz, whom they obviously wished to get rid of, and they just expelled from Azerbaijan an American representative of the Food and Supply Adviser who had been trying to prevent famine in the province. Further, they had placed obstacles in the way of the operations of General Connolly's force, which was dedicated to the transportation of supplies to Russia. They had not yet even expressed their assent to the presence in Iran of this force. (In this latter connection, Mr. Murray remarked that it was unfortunate the British Government had not advised the Soviet Government of the plans to bring in American troops. We felt that since the British were in control of southern Iran, it was their responsibility to clear a matter of this kind with their Ally, instead of which we had been placed in the position of making explanations to the Russians which should never have had to be made. We now understood that the British minister at Tehran had offered to provide full information to

the Soviets, but we did not know whether he had done so. (Mr. Lang said he had no information on this.)

The general Russian attitude, Mr. Murray said, was reminiscent of pre-1914 period, when Morgan Shuster was forced out of Iran by Russian pressure. The Department had been thinking, therefore, that it might be advisable for the American and British Governments to open parallel or joint conversations with the Russian representatives in Tehran, with the idea of enlisting active Soviet cooperation in solving Iranian problems. Mr. Strang commented that it was impossible to talk to the Soviet authorities except at Moscow, and Mr. Murray replied that we realized the Ambassador at Tehran would not be able to make any important decision but we felt it would be well to begin by taking soundings at that point.

Mr. Murray alluded to the question of "disestablishment" of the Allied powers in Iran which would arise at the end of the war. He felt that American influence and activity in Iran would be helpful at that time. In this connection, he felt we should keep in mind the strong personal interest of the President in the general Iranian question, and he referred to the exchange of messages which had taken place between the Shah and the President at the time of the Anglo-Russian occupation. The President had taken note of the assurances given by the British and Russian Governments that Iranian independence would be respected. Mr. Lang asked how much of the foregoing had been sent to London. Mr. Murray replied that we had advised London fully by telegraph of our general attitude toward the Iranian situation and had also been in close touch with the Foreign Office regarding specific problems which had arisen. In addition, we had discussed matters with Mr. Casey on the occasion of his visit to Washington. We had not, however, been in communication with London with respect to the Russian attitude, which had only become alarming in recent weeks, although the matter had been mentioned in passing to Mr. Casey.

In the course of our interchanges with London, we had received the impression that there was a complete meeting of the minds between the Foreign Office and the Department, but there seemed to be a hiatus between the views of the Foreign Office and the actions of the British authorities in Iran. There also seemed to be an impression that the American Minister at Tehran was anti-British and he was not cooperating with his British colleague. Mr. Murray felt that this was unfortunate, in the first place because he was sure it was not true. He emphasized that the Minister had been in very close touch with the Department throughout the recent difficulties and had been acting in precise accord with the instructions of the Department. Mr. Strang said that he did not himself deal with Near Eastern affairs and could not comment on Mr. Murray's remarks. However, he had made careful notes and would report our views to the Foreign Office.

Franz Mayer Documents

The discovery in November 1942 by the British of documents concerning a pro-Axis plot was reported above. Dreyfus has a report dated March 25, 1943, and entitled "Franz Mayer Documents: A collection of papers allegedly seized by the British and published by them to show a widespread Axis plot in Iran" (Dispatch 495 and enclosures, 891.00/2008). On the discovery of these documents, the American Military Attaché writes:

> The history of the discovery of these attached documents is as follows: On November 2, 1942, in Isfahan during mid-morning hours, Franz Mayer himself is reported to have had an altercation with his servant. This reputed wiry, wily, spy is said to have lost his head and tried to fire at his servant with his pistol. The pistol, according to reports, jammed; he then threw the pistol at his servant and it is not clear whether his servant returned any fire. Sufficient to say that Franz Mayer ran out of his house instantly and the servant likewise ran out making a direct line for the English Consul's residence in Isfahan. Here the time element is confusing as it was reported that the Consul took an escort of British troops and immediately went to the house occupied by the said Franz Mayer before he, Mayer, could remove his belongings. Not knowing the time element in this operation, I am unable to state the feasibility of such an action, i.e. (1) Distance from Consul's home to point of British escort. (2) Distance from Franz Mayer's residence to point of British escort. (3) Mode of transportation used. (4) Any pertinent combination of time, distance, and rate. However, upon entering the residence of Franz Mayer a search was made and a brief case with an attaché case full of letters was seized and the translation of these letters are the documents herein attached. Such are the brief, sketchy, and all too meager facts concerning the recovery of these documents.

Dreyfus comments on these documents:

> I have the honor to enclose herewith in single copy a set of papers known as the "Franz Mayer Documents" together with an analytical report on them by Major John G. Ondrick, formerly Military Attaché at Tehran. These papers . . . have been widely used by the British authorities in Iran as evidence of a widespread and highly organized Axis plot. It was on the strength of the "evidence" contained in these papers that the British last December arrested General Zahidi, Governor General of Isfahan. The peculiar circumstances surrounding the seizure of these documents, the complete confusion of the order of presentation, the prevalent amount of trivial correspondence, and the manner in which the British used these papers make any definite conclusion as their authenticity and importance extremely difficult. It will be noted that Major Ondrick was unable to reach any positive conclusion although his analysis and reasoning show a thorough study of the papers and sound reasoning. His statement that some of the papers are authentic and some manufactured can not be questioned although the motives for the forging of such trivial material may seem rather obscure. In my opinion the British authorities did lay their hands on certain correspondence belonging to Franz Mayer and used them to spread the legend of a widespread plot. I do not mean to imply that there was no plot nor that Franz Mayer and certain others mentioned in the documents were not engaged in an undertaking perhaps even directed by the appropriate authorities in Berlin. I can not accept, however, the enclosed documents as evidence of a dangerous conspiracy against the security of Iran. I feel that one reason for the complete confusion and lack of chronological sequence with which the papers are presented was to hide the essential weakness of the "plot" they reveal. It is interesting to note that the Soviet authorities in Iran apparently took no action on these documents and gave the British no material support in their arrest of persons involved. No one can accuse the Russians of neglecting counter espionage where needed. Russians are refusing to deliver to British certain Iranians who have taken refuge in Soviet occupied zone.
>
> By and large, I believe that the British have been guilty of over-emphasis rather than deliberate fabrication, though as I have stated above there is considerable evidence of that. No one can question the fact that a great majority of Iranians are anti-British and anti-Russian and, being born intriguers, a certain number were bound to engage in some sort of pro-Axis activity. A great number of the letters involved appear

to be merely those of certain Iranians who went off "half cocked" believing the Germans would soon be in Iran and desiring to climb on the band wagon in plenty of time to assure their positions when the invasion occurred. Vaziri, the Irantour employee whose correspondence with Mayer constitutes the great bulk of the documents, is a typical example of this. Vaziri, incidentally, is still at large and all British efforts to capture him have been fruitless. A great part of the Vaziri correspondence is probably authentic although, we may question his letters involving name of his fellow conspirators in any considerable number. Although the British spread the word throughout Iran that they had obtained evidence of a serious axis plot, they have to date failed to take any vigorous action against a great many of the people involved. While they did arrest General Zahidi and a few others on the strength of the Franz Mayer documents, certain persons whose names occur again and again in them have been left unmolested. The outstanding example of this is Deputy Nobakht, the "N2" of the papers who not only is at large, but attends the Majlis everyday vigorously defending Naser Khan Qashqai and constituting a constant thorn in the allied side. General Aghevli is another. It would seem that even the British feel that the evidence provided by these documents would not stand very close scrutiny. Furthermore the fact that the papers do not contain more important names than they do may very well indicate that the British did not feel the evidence was strong enough to make arrests of important persons on a large scale. This is perhaps the principal reason for believing in the authenticity of many of the papers since if they had been wholly fabricated it would have been logical to include practically everyone of importance known to have pro-German sympathies.

The fact that Franz Mayer would abandon such documents for the British to pick up at will lends little credulity to them although it is not difficult to imagine a German living in hiding as Mayer has been, abandoning his Iranian accomplices if he saw fit.

It is not beyond the realm of possibility that Mayer, concerning whose existence there is little doubt, encouraged various Iranians to organize pro-German groups, to make plans such as those mentioned in the enclosures, to communicate with each other and with him, and by and large consider themselves a great fifth column movement. . . . Surely, the Germans did not take this "plot" seriously or they would, as Major Ondrick points out, have lent it greater support, guidance, and equipment. The sloppiness of the organization and the abandoning of the documents by Mayer are fairly conclusive evidence that this is not primarily a German undertaking. My opinion is that the British did discover a certain number of documents, possibly not under the circumstances described in the Military Attaché's opening paragraph, edited them, added certain material to suit their own purposes, such as the Zahidi letter, No. 190, and printed them in a deliberately garbled order so that their weakness would not be apparent. The organization charts, the military plans for the treatment of Jews and foreigners, and the letters involving a large number of personalities do not ring true. In any event, the documents failed to serve their purpose since practically no one believed them and it was not possible to make large scale arrests of the persons involved. Even if every paper in the collection were bona fide, there is still no evidence of a serious fifth column plot but rather of a small group of pro-German Iranians playing at being spies and saboteurs.

Chapter 18

American-Iranian Relations and American Policy on Iran

While Americans remained popular, with deteriorating conditions, strains had surfaced. Dreyfus on October 26, 1942 (Dispatch 363 and enclosure, 711.91/90):

> I have the honor to enclose a leading editorial from the *Journal de Teheran* of October 20 regarding American-Iranian relations. Press comments on the United States, as indicated in this editorial, continues to be favorable. There is, however, as I suggested in my telegram No. 340 of October 24, a growing tendency to classify the United States with the allies and to blame us increasingly for Iranian woes. I am afraid we will have to expect this tendency to grow during coming months as Iran feels ever more the pinch of war. It is remarkable that the press has not been more critical of the United States at this time when criticism of the allies, in the Majlis and press and among the public, has reached a pitch of intensity and bitterness. The important subject of press and public feeling toward the allies and the United States will be given further and more detailed consideration in early despatches.

In a report of March 9, 1943, Dreyfus discusses American-Iranian relations (Dispatch 480, 711.91/92):

> I have the honor to submit the following discussion of current American-Iranian relations. The Department is well aware of the friendly attitude toward the United States which has been shown during the last

year or so by the Iranian people and press. The purpose of this despatch is to consider how these cordial relations have been affected by our increased activity in Iran and by the deteriorated internal situation of the country. I suggested in despatch No. 363 of October 26, 1942, that there is a growing tendency on the part of the Iranians to classify the United States with the British and Russians and, at least by inference, to blame us increasingly for Iran's woes. While this tendency is still noticeable to a certain extent, the press and public continue on the whole to treat the United States in a friendly and favorable manner. It would seem not unlikely, however, that Iranian criticism of the United States will grow as our complex problems in Iran multiply, as the Iranians feel more and more the inevitable pinch of the war, as some of the more difficult Iranian problems continue unsolved, and as Iranians begin to find that American advisers are human beings capable of error. The following paragraphs will examine some of the problems which are, or may become, points of irritation in our relations with the Iranians.

The presence of American troops in Iran is a potential source of difficulties. As indicated in my telegram No. 198 of February 22, the Prime Minister was interpellated in the Majlis on the subject of the presence without consent or agreement of American forces in Iran. The newspapers have also taken up this point but in a very mild and restrained way. There follows a typical example of newspaper comment on the subject: *Keihan* Feb. 21. "We have very happy relations with the United States Government. But things should be done according to principles and regulations. They (the Americans) should not have entered this country in violation of principles and without previous authority. The Iranians did not protest because of the extreme friendship existing between the two countries. I request the cabinet of Mr. Soheily to maintain relations on the basis of principles. If the Americans wish they may also participate in the Treaty (tripartite pact)."

The Prime Minister, in answer to criticism on this score, replied in the Majlis on February 21 as follows: "In the meantime I wish to bring to your attention the information I have obtained concerning the Americans. I will read to you the text of a letter received from the Foreign Office: 'Whereas the American Government assumed the position of sending armed forces to Iran, stating that the action is essential to expedite transport on the Iranian railway; whereas on the strength of the Atlantic Charter and the democratic principles which form the basis of the policy of the United States Government, the Iranian Government has always been certain the American Government will not take any action inconsistent with the independence and integrity of Iran; Therefore, in order that the dispatch of these troops to Iran on the basis of the Atlantic Charter and with the consent of the Iranian Government should be based on an agreement with mutual consent, the Iranian Government requested the United States Government to enter into an agreement in this matter. A reply has been received from the Legation in Washington to the effect that the American Government is in principle in accord with the Iranian Government that this matter be put in order. For this reason it is contemplating an agreement between the two Governments in this respect. We hope that this project will be prepared and the agreement will be concluded.'"

The conduct of American forces in Iran leaves something to be desired. Iranians are apt to notice and remark on the drunkenness and disorder on the part of foreign troops. They have been impressed by the superior conduct of Russian soldiers as compared with American, British, and Polish. There is circulating an apparently authentic story of a Russian officer who was first broken in rank and later in the day executed for drunken conduct in the Palace Hotel. In contrast to this British troops, and to some extent American, receive little disciplinary action for their rowdy and sometimes drunken conduct. The question is receiving serious attention by the American military authorities in Tehran and there is, I believe, some improvement. It should be mentioned that the American forces here are raw and untrained technical forces. Motor accidents and occasional incidents are unavoidable where there are concentrations of troops. There have been several motor accidents, one or two fatal, involving American drivers and Iranians, but so far they have been settled with a minimum of friction, usually on the payment of "blood money." A serious incident, which has given rise to public criticism, has just occurred. An American sentry at Camp Atterbury shot and killed an Iranian whom he was endeavoring to dissuade from defecating in or near the water supply. Warning shots were fired in the direction of the man and one appears to have deflected from a stone and caused his death. The sentry has been arrested and held for trial and the Iranian Foreign Office furnished full details. The incident has led to widespread misstatements that American soldiers have fired on many Iranians. The following statement in the Majlis is typical. Deputy Amir-Teimur in the Majlis on March 4: "I have a question to ask the Prime Minister, who is also the Minister of Interior, and I request him to come here and answer it. The question is this: it is understood that American soldiers have opened fire on a number of innocent people and have killed several. I should like to know how many have been killed and why no action has been taken. If the matter is not true he may deny it, and if it is true the offenders should be punished." I have furnished full and correct details to the Prime Minister to enable him to answer the interpellation in the Majlis. In this connection I am promised by the Iranian Government that its agreement to permit jurisdiction by American military authorities over offenses committed by our forces will be forthcoming in the immediate future. I feel certain that the Iranians will not question American jurisdiction in the present case. The entire matter will be reported to the Department by separate despatch.

There is an increasing tendency on the part of the Iranians to think of the United States as one of the allies when they heap abuse and blame on the allies for Iran's unfortunate food situation. I greatly regret the delays which took place in getting the 25,000 tons of wheat from the United States under way since it is arriving too late to meet the winter famine. However, it is certainly no fault of this Legation or of the Department of State, both of which moved heaven and earth to see that Iran's wheat shortage was met. I am constrained to repeat that the fault must rest on the shoulders of the British who, even if well-intentioned, delayed the matter consistently because they were of the opinion that wheat hoards existed in the country and could be brought to light if sufficient pressure were put on the Iranians. The press takes the view that Iran has been pillaged by the allies, who now look blandly on while Iran starves. British propaganda in this matter of food has, in true style, tripped itself up and smashed its nose on the curb stone. In a radio broadcast and press release, to prove to the Iranians that the allies are actually in the process of helping Iran with wheat supplies, the British gave the opposite impression. Their statement repeated that there are hoards of wheat in various parts of Iran and declared that the reports being circulated to the effect that 10,000 tons of wheat from the United States have arrived are false. They failed for some mysterious reason to make known that several thousand tons of wheat have in fact arrived or about to arrive at Persian Gulf ports. This broadcast was, I am told, the work of Counsellor Squire, that Indian civil servant par excellence, whose main preoccupation is to justify his consistent contention that there is sufficient wheat in Iran to feed the people. I have decided to take the matter in hand and see personally that newspaper editors are told the truth about allied aid to Iran in wheat, transport and other matters. The following excerpts from a leading editorial of *Mehr-i-Iran* of March 4 are typical of the bitterness Iranians feel about the wheat matter. They also reveal the potential danger to our own relations with Iran inherent in the wheat situation. "According to the broadcast, the Allies have not as yet lent Iran any assistance. But they admit that we have faithfully lived up to all of our undertakings. This is one kind of friendship, the story of which will be read by future generations, who will pass judgment on such friendships. In this broadcast they insist on the existence of wheat in various parts of the country. . . . You say there are large quantities of wheat and we say there are not . . . if the wheat is not there why do you insist on creating illusions? You have all the lines of communications in Iran in your hands. We do not believe it will be impossible for you to ship these huge quantities of wheat. . . . Existing evidence shows that whatever provisions existed in Iran have been consumed, that is to say the noble Iranian nation offered their allied guests whatever they had. Now the guests claim that we owe them. They say we owe the British army and Polish refugees 3,000 tons of wheat. The net result of the broadcast is that the allies cannot help us and we must solve our own problems. . . . This is the meaning of friendship and alliance with Iran and this is what is meant by the Pact of Alliance which was signed between Iran and the allies. If political and economic pacts and international treaties of friendship are so flimsy why do you take the trouble to sign them? Imagine the great British Empire which holds the belt of the globe, which has dominion over such large portion of the earth, which would not stand for the occupation of Danzig, which declared war to safeguard her pledged word, a Government which is world famous as a partisan of the principles of justice and freedom! It is a pity that such a Government should, fourteen months after the signing of the Tripartite Pact and four months after signing the Food Declaration, make such a broadcast in reply to Iranian public opinion which has been calling for Iran's right to reciprocal assistance."

Americans are being blamed to some extent by the Iranians for the acute kerosene shortage in Tehran, a matter discussed in my telegram 253 of March 10 and which will be covered in a separate despatch. They believe, erroneously, that Americans are already in charge of railway movements control, whereas the British have not yet relinquished allocations on the southern section of the Trans-Iranian Railway. I am somewhat preoccupied at the lack of understanding on the part of the American military authorities of the necessity, both political and practical, of taking care of the needs of the Iranian civil population. Military men usually take the view that they are here to "do a job of war work" and that nothing can be permitted to interfere with this primary task. The railway allocation northward to Tehran from the Gulf for Iranian civil use is only 200 tons a day, an absurdly low figure. The program of moving 25,000 tons of American wheat to Tehran from the ports will consume the 200 tons of railway capacity daily, leaving nothing for Iranian needs or for the reduction of 20,000 tons of goods piled up at warehouses in the South. British allocations officials will agree to a sharp upward revision of the Iranian civil allocation and put it into effect before the Americans take over movements control. I will keep the Department fully informed of developments.

The conduct and activities of American advisers is the fulcrum in our relations with the Iranians. . . . Briefly, the Millspaugh, Ridley, and Schwarzkopf missions have got off to a good start and popular reaction to them has been satisfactory to date. Mr. Timmerman has been kept somewhat in the background pending the signing of his contract now under consideration in the Majlis; his mission is still being weighed in the balance. Mr. Sheridan has been the subject of most bitter attacks and has, on the whole, done the cause of American advisers in Iran little good. . . . There are those who believe the existence of undercover efforts on the part of the British and Russians to discredit our advisers and American efforts in Iran. I see no evidence that the British are indulging in any kind of propaganda or whispering campaign to discredit us. They are undoubtedly aware that, considering their own low repute, any such program would fall on sterile ground and operate only their harm. As the Department knows, the British have in some cases requested that American advisers be sent to Iran. However, I have a feeling that the British readily agreed to our adviser program in the hopes that American prestige in this country, which they know has been at a peak, will fall considerably when the Iranians discover advisers are ordinary human beings and not yet supermen. The British know from bitter experience how difficult the Iranians are to deal with and perhaps take secret delight in letting the Americans have their round. As to the Russians, I have received several indications that they are beginning to resent the American adviser program. The Russian Ambassador has let drop a number of remarks which would indicate he is not entirely pleased. The Foreign Minister told me, for example, that the Ambassador had in conversation with him inquired pointedly as to why the Iranians are employing American advisers when it is well known that the Russians are the best administrators in the world. While these are straws in the wind future Russian reaction to our program should be carefully observed. . . . The press, public, and Majlis continue to treat us, on the whole, in a most friendly and flattering manner. Scores of press items monthly deal with America, principally with our war effort. They give stories of leading American personalities, reproduce pictures of planes and ships, print facts regarding American war production and generally deal with the American war effort in a favorable light. Let me quote, in closing, excerpts from a few of many editorials which have in recent weeks presented America to the Iranian public in a most favorable manner.

Keihan Jan. 14. "At present military needs and war exigencies require that we should have more contact with Americans. In our opinion even if the war has brought about several great catastrophes for Iran at least it has brought about the opportunity to know the American people better than in the past and to benefit from the high ideals which the people of that land have given to the world. . . . All the well-informed and well-meaning people in Iran earnestly hope that after the war the extensive oceans and the vast continents which separate Iran from the United States will no longer be a barrier and that in addition to ordinary economic transactions and apart from the happy political relations the liberty-loving people of the United States will be the best of friends with Iran."

Bakhtar Jan. 24. "In the famine of 1918 when several thousand people starved and died of influenza, the good-hearted humanitarian people of the United States again came to our help. They gave us bread and medicine. We will never forget the good they did for us. . . . We have two requests to make of the Americans. First, that they shall not forget us in peace but protect our rights, and second, that they should help us during the war with food and medicines. Oh, gentle breeze, thou art the most truthful and unbiased of messengers. Cross the oceans, kiss the Statue of Liberty and tell the brave people of that great land that their Iranian friends send them greetings and this message: The men you send to our land are safe and sound. Do not be worried but think of our future."

Nobahar Feb 28. "We are still greatly attached to the respectable Americans serving in Iran. The Iranian people like America and the Americans. The Iranian people have good memories of the Americans. In this war of nerves when humanity has naturally become irritated and nervous, we find it necessary every few days to say and to prove that we like America and the Americans. If in certain cases grievances are expressed with regard to certain advisers or the unauthorized landing of American troops in Iran, this does not mean that the fondness and confidence of Iranians in the Americans have been diminished. We have hopes in the American Government and people."

Murray's comments on the above dispatch are given in a memorandum of April 2, 1943, to Berle and Welles (Memorandum, 711.91/102):

> The attached despatch from Tehran gives a valuable picture of certain developments in Iran related to our policy in that country. Minister Dreyfus reports that American prestige remains high and that we are popular with the Iranian press and public. There have appeared, however, certain as yet minor notes of criticism, and the Minister suggests that these may grow in volume as American activity and problems increase, as the pinch of war is felt more severely, and as familiarity with American advisers dispels the romantic notion that they are super beings immune to error.
>
> 1) Although there seems to be no opposition to the presence of American troops in Iran, considerable criticism has been voiced at their coming without a prior formal agreement between the two governments. The Prime Minister was attacked in the Majlis on this score. 2) Incidents have occurred between American troops and Iranian civilians. None of these has been especially serious as yet, except for the accidental killing of a civilian by a warning shot fired by an American sentry. They have, nevertheless, given rise to exaggerated reports and are a potential source of danger. 3) The Iranians increasingly tend to lump America with Great Britain and Russia when they abuse the Allies for the food shortage. As has been previously reported, the Iranian attitude is that the Allies have plundered Iran and now do nothing to help her. British efforts to refute this thesis have been rather inept. A recent British broadcast insisted that there is plenty of hoarded wheat in Iran and denied reports being circulated that 10,000 tons of wheat from the United States had arrived. (The reports were substantially true, and it is not clear exactly why the denials were made. In any case, it has produced an unfortunate effect on Iranian public opinion.) From this and other reports, it appears that the British Counselor of Legation, an Indian Civil Service product, is the cause of much British blundering and obstinacy in Iran. 4) Popular opinion also blames the United States to some extent for a recent shortage of kerosene in Tehran, because of a belief that our forces were in control of transportation. This was not then true, as the British still handled movement control and were responsible for an insufficient allocation of space for Iranian civil needs. They have now agreed to a larger allotment.

> 5) The success or failure of the American advisers is the key point in our relations. Mr. Sheridan, the Food and Supply Adviser, has come in for severe criticism. Whether this is justified is not made clear by the despatch. Dr. Millspaugh (Financial Adviser), Colonel Schwarzkopf (Rural Police), and General Ridley (Military) have gotten off to a good start and popular reaction has been satisfactory so far. Mr. Timmerman (Municipal Police) has not been in the limelight and his work is still being weighed in the balance. Mr. Dreyfus suspects that the British may be taking secret pleasure in the difficulties encountered by the Americans, knowing how difficult it is dealing with the Iranians. He does not believe, however, that they are in any way working against our people. As for the Russians, there have been several indications that they are beginning to resent the American advisers. Among other things, the Russian Ambassador recently asked the Iranian Foreign Minister why Iran was employing Americans when it was well known that the Russians were the best administrators in the world.

Iranian dissatisfaction with America was on the rise. Dreyfus on April 22, 1943 (Dispatch 528 and enclosure, 711.91/96):

> I have the honor to enclose, for the Department's information and records, a memorandum of conversation which took place between Secretary of Legation Bertel E. Kuniholm and Allah Yar Saleh, Iranian Minister of Finance. This memorandum should be read in connection with the Legation's telegrams 355, April 6, and 384, April 14.

The conversation took place on April 5, 1943:

> I called on Mr. Saleh this morning at his request. In a conversation lasting just over an hour he made comment substantially as follows. The good will which has been manifest toward Americans for so many years is now at an all-time low. Principal among the reasons for this are: the hostile attitude against the Allied occupation forces in Iran; the failure of American advisers to effect reforms with any kind of despatch; the operation of the lend-lease agreement, which has produced nothing tangible as yet for Iran; the delaying tactics of both Britain and America in shipment of grain to Iran; and, finally, the failure of the American Government to stand up to the Russians in an endeavor to ease the pressure now being exerted on the country by the Soviet Government. The combination of all these factors has set in motion an anti-American movement which, quite frankly, is acquiring substance with each passing day.

The present status of the American advisers is precarious. It would take very little more to make the situation virtually hopeless. The majority of Iranians are not convinced that Americans are especially gifted to reduce the ills of the country; there is a strong movement against the particular Americans who are in the country now. I personally advised the Department of State, and Mr. Sumner Welles in particular, that it would be useless the send American advisers to Iran unless the American Government was prepared at once to extend aid and to ship goods and raw materials urgently needed. The situation at the moment is that the American advisers begin to look ridiculous, for they are able to do nothing more than present blueprints of what should be done, with no power whatsoever of carrying policies into effect. Attacks against these advisers will not lessen in the near future; in fact, they are bound to increase. The only possible means of alleviating the situation is for America to make immediate shipment of necessary supplies to Iran, even if these shipments are on a relatively minor scale. What is necessary is visible and concrete proof of American concern as to the needs of Iran. To hold out promises over a period of time is like stretching a metal to the point of permanent set. The breakdown of American prestige in Iran would be fatal; it would affect the American position throughout the whole of the Middle East. I am particularly disturbed about Dr. Millspaugh; he is under such constant attack, and the object of so many malicious and pernicious cabals, that I am not at all certain that he is going to be able to weather the storm.

As constituted at present, the Majlis is one of the worst influences operating in the country. All of its members are Reza Shah's men, and do not represent the spirit which is prevalent among the people now. New elections will be had in a few months. New deputies must be brought in, and new blood injected into the body politic. . . . The attitude of most members of the Majlis is that America is simply using Iran as a highway to Russia, and hopes to put off the Iranians indefinitely, with vague promises of assistance in the dim future. As month succeeds month, and action is not forthcoming, the attacks against the Allied Governments, and particularly the American advisers, will become more and more acrimonious.

Iran's needs have been indicated time and time again. The most essential needs to be satisfied are those of grain and transport. Among the latter are buses, trucks, tires, and railway rolling stock. The demands are not great; they are, nevertheless, urgent, and some attempt should be made at once to alleviate them. My efforts in America, prior to departure for Iran, were certainly not crowned with success, and I must confess, quite frankly, that the whole business of wheat was disappointing in the extreme. Surely the sacrifice of shipping space for us, if nothing more than indication of good will, would be worthwhile at the present difficult conjuncture. All that we expect is an earnest display of American good faith and sincerity; words and declarations will have no effect any longer.

Dreyfus tried to slow the decline in American popularity. In a report of May 3, 1943, he writes (Dispatch 543, 891.24/442):

> I have the honor to call to the Department's attention an objectionable editorial in the *Providence Journal* quoted in Radio Bulletin No. 104 of May 1, 1943. This summarized editorial was copied by the Legation's radio operator as follows: "A little over a year ago American railroad crews set out to make the Persia corridor the main war supply route to Russia. . . . They have laid fourteen hundred miles of tortuous track uphill and down dale . . . into the regions of the Caspian. . ." Compares our up to date methods with old Persian methods of construction and says that old methods will undoubtedly survive "but we'll have got the stuff to the Russians, by George. And on time, too."
>
> I have often remarked to the Department on the harmful effects of this "holier than thou" or "aren't we wonderful" kind of propaganda when used in Iran by the British. Disregardful of facts and based on the assumption of the depravity and incompetence of the "natives," this mistaken philosophy can do a great deal of harm. It has, in fact, been one of the primary causes of British unpopularity in Iran. I am sure that we shall not be foolish enough to fall into the same unfortunate error, especially when we learned by bitter experience in Latin America that this haughty attitude pays poor dividends.
>
> The statements in the editorial are, of course, incorrect. The Trans-Iranian railway was built by the Iranians; the Americans have just taken over the last link of the southern section of this railway; Americans have not laid 1400 miles of track in Iran; and Americans do not operate the railway from Tehran to the Caspian Sea. The facts, however, are not as important as the disdainful and uninformed assumption that "native" peoples are incompetent. I am not at all sure that native methods are so incompetent, but even if they are it does no good to call attention to the fact. I have suppressed this item from the Legation's mimeographed radio bulletin to make sure it does not come

to the attention of the Iranians. I shall find occasion to discuss the matter with General Connolly with a view to insuring that articles of this kind are not encouraged or inspired by military circles in Iran.

American Policy on Iran

In a memorandum to Assistant Secretaries Berle and Acheson, Under Secretary Welles, and Secretary Hull, dated February 11, 1943, Murray gives an outline of American policy on Iran (FW711.91/98):

> The attached memorandum is a summary of the thoughts of NE and myself regarding the general bases and direction of our policy toward Iran, which we should like to submit for your consideration. If you approve, we shall guide our actions accordingly and shall send appropriate instructions to our Minister at Tehran. I have also in mind the possible desirability of asking the planning organizations under Mr. Pasvolsky to give special attention to Iranian problems along the lines indicated. Briefly, the memorandum sets forth the following points:
>
> 1) The past and present attitudes of Great Britain and Russia toward Iran, together with the current weakness of the Iranian Government and disorganization of the country's internal structure, justify fears that Iran may prove a danger point when we come to the post-war settlement. 2) The best hope of avoiding trouble in this regard lies in strengthening Iran to a point at which she will be able to stand on her own feet and in assuring both of the interested Great Powers that neither one need fear the acquisition by the other of a predominant position in Iran. 3) The United States is the only nation able to render effective assistance to Iran without rousing the fears and opposition of Great Britain and Russia, or of the Iranians themselves. 4) Since we have a vital interest in the fulfillment of the principles of the Atlantic Charter and the establishment of foundations for a lasting peace throughout the world, it is to the advantage of the United States to exert itself to see that Iran's integrity and independence are maintained and that she becomes prosperous and stable. 5) Therefore, the United States should adopt a policy of positive action in Iran with a view to facilitating not only the war operations of the United Nations but also a sound post-war development of the country which would eliminate the need or excuse for the establishment of any sort of "protectorate."

The memorandum entitled "American Policy in Iran," is dated January 23, 1943:

This Government has come during the past year or more to play a relatively active part in Iranian affairs. In the past, the United States had no important political interest in Iran and has been seriously concerned with events in that country only from time to time. Our recent activity, therefore, is rather a new departure and has arisen primarily out of our participation in the war and natural concern that political matters in all theaters of war operations should develop favorably with respect to the United Nations. Iran has been, and is, important in this connection because of its value as a supply route to Russia, its strategic location and its vast production of petroleum products. When occasion has arisen to set forth our policy, we have based it upon the foregoing considerations, and I feel they constitute ample justification for the attitude we have adopted. I believe, however, that it is worthwhile at this time to put down on paper certain much broader considerations which, it seems to me, should likewise impel us to follow a positive policy in Iran, not only while the prosecution of the war is still foremost in our minds but also in the period when victory is in our grasp and we come to the conclusion of the peace.

I should like to suggest that Iran constitutes a test case for the good faith of the United Nations and their ability to work out among themselves an adjustment of ambitions rights and interests which will be fair not only to the Great Powers of our coalition but also to the small nations associated with us or brought into our sphere by circumstances. Certainly, nowhere else in the Middle East is there to be found so clear-cut a conflict of interests between two of the United Nations, so ancient a tradition of rivalry, and so great a temptation for the Great Powers concerned to give precedence to their own selfish interests over the principles enunciated in the Atlantic Charter.

For considerably more than one hundred years, Russia has been pressing down upon Iran from the north, repeatedly threatening new annexations of territory, repeatedly attempting in one way or another to dominate Iran. Three times in the present century alone Russian troops have entered Iranian territory against the will of the Iranian people. For the same period of time, Great Britain has opposed the Russian movement southward, fearing for her own position in the Persian Gulf and Indian Ocean and especially fearful of the potential threat to India. British troops have been on Iranian soil at least twice since the turn of the century and British influence has been exerted over and over again to counter the Russian expansion. Although Russian policy has been fundamentally aggressive and British policy fundamentally defensive in character, the result in both cases has been interference with the internal affairs of Iran, amounting at times to a virtually complete negation of Iranian sovereignty and independence. It is superfluous to point out that this has created an ingrained distrust of both powers in the Iranian people and has not been without effect upon the attitude of the other weak peoples of the Middle East.

If this were merely history, it would be of no importance. Unfortunately, there are signs that history may be in the process of repeating itself. The basic factors are unchanged: Russia is still without a warm water port; Britain still clings to her predominant position in the Middle East and east of Suez. Even if we assume the eventual independence of India and Burma and a British withdrawal from Iraq, Palestine and Egypt, there is every reason to suppose that Britain would not welcome an advance into that area by Russia. Once again Russian and British troops are in Iran, the former in the north, the latter in the south and center. It is true that their presence is made necessary by the imperative considerations of military expediency and their withdrawal at the conclusion of the war has been solemnly promised, but I need not recall the hundreds of instances in which the forces of a Great Power have entered the territory of a weaker nation for one purpose and have remained, indefinitely, for other purposes.

Largely because of this occupation of Iranian territory, the governmental machinery of Iran, and its economic structure, have been seriously weakened. This has become both a reason and an excuse for direct intervention by the Russian and British authorities in Iranian political matters. At the present moment, no Iranian cabinet can survive without direct support of the Allied powers. While it is obvious that the United Nations could not permit a hostile government to function at Tehran, it is equally obvious that the Iranian political and economic organization must be strengthened to a point at which it will be able to function efficiently by itself, if Iran is to survive as an independent nation. It is unnecessary to point out that a political vacuum is as impossible as a physical vacuum; if Iran fails into a state of anarchy, some power must assume responsibility for its government, and it may be assumed that the first to offer themselves for this task would be one or both of the present occupying powers.

Apart from the general situation in Iran, I believe we should be fully alive to the character of the present Russian occupation of the northern provinces. In Azerbaijan, the Soviet authorities have greatly restricted the operations of the Iranian civil authorities and have virtually immobilized the small Iranian military forces which they have reluctantly permitted to return to the area. They have alternatively encouraged and discouraged the restive Kurds, always a thorn in the flesh of the local government. More important still, they have been so successful in propagandizing the population that our Consul at Tabriz has reported that a soviet could be established overnight in Azerbaijan if the Russians gave the word. In this connection, it is well to remember that Azerbaijan is inhabited largely by Turkish-speaking population whose cultural ties with the Soviet Transcaucasia and Turkish Kurdistan are almost as strong as those with the rest of Iran. It is also the most important grain-producing region of Iran and would be a welcome addition to the food resources of Transcaucasia. There are other items which might be mentioned: the strained relations between the Russian and British authorities in Iran; the suspicion with which the Russians appear to view every move made by the British or Americans, for example their obvious hesitancy in agreeing to our operation of the southern section of the Trans-Iranian railroad; the apparent attempt by the Russian government to weaken British influence by leaving the British to bear the brunt of Iran's economic problems; the continued refusal of the Soviet authorities in Iran to permit transportation of grain from Azerbaijan to meet the urgent needs of Tehran; the impending move by the Russians to take control of Iranian arms plants. On the British side, the blunt, uncompromising attitude which has characterized British policy towards Iran does not augur well for a future amicable adjustment of Anglo-Iranian relations. Nor is it reassuring to recall the recent British proposal to arrogate to the Allies the power to modify the Iranian cabinet at will.

It may be that the situation outlined above represents nothing more than the inevitable result of the stress and strain of coalition warfare and that once the victory is won all parties will be glad to revert to their former positions, leaving Iranian sovereignty as intact as it was before the Anglo-Russian occupation. Both Britain and Russia have repeatedly promised to do so, and both powers, and Iran as well, have adhered to the principles of the Atlantic Charter. I should like to submit, however, that the United States has a vital interest in seeing to it that the United Nations do live up to the Atlantic Charter and, consequently, in making it as easy as possible for them to do so.

What I have in mind is the situation which will arise when the war is won, or nearly won, and the time comes to think of British and Russian withdrawal from Iran, with consequent full rehabilitation of Iranian self-government. Have we not some reason to anticipate that the respective British and Russian forces may remain suspiciously eyeing each other, each proclaiming its entire willingness to withdraw as soon as the other has done so? Is it not possible that one or both powers will allege, perhaps with reason, that Iran is in such a state of confusion that she must be "protected" for a time? And is it probable that either will withdraw and allow the other to carry out this "protection"? Carrying this thought one step further, if Russia should really harbor ambitions for expansion in Iran, is it not at all too likely that she would insist upon Iran's need for Soviet guidance, and that she would violently oppose the interposition of another interested power in the role of tutor? And if Great Britain should give way on this, would not Britain all the more cling to her position in Iraq and other parts of the Middle East, as protection against future Russian thrust toward Suez, thus checking the progress which we hope to see in the direction of independence for all Near Eastern peoples?

I think we may assume that the Iranian Government has long since thought of all the foregoing considerations and that its ever-stronger appeal for American assistance is based upon them. So far, we have rested our response to this appeal primarily upon our interest in winning the war. I wonder if we should not also begin, privately, to base our response upon our interest in winning the peace? The United States, alone, is in a position to build up Iran to the point at which it will stand in need of neither British nor Russian assistance to maintain order in its own house. If we go at this task whole-heartedly, we can hope to remove any excuse for a post-war occupation, partition, or tutelage of Iran. We can work to make Iran self-reliant and prosperous, open to the trade of all nations and a threat to none. In the meantime, we can so firmly establish disinterested American advisers in Iran so that no peace conference could even consider a proposal to institute a Russian or British protectorate or to "recognize the predominance" of Russian or British interests. If Iran needs assistance of a material character, we can provide it and so remove any cause for claims for compensation by other powers. We can forestall loans carrying with them control of the customs or any other servitudes upon the Iranian Government. If railroads, ports, highways, public utilities, industries are to be built, we can build them and turn them over to the Iranian people free of any strings.

I realize that objections can be raised to such a policy. Some which occur to me at the moment are: (a) it is unprecedented in our relations with the Middle East; (b) it impinges on "spheres of influence" hitherto considered exclusively British and Russian; (c) there is no guarantee that it will succeed; (d) it might involve expenditure or loss of money; (e) if it came to public notice, it might arouse domestic criticism on the part of isolationists. To answer these seriatim:

(a) The present war and the problems of future peace for the United States are likewise unprecedented. We have now realized, and publicly stated over and over again, that we cannot be indifferent to the welfare of any part of the world, no matter how remote, because sooner or later it will affect our own peace. (b) The very fact that Iran has been a "sphere of influence" in dispute between two Great Powers, makes it all the more desirable that a third, disinterested, power should be called in to eliminate dispute. Both Britain and Russia would be relieved of an anxiety and constant source of friction if each could be assured that the other would have no special position in the area, and it is not inconceivable that both would regard this assurance as worth whatever ambitions might be given up. In this connection, it seems hardly possible that either could suspect the United States of having imperial designs in a country so far removed from us and where we could never hope to employ military force against an adjacent Great Power. (c) If war cannot be waged without taking risks, I submit that the same is true of the making of peace. In any case, if we try and fail, we shall have lost nothing than if we do not make the attempt. If the ambitions of Britain and Russia, their mutual distrust, or their established interests, are so strong that they would override a purely disinterested effort on our part to improve conditions in Iran, than we may assume that peace, in that part of the world, was doomed from the beginning. (d) The expenditures involved, even if all of them should be a total loss, would be insignificant by contrast to the cost of the present war, and infinitesimal beside the material and human cost of a failure to make a satisfactory peace throughout the world. (e) This objection will be met with in connection with any effort by the United States to participate in a cooperative post-war settlement, and we must be prepared to accept it. In the case of Iran, it could be countered by emphasis on the humanitarian aspects and should appeal to the normal American sympathy with anything savoring of assistance to the underdog. If properly presented, a policy of help for Iran might, indeed, receive the same sort of popular approval as has been accorded to our support of China.

Finally, I should like to reiterate the conviction previously expressed that if the principles of unselfish fair-dealing enunciated by the Atlan-

> tic Charter are ignored when it comes to Iran, or any other country in similar circumstances, the foundations of our peace will begin to crumble immediately. In my opinion, this is the overriding argument which should lead us to seize every opportunity to direct events in such a way that there will be no occasion for power politics or conflicts of interests among the United Nations in their relations with Iran.
>
> If this conclusion is sound, I believe that we should not only comply to the best of our ability with Iranian requests for advisers and supplies but should also take the initiative in suggesting the employment of American specialists and application of American methods in various fields; further, we should not be content merely to support or oppose British or Russian policies and demands in Iran, but should put forward positive suggestions of our own for the improvement of conditions. To this end, we should regard ourselves as at least equally responsible with the British and Russians for the solution of Iranian problems and need not, in any way, leave the initiative to them merely because they happen to be the occupying powers. Moreover, here in Washington we should actively enlist the cooperation of all appropriate agencies of the Federal Government in support of this policy, and we should not confine ourselves solely to steps whose close connection with the war effort can be clearly demonstrated. If necessary, we should make it clear to the other agencies that we regard measures to see satisfactory ultimate settlement in Iran as being only slightly less important than those immediately directed towards the winning of the war, and that we consider it most unwise to defer all such measures until the war is over.

The above memorandum was forwarded to Dreyfus by Welles on March 13, 1943 (Letter and enclosure, 711.91/91):

> There is enclosed herewith a copy of a memorandum which represents the view of the Department on the general policy to be followed by this Government with respect to Iran which you may, accordingly, take for your guidance in this connection. The Department would be glad to have any observations you may care to make, in the light of your knowledge of conditions on the spot, regarding the practicability of putting into effect the line of policy laid down in this memorandum. You are also requested to suggest, from time to time, whatever measures may seem to you likely to be effective in attaining the objective set forth, namely, the development, with American assistance, of a stable Iranian Government and a strong Iranian economy. In working

toward this objective, the Department considers it essential to avoid any appearance of conflict with Great Britain or the Soviet Union, and it is believed the safeguarding of legitimate British and Russian economic interests in Iran is a requisite for the success of our efforts.

Dreyfus' comments are given in a dispatch of April 14, 1943 (Dispatch 517, 711.91/95):

I have the honor to offer the following comments on American policy in Iran, comments which were suggested by the statement of policy set forth in a memorandum enclosed with the Department's instruction No. 202 of March 13, 1943. I welcome the Department's statement of policy with regard to Iran as constructive, statesmanlike and especially timely. I hardly need to declare that I am in full agreement with the Department's exposition of our aims and objectives in Iran; the telegrams and despatches of this Legation, I believe, bear evidence of this complete accord. I am happy that the Department has been able to arrive at so clear cut an understanding of the issues involved in our relations with Iran and to crystallize the whole into so simple and straightforward a representation of the American viewpoint. For my part, I will endeavor, as requested by the Department, to suggest from time to time measures which may assist in implementing our stated policy and to report fully on matters which may affect the attainment of our goal.

The Department's reference to Iran as proving ground for the Atlantic Charter struck me as particularly timely and interesting. The same thought had occurred to me and was expressed at the end of despatch No. 511 dated April 7, 1943 on the subject of the operation in this country of the Middle East Supply Center. I suggested in that despatch that we go in for some honest introspection to determine whether or not we are living up to the ideals of the Atlantic Charter in our daily actions and long range aims in Iran and I stated the belief that we could indulge in this soul-searching operation without a severe twinge of conscience. I expressed regret, however, that it has been found necessary to associate ourselves in this country with a MESC program based on compulsion and monopoly. It seems to me that it would be preferable for us to adopt a purely American approach to the Iranian problem, always bearing in mind, as aptly suggested in the last paragraph of the Department's instruction, that the safeguarding of legitimate British and Russian interests in this country is a requisite for the success of our mission. Some of the obstacles in the way of the attainment of our Iranian objectives were discussed in my despatch No. 480, March 9th. They may, it occurs to me, be divided roughly into the four sources from which they may possibly spring—(1) the Soviets (2) The Iranians themselves (3) the British and (4) the Americans. While I have discussed these obstacles in various recent despatches and telegrams, it may be useful to recapitulate them briefly in this despatch.

(1) The Soviets. I have reported in a series of telegrams and despatches in the last month the effort which is being made by the Russians to ensconce themselves securely in Iran, by means of astute propaganda, by socialist indoctrination, by good example of their forces and by a policy consisting of a strange mixture of kindness and strong arm methods. Soviet policy in Iran continues to be, as recorded in the Department's memorandum, positive and aggressive. . . . An amazingly obvious bid for Iranian sympathy came to light only the other day when it was officially announced that the Russians are making available at a Caspian Sea port 25,000 tons of Soviet wheat to feed the people of Tehran. The Department is well aware of the background of the Iranian wheat affair, how we have agreed to make up Iran's wheat deficit, how at great cost to our shipping position 30,000 tons of wheat have been sent, and how the Iranians have complained that the wheat is not forth coming or in any event will arrive too late to be of great benefit. The Soviets, holding their punch until the last round, now come forth as the saviors of Iran and make wheat available where the British and Americans are popularly believed failed. The Iranians cannot be made, or do not wish, to understand that some 8,000 tons of the wheat from the United States have arrived in Tehran and much more at Persian Gulf ports. In fact, the Soviets have stepped in when the wheat crisis in Iran is virtually over and offered wheat which is not presently needed. One must ask, also, where the Russians will get the grain they are offering to Iran. They do not have it in Azerbaijan for, as I have reported, the authorities in that State are having difficulty in carrying out their contract to deliver 5,000 tons to the Russians. I am under the impression that large quantities of grain are being supplied to Russia from the United States so surely they do not have it to spare in Russia. In any event, it would appear that the gesture will have the intended effect – to increase Soviet prestige in Iran at the expense of the Americans and British just when the Majlis elections are coming up.

(2) The Iranians themselves are perhaps the greatest possible source of danger to our position in Iran. The Iranians, as I have so frequently pointed out to the Department, are not an easy people with whom to

deal. Basically anti-foreign, obdurate, super-sensitive, hyper-critical, completely lacking in social consciousness, corrupt, selfish and given to exploitation of their own helpless masses, they "keep the noiseless tenor of their way." Recent arrivals here and those who have only a superficial knowledge of Iranian culture and mode of life often ask whether the Iranians are really worthy of our help. Personally, I believe that they are. I feel that there is a basic common sense and germ of goodness in them which should be protected and nourished. This again brings to mind the Atlantic Charter. Surely, the supreme test is whether we can live in peace and understanding with peoples who are so basically different from us and with whom we have so little in common, not whether we can live in amity with our own family and those of whom we fully approve. Our task should be, therefore, to assist the Iranians to overcome their faults rather than to abandon them because of the very existence of their shortcomings. As I indicated in my telegram No. 355 dated April 6, there is evidence of concerted and deep-rooted campaign against our advisers. This springs undoubtedly from corrupt and selfish political elements in the Majlis who stand to lose personally with the institution of the kind of regime our advisers contemplate. This campaign may well be, as is commonly thought here, abetted by the Russians. I have suggested to the Department the necessity of adopting a strong line in dealing with the Iranians in this matter. Unless we can require that our advisers be supported and given powers, their efforts will fail and the whole program will fall to the ground. The result of such failure would be not only to let down the Iranians but as well to cripple our own prestige. Our policy should be firm but kind, forceful but friendly, insistent but considerate. The Prime Minister, a few days ago in a conversation concerning the delay in granting Millspaugh's powers, remarked smilingly that foreigners are apt to forget that Iran is an oriental country and that things here are not done in a day. This is a statement of fact which is too often overlooked by foreigners who think of Iranians as westerners simply because they have adopted western clothing and strive to emulate us in things material.

(3) The British. There is no evidence that the British have offered any great degree of obstruction to our adviser program or the development of our influence in Iran. On the contrary, they have encouraged and sometimes suggested the appointment of Americans. However, at the risk of seeming to be an alarmist who sees a burglar behind every tree, I venture the opinion that the British have two factors in mind in supporting our program—first, if given enough rope we might hang ourselves by making failure of the adviser program and second, to use us,

as do the Iranians, as a buffer to counter the growing menace of Soviet domination of the country. I have not the slightest doubt that British enthusiasm for our program will wane if the Russians withdraw or if their influence becomes sufficiently reduced.

(4) The Americans. We must, finally, be sure that our own house is in order. We should, first, select competent and well balanced advisers and, second give them the advice and support they require. On the whole, as I have reported in a series of despatches dealing with the work of the various missions, our choices have been good. The Millspaugh, Ridley and Schwarzkopf missions are composed of able and sensible men. Sheridan, I am unhappy to report, has harmed our position in Iran. His penchant for taking ill considered action and his babbling tongue keep him and the Legation in constant hot water and embarrassment. I am informed that the British, neither agreeing with his methods nor appreciating his accomplishments, would welcome his departure. Notwithstanding this, our batting average is high.

An ever present source of friction is the presence of American troops on Iranian soil. While from our point of view our forces have been reasonably well behaved, the Iranians complain that their conduct is bad. The American military authorities are trying to keep them out of Tehran as much as possible by building barracks on the outskirts of the town. There are naturally incidents that have unfavorable repercussions on our relations with the Iranians and we must expect the increasing criticism these must inevitably bring. It appears evident that the Iranians, basing their ideas of Americans on the few missionaries and government officials they have known, are surprised at the poor conduct of some of the members of the American forces in Iran. Perhaps, having tended to look upon us in recent years in an idealistic light, they are shocked to find we are human beings. Part of our military men, I am afraid, have adopted the typical and unfortunate attitude of the casual foreign observer that the Iranians are corrupt and backward race not worthy of help. Most of them feel, too, that they are here to do a job of war work involving moving the maximum amount of war supplies to Russia and that the needs of the Iranian civil population must not be allowed to interfere with their program. As incidents involving American troops, such as shooting of Iranians by American sentries, alleged acts of mistreatment of Iranians, traffic accidents and misunderstandings increase, a growing note of asperity creeps into communications from the Foreign Office. For example, a Foreign Office note of April 6, complaining about the removal of fire bricks from the Keredj foundry by American forces, used the following severe language: "If the American Government and officials sent here consider themselves within their rights to be able to seize and take away property belonging to the Iranian Government, it is requested that the Ministry of Foreign Affairs be advised, to the end that the Ministry may advise the Imperial Government of this undesirable attitude of American officials and the necessary decision be taken." In this case, the Minister of Foreign Affairs, a capable and friendly, although nervous and precipitate, individual, went off "half-cocked" since the investigation revealed that the bricks were removed by the Americans on the written request of competent Iranian authorities. The Foreign Minister made amends by calling me to the Foreign Office to express regret that he had acted without investigation. However, the incident serves to show the increasing tendency of Iranian officials to be critically conscious of the activities of our forces.

In conclusion, it seems to me imperative that we should continue on our way with patience and balance, with our objective ever in view. We must not be discouraged. The Iranians oscillate politically between dictatorship, democracy and chaos in almost perfect keeping with Plato's theory. They have remarkable resiliency, powers of recovery and ability to throw off foreign invasions, conditions which are apt to keep them going when States considered stronger and more modern have succumbed.

The Work of Grace Dreyfus

An account of American-Iranian relations would be deficient without a mention of the charitable work of Grace Dreyfus, the wife of the American Minister. On July 30, 1943, J. Hall Paxton, Second Secretary of the Legation, had written to Paul Alling, Chief of the Division of Near Eastern Affairs (Letter and enclosures, 123 D 82/562):

I enclose a few of many quotations from articles published in the local press which you will be interested to read and which I feel might well form a part of the files of the Department. They concern the notable work of Mrs. Dreyfus for the poor people of Tehran which, done though it has been without fanfare, has not passed unnoticed by the Iranians. This work has entailed a great deal of effort on her part and she has had to do it almost single-handed. Although it has been motivated purely and simply by reasons of sympathy for human suffering and without any political purpose, its implications have not escaped

> the local public, who, already favorably impressed by American philanthropy in this country, now have this feeling deepened by the unusual sight of the leading American lady seeking to alleviate the sufferings of the otherwise friendless poor of this city. The fearful risk of infection by some of the many diseases that afflict these people, especially typhus, has in no wise deterred her; she has given generously of her time, effort and money to do what one devoted soul could to give them not only material assistance but the even more important benefit of her deep human sympathy with their suffering, which has been so much appreciated by Iranians of every class.
>
> I am so sure that the Minister would not permit these matters to be made the subject of an official despatch over his signature that I am not even showing him this letter until it has been mailed, when I am prepared to risk his possible displeasure in order to get the facts on record because I consider that they will constitute a most significant factor in Iran-American relations for some time to come. The Iranian people have a memory as long as that of the proverbial elephant and will not soon forget what this gracious lady has done for them by her generous spirit, even more than by her considerable efforts.

The *Keyhan* of July 25, 1943, has a piece entitled "The Iranian People Are Grateful," with a photo of Mrs. Grace Dreyfus. The translation reads:

> It will be no exaggeration to say that one of the outstanding qualities of the Iranian, an inborn quality, is his gratitude. An Iranian appreciates any act of kindness and benevolence. He feels indebted and does not give up until he relieves himself from the burden of obligation by reciprocating the favor. . . . This is one of the natural idiosyncrasies of the Iranian. The kind and philanthropic lady who spends her time with the greatest pleasure on our sick children and women, that high-grade lady, the lover of mankind, who calls the poor Iranian children as her own children, the respected lady whose brilliant eyes radiate altruism, who does good for the good itself, whose action is even loftier than what the famous Iranian poet said, "Do good and throw it in the Tigris, God will return it to you in the desert"; she should remember that the Iranian will never forget her work of charity and her efforts to help the poor. Up to this date we hesitated to voice the sincere appreciation of the people of Tehran because we are sure that this honorable lady is by no means willing to see her name and her good work reflected in the press. But that benefactor must know that her reputation is so high in

the capital of this ancient land that it is without bounds and beyond description. The good impression left by her unparalleled work in the service of humanity is so deep that the heart of every Iranian beats with gratitude.

On April 19, 1943 (Farvardin 29, 1322), the newspaper *Mehr-e-Iran* published an article entitled "An Example of Service to Mankind" discussing some of the relief extended by this lady to the sick children and women of Iran. On July 14, 1943, the newspaper *Ettelaat* printed a long article under the caption "For the Sake of Service to Humanity," reproducing the picture of this kind-hearted lady who is so sympathetic to the poor. We shall not repeat the facts published by the said papers. . . . This worthy lady is Mrs. Dreyfus, the wife of the Minister of the liberty-loving United States in Tehran. A part of her life was spent in Peru on humanitarian services. Mrs. Dreyfus is a member of the Irano-American Relief Society. Because of her inborn humanitarian sentiments she proceeded with her work of charity before the Society was created. She has been most enthusiastically continuing this work. She has visited 4,814 patients either at their homes or in the clinic she established on March 18, 1943 (Esfand 27, 1321). She has paid these visits either alone or accompanied by the physician placed at her disposal of the Society by the Ministry of Health. She has offered them medical care. She has distributed two thousand healthy meals between the poor and the sick, meals consisting of rice, fruits, compotes and other provisions suitable for patients. She has furnished more than 200 needy women and children with clothing. Furthermore she has arranged a school where a number of women and girls are learning handiwork. The Irano-American Relief Society has found her work worthy of the highest commendation and in order that it be extended to cover a larger number of the poor people it has recently allocated 50,000 rials to be spent under the auspices of Mrs. Dreyfus to extend the clinic and the school and other activities mentioned above.

Mrs. Dreyfus should know that the Iranian nation and the people of Tehran in particular will never forget her kind efforts for the sake of humanity and her relief to the sick children and poor women of Iran. (Paragraph in bold type) B. Shafazand.)

Chapter 19

Russian Policy in Iran: Propaganda and Pressure

Russian policy, as noted, combined political and economic pressure with skillful propaganda spread by the socialist and communist newspapers that appeared after Reza Shah. The first communist and socialist newspapers had appeared in early 1942. "Appearance of Communist Newspaper *Mardom* and Socialist Newspaper *Siasat*," is the title of a report by Dreyfus dated February 25, 1942 (Dispatch 216, 891.911/104):

> I have the honor to inform the Department that a communist newspaper, *Mardom*, began circulation on February 1, 1942, and a socialist journal, *Siasat*, on February 23, 1942. *Mardom* (people) takes a rather strong communist line as will be shown by the following cross section of its recent articles: February 2, article "Brokers of Death" advocating the cutting off of hands of hoarders; same day, an article "I am a laborer" depicting the pitiable plight of a laborer; February 3, article on the terrible life of a peasant who toils to raise wheat to turn over to others; February 7, letter from a government employee depicting the unhappy condition of his class; February 8, article entitled "Carpet Weaving Girl" painting a miserable picture of the life of a poor tubercular child weaving rugs for almost no wage; February 14, article showing the miserable life of a school teacher; February 12, article on a journey into a village, showing the pitiable and filthy condition of the peasants and the oppression of the landlords; and an article on February 16 entitled "Cut the hands of the despotic government." The newspaper takes a stand in favor of the communistic movement in Iran and

strongly against Hitler. On February 16 it printed an article clearly in favor of the Atlantic Charter, printing the photographs of Mr. Churchill and President Roosevelt.

This communist newspaper is edited by Abbas Naraqi, who was imprisoned by Reza Shah for communistic activities and only recently released. It will perhaps come as a shock to the Department, as it did to this Legation, to learn that the newspaper is secretly owned by Mustapha Fateh, a leading official of the Anglo-Iranian Oil Company. When it became rumored about Tehran that Fateh was the real owner of *Mardom*, I went to the British Minister to inquire what interest the Anglo-Iranian Company could possibly have in communism and was informed confidentially that Fateh interest in the paper is personal and not official. I happen to know that Fateh in the past has expressed some mild interest in socialism, for example that he once wrote a thesis on the need for socialized medicine, but I was not aware that his affection was so deep. If he has some ulterior motive, it is not yet evident. However, since articles on communistic subjects in *Mardom* are dwindling in number while those against Hitler and fascism are increasing in number and violence, an outside possibility is that the communistic attitude is a pose to gain favor with the masses in order to put effective propaganda against Hitler.

The socialist newspaper *Siasat* (politics) began publication on February 23, 1942, under the editorship of Abbas Eskandari. Organ of the Masses party, its policy is actually dictated by Soleiman Mohsen, former Minister of Education, leader of the party and known for many years as a socialist democrat. For example, at the constituent assembly which elected Reza Khan as Shah, Mohsen objected strongly to a clause permitting the passing of the crown to the Crown Prince on the ground that people should be free to elect their rulers. The policy of the paper is stated to be maintenance of the territorial integrity and independence of Iran; in favor of democratic government and against despotism; establishment of individual and collective rights; freedom of expression, of thought and of the right to gather; free and compulsory education; improvement in health; adjustment of taxation in regard to the masses; and disposal of the properties of the former Shah in the interest of the Iranian people. It may be stated that Mohsen was last seen Monday evening at a large cocktail party at the Soviet Embassy surrounded by Soviet officials and engaged in earnest conversation. There are those who believe he might be a Soviet candidate for Prime Minister or even for President of Iran.

In a report entitled "Increase in Socialistic Proselytism in Iran," dated March 8, 1943, Dreyfus enlightens the reader (Dispatch 478, 891.00/2003):

> There has been, I have the honor to inform the Department, a noticeable increase in socialistic and communistic proselytism in Iran during recent months. This despatch will deal briefly with the subject in its political, press and social aspects. Perhaps no country in the world today is more ripe than Iran for socialistic indoctrination. The recent history of this country has been one long recital of abject misery and harsh exploitation. The political system of Iran is unique, the word "nation" denoting the one percent of capitalists, large landowners and rich merchants while the toiling and underfed masses are hardly taken into consideration. A very brief glance at the social history of the last fifty years may be helpful before proceeding with a consideration of present conditions.
>
> Iran in the latter part of the last century was under the despotic heel of the Qajars. The Shah, "the shadow of God" or "altar of the world," supported by a limited class of vazirs and lackeys, ruled under the dictum that the Shah's word was the word of God. The masses, blissfully unaware of the great changes taking place in the social order of the outside world, bore their miserable plight with equanimity under the spell of the Islamic doctrine that such a state of affairs must be the will of God. Governments, in their desire to perpetuate the system, kept the people in illiterate ignorance. It is said that Nasr-u-Din Shah boasted that he did not want his people to know whether Brussels was the capital of a country or a kind of vegetable. However, after the turn of the century enlightened persons returned from travels in Europe with more advanced ideas and began to agitate for a better way of life. This movement was heightened by a similar movement in the disintegrated Ottoman Empire. It was further aided by the British who desired to reduce Czarist influence in Iran by contributing to a constitutional movement. Liberals were made more bold by the murder of the despotic Nasr-u-Din Shah by one of their group in 1896 and they were encouraged by the weakness of the next Qajar, Mozafar-u-Din Shah. Conditions, such as exhaustion of the treasury and decline in the prestige of the court, played into their hands. The constitutional movement, which culminated in the Constitution of 1906, was a success only in that it brought the political and social ills of the country into the open and put on record a document which might well form the foundation of a better political system.

However, it did nothing at all to improve the condition of the masses. Rascals, politicians and land owners flocked to the constitutional standard for the purpose of protecting their own interests and Persia continued calmly on its former path. The liberals were discouraged almost to despair by the Anglo-Russian agreement of 1907, which seemed to remove any possibility of improvement in Persia's political order. They received, however, more help than they had expected from the British liberals and Russian socialists. Their hopes were revived with the dethronement of Mohammad Ali Shah but were dashed by a period of four years without a Majlis or representative government. The World War brought further hardships to an already overburdened people who suffered without knowing the reasons therefore. With the fall of the Czarist regime in Russia and the failure of the British to make the treaty of 1919 stick, liberals again took heart and had reason to hope that the great reforms of Reza Khan, especially the establishment of security and the elimination of ecclesiastical influence, might usher in a new era.

In this they were sadly wrong, for the "golden era" of Shah Reza resulted in even greater exploitation of the masses. They were oppressed and mistreated by the police, military and government officials, who, aping Shah Reza, vented their spleen on a helpless people. An important result of this government persecution has been that every Iranian peasant considers the government his personal enemy and expects nothing in the way of help from it. This will make difficult the inauguration of a proper regime in Iran. The army was a good example of this exploitation. A common soldier received a monthly wage of less than 10 rials (less than 50 cents in exchange and less than $1.00 in purchasing power) and of this he was robbed of a substantial part by his dishonest officers. In addition, he was subjected to all sorts of humiliation, including flogging. The masses lived an even harder life than before, booted about by the government, oppressed by new and heavy taxes, relieved of their lands by the greedy Shah and having no part in the political life of the country. Taxation, then as now, fell on the poor and the middle classes in indirect taxes while the upper classes were almost entirely free from taxation. Cost of living increased as the artificial industrialization of the country proceeded and the fine buildings and paved streets in the towns were paid for by the sweat of the masses. Not content with this treatment of a submissive population, Shah Reza impressed 150,000 of the people into the army where they lived in a condition of semi-slavery. Despite such a treatment, or perhaps because of it, communistic teaching thrived clandestinely but adherents of this heretical faith were ruthlessly punished when caught. Thousands found their way to death or prison but some have lived to see the light of day again. Shah Reza's house of cards came tumbling down with a slight shock when the country was invaded in August, 1941. The day of the masses had perhaps arrived.

Something resembling a democracy has been instituted. There is freedom of press, freedom of speech, a firm regard for constitutional procedure and, in all outward aspects, a constitutional and democratic form of government. Again, however as in 1907, the people have not benefited. While giving lip service to democratic ideals, the government continues to represent the entrenched classes of large landowners, unscrupulous merchants and dishonest politicians. The Government plays about on the brink of the pool of democracy without having the courage, or apparently even the desire, to take the final plunge. The situation today, however, is different from that of 1907 in several respects. First, there is now freedom of speech and action which enables the socialists to come out into the open without fear of punishment. They can sow the seeds of rebellion with the hopes that it will pay a higher return than wheat, which gives only six grains for every one sown. Secondly, the presence of Russians in the country introduces an entirely new element into the picture. Third, the masses, driven almost to starvation by the wheat shortage and soaring cost of living, have everything to gain and nothing to lose. The second of these points requires some elaboration.

The Russians, when they invaded Iran a year and a half ago, were regarded as exploiters and savages. It was amazing to those of us who were in Tehran at that time to see Iranians run for cover as the Russians approached, to see them hide their women-folk and their goods in the certainty that the dreaded Russians would abuse them in every conceivable sort of way. Imagine their astonishment and relief when they came to realize that the Russians were well disciplined and kindly intentioned toward the people. Russian action in Iran has been a masterpiece of constructive propaganda. It is almost certain that strong-arm tactics on the part of the Russians would have repelled the Iranians who, like the Chinese, have a historic facility in throwing off foreign invasions. It is true that the Persians were successfully invaded on one occasion—by the Arabs who brought the great and appealing religion of the desert—Islam. It is possible that the Russians, who came bearing a philosophy of equality and brotherly love will succeed in a second invasion of Iran? The Russians have played their cards well, refraining from overt interference in the political life of the country, propagandizing by personal example, teaching through the individual good conduct of their troops in contrast to the reprehensible and drunken conduct on the part of the other occupying forces, and feeding the people of their zone in distinction to the hunger of the masses in the British zone.

This does not mean that the Russians have all of a sudden become popular or loved by all the people. The upper classes, viewing this movement of the masses toward the Russians, are alarmed but helpless. The Prime Minister in speaking to me about it the other day said he has long realized the great and growing danger to Iran. However, he and other Iranian officials appear to be impotent in the face of the Soviet menace. They acceded to Soviet demands after a brief and futile struggle. Instances of these are the signing of the agreement for the operation of the arms plants by the Russians and the contract for the operation of the canning plant at Shahi, both of which the Iranians desired to avoid. At the present moment, they wish to escape the signing of the proposed Soviet-Iranian financial agreement, which is unfavorable to Iran, but in the end they will probably accede gracefully.

The Soviet occupation has come at a time when the masses are hard pressed. Iranians dwell in the same miserable mud huts and exist in the same superstitious and ignorant circumstances. They still wear the same ragged clothing which breeds typhus bearing lice in the winter. In the south of Tehran, people live like animals in cellars, hovels and chicken houses or sleep in the streets with the dogs. In the villages or in the country they continue to slave for the rich landowners with bent back and careworn face. In the factory children toil, for wages that will not even buy food, for the benefit of capitalists who are able to pay as much as $20,000 for a Buick automobile. These conditions, one may say, have always existed in Iran. That is true, but today there are numerous new elements. First and foremost, the Iranians in Tehran have suffered this winter as seldom before. Bread, their only staple food and the only one their limited funds can buy, has been scarce and at present is almost not to be had. Due to allied exploitation of the railways for aid to Russia, the vital commodity kerosene is so scarce that women and children wait in block-long queues for hours to get it and then are often disappointed. This is in a country which exports petroleum and in a world which talks of Atlantic Charters, a better world and a new order. Is it any wonder that the Iranians are being swayed by the promises of the teachers of socialism?

Communistic doctrine is being spread in Iran most effectively by the Russians by personal good conduct, a system which is effective in dealing with a people who have never been deluded by the foreigners who have dealt in kindly words accompanied by obnoxious deeds. Iranians are beginning to say more and more, to the constant irritation and embarrassment of the British, that the Russians in the northern zone of the country are feeding the people and caring for them in a paternal fashion, while the British in their area are starving the masses. This is having a telling effect.

The socialist press (whether openly aided by the Russians or merely encouraged by Russian implied blessing is unimportant) is taking an even more open and inciting line. The two principal socialistic newspapers are *Rahbar*, organ of the Tudeh (Masses) party and an out and out communistic journal, edited by Iraj Eskandary, and *Nobahar*, a leftist paper edited by Mohammad Taqi Bahar. *Nobahar* is having a deep effect on the people because it is edited by a man who is perhaps Iran's greatest living writer and is considered a poet laureate. This should be emphasized because Iranians, even the illiterate masses, are more swayed and influenced by beautiful prose and poetry than are the peoples of other countries. Just how Bahar became converted to socialism is not clear but the fact of his conversion shows the extent of the penetration of this philosophy. Other newspapers, particularly *Eqdam* and *Mehr-i-Iran*, preach subversive doctrine, but probably unwittingly, in their tirades against the Government. Let me quote some typical press items:

Nobahar Feb. 25. "You millionaires with your sham relief work are only trying to win the hearts of the poor in order that when the time comes they may have mercy on you; in order that they may not plunder you; in order that they may not murder you. Before you win their hearts you take their lives. Your millions are their souls. Your automobiles have broken their thin limbs. Your red carpets, the 1500 rials red shoes which you put on and walk on these red carpets, the red color of the rugs and the shoes is the red blood of the poor! Do not set up false relief! Do not tell lies! Get busy with your gambling and speculation. Get together with the contractors and brokers. Build high mansions. Heap up your dollars and sterlings. Store the provisions. You store them up and let the poor people shed tears at bakeries and kerosene shops. Scholars and educated people are losing their health because of poor nourishment and public misery. Let them die and you lean back on your armchairs in your palaces. Be a Cabinet Minister, and a Deputy, and make fun of penniless masses! But remember you will not take the spoils home. This light will be put out. To the end that there should be no poor any longer, there will be no more wealth."

Rahbar Feb. 2. "Lands belong to the peasants. Some nine-tenth of the people of Iran are peasants. They are the wealth producing classes yet they are the most unfortunate." The paper then goes on to urge the abolition of landed estates and division of land among the peasants. *Mehr-i-Iran* Feb. 7. "It is indeed surprising in a country where the moanings of the people can be heard up to the skies, where the pressure of exorbitant prices has broken the backs of the people, Ministers quarrel with each other. . . ." *Nobahar* Feb. 22. "Passengers from the north say that bread is abundant in those places. There is sugar and tea and no clamoring for kerosene. We have a right to call on the Government to give us a balance sheet of what has been delivered to the allies since the tripartite pact and what has been given to the people." *Mehr-i-Iran* Feb. 25. A leading editorial calls attention to the appalling mortality rates and gives pointed warning that the day will come when the people lose their patience. *Rahbar* Feb. 28. "The mud brick bats produced by the silo in place of bread do not require such pomp and circumstance as one finds in the Ministry of Food, especially when this organization is unable to distribute the mud brick bats properly among the poor."

Eqdam March 1. "Oh God Almighty, to show that thou hath the power to do anything, take this burden of the Ministry of Food off our shoulders in spite of the Allies. Plant this sacred adviser (Sheridan) in Abyssinia or Zanzibar. . . . We are not worthy of a person who is leading us to death. . . . Oh God, give Mr. Sheridan a lovely child so that he may hurry away to see him. . . . Do not place the poor people any longer in the hands of the executioners, who think they are the creators of the people. . . . No bread, no kerosene and widows crying in the dark of the night over their dead husbands. Hungry children are moaning. Look at the orphans and at the parents who have lost their children. Cold, hunger, sickness, disaster, distress! Everything in this country has a high price except human life." *Bakhtar* March 2. "The people have seen that their bread has been converted into luxurious cars and furniture. Naked and hungry people do not need high mansions. Put up to auction those unnecessary desks and provide the people with food." *Khorshid-i-Iran* March 2. "There is no use in weeping. Let us rise! Weeping is fruitless. Courage and action are necessary. We must not submit to oppression, no matter who the oppressor. . . .

The life of the country today is at stake. Profiteers, contractors and merchants have taken advantage of the Government and have become millionaires in a few months. They have acquired extensive lands and luxurious automobiles. This state is absolutely untenable and should be corrected by a national insurrection. How much better it would be if this should spring from the wealthy and intellectual classes. . . . When people are starving in multitudes in the cold you have no right to be living a life of luxury and debauchery. This is not right. By decree of God, religion and nature this system will be overthrown and you will be deprived forever."

There are two socialistic parties in Tehran but they are poorly organized and have not as yet exerted a very great influence. They are the Tudeh (Masses) Party headed by Soleiman Mirza and the recently organized Hamrahan (Socialist) Party headed by Mostafa Fateh, that strange combination of preacher of socialism and representative of the capitalist class in daily life. His socialism appears to be of the Fabian or parlor variety. His program begins like this: "The chains of slavery for the mass of Persian workers are being tightened day by day and the burden of oppression becomes heavier upon them. During the last half century any event or change which has been brought about in this country has been detrimental to the interests of the Persian people. Today conditions of life for the inhabitants of this land have entered a phase when endurance of their misfortune is beyond human power. A way must be found to break these chains of poverty and misery, to free the people forever from these ties of bondage. The longer the delay in finding a way, the tighter the bonds of oppression and the heavier and stronger will be those chains. These hungry and plundered folk will only succeed in breaking their chains of servitude when they realize their true and natural rights and come to understand their countless deprivations." It ends with the following call to action: "The time has come to put an end to this sham; if we ourselves fail to take the necessary steps the deluge of post-war civilization will sweep away this precarious foundation. We the people of Iran know that it is wrong to expect generosity from groups of people who have been reared in selfishness. If we expect to see the walls of our prisons, where our bodies and souls are confined, fall in, and the chains of poverty and ignorance in which our hands and feet are bound, broken, we must first reject our gaolers of heretofore and keep their hands from Government affairs. . . . For a life in which a large number of men drudge to gain a morsel of food while a small number of another class indulge in ease and vice is very transitory and unstable. A true life means the

> enjoyment of social justice, knowledge, the beauty of nature, free work, free thinking and evolution. We should endeavor to obtain such a life. The Hamrahan (Socialist) Party, who aim at providing all Iranians with that true life, as described above, hereby address their countrymen: Wake up from the deep sleep of centuries; seek your rights and obtain them, for rights are not given but taken."
>
> The above discussion is intended to indicate a trend and explain the manner in which it is being developed and not to suggest a solution. The Iranian Government has a golden opportunity to begin to correct the ills of centuries and to bring Iran into line with modern social trends which have long been developing in other countries and which after the present war will almost certainly come to full flower. If the Government fails, and there appears to be little evidence that they are awake to the great call, the solution will be found by others. The decision is in the lap of the gods.

Ahy's Conversation with Stalin

Dreyfus on June 14, 1942, reports the recall of Mohammad Saed from Russia and his replacement by Majid Ahy (Telegram 197, 701.9161/16): "Rumor has it that Ahy left Cabinet voluntarily because he did not get along well with Prime Minister. He will be missed in the Cabinet as he is a man of ability and integrity." Dreyfus on June 22, 1942 (Telegram 210, 701.9161/17):

> Reference my 197 June 14. Saed yesterday assumed office as Foreign Minister. It now appears that agrément for Ahy as Ambassador to Russia was sought and given without his consent and that he is reluctant to accept the post. Tendency toward political intrigue and uncertainty reported in my 186 June 3 continues to develop.

Standley on September 5, 1942 (Telegram 749, 701.9161/18): "The new Iranian Ambassador Madjid Ahy arrived in Kuibyshev by air from Tehran September 2."

Henderson on December 9, 1942 (Telegram 1071, 740.0011 EW 1939/26440):

> During a conversation which I had yesterday with Ahy the Iranian Ambassador, he talked at some length the present situation of Iran and Soviet-Iranian relations. Ahy has been in the Soviet Union about four

months. During recent years he has held several Ministerial posts in Iran and I understood from him that he was in charge of the construction of the Caspian Sea-Persian Gulf railroad. I am convinced that he is both genuinely friendly to the United States and sincerely anxious that we should play a progressively more important role in Iran. A summary of some of his statements is set forth below.

(One) In the early part of October he had protracted conversation with Stalin who was extremely cordial. Stalin expressed regret that the Russians had found it necessary to occupy northern Iran, pointed out that the war situation rendered occupation obligatory, and stated categorically that upon the conclusion of the war not one Russian soldier would be left in Iran and Iran's complete independence would be restored. He also said that he would undertake to reduce to a minimum the inconvenience which Soviet occupation might cause Iran and the local population. He appeared sympathetic in discussing Iranian economic difficulties and promised to investigate for the purpose of ascertaining whether steps could be taken to alleviate conditions. Molotov, with whom the Ambassador also talked, was likewise very friendly.

(Two) Unfortunately the assurances and expressions of good intentions of the Russians at the top have thus far not been reflected in the attitude of lower ranking Russian officials who make decisions with regard to current problems in Soviet-Iranian relations. Not only have Soviet authorities turned down an Iranian request for grain, but they have continued to export foodstuffs and raw materials from northern Iran to the Soviet Union. Those in charge of local communications and transport still failed to give due consideration to civilian needs. On the other hand, the Russians apparently had abandoned, at least for the present, attempts to Sovietize the Iranian population. The Russian soldiers were well disciplined and in general showed more consideration towards the local population than the soldiers of any other country. They stayed for the most part in their camps or barracks, and when they went out they rarely annoyed or molested Iranian civilians.

(Three) As a result of Russian exports from the north, British exports from the South, and consumption by occupying forces, the situation in Iran with regard to food was still extremely critical. The Iranian Government was hoping that the United States would relieve the situation by exporting foodstuffs to Iran. A few shiploads of carefully selected food and other necessities would have a tremendous effect upon Iranian morale and would strengthen materially the currency system. At present many Iranians had the impression that the Allies considered Iran merely a highway to Russia and little interest in the people for the welfare of whom they had become responsible when they seized control of the highway. They felt that the diversion of an insignificant percentage of supplies through Iran to various destinations would amply repay the Allies for the sacrifices involved in increasing the goodwill of the population and stabilize the economic life of the country.

Four. Iranians in general were hoping that the United States would greatly extend its activities in Iran. They trusted the United States because they knew that it had no national or imperialistic ambitions in the Near East. They also believed that the Americans in general were inclined to be considerate of the welfare of the people dependent upon them.

Five. It is my understanding that arrangements have recently been entered into between the Iranian Government and the American and British Governments which may alleviate to an extent at least economic conditions in Iran. He did not refer to them, however, and since I did not know their exact nature I did not call them to his attention.

Six. The Iranians had full confidence in the American Minister in Tehran, who they feel thoroughly understands the situation and whose efforts on their behalf are deeply appreciated.

Seven. First five numbered paragraphs are being sent by courier pouch to Tehran.

Bullard's Note to Smirnov

Having purchased 20,000 tons of wheat and barley in Azerbaijan in December 1942, in April 1943, as noted in chapter 18, the Soviet government had offered 25,000 tons of wheat to help feed Tehran. The offer had greatly surprised the American and British governments, prompting Bullard to send a sharp note to Smirnov. Dreyfus on May 14, 1943, in a report entitled "Enclosing a copy of a Communication Addressed by the British Minister to the Soviet Ambassador Concerning the Iranian Cereal Situation in Azerbaijan." (Dispatch 552 and Enclosure, 891.5018/24):

I have the honor to enclose a copy of a note addressed by the British Minister in Tehran to the Soviet Ambassador concerning the Iranian cereal situation in Azerbaijan and suggesting closer coordination of allied efforts in matter of Iranian food supplies. The Department is already well informed of the background of this general question of the cereal position in Azerbaijan. I have reported how the Azerbaijan grain surplus failed to find its way to Tehran and how the Russian grain purchases in that zone adversely affected the general Iranian food position. The note is submitted to the Department less for its factual recapitulation than for its political implications. It is just another example of the British Minister going out of his way to irritate the Russians with this shopworn subject at a time when we are striving to gain Russian confidence and bring about closer allied cooperation in this country. Again, as is so often the case with the British in Iran, it is the manner of approach rather than the basic soundness of the idea which is at fault. The note might, for example, have begun with an expression of a desire on the part of the British to effect close cooperation and coordination of efforts on the part of the allies and an offer of full British participation in such a move. It might then have gone on to show the harmful effects of lack of full allied consultation by citing the Azerbaijan grain situation as a case in point. "Pin prick" notes of this kind often serve to irritate and usually fail to accomplish the purpose for which they were written.

I talked at some length on the subject with Sir Reader who stated that his purpose in writing the note was to establish for the record that the Russians had not allowed grain to come out of Azerbaijan and that their action had been harmful to the general Iranian food situation. To use his own words, he did not intend to let the Russians "get away with it." While I did not commit myself to Sir Reader on the subject of sending the note, I urged strongly the desirability of more effective coordination and consultation between our two Legations and the Russians in matters of this kind.

Mr. Smirnov, when I spoke to him about the note, denied, as he has always done, that the Russians have prevented grain from coming out of Azerbaijan. He referred to the considerable amounts which the Russians have not only permitted but have expedited from Gorgan, Zenjan and Khorassan. He will not admit that as little as 250 tons of wheat were sent from Azerbaijan to Tehran during this crop year. I have heard, in support of his contention, that some wheat which arrived here from the Zenjan area probably originated in the neighboring Azerbaijan zone. However, on the whole, I subscribe to the facts as set forth by Sir Reader and I have from time to time made known to the Ambassador my preoccupation that more cereals were not forthcom-

> ing from this surplus producing area. I thought it best, in view of our efforts to cooperate here with the Russians, not to give to Mr. Smirnov the impression of backing the British view as opposed to his. Rather I took the line that we should indeed have more full consultation and cooperation on the part of the allies in all matters of mutual interest in Iran. To this he readily assented but I am not sure how far in this direction he is willing, or in fact permitted, to go. I told him that it is the policy of my Government to help the unfortunate Iranians in every way possible to institute a strong Government and get on their feet economically. For this reason, I added, we have permitted our advisers to come to Iran at Iranian request. His answer to this was to the effect that it hardly seems necessary to help a people who refuse to help themselves. I do not believe that this is his honest view. His remark should perhaps be paraphrased to read "Why should the Americans send advisers to help the Iranians when the Russians can do it so much better?"

Bullard's note to Smirnov (No.G.159/28/43) is dated May 3, 1943, and begins: "I have been re-reading Your Excellency's letter No.469-B of November 4h, 1942, on the subject of the food situation in Persia and should like, if you will allow me, to offer certain comments thereon, especially in the light of more recent developments." It then continues:

> 2. Your Excellency referred to the readiness of the Soviet Government to render assistance to the Persian Government in transporting to Tehran from Persian Azerbaijan up to 35,000 tons of wheat out of a surplus which this Legation had estimated at 40,000 tons and you argued that the export to the USSR of only 5,000 tons of wheat from Persian Azerbaijan could not cause a deterioration in the food situation in that province or create political difficulties for the Allies. In this connection, I would only remark that, while it may be true that no deterioration of food supplies or political difficulties have occurred in Persian Azerbaijan, it is unfortunately the case, and will not have escaped Your Excellency's notice, that for one reason or another hardly any of the expected 35,000 tons of wheat actually reached Tehran, with the result that serious political difficulties did, in fact, arise here. The exact amounts of wheat and barley supplied to Tehran from the Azerbaijan area up to March 6th were, according to statistics supplied to this Legation by the Persian Ministry of Supply, 242 tons only.
>
> 3. Your Excellency was also good enough to say that you did not think that the purchase of 15,000 tons of barley for the needs of the Red

Army in Persian territory could be considered as prejudicing the food situation in Persia and you mentioned that barley was not usually used as food but only as forage. I do not know what effect these purchases of barley may have had on the situation in Persian Azerbaijan, but Your Excellency will be aware that there has been an acute shortage of barley in Tehran and other parts of the country, not only for forage but also for use as an adulterant in bread, with the result that large quantities of barley, amounting on April 21st to a total of 14,895 tons, have had to be dispatched to Persia from Iraq.

4. As regards to rice, of which commodity 30,000 tons were, according to Your Excellency's letter, being purchased for export to the USSR, I observe that Your Excellency drew attention to the offer made by the Persian Government to supply as much as 50,000 tons from the harvest of the current year. Unless my recollection is at fault, however, this 50,000 tons of rice was only offered to the Soviet Government in exchange for an equivalent amount of wheat, and the proposed arrangements for this exchange were not eventually put into effect.

5. In conclusion I may add that I fully subscribe to the sentiments expressed at the end of Your Excellency's letter concerning the desirability of solving the financial, economic and political problems arising in this country by means of an exchange of information and mutual aid, and I can only record my regret that Your Excellency did not feel it necessary to inform me in advance of the arrangements recently announced for the importation into this country of 25,000 tons of wheat from the USSR, which I should much have liked to report to my Government at the earliest possible moment with a view to the efficient co-ordination of our respective efforts in the interests of the food supplies of Persia. In order to effect this co-ordination, I would request that Your Excellency and myself should discuss the food situation periodically. I am sending a copy of this letter to my American colleague.

Soviet Economic Pressure

Following the financial accord with the British in November 1942, the Russians had also demanded an agreement. Dreyfus on December 17, 1942 (Telegram 446, 891.24/325):

Soviet Ambassador is pressing Iranian Government to agree to financial accord. . . . Russians estimate their rial needs for next twelve months at eighty five millions a month. In addition they will need a credit spread of over next few months of some 340 million rials to carry out projected plan of taking over and operating Iranian arms factories (my 421, December 7). Iranians object to proposed agreement because (one) rials would be given without foreign exchange being immediately delivered; (two) gold would be held in Moscow or transported at full risk to Iran Government and (three) dollars would be held in blocked account usable only if Iran had no other dollars available. Qavam called me to say that Iranians feel they are being forced into making the agreement since Soviets threaten otherwise to cut off shipments from the north of wheat, coal and other urgently needed products. Russians will need rials at once since Sheridan has promised to sell them thirty thousand tons of rice, fifteen thousand tons of barley, five thousand tons of wheat and two thousand tons of potatoes to total value of two hundred million rials. . . . These new Russian rial demands taken together with greatly increased American rial needs (my 438, December 14) place Iran in a perilous financial position. In appealing to me for aid Qavam said he would appreciate anything Department may be able to suggest looking to solution of this difficult problem.

Dreyfus on January 9, 1943 (Telegram 25, 891.24/344):

Prime Minister informs me his Government has signed contract with Russians by which latter take over operation of canning plant at Shahi. 80% of production will be taken by Russians and remainder by Iranians. Because of Iranian insistence Russians agree in slaughtering animals to consider carefully Iran's food requirements and economic needs. Prime Minister states Iranians were reluctant to sign contract and it was done solely to appease Russians who are pressing them on other more objectionable questions, most important of which are the financial agreement (my 446, December 17) and taking over the arms factories (my 7, January 4). Iranians are indulging in delaying tactics in these two matters but are apprehensive of carrying this policy too far.

Dreyfus on March 20, 1943 (Telegram 295, 891.24/405):

There is mounting evidence of (one) increase Soviet domination of Iran and obnoxious pressure to obtain their ends and (two) Soviet resentment and suspicions of American advisor program and of general American action in Iran. Dr. Millspaugh expresses deep concern at what he considers Soviet exploitation of Iran, particularly in matters of

> arms contract (see my 58, 891.113/20, January 18) and the Iranian-Soviet financial agreement which was signed yesterday. He believes these agreements are harmful to Iran and were negotiated virtually under virtual duress. He is of opinion that question of Iran's involuntary subordination to Soviets must be clarified. He believes Iran Government is too weak to withstand Soviet pressure unless it feels assured of positive and immediate American and British support. Soviet authorities here are cordial but wholly uncooperative. General Connolly has had difficulties in obtaining Soviet permission to establish service stations and accommodations for convoy drivers in the Soviet zone. As result he is dumping war supplies at Kazvin until his reasonable demands are met.

As reported in chapter 18, the Minister of Finance, Allah Yar Saleh, had a long conversation with Vice-Consul Kuniholm on April 5, 1943 (Dispatch 528 and enclosure, 711.91/96). Referring to the upcoming elections to the 14th Majlis, Saleh stated: "We are all very concerned about the occupied territories, of course, and expect that the new deputies from Azerbaijan, Mazenderan, Gilan and Khorassan will be quite leftist, and under the influence of Moscow. In general, the composition of the new Majlis is bound to be 'pink.'" Saleh adds:

> The cabinet has been subjected to a constant pressure from Ambassador Smirnov and the Soviet authorities in this country. The Russians are the most uncompromising and inflexible people with whom we have had to deal; they are never prepared to make any concessions whatsoever in any negotiations undertaken between our two countries. In fact, it is a question in practically every instance of "take it, or leave it." The agreements and contracts effected are never in our interest, but unfailingly in the interest of the Soviet Union; we get no benefit whatever. As this Soviet pressure increases, the leaders of our Government become more and more sour and feel more and more disenchanted and disillusioned. The prevailing feeling now is that, unless the Allied Governments can bring about an easing of the Soviet pressure, the Iranian Government will be forced to knuckle under to the Russians.

A week after Saleh's conversation with Kuniholm, the Russians had announced that they were shipping 25,000 tons of Russian wheat to Tehran. Also, at this time the Iranian government was faced with complete financial collapse. Despite the fact that they owed Iran large sums from earlier transactions, the Russians were insisting on immediate payment for the wheat. Dreyfus on May 21, 1943 (Telegram 526, 891.24/440):

> Department's 243, May 20. Iranian Government considers sale of grain to Russians in Azerbaijan and purchase of 25,000 tons of wheat from Russians to be separate transactions. My investigations fail to reveal that barter was either effected or contemplated. Rice referred to by Russians is same 30,000 tons referred to in my 331, October 23. Facts are as follows: Russians and Iranians signed in December contract for delivery by latter to former of 5,000 tons of wheat, 15,000 tons of barley and 30,000 tons of rice. To date about one third of wheat and barley and 22,000 tons of rice have been delivered. Russians owe Iranians about 63,000,000 rials for these grain purchases. Russians out of clear sky in mid-April offered to sell Iran 25,000 tons of wheat to help feed Tehran. Offer was accepted and grain is coming forward at rate of 7500 tons a month beginning in May; small amounts have already arrived. Millspaugh states that Russians are demanding 32,000,000 rials in partial payment for this wheat. While Russians did not mention barter to Iranians, it is possible they intended that the two transactions would ultimately cancel each other. If this is the case, it is difficult to understand why they press for payment for wheat sold when they owe a great deal more for their own purchases. It should be noted also that the 25,000 tons of wheat were not needed since wheat from United States is arriving in sufficient flow to feed Iran up to the next harvest. Iranians agreed to purchase Russian wheat because they were not sure of wheat arrivals from United States in view of the great delays in shipments already encountered. Repeated to Moscow in reference to its 458 May 15.

Dreyfus on May 26, 1943 (Dispatch 560 and enclosure, 861.24/1524):

> I have the honor to enclose a copy of a list of goods which the Russians desire to purchase in Iran for export to Russia during the present year. This information was furnished to me confidentially by Dr. Millspaugh. The Department will note that the amounts requested are substantial and considerably greater than those exported during the previous year, statistics for which are also included in the table. This brings up a question which has long bothered me and is beginning to preoccupy Dr. Millspaugh – that of purchases in Iran by allied authorities. I have always felt that Iran owes to allied purchases to a very considerable extent the present scarcity of goods, high prices and inflationary con-

> dition. The Poles, British and Russians vie with each other to purchase Iranian goods, whether or not surplus to the needs of the country, while maintaining for the record that they are not purchasing in quantity sufficiently great to harm the economy of the country. The American army happily brings with it most of the goods it consumes, a fact which has been noted by a great many Iranians.

In 1321 (1942/43) the Russians had purchased and exported 50,000 tons of rice, 100,000 sheep and 6,000 head of cattle, and 5,000 horses. In 1322 (1943/44) they desired to export 50,000 tons of rice, 10,000 tons of dates and raisins, 3,000 tons of legumes, 20,000 head of cattle, 25,000 sheep, 5,000 horses and 1,000 mules. Their shopping list also included 1.4 million meters of canvas cloth and bags, 600,000 meters of woolen piecegoods, 50,000 blankets, 1.75 million cartridge belts, 200,000 pairs of boots, and 5,000 tons of wool.

Dreyfus in a report of July 5, 1943, entitled, "Enclosing Memorandum Prepared by Dr. Millspaugh on Subject of Financial and Economic Relations Between Iran and Soviet Government; Discussion of Soviet Position in Iran." (Dispatch 606 and enclosures, 761.91/257):

> I have the honor to enclose a copy of a memorandum in which Dr. Millspaugh, Administrator General of the Finances, sets forth in some detail the harmful effects on Iran of Soviet financial and economic action in this country. Dr. Millspaugh has become firmly convinced that Iran is suffering considerable financial and economic exploitation by the Soviet occupying forces. His memorandum gives formal expression to these views. In it he faces a difficult and potentially dangerous situation with courage and realism. He brings out into the open, for the first time, a problem which has long preoccupied the Iranian Government but from which Iranian politicians have fought shy because of their great fear of the Russians. The memorandum was prepared as a statement of the Iranian case for the information of the Iranian Government and to form the basis of eventual approach to the Soviet Government to seek correction of the abuses. It was also intended to prove the validity of the Iranian case to the British and American Governments in the hope that they will be willing and able to bring about an improvement in a situation which is harmful to Iran in an economic and financial way and which directly threatens Iranian sovereignty and independence. Dr. Millspaugh furnished this Legation a copy of the memorandum and also handed a copy to the British Minister. He has not given a copy to any Soviet official nor has he made any

approach to the Soviet Embassy in the matter. It is suggested that the Department read this memorandum in connection with my despatches Nos. 478 March 8, 499 March 27, 504 April 2, and 513 April 8, and my telegram No. 672 June 29.

It is hoped that the great length of the memorandum will not deter the Department from reading it with care and giving the matter the attention it merits. The importance of the question is out of all proportion to the small financial and economic issues involved. Almost for the first time the allies are faced with the problem of one of the United Nations exploiting an occupied country in a manner hardly in keeping with the spirit of the Atlantic Charter. If, as many believe, Iran offers an ideal proving ground for the Atlantic Charter, the other allies can hardly close their eyes to such action. The question is, however, a complex and difficult one which cannot be approached with haste. The Soviet authorities, when they are approached on the subject as they eventually must be, are sure to deny any exploitation of Iran and beyond doubt will have ready answers on all counts. They will perhaps point to the superior conduct of their forces, to their kindly attitude toward the Iranian people, to their lack of interference in the internal affairs of the country and to many other things to prove that, far from exploiting the country, they have adopted a friendly and cooperative policy.

The Russians appear to have, as a matter of fact, two policies in Iran. On one hand they treat the people as individuals in a considerate and kindly manner, an effective and very astute means of proselytism. On the other hand they have the most utter contempt for the corrupt and inefficient Iranian system of Government by and for the entrenched classes and robber barons. When dealing, therefore, with the Government, as distinct from the people, they give no quarter and resort to the most selfish methods of exploitation, some of which are enumerated in Dr. Millspaugh's memorandum. The Russians are also apt to point to what they consider Anglo-American trade and political penetration through such agencies as the MESC and the American designs on Iran in the form of the adviser program. Some blame does attach to British action in Iran and to a much smaller degree to American action. However, both the Americans and British are fair and reasonable peoples and nations with whom such matters can be discussed with hopes of arriving at proper settlement. But dealing with the Russians, in Iran at least, is a form of futility which almost invariably leads to a dead end. Thus, obtaining relief from the abuses Dr. Millspaugh enumerates will not be easy. We must also take into consideration the probability that

> the Russians will receive the Iranian view as expressed by Dr. Millspaugh with some resentment. They may become even more suspicious of our adviser program and the matter may lead to strained relations between the Soviet Embassy and Dr. Millspaugh. Dr. Millspaugh's interest in the entire question is a purely practical one of obtaining relief from Soviet financial exploitation of Iran, especially in view of the present desperate financial situation of the country. Dr. Millspaugh will probably wish to await the return of the Soviet Ambassador from leave in Russia before presenting the Soviet Embassy a copy of this or a revised and specially edited memorandum. I will keep the Department informed of developments.

Soviet economic pressure was unrelenting. In the fall of 1943, after long negotiations the Soviet government undertook to deliver 40-50,000 tons of wheat from northern Iran for Tehran, provided the Iranians could supply the needed road transport to the nearest railhead. In exchange, the Soviets obtained rice and exchanged other goods. Ford in a report of December 29, 1943 (Dispatch 775 and enclosures, 891.6131/4):

> I have the honor to refer to the second and third paragraphs of the Legation's despatch No. 693 of October 16, 1943, regarding negotiations then in progress between Soviet and Iranian authorities for the division of the Iranian rice crop. Those negotiations were finally brought to a conclusion during November by the signature of two contracts for the sale of rice to the USSR by the Iranian Government and the other for the sale of certain manufactured goods to the Iranian Government by the USSR. Although in fact related to each other, the two contracts are understood to be legally separate. Both call for payment in cash, and the transaction is not, therefore, a barter agreement in the strict sense of the word. The Legation has as yet been unable to obtain copies of the contracts, but Mr. Bernard lamb of the Millspaugh Mission, who conducted the final negotiations, has furnished the following information regarding the general terms of the arrangements made:

> Sale of Rice. (1) A syndicate of six or seven Iranian commercial firms will act as agents for the Iranian Government to purchase 60,000 tons of rice at prices averaging 6.50 to 7.00 rials per kilogram. These agents will receive a commission of five per cent on the purchase price. (2) Of the total purchased, the Iranian Government will resell to the Soviet authorities 36,000 tons at prices averaging about 3.00 rials per kilogram. The remaining 24,000 tons will be moved by Russian transport, but at Iranian expense, to Tehran for distribution to the Iranian public

at prices and through agencies yet to be definitely determined. (3) Deliveries of the rice to the Soviets are to be made during the period December, 1943 through April, 1944 in quantities of roughly 7,000 tons monthly. Proportional deliveries to Tehran of the Iranian share are to be made simultaneously. (4) Payment by the Soviets is to be made within twenty days after each delivery, but they have the right to move the rice to Baku for inspection before acceptance.

Purchase of Goods from USSR. (1) The Iranian Government will buy from the Soviet Union goods of the total value of 115,000,000 rials. Eighty million rials of this total will be represented by approximately seven million meters of cotton piece goods, and the remainder by newsprint, glassware, and miscellaneous items. (2) Deliveries of these goods will be made at the Irano-Russian frontier, and payment must be made by the Iranian Government within three days after notification that the goods are at the border ready for delivery. If payment is delayed, a 10 per cent penalty is payable.

It is obvious that the foregoing terms of the two contracts are decidedly unfavorable to the Iranian Government. The immediate loss on the 36,000 tons of rice sold to the Russians can hardly be less than 135,000,000 rials ($4,200,000 in round numbers) and more probably will be about 150,000,000 rials, (say, $4,690,000). On the other side, the prices of the cotton piece goods to be sold to the Iranian Government average about 11.40 rials per meter, which is four rials per meter higher than the Soviet price last year and more than five rials higher than the current price of cotton goods from India, CIF Persian Gulf port, according to Mr. Lamb. Likewise, the terms of payment for both rice and the Russian manufactured goods clearly favor the Soviets. The Legation is informed that the original Soviet proposals included other minor provisions which would have imposed additional hardships upon the Iranians but which they were successful in having eliminated.

The reasons for Iranian acceptance of so inequitable an arrangement were primarily political. According to Dr. Millspaugh and Mr. Lamb, the Russian authorities were unyielding in their demands, and the Iranians feared that unless an agreement was reached the Soviets would simply take the quantity of rice they wished, using their own agencies and, perhaps, disregarding the needs of the Iranian population. For obvious reasons, the Iranian Government preferred to have the purchase and distribution of the rice crop carried out under its own auspices, even though it might have to suffer a financial loss. Furthermore, it was hoped that if the Russians were satisfied on this point, they might be more inclined to take a cooperative attitude with regard to other matters notably the collection and distribution of wheat and barley in the northern zone, which are of greater importance in the Iranian picture. The Iranian Government does not expect to suffer any substantial direct loss on the over-all transaction. Mr. Lamb hopes to recoup the loss on the rice sold to the Soviets by means of the profit to be obtained by sale in Iran of the goods received from the USSR. (He admits, of course, that the high price of Soviet goods will result in an indirect loss, not appearing on the books, since most of the articles in question could be obtained more cheaply elsewhere.) The first delivery of Russian goods has already been made at the Azerbaijan frontier, and payment was made immediately by the Iranian Government. Mr. Lamb states that he is very anxious to fulfill the terms of the contracts to the letter, not only to avoid the invocation of the penalty clauses but also to place the Iranian Government on a better business footing vis-à-vis the Soviet authorities in the future. Dr. Millspaugh has just made a brief trip into the rice producing area of northern Iran, principally to look into measures being taken in connection with the rice contract.

Ford on January 24, 1944 (Dispatch 811 and enclosure, 891.6131/7):

I have the honor to refer to my despatch No. 775 of December 29, 1943, reporting two contracts made between the Iranian Government and the Soviet authorities for the sale of Iranian rice and the purchase by Iran of certain Russian manufactured goods. There are transmitted English translations of the two contracts in question. . . . Some points worth of note are: a) The Soviet authorities have a leeway of 10 days for taking delivery of rice, as compared to only 3 days granted the Iranians for taking delivery of the Russian goods. b) The Iranians are charged with responsibility for storage and safekeeping of the rice at the Caspian ports until it has been shipped to the USSR, even after formal delivery has been made to the Russians. c) The average price of rice sold to the Soviets would appear to work out at about 3.37 rials per kilogram, rather than 3.00 rials as stated by Mr. Lamb. d) Examination of the rice for quality is to be made at Pahlavi, within Iran, rather than at Baku as stated by Mr. Lamb. e) The Soviet authorities are granted a leeway of 30 days for delivery of goods sold to Iran, without payment of any fine or damages (note paragraph 5 of the contract), whereas for each day's delay in accepting delivery, the Iranians must pay a penalty equal to 10% of the value of the goods involved. (Paragraph 11 of the contract).

Chapter 20

Russian Policy and Conditions in Azerbaijan and Khorassan

In a letter to Dreyfus dated February 10, 1943, the US Consul in Tabriz, Bertel E. Kuniholm, comments on the Iran-Soviet grain agreement of December 1942 (OSS Report 35587):

> The problem has now resolved itself into the delivery of grain to the Soviet forces in Iran, to the exclusion of the needs of the people of Tabriz. We have two weeks' supply of wheat here, and little likelihood that we can see the spring through, much less the summer. I have accompanied Vivian (an American Adviser to the Ministry of Food stationed in Tabriz) to the local silo, to the ambars (storage) near the Soviet border, and to the Kurdish ambars at Maragheh. The picture is gloomy. As I have reported to you before, the wheat is simply not here. In our talks with officials in the outlying areas, as in Kurdistan, it is clear that the wheat has gone, where, it is anybody's guess. The biggest potential grain reserves are at Ardebil and Maragheh, but in both cases the principal ambars are located in distant mountain districts, with little prospect of being able to move any substantial portion before June, because of the dearth of camels and donkeys. You know how slowly grain moves by caravan. Incidentally, in connection with Ardebil, Vivian has received two telegrams from the Prime Minister (Qavam) requesting the immediate delivery of 4,000 tons of wheat from Ardebil (there are 300 tons there now). The Prime Minister, it seems, had obtained this figure from Forouzan, who had in turn picked it up as a rumor current in the Tabriz bazaar. Vivian believes that the Prime Minister signed the grain agreement with the Soviets on the

basis of incorrect data submitted to him by Forouzan, Vivian's predecessor, and partly due to political pressure.

Letter of February 14, 1943, from an American in Tabriz to New York (MID-Iran, 5970): "Since I wrote the general letter to Francis things have again been going up leap after leap. I don't know what is going to happen here. There is food and plenty. But hoarding and speculation has brought about a terrible condition. The suffering of the poor is great indeed." Letter from Tabriz to New York, February 27, 1943: "The one subject of conversation—prices. They just keep on going up and up. One cake laundry soap is now 24 rials. . . . Iran is certainly on the verge of something terrible if relief doesn't come soon, change of some sort."

Another letter from Kuniholm to Dreyfus, February 23, 1943 (OSS Report 35587):

> The Soviet-Iranian grain agreement, as I have stated before, should never have been made, for if it is carried out according to plan, there will be famine in Azerbaijan. The Iranian Government, in my opinion, would do well to invoke the penalty clause of its contract, pay the fine provided, and proceed to try to feed its own people. . . . Today a large and unruly crowd of Armenians descended upon the Consulate, and demanded my intervention with the Iranian authorities in the hope of obtaining bread. They said the Moslem bakers would not sell them bread, and that Armenian bakers could not obtain flour. They repeated several times that they had been informed by the local authorities that "the Americans" were in control of bread rationing, and that it was up to me to see justice rendered. I am sure that they were "sicked" on to me by the Governor General or his henchmen. We finally prevailed upon the crowd to disperse, after about an hour of haranguing. As the situation deteriorates, these incidents will be repeated and will become more menacing in nature. . . . After repeated previous refusals, the Red Army has now furnished trucks for hauling grain from the Ardebil area. The latter, as you know, is dominated by the Shah Sevans, a people as fierce and war-like as the Kurds, and it would have been quite impossible for Vivian and his administration alone to have effected grain deliveries there. The movement of grain from Ardebil, however, is for the Red Army only, and, at best, is only a stop-gap. In another month or two, with the present crook of a Governor General and his gang of incompetents on the scene sabotaging Vivian's every effort, we are headed for bread riots and grave disturbances in Tabriz.

The difficulties of Rex Vivian increase with each passing week. I am confident that, unless the present incompetent Governor General is removed without delay, a crisis will develop in this area soon, which will defy the best efforts of any of us. The Governor General is exerting all possible pressure to have Vivian removed. . . . A whispering campaign against Vivian is now in full spate in the bazaars, and feeling is running high. There is, also, collusion on the part of the local police, which receives the tacit approval of the Governor General. . . . We are all convinced, of course, that certain amounts of grain have been hoarded by the more opulent proprietors, but it will be next to impossible to disgorge any substantial quantities of this grain. As long as we have a democratic regime in Iran, it will not be possible to take really effective disciplinary measures against proprietors. In the days of Shah Reza there were the bastinado, the knout, and all the refinements of Persian methods of persuasion, but those days are gone. Now, the proprietors know that they will suffer no corporal punishment, and are not particularly concerned about going to jail. Most of them put up their bail with nonchalance, or submit docilely to imprisonment, stating that they would rather rot in prison than submit to oppression by the "American gaoler."

The Russians have been doing their best to make a "Stakanovite" out of Vivian, without apparent success. Kuznetsov, the Soviet Consul General, always begins his talks with a long harangue about the necessity for all of the allied representatives here to take a firm action with Vivian to the end that grain deliveries shall be made to the Red Army in conformity with the Soviet-Iranian grain agreement, like the stereotyped addresses of the Polit-commissars at Communist Party meetings. We have tried to prevail upon Kuznetsov to take a firmer attitude with the Governor General, since the executive function reposes in the latter as senior Iranian Government official in the area, and not Vivian who is merely an administrator with no power whatever over the municipal police or the gendarmerie. So far we have gotten nowhere.

Expulsion of Consul Kuniholm and Vivian from Azerbaijan

Cable to Dreyfus on March 12, 1943 (Telegram 123, 891.24/370): "Kuibyshev's 241, March 8, to Department regarding Soviet complaint against Kuniholm and Vivian. Department assumes you will consult Kuniholm in this connection, and we shall, of course, await your comments before considering a reply." Dreyfus replied on March 20, 1943 (Telegram 295, 891.24/405):

> Department's 123, March 12. Kuniholm reports that bread riots took place in Tabriz Tuesday. He is of opinion that Azerbaijan's problem can be improved only by (one) strong government action against recalcitrant landlords, (two) dismissal of dishonest and unreliable Governor General Mugadam and (three) cancellation of Iranian-Soviet cereals contract even if penalty clause be invoked. He reports great Soviet pressure for removal of Vivian, who he considers has done a heroic job against hopeless odds and in spite of lack of Iranian or Soviet cooperation. Prime Minister informs me he is sending Tadayyon to Tabriz to investigate. This turn of affairs in Azerbaijan brings to a head the general question of Soviet policy in Iran.

State Department Information Series for March 1943 (MID-Iran, 5940):

> Reports from Tabriz stated that bread riots had taken place in that city on March 16. Iranians allege that Russian purchases of grain were at least partly responsible for a food shortage in this area, and that this was only one evidence of Russian disregard of Iranian interests. . . . Russian resentment and suspicion of American involvement in Iranian affairs was resulting in an uncooperative attitude. . . . It was felt necessary to call Soviet attention to the fact that American assistance to Iran had been offered in the interests of the United Nations cause and not for American aggrandizement, and in particular to facilitate the sending of supplies through Iran to the Soviet Union.

On March 27, 1943, Dreyfus reports on the Vivian and Kuniholm affair and on Soviet position and policies in Iran (Dispatch 499 and enclosures, 891.24/429):

> I am of firm conviction, after having studied these reports and after having discussed the matter with Kuniholm, the Russian Ambassador, and the Prime Minister, that neither Kuniholm nor Vivian has been engaged in any kind of anti-Soviet activity. Their activities in Azerbaijan have no doubt clashed with Soviet policy and out of this perhaps arose the resentment and suspicion on which the complaint seems to have been founded. The complaint appears to have originated with two persons—Koussenitzoff, the Russian Consul General, and Mugadam, the Iranian Governor General of Azerbaijan. While the ostensible cause was wheat, there is a deeper and more real political basis, a matter

discussed below. Kuniholm and Vivian have, in my opinion, done excellent work in Tabriz, both for the United States and in the interests of Iran; the complaint against them may arise out of this very fact. Kuniholm was not expelled from Tabriz and is the bearer of a valid Soviet permit to return there. Vivian, on the other hand, was virtually expelled from Tabriz by the Russians, who gave him 24 hours to leave the city on the grounds that his permit had expired. As I pointed out in my telegram, this action was not only a derogation of Iranian sovereignty but was also based on false grounds, since Vivian's permit was a mere laissez passer to travel through the Soviet lines and in no sense a residence permit. In any event, Vivian's expulsion was objectionable from the Iranian point of view since it represented unwarranted and summary action against an Iranian official; it is to be deprecated from the American standpoint because it tends to reflect on an American adviser. Tehran is already bussing with the story and Iranians eagerly await the next installment. There is some hope, I should add, that as a result of conversations taking place in Tehran it may still be possible to obtain Soviet permission for Vivian to return to Tabriz.

The Department is well informed regarding the Iranian wheat situation. A few words as to the Azerbaijan angle may be helpful here in explanation of the present Soviet complaint. Azerbaijan is one of Iran's principal wheat growing areas and in normal times has a surplus production of from 20,000 to 40,000 tons. Had it been possible to obtain possession this year of the estimated 35,000 tons surplus, as British officials and the more sanguine Iranians hoped, it would not have been necessary to import wheat from the United States to feed the Iranian civil population. This Legation long since took the view that little, if any, wheat would come to Tehran from Azerbaijan. After much discussion, the British were brought reluctantly to consent planning wheat imports on this basis. To date, less than 300 tons of Azerbaijan wheat has been received in Tehran! What has become of the surplus? First, it escaped over the borders into Iraq, Turkey and Russia; second, it trickled into the black market and some of it may have found its way clandestinely into the Tehran area; thirdly it was delivered to the Russians under a contract made in December; fourthly it was hoarded by unscrupulous landlords who are holding it for black market prices; and fifthly it still exists in places from whence its transport is almost impossible because of lack of trucks and camels. The combination of these factors account, in my opinion, for the present Tabriz shortage. In December Mr. Sheridan, in the hopes of being able to appease the Russians into letting grain from Azerbaijan come to Tehran, signed a cereals contract providing for the delivery in Azerbaijan by the Iranian

Government to the Russians of 30,000 tons of rice, 15,000 tons of barley and 5,000 tons of wheat. This grain contract is the root of the present difficulty and explains the Russian objection to Vivian. The Soviets, through Consul General Koussenitzoff, insist on their pound of flesh while Vivian, standing alone for the Iranians, takes the view that to carry out the contract will cause a bread shortage in Tabriz. His view in this respect has been vindicated by the actual shortage which has developed. It is also borne out by the fact that Vivian in spite of all his efforts has been able to deliver to the Soviets only a small part of the cereals covered by the contract. (Circa 1500 tons of wheat and 3500 tons of barley). The situation is the more tragic because sufficient wheat perhaps actually exists in Azerbaijan to feed Tabriz and fulfill the above mentioned Russian contract. Unfortunately, however, the only wheat immediately available, in the nearby accessible places such as Ardebil and Maragheh, is sufficient to meet one of these objectives but not both. The wheat in more distant places simply cannot be moved in time and that from some possible nearer sources cannot be extracted from the greedy landlords.

Governor General Mugadam's desire to get rid of Vivian was beyond question based on the fact that Vivian's program of endeavoring to make the dishonest and grasping landlords disgorge their hoarded wheat threatened his pocket books, being himself one of the largest landlords in Azerbaijan. Vivian's action against the landlords was as heroic as it was futile. The situation was not peculiar to Azerbaijan, Sheridan having had a similar experience in the zones outside Soviet occupation. The Iranian Government, subservient to the entrenched classes, simply will not take strong action against landlords, speculators, merchants, profiteers and hoarders. While Sheridan and Vivian have succeeded in pushing the Government into arresting some of them, they are mostly "small fry" and none has been severely prosecuted. Thus, Vivian had to fight the Russians and his own colleagues single handed!

The complaint against Kuniholm is yet another manifestation of the evident and growing desire of the Russians to prevent foreign eyes from prying too closely into their affairs in Azerbaijan. While there may have been, as suggested to me by the Russian Ambassador, some Soviet feeling against Kuniholm because of his Finnish ancestry, I consider this as incidental to the main political issue. There are numerous indications of Soviet resentment of the American advisor program and suspicion of American motives in Iran. General Connolly has been unable as yet to obtain Soviet permission to establish truck service stations and accommodations for convoy personnel in the Soviet occupied part of Iran. At the moment, in the absence of such permission, he is dumping supplies destined for Russia at Kazvin. It is unbelievable that the Russians can fail to facilitate American aid to them on such flimsy political grounds. There are those who believe that the Russians want to keep the population of Azerbaijan from seeing these happy and well fed Americans. It is indicative, too, that the Russians have on many occasions complained to Kuniholm about the poor quality, bad conduct, and laziness of American troops carrying supplies to Russia. Dealing in almost any matter with the Soviet authorities in Tehran is a form of futility and usually results in what is known here as the "run around." This is experienced particularly in applications for visas for Russia, permits for American airplanes to proceed to Kuibyshev and permits for Americans to visit the Soviet occupied sections of Iran. Soviet officials are pleasant and friendly but their action appears to be designed to cause such delay that the petitioner tires and eventually gives up. Colonel Schwarzkopf, American head of the Iranian Gendarmerie, has been endeavoring for a fortnight to obtain a Soviet permit to go to Resht on an official inspection trip. Up to the present, in spite of my assistance, he has been unsuccessful.

Dr. Millspaugh is much perturbed at the Soviet pressure on the Iranian Government and is of the opinion that this situation needs immediate clarification. He is particularly disturbed that the Soviets have been able, against Iranian wishes, to force the signature of such objectionable documents as the arms agreement and the Soviet-Iranian financial agreement. These two subjects are being taken up by separate despatch. Dr. Millspaugh believes, and I concur, that the Iranians are too weak to withstand Soviet pressure and as a result will fall increasingly under Soviet domination. Dr. Millspaugh observes this pressure in his daily work. For example, he told me the other day that he received a routine request from the Iranian Treasury to advance 200,000 rials out of public funds to repair a private house in Kazvin for occupation by Russians. Since the payment is not covered by law, he intends to refuse.

I discussed the situation in Azerbaijan yesterday with the Prime Minister, who declared that he intends to remove Governor General Mugadam without delay. He promised to endeavor to ascertain whether the Governor General was guilty of acting as an informer to the Russians against Kuniholm and Vivian. He is also sending a commission to Azerbaijan to investigate the general situation and examine into the Mugadam "reign of terror" which resulted in the severe beating of the Mayor.

The Prime Minister in the strictest confidence volunteered the interesting statement that it is being widely said in the bazaars that the growing criticism of the American advisers in the press and Majlis is inspired not only by the Russians but as well by the British. This seems to me an important fact, for the evil effects of the inevitable criticism of our advisers will be somewhat attenuated if the people believe it is inspired by the Russians and British. The following amusing story bearing on the wheat situation in Azerbaijan was told me by the Foreign Minister. Minister Farrokh was decorated by the Shah as a reward for his wheat inspection trip to Azerbaijan, an undeserved action for the Minister came back with completely false information. At the ceremony of decoration the Soviet Ambassador whispered to the Foreign Minister, "He should be decorated with the Order of Lenin, not the Order of Homayoun."

The Russians are suspicious of American actions and motives in Iran. This is not unnatural in view of the fact that Iran has since the time of Peter the Great been considered by the Russians as their actual or potential field of expansion southward toward the Persian Gulf. I must, in all frankness, admit that there is some justification for this Soviet preoccupation. For example, I know that the Soviet Ambassador views with alarm the octopus-like grasp the British and Americans are getting on Iran through the UKCC and MESC. We, the Americans, are certainly inspired in these matters by no long range political or trade motives but I am sorry that I cannot say as much for the British. I, myself, look with dislike and apprehension on the monopolistic tactics of these organizations and can readily appreciate that the Russians see in them an Anglo-American bid to seize trade and political power for post-war use. Perhaps the Russian arms agreement is an answer to their apparent Anglo-American trade infiltration! MESC action in Iran will be made the subject of a separate confidential despatch.

Realizing that this problem of the Soviet position in Iran is only one facet of the larger question of Soviet relations with the allies, I do not suggest any precipitate action which might adversely affect the general picture. However, I do feel that clarification is needed as soon as possible if Soviet domination of Iran is to be avoided. In this regard, please see my despatch No. 478 dated March 8, 1943, entitled Increase in Socialistic Proselytism in Iran. The Iranian attitude was aptly summed up as follows by Dr. Mbassar, an Iranian judge, in a conversation with me last evening: "The Iranians believe that unless the British and Americans take some action *now* to restrain the Russians in Iran they may well be too late."

Politics of Hunger in Tabriz

US Vice Consul Rudolph W. Hefti's report of April 2, 1943, on the New Year "festivities" held in the Office of the Governor General in Tabriz (OSS Report 34466):

> The Noruz reception at the Ostandari last Monday was a cold and mournful affair. The atmosphere was tense and everyone appeared uncomfortable for one reason or another. There were numerous inquiries regarding the sudden departure of Vivian and Kuniholm. I said that as far as I knew, Vivian was making a routine trip for the purposes of consultation, and that he was expected back shortly. As for Kuniholm, he had been planning a visit to Tehran for some time, and Vivian's trip offered him a means of transportation. To our monshi, people were less reserved in their comment. The prevailing opinion, as maliciously nurtured by the rumor-mongers of the Governor General and the Soviets in the bazaars, was that Vivian had fled in disgrace. However, there was a small minority of honest and intelligent individuals, who appeared to see through the fabric of local corruption and deceit. . . . Other tongues were tied, however, by fear of the bastinado, in the application of which the Governor General and his gang of ruffians are expert, and you will recall from the recent beating administered to the Mayor of Tabriz (see the Consulate's letter of March 10, 1943). The Mayor, incidentally, was among the guests at the reception, although he remained quietly in a corner and was quite uncommunicative. The violent campaign against Vivian, and indirectly his associates, which has been sweeping the bazaars and government offices, has undoubtedly been instigated by the Soviets, the Governor General and the landlords for their own several purposes (see my telegram of March 30, 11 p.m.). . . . Meanwhile, the Governor General is becoming more and more entangled in his own machinations with the Soviets. I think, however, that the charge against him of pro-Soviet sentiment is probably a distortion of the true situation. . . . The Soviets are in the saddle here, and therefore he is courting them. But it certainly does not follow that he is pro-Russian. In truth, Mugadam is the antithesis of everything Soviet, except possibly his propensity for double-dealing, at which he is hopelessly outwitted by the Russians. . . .
>
> Of all those present at the Ostandari, none appeared more miserable than the Governor General himself. His face was lined with fatigue and beset with worry, and it was obvious that his thoughts were far from the scene of "festivity." In his conversation with me, General

Mugadam confined himself to banalities, which he accompanied with a pained smile. Even such an innocuous discussion, however, was sufficient to reveal that the weather has also been against him. The unseasonable cold spell had continued to block the roads with snow well past the time when blossoms ordinarily begin to appear. Five hundred tons of wheat is said to be available in Ardebil, but the Suyun Pass on the road from Tabriz has been buried under three meters of snow, and a large caravan of camels has perished. There is another 1000 tons at Takan Tape (Tikhat) about 150 kilometers southeast of Miandoab, but the road will not be open for another five weeks. Likewise, a further 2000 tons in the Moghan district in the northeastern corner of the province must wait at least a month before it can be moved here.

The Governor General evidently had hoped that he would be able to win the favor of the population, after Vivian's departure, by at once restoring the 500 gram bread ration which had been halved following the bread riots of March 17, but this has been virtually impossible, since wheat deliveries to the Tabriz silo last week averaged less than 36 tons daily, or a little more than half of the city's normal requirements. Thus, during the Noruz holidays, only 250 grams of bread per person was distributed with an additional 250 grams of potatoes on two occasions. On March 30, however, Mugadam could no longer resist popular pressure, despite no material improvement in the situation, and so he drew upon the city's meager 190 ton reserve of wheat and flour, in order to permit the reestablishment of the 500 gram ration. It is not to be denied that this irresponsible act of jugglery created a favorable impression among the public at large, but it was short-lived, for yesterday the ration was again cut to 250 grams, and deliveries have dropped to less than 10 tons per day. Consequently, Tabriz must somehow survive the coming weeks on a bare hand-to-mouth basis, unless some of the recalcitrant landlords are compelled to disgorge their hoardings. . . . Both the Persians and Armenians have repeatedly emphasized to us that only brute force will establish respect for government among the local population . . . thus saving the lives of thousands of the starving poor. To the Soviets, however, the starvation of the public is but a minor consideration. What they principally want at the present time is wheat, and they have no particular scruples as to the manner of obtaining it. Undoubtedly, Mugadam and the Russians have reached some mutually profitable understanding in this respect, whereby the Iranian Government will inevitably be the principal loser.

Hefti's letter of April 15, 1943, to Dreyfus (OSS Report 35398):

Since my last report of April 2, 1943, the Minister of Food, Mr. Taddayon, has visited Tabriz ostensibly to make a spot examination of the food supply problem in Azerbaijan. His arrival was preceded by a fanfare of rumors to the effect that he would be accompanied by Sheridan, Vivian and a miscellany of other officials, although there were many who insisted that Vivian would not return. When the Minister turned up alone, or at least without a distinguished suite, Tabriz was plainly disappointed. . . . The public has learned to expect nothing good from the comings and goings of a cabinet minister . . . and for the present Tabriz must struggle along on a half ration of bread. I told the Minister that there were persistent reports in the Bazaar that the Russians had compelled Vivian to leave Tabriz, because they considered him to be anti-Soviet. Such a charge, I said, would be a grave injustice. Vivian had been appointed here primarily to assure the food supply of Azerbaijan. As an Iranian official, his first obligation was to safeguard the civil population from starvation. If at the same time he was unable to deliver grain demanded by the Russians under the Treaty, that in itself was surely not an indication of anti-Soviet sentiment. By a similar process of faulty reasoning, Kuniholm himself might be labeled anti-Soviet, just because in the passive role of interpreter he had echoed Vivian's views on wheat. But that would be ridiculous. Kuniholm had time and again expressed to me his admiration for the Russians in their great struggle, and had stressed the importance of all-out aid to Russia. But the Soviets must appreciate that it is in their own very interest to assure the food supply of the province, in order to avoid famine and its attendant disorders, which, if they occurred, would certainly play in the hands of enemy propaganda. I added that if only all interested parties would whole-heartedly cooperate in solving the food supply problem in Azerbaijan, there would be more than enough to go around for everyone. . . .

General Mugadam then went on to complain, as had the Minister of Food, that Russian commission agents were buying up all available food supplies in Azerbaijan, which of course we have known and reported to you from time to time. Meat, vegetables, cheese and dried fruits have been shipped across the Soviet frontier in sealed cars, which Marzaban, the local Director of Customs says he has been powerless to prevent. The resulting scarcity of food has sent the cost of living sky-high. Meat, for example, has doubled in price, just since Kuniholm's departure some three weeks ago. I have also heard that a certain amount of wheat outside the Grain Treaty has been slipping across the frontier, although Urquhart (British Consul) says he has no definite information confirming this. The Soviets, of course, tell quite a different story, in an effort to play up the food situation here to their advantage. When Marchenko came to me after Vivian's departure to clear the Soviets of complicity in the plot against him, he simultaneously insinuated that the British must bear much blame for the grain shortage which had developed in Azerbaijan. It is true, he said, that perhaps 2,000 tons of contraband wheat had gone to Turkey, but another 5,000 tons had been smuggled out of the province to Iraq and 20,000 tons to Tehran, without any interference whatsoever from the British authorities, who were in control in those regions. It is interesting to recall that at the end of last year there were reports that contraband rugs were being shipped from Azerbaijan to Iraq, whence they were finding their way through Turkey to Germany, where it was said they were being unraveled for the wool. At the time, Urquhart said that their people in Iraq knew of this traffic and had the matter well in hand. As to the 20,000 tons of wheat to Tehran, he smiled and said the Soviets were evidently engaging in astronomy and not mathematics; that the very maximum which might have slipped through was 5,000 tons.

I heard nothing more from Urquhart on the subject until yesterday, when he called with an excerpt from a note which Maisky had sent Eden some time in February. In it, the Soviet Ambassador discussed the very problem of food supply in Iran, and specifically Azerbaijan. Here again appeared the same 20,000 figure, with the rather blunt comment that it was evident the Allies should strive for greater cooperation in solving the food question here. (As though we have had any cooperation from the Soviets!). Furthermore, Maisky called attention to the 30,000 or more Poles in Tehran, who were eating up valuable supplies. The note went on to say that it was erroneous to assume that Azerbaijan in the past had been the principal source of wheat for Tehran, because Soviet investigations had revealed that the city actually obtained 30,000-40,000 tons annually from central and western Iran. This statement fits in well with the Soviet propaganda in Tabriz, which has been responsible for widely circulated reports, that if there is starvation in the British zone of occupation, it is only because the British are burning large food supplies in the southern and central sections of the country. The Soviets, on the other hand, have always defended the interests of the population under their protection. The British would have drained Azerbaijan of its entire wheat supply, if the Russians had not intervened and actually turned back trucks on their way to Tehran.

> That's the story the Soviets have been handing out to the merchants in the Bazaar, much as ward politicians distribute cigars at election time. But they have gone further than that in their campaign against the British. They now say that it is the Indian convoy drivers from the south, who have brought the typhus to Tabriz.

In the summer of 1943, the situation had greatly deteriorated following disorders in the southern tribal regions. In contrast, the situation in Azerbaijan remained relatively calm, despite the bread shortage. Samuel G. Ebling, US Consul in Tabriz, on July 15, 1943 (Report No. 44, 891.00/2038):

> The ability of the Governor General to restrain destructive criticism has influenced the tone of the local press which in general has maintained a sympathetic attitude toward the difficulties of the administrative officials. In comparison with other parts of Iran, there seems to be order and tranquility in Azerbaijan. It is difficult to attribute this apparent complacency to the real contentment of the people. In other words it might be said that the people through their fear of the present administration have limited to a minimum their complaints against unsatisfactory conditions. The adherents of the Governor General also emphasize his ability to find a mode of operation with the occupying Soviet forces. A certain apprehension has been manifested by responsible residents as to the problems of administration in case of removal of the present Governor General. . . . On July 12, 1943, a crowd of about 200 persons assembled at the Municipal Building to complain about the reduction to 200 grams in the daily bread ration. On that day the people were unable to buy bread, as flour had not been delivered to the bakeries. Governor Ahmadi, at present in charge of the Administration of the province during the absence of the Governor General, endeavored to explain to the crowd that the supply of flour would shortly be made available to the bakeries. The Governor, being mistaken for Director Gahramani of the Supply Department, was attacked and manhandled so that he was forced to withdraw to his offices. The crowd later proceeded to the Supply Department but was unable to located Director Gahramani. Upon the arrival of the police and military officers, the crowd dispersed. In the afternoon flour was delivered to the bakeries and the agitation ceased. This demonstration was far from convincing and older residents allege that such disorders only occur when instigated by outside elements. It is alleged that the present incident was instigated to show the urgent need of the absent Governor General to return to Tabriz for the maintenance of order.

Ebling on July 24, 1943 (Dispatch 45, 891.00/2039):

> Continued observation of Soviet officials stationed in Azerbaijan fails to disclose any definite activities which would indicate the determination of the Soviet Union to remain in permanent occupation of Northern Iran after the cessation of hostilities. . . . During recent weeks it has been noticed that Soviet officials take particular pains to emphasize that they have no desire to interfere in the internal administration of the province. . . . In this connection attention is invited to the incident which occurred on July 12, 1943, when a crowd of about 250 persons staged a demonstration in connection with the reduction in the daily bread ration. This latter demonstration was also apparently arranged in order to illustrate the great service which the Governor General is capable of rendering with respect to the maintenance of public security. The price of wheat is now rials 12,000 ($375.00) per metric ton. The announcement was made at Tehran that the Ministry of Food has been abolished and transferred as a Division in Dr. Millspaugh's organization in the Ministry of Finance. . . . Regarding the harvest, which will begin within the next few weeks, the present plan of the Governor General provides that 80,000 tons of wheat will be collected from individual landowners, as agreed. The collection of wheat from each village will be established according to the last census of 1939. The Ministry of Finance has abandoned the practice of sending agents through the province to assess the amount of wheat which can be collected from the different villages.

Shortly after, the Iranian government had recalled the Governor General, Soviet displeasure notwithstanding. Dreyfus on September 17, 1943 (Dispatch 675, 891.00/2053):

> I have the honor to report the following information, furnished to me in the strictest confidence by the Prime Minister, regarding the recall of the Governor General of Azerbaijan, General Hassan Mugadam. . . . The Prime Minister told me that the Soviet Chargé had asked him not to take any further action to bring about Mugadam's departure from Tabriz until the Soviet Government has had an opportunity to instruct the Embassy in Tehran in the matter.

Looming Fall Crisis

The wheat situation in Azerbaijan, similar to the rest of Iran, remained precarious, even at harvest time. Consul Richard Ford from Tabriz on

August 11, 1943 (Dispatch 3, 891.00/2047):

> The government granary in Tabriz is reported to be fresh out of wheat, and thus local bakeries are having to find their own grain. This has created something of a local shortage in this district, but thus far there has been no rioting. It is reported that no improvement in the situation may be expected until grain from the new crop starts arriving.

Ford on August 23, 1943 (Dispatch 7, 891.00/2048):

> The current condition of the grain harvest, with its inevitable bearing on the general political situation, appeared until Friday, August 20th, to offer excellent prospects for a more than average yield. However, a severe electrical storm, accompanied by a heavy precipitation of hail and rain, struck the Tabriz district Friday afternoon and has been followed since by other heavy unseasonal rains, and while early reports indicate that the storms have not been widespread, some damage has undoubtedly occurred in this immediate vicinity. Much of the grain in this area has of course been gathered, but a considerable portion of this was still on primitive threshing floors, and thus the unexpected rainfall might well have soaked most of this beyond recovery. Thus far no estimate is available as to what total losses may be, or even whether they will reduce to any appreciable extent the total grain yield of Azerbaijan. However, as is inevitable, various gloomy forecasts are being heard in this community due to the storms, most of them predicting darkly that the grain situation, so rosy a few days ago, has now taken quite a different complexion.
>
> During the past three or four days delegations of bread-shy citizens have waited on the Governor General, both at his home and at his office, demanding relief from the current bread shortage and also the increased cost of this highly essential commodity. The Governor General has handled the situation by (1) rebuking the people for their undignified action in invading the privacy of an Iranian government official's home, and (2) instructing the gendarmerie guarding his office to make sure that no undue gathering of people is permitted to congregate in or near the government offices. The announced increase in the price bread, is to take effect August 24, 1943, (Shahrivar 1, 1322), amounts to one rial (about 3 cents) a kilo, and considerable murmuring about this is being heard locally. The people say of course that in the midst of one of the largest harvests ever realized in Azerbaijan the idea of increasing prices and rationing bread may only be attrib-

> uted to government trickery, and they appear determined to resist such action. However, except for the above-mentioned delegations, consisting generally of 40 or 50 hungry men, women, and children, no action has been taken by the people to implement their determination. . . . Not a few accusations in connection with the general food situation in this general area are being aimed at the Russian military occupation. It is claimed repeatedly that these troops are making serious inroads on the food supplies in Azerbaijan, including cereals, meat, fruit, vegetables, etc., and that furthermore the Soviets have been directly responsible for the fantastic increases in the prices of fire-wood in this district. Finally, it is claimed that the unusually large consumption of water, over and above normal uses, is an indication of the increased numbers of Russian soldiers now quartered in this area, while some complaint has been heard that the Soviet action in buying up large numbers of horses for their military activities both here and in Russia has created an acute local shortage in the supply of work animals available for agricultural purposes. The Soviet action in reminding Iran that she still owes her northern neighbor 10,000 tons of wheat from last year also has been unfavorably commented upon here.

The grim outlook in Azerbaijan is described by Ford in a report dated September 2, 1943, and entitled, "Tabriz Faces Bread and Fuel Famine" (Dispatch 15, 891.5018/28):

> I have the honor to report that careful inquiries in this community indicate beyond any doubt that Tabriz is headed for an extremely bad winter and that under the present regime of corruption and complete lack of management the scenes of 1919, when according to reliable residents then living here carts went through the streets each morning collecting scores of human corpses from doorways and gutters, will probably be repeated here this winter, particularly should it prove to be a typical sub-zero Tabriz winter. In fact, the indications of an approaching famine are said to be far more apparent today than they were during that grisly period twenty four years ago. Although fully a month has elapsed during which the government's so-called grain collection service should have been in operation throughout Azerbaijan, the 16,000 ton government grain elevator in Tabriz remains virtually empty. One authoritative source reports that this winter storage warehouse at present contains some twenty tons of wheat. The normal daily wheat requirements of the city of Tabriz are between 60 and 63 tons, although because of current alleged shortages this quantity has recently been reduced to around 50 tons per day. It is thus all too tragically

apparent that to date this city has been living on an almost hand-to-mouth basis and that little if any provision has been or is being made for the winter months ahead. And already a good four or five weeks have been lost during which the normal collections of grain might have been made, while there remains at most another two to three months in which to effect these collections. Between the first and the middle of December the dirt roads and camel trails connecting outlying villages with larger centers of secondary collection are rendered impassable by weather conditions, and they may remain so until the following spring.

The fault is reported to lie, first, with the Government's failure to provide the necessary transportation serving these remote centers of collection to supplement the local limited means of transport, and second, with the unlawful practices of local officials and village proprietors in utilizing these existing means of transport for their own nefarious ends; namely, for illegally bringing grain to Tabriz for private or black-market sale either to local buyers or to purchasers for markets outside of Azerbaijan. In a town such as Maragheh, for example, it is estimated that from 15 to 20 government trucks are needed during the height of the grain harvesting season to augment local means of transport in relaying the grain of surrounding villages from its temporary storage in Maragheh and vicinity to Tabriz. A similar if not greater need exists in the important grain producing region of which Ardebil is the center, while other points of secondary collection must also be considered. Altogether a total of around one hundred additional trucks is estimated as being the minimum requirement adequately to meet or to have met the situation. Thus far these trucks, although long since requested, have not been supplied, or the ones supplied have all too often been put to private use of the corruption which is officialdom in Azerbaijan. One dependable informant states that there are at present in the Tabriz vicinity 25 government trucks and another 40 on lease engaged in bringing grain to this city, but that their combined capacity is no more than sufficient to keep this city's daily needs supplied, and that an additional hundred trucks are essential at least during the next two months if any surplus wheat for winter consumption is to be brought from outlying points. This informant further stated that due to the heavy purchases of farm animals, including horses, donkeys and oxen, by the Soviets the movement of farm produce from the villages themselves had been gravely disrupted and that in some localities as much as 90 percent of the animals used in this initial step in the transport of grain from villages to nearby towns and hence to Tabriz had been irretrievably lost.

At the present time just at the close of a plentiful harvest, the bread ration in Tabriz, ostensibly 400 grams per person per day, actually ranges from 200 to 350 grams per person, the lower figure being the more frequent than the higher one. And, to reiterate, this reduced ration is being supplied by newly harvested grain deliveries made from day to day, with nothing being set aside for the rapidly approaching winter months. The quality of the bread being supplied the Tabrizi is something else again, although to complete the sorry picture it is somewhat revolting to note that, according to the Director of the Government grain elevator in Tabriz, whereas the 94 bakers in this city are each day supplied a total of about 50 tons of flour, their customary practice is to sell at least half of their respective portions on the black market and then to mix barley, hay, straw, dirt and rather more unspeakable ingredients with the remainder which is used in making bread for the people. The Government sells the flour to the bakers at 200 tomans a ton and they are able to sell it on the black market for around 600 tomans a ton, which insures them a very nice profit and satisfies the shrunken bellies of their customers with straw.

The Fuel Situation. This dangerous situation is said to have no basis in official corruption or in the profiteers' cupidity. It appears to be attributable instead to the enormously increased prices of all types of fuel in this community due in large part no doubt to the decreased purchasing power of the rial, or rather of the tomans, since rials have virtually ceased to have any significance here as a medium of exchange, although incomes unfortunately are still figured on a rial basis. Some reports suggest, probably with considerable accuracy, that the increase in local consuming power resulting from the Russian military occupation is an important contributory factor in the current fuel shortage and high prices. Be that as it may, it is a hard cold fact that the price of fire wood in Tabriz has increased from 30 tomans per kharvar (about 1000 pounds) to 70 tomans, with the trend still upward. (The toman at present is worth about 31 cents US). Charcoal, the common people's fuel when they can't get wood, is at present selling for 250 tomans per kharvar with predictions being freely made that this will be nearer 500 tomans with the advent of cold weather. The local type of coal, which contains more dirt and stones than combustible material, is at present priced at 20 tomans a kharvar. Coal of better quality from Maragheh, which incidentally is virtually unobtainable because there is no cheap way to get it to Tabriz, is presently priced at 75 tomans per kharvar, which automatically places it out of reach of fully ninety-five percent of the inhabitants of this city. The foregoing prices in a community in which the average wage earner's income is probably not much more

> than two tomans a day (which with the usual five mouths to feed and five emaciated bodies to clothe and keep warm works out at about four rials per day per person) requires no further comment in proving that they spell disaster for a people faced with a normal Tabriz winter when the temperature hovers around zero Fahrenheit for weeks on end.
>
> This information is for background purposes only, since the conditions outlined unavoidably have grave political repercussions locally during the coming winter. There is probably little if anything to be done about the situation, since even if the Iran government could be induced to act in relieving the people of Azerbaijan, the unspeakably crooked nature of the officials and wealthy groups of this province would undoubtedly nullify any beneficial action which might be undertaken.

A Combined Intelligence Centre Iraq (CICI, a British agency) report, September 18, 1943, reads (MID-Iran, 4220):

> There is no reported change in the general economic situation in Iran during the week. The grain collection program is proceeding, but not very successfully. In Teheran, the wheat stocks are falling to a dangerous level; in Azerbaijan, food prices have risen to a level which puts them beyond the means of the very poor; wood and charcoal have also sky-rocketed in price.

Ford on September 21, 1943 (Dispatch 22 and enclosure, 891.5018/29):

> I have the honor to refer to my despatch No. 15 dated September 2, 1943, regarding the failure of local officials to inaugurate grain deliveries to the Tabriz elevator in preparation for the winter needs of this community, and to transmit herewith a translation of an editorial bearing upon this subject which appeared in the September 17th issue of the Tabriz newspaper *Shahin*. The reference to the generosity of the Allies and particularly of the Soviets in connection with the wheat needs of Iran and especially of Azerbaijan is perhaps the most significant point in this editorial comment. The editorial statement and interrogations relative to the continued failure of the competent authorities to make provision for winter wheat storage in Tabriz do not appear to be wholly borne out by the facts. A reliable informant who is connected with the Tabriz grain elevator advised me today that, whereas the situation was extremely serious up until a fortnight ago, during the past ten or twelve days wheat had started flowing into Tabriz at the rate of between seventy and a hundred tons daily. He explained that while between fifty

and sixty tons of this are distributed each day to local bakers to meet the city's current needs, the balance is being placed in the grain elevator for the winter, and that this winter storage now totaled some 500 tons, largely representing deliveries received during the past ten days.

The *Shahin* editorial of September 17, 1943, reads:

The provisioning of this city is going to be very critical when the roads are blocked with snow. There is no news of the trucks promised by the Government to provision the city. The representatives who had gone from this city to supervise and make sure of the 24,000 tons of wheat which was allotted to Tabriz have returned and have stated plainly that with the present difficulties and obstacles being placed in their way there is no hope of their being able to perform their duties, and they see worse conditions in this city than prevailed last year. In view of the above we ask the Government authorities and responsible officials of the Department of Provision what the unfortunate people are going to do? How are they to live during the six or seven months when the roads are blocked by snow? Although Azerbaijan produced enough food for two years, are we again to endure a famine? Where is the difficulty, and why are the unfortunate people not told of it? Are you again, as last year, going to attribute your own carelessness and negligence to the Allies, the Allies who are bringing us wheat from other parts of the world? Are you again going to say that the Russians are taking our wheat away from us? These same Russians, although they need it themselves, have supplied 32,000 tons of wheat to Tabriz, Tehran and Khorasan, and thereby saved us from famine. Of this debt of 32,000 tons, we have repaid the Russians only 11,000 tons of barley and wheat, and this in order that we ourselves should not encounter difficulties and embarrassment. Even the 50 trucks which were especially designated by the Iranian Government to be used in returning to the Russians the debt of grain which we owe them have been placed at our disposal by the Russians to help us get our wheat to Tabriz.

The deplorable conditions in Azerbaijan are further described by Ford in a report of October 2, 1943. Of course, conditions were far worse in the less favored regions of Iran (Dispatch 24 and enclosure, 891.00/2063):

Society in Azerbaijan, instead of being divided roughly into an upper, middle, and a lower class, is separated very sharply into two groups; namely, the affluent and the destitute. The former, from the baker, the butcher and the bazaar owner, on through the minor government official, and up to the governor general himself, appear to be in a constant process by hook or crook of becoming yet more affluent. The latter have nothing, and under the economic system in which they exist, are not likely to get anything. . . . The conditions under which a considerable proportion of the population must live in a town such as Tabriz, capital of Azerbaijan and second largest city in Iran, are indescribably bad. The antiquated drainage system of Iranian towns is of course proverbial. It is sufficient to note that its open nature permits it to serve simultaneously as both a fresh water supply and a sewage outlet. The congested residential districts of this town are built somewhat after the disorder of very insanitary rabbit warrens, being composed almost entirely of one-story mud houses and hovels. Their furnishings are scant, neither heat nor water is provided, the only water, running or still, is of course in the open drain in the street, although in some sections this water supply dries up completely during certain months of the summer season. In these humble homes families of five to fifteen or more somehow live. During the long cold winters the larger families are probably more comfortable.

The clothing of this destitute group is more in the nature of rags and tatters than whole garments. Some of the costumes in fact are really masterpieces of patches, the patches frequently having completely devoured the original garment and themselves being in process of devourment by yet more patches. Many of the younger children wear few if any clothes at all, particularly from the waist down. Moreover, these costumes, or the lack of them, are frequently worn the year round, whether it be during the hot summer or the zero weather of winter. In this connection it is stated that the custom, particularly among the poorer women, of continuing to wear veils in spite of government edicts to the contrary, is more to their desire to cover their rags than to religious convictions.

The chief food of these people is bread. It comes not in the form of loaves but in long pliant sheets and strips, generally about a yard long, not quite half that wide, and as thick possibly as a damp waffle. It is brown in color, coarse in texture, rather gritty to eat, and while its base is wheat flour it variously contains other ingredients of questionable wholesomeness. It is baked briefly on beds of hot pebbles in privately owned bakeries throughout the province, there being 94 of these establishments in Tabriz alone. During the Azerbaijan summer of good weather and lush production, this bread is supplemented by a wide variety of fairly cheap fruits and vegetables and, when available, small quantities of rice and other staples, although meats, eggs and butter are rather out of the financial reach of many of these people. A limited quantity of milk is kept inside goats and sheep tethered along the sidewalks of many city streets. In general, however, and particularly for year-long consideration, a portion of a sheet of bread, washed down by a little drain water, constitutes most of the food intake of most city dwellers during any given period of twenty four hours. When there is a shortage of flour, as frequently happens, and the daily ration must be cut, quite a number of the poorer people remain hungry. As a footnote to this condition: I was particularly struck during the first days and nights of my residence in Tabriz by the number of screaming infants who seemed to inhabit the mud houses surrounding the consulate's compound, and I concluded that Iranian parents must be very cruel to their children. Closer inquiry, however, developed the probability that many of these cries were merely hungry cries emanating from homes where the day's bread supply had not stretched quite all the way around the family circle.

One is rarely out of sight or smell of insanitation in the cities and towns of Azerbaijan. However, it is difficult to describe and impossible to cite figures which might prove the actual conditions which exist here. An American medical missionary who has lived in this neighborhood for well over a quarter of a century and who is at the head of the American Presbyterian hospital in Tabriz, states that he has never seen any published statistics regarding the health conditions in the province. In this connection, he reports that some years ago, chiefly for his own interest and information, he undertook to compile some informal figures covering infant mortality in Tabriz, his method being to question the mothers who came to him for medical treatment and advice. He states that his conclusions based on data obtained over a considerable period indicated that from sixty to sixty five out of every hundred babies born in this city die before their fourth or fifth year. He of course disclaims any accuracy for his findings, and stresses their informal, inconclusive nature. He adds, however, that if this percentage of deaths or anything approximating it occurs before the fifth year, it is reasonable to suppose that another fifteen or twenty of the original hundred babies die before their tenth year. This same informant reports that at present, of the three hospitals in Tabriz with its 200,000 souls, the American mission hospital is the only one in full operation, one being unable to accept any in-patients at all because of lack funds and the other undertaking only a limited service for well-to-do-patients.

No object would be served in detailing the dirt, filth and squalor in which most of the poorer classes of this province must exist throughout their lives. Such conditions, of course, are not peculiar to Azerbaijan, and in fact it is probable that the situation here is, if anything, better than in other parts of Iran and possibly the average Middle Eastern community. Certainly, the summer months in this region, with their deodorant and disinfectant of hot sunshine and their comparatively abundant production of food, are not too bad. It is when winter comes that not only is spring far behind but real suffering dwells in the homes of these people. The winter just now approaching promises to be especially bad since the prices of all fuels have recently advanced to unprecedented levels.

Letter dated October 30, 1943, from G.L. McKinney, an American missionary in Tabriz, to L. McKinney, Wingate, Indiana (MID-Iran, 5070):

When war started inflation came to Iran. Also she has been drained of vast quantities of needed staples. Living cost has risen over 500%. When I returned from furlough six years ago 1000 lb. of wood for fuel was 80 rials, now it is 700 rials. A meter of calico 2 rials, now 70 rials. Food prices also go continually higher. How the really poor exist I know not. We pray for a mild winter. Fuel a prohibitive price for the poor. . . .

Conditions in Khorassan

Letter, December 27, 1942, from Patman, AIOC, Shahrud, to Miss M. Moss, Ivy House Farm, Pilley Village, Barnsley, Yorkshire, England (MID-Iran, 5970):

Things have become very bad in the country. There are serious shortages of essential bread supplies, not because there is no wheat, there is plenty, but it is locked up in the stores of the rich people. The local Government is incapable of dealing with the situation, because if they made any restriction or brought in any measure against the hoarders of wheat, they would be condemning themselves, because the members of parliament are the worst offenders. Consequently the poor people are starving whilst prices soar. Serious riots have broken out in Teheran and all the principal shops were looted, and order was only restored by our troops occupying the city. A strict military curfew is now in force. . . . It is these rich people who are pro-Nazi and cause us

> trouble. . . . Many of the better class of Iranians have expressed the hope that we never leave the country and that it becomes a mandate or even colony.

An OSS report, December 28, 1942, on road conditions between Birjand and Duhak, distance of 123 miles in eastern Iran, gives the following (MID-Iran, 4610): "No supplies of food are obtainable. Water is unobtainable except from hauzes. Wood from neighboring hills can be collected with difficulty. No gasoline is available." Letter from Mashad to New York, January 14, 1943:

> This trip I spoke of was taken with the Manager of the Oil Company, an inspection tour to three cities to the Southwest of here. Transport from Shahrud, the rail head, is so scarce that stocks cannot be brought here, and from here distributed to these outlying places, so that in many of these places it is being rationed. And here, where stocks are low, it is being sold to retail merchants who in turn sell it at very high prices. So there is much unrest in the city. Prices of foodstuffs have doubled, trebled, and quadrupled in some instances. Imported things are of course out of sight. . . . Drugs are almost prohibitive in prices, and we should have to stop dispensing altogether if we depended on the open market. All prices have gone up from 300 to 800 per cent..."

Mrs. Skrine, wife of the British Consul in Mashad, blamed the Iranian Government in a letter of June 5, 1943:

> We know that the military occupation superintend posts, railways and such like, but leave the administration to the Persian officials, and from top to bottom there is corruption, graft and dishonesty. Food, fuel and all necessities are in the hands of "rings" co-operating one with another. There is no social sense or public opinion and laws are not enforced, because the police are the biggest racketeers.

Not even the wife of the British Consul was immune from censorship.

Report by Richard Lowe of the OSS, dated July 23, 1943 (Report No. 38, 891.00/2034–1/2):

> The harvest of wheat and barley all the way from Tehran to Meshed is one of the best for several years. Threshing is now in progress. Reports from other grain-producing sections of the country show similar excellent crops. A relatively small number of government trucks, say

30, were seen on the Tehran-Meshed road. If the government can collect and keep the harvest, the days of inedible bread should be over. However, the government's trucking facilities are still very limited and the railroad continues firmly in Allied hands. The attitude of the Allies toward the bumper grain harvest is also not yet apparent. It is probable that this year, as last, part of the crop will be taken by the Russians and the British, though there is a possibility that this year it may be done through the Iranian authorities, thus supporting the government's attempts to enforce a strict monopoly of grains. Some smuggling to Turkey and Iraq is also probable, because of the continued weakness of the government on the frontiers. . . . From the Persian point of view, it is therefore important to keep the grain surplus in the country. Gasoline at Meshed costs 75 rials or $2.25 for a five gallon tin.

The daily wage of an ordinary laborer in the Meshed area has risen during the last three years from 3 rials a day to 12 to 15 rials. Merchants and artisans have raised their prices accordingly; any landowner or cultivator with surplus crop is not disturbed by the rising costs. Although he is legally bound to sell his surplus to the government, he, in practice, bribes the officials, keeps back a portion of his surplus and sells it in the black market. The black market price for wheat in the Meshed area is now between 5000 to 6000 rials a ton ($150 to $200) as against 2100 rials at this time last year. A 1 pound tin of Borden's Klim sells in Meshed for $6.60; a similar tin of Quaker Oats sells for $3.00; a 12 oz. tin of Armour's corned beef sells for a dollar. Four brothers in Nishapur made from their wheat crop last year a profit of $300,000 which is just sitting in the bank. Those who are making money here are making so much that for them, money has lost its value. The group between millstones consists of people unable to work, unable to secure steady work, or living, like all government officials, on a fixed income. It is this class, though largely powerless, which would welcome any governmental or social changes.

Letter dated August 7, 1943, from R.E. Hoffman, American Hospital, Mashad, to Mary E. Hoffman, R.F.D., Leipsic, Ohio (MID-Iran, 5970):

This country has gotten into a bad condition, with food exploiters and hoarders; prices are higher than we ever saw, and still rising. The Board has given all workers in Iran an increased salary allowance, and we have really more than doubled the wages of hospital workers; but

> even at that it takes all we can scrape for food and fuel. Fire wood is ten times the price of 4 or 5 years ago; bread more than ten times as much, meat 6 or 8 times as much, etc. There was a big crop last year; and we have had so much rain this winter and spring that crops should be very large this year also. But whether food is being shipped out of the country, or just hoarded, we have no means of knowing. But thank God we have enough to eat, and our clothes will last pretty well a couple of years more at least. Of course there are plenty of sick folks, the many of them are half starved or worse; and the hospital is full at the time.

OSS report by Lowe on his trip to Mashad during October 26 to November 10, 1943 (Report 74, 891.00/2091):

> According to the American Mission doctors in Meshed, there is a large increase this year in the number of sick people and several cases of typhus have already appeared. The explanation is general under-nourishment and exposure last year to the cold. The doctors anticipate a large number of deaths in the area this winter due to the fact that the large majority of the people cannot afford to buy either adequate food or clothing; nor can they buy fuel. The result will be overcrowding and the spread of disease. The explanation for the high price of fuel is the lack of transportation and heavy Russian purchases of wood for cooking and heating purposes of their troops in the area. The high price of food is partly attributed to large Russian purchases, though the countrywide increase of prices also plays a large role. It is reliably reported that in the region of Quchan the Russians purchased during a period of six months, ending six months ago, 70,000 head of mutton, 8000 head of cattle and 700 horses.

CICI report, January 4, 1944 (MID-Iran, 5070): "With the arrival of winter the cost of living in Meshed has increased. Piece-goods are scarce and Russian purchases have pushed up the prices of animal products."

Chapter 21

Allied Failure to Deliver Wheat on Time

From the beginning, the program to ship wheat to Iran under the Tripartite Declaration of December 4, 1942, was on shaky ground. With an agreement in sight, on November 19, 1942, Secretary of State Cordell Hull had written to the Chairman of the Joint Chiefs of Staff. A similar letter had been sent by Assistant Secretary Dean Acheson to the War Shipping Administration (WSA). Hull's letter (891.24/280):

> As you may be aware, there has arisen in Iran during the past few weeks an acute political and economic situation, largely caused by a serious shortage of grain. Because of the food shortage, and generally unsatisfactory economic conditions, the Iranian Majlis (parliament) has been reluctant to make available Iranian currency needed for operations of United Nations troops, and even more serious difficulties have appeared to threaten the Anglo-American position in Iran. The Department of State, the British Foreign Office at London, and the British and American Ministers at Tehran have been endeavoring to work out a solution to this problem, and it has now been agreed that the American and British Governments shall undertake, under certain conditions, to make up any deficit in the domestic Iranian grain supplies which may be found to exist prior to the gathering of the 1943 harvest. These Governments will also undertake to provide transport for the movement of grain from surplus areas in Iran to the deficit areas in that country. A copy of the agreement, which it is hoped will be signed and made public within a few days, is attached herewith. Apart from the undertaking explained in the agreement, the British Government is endeavoring to arrange for the early shipment to Iran of 20,000 tons of

wheat as a replacement for an equivalent quantity of Iranian grain reported to have been purchased by the Soviet Government. The Department of State has given its approval to this shipment, which is expected to be made as follows: 5,000 tons during the month of November, 5,000 tons during the month of December, and the remaining 10,000 tons as soon as possible thereafter.

In this connection, the Foreign Office has stated that the despatch to Iran at this time of 20,000 tons of wheat will necessitate a corresponding reduction in other commodities programmed for shipment to the Persian Gulf and forwarding overland through Iran. Mr. Eden has informed the Soviet Ambassador at London that shipments to Russia via Iran will necessarily be reduced, and the appropriate British authorities are also being advised of the situation. The Foreign Office has requested that the Department do likewise in Washington. Accordingly, it would be appreciated if you would take the matter under consideration and inform all interested agencies in this country, such as the Office of Lend-Lease Administration and the War Shipping Administration. I should like to emphasize that, in all probability, additional wheat shipments to Iran will be necessary during the coming year, if famine conditions in that country are to be avoided. I assume that such later shipments will also necessitate a revision of shipping programs for other commodities, in the light of available shipping space and the capacity of Persian Gulf ports and the Iranian transport system. Consequently, it is hoped that the Joint Chiefs of Staff and other interested agencies will keep this factor in mind.

By way of background, I should explain that grain, wheat and barley, is the staple foodstuff of the Iranian people. For this reason, an adequate supply of grain for the people has always been the touchstone of success for any Iranian Government. It is significant that upon his recent accession to power, the present Prime Minister publicly declared that if he could assure the provision of bread to the public, all other problems would solve themselves. His relative lack of success in this undertaking, which has been signalized by recent bread riots in Iran, has resulted in weakening the position of the cabinet to a point at which its fall is threatened. The Department of State feels that the United Nations should do everything possible, consistent with their urgent military needs, to see that the minimum food requirements of the Iranian people during the current crop year are fulfilled. The considerations which have led the Department to adopt this position may be summarized as follows:

(1) This Government has proclaimed that a power which is in occupation of the territory of another is responsible for the well-being of the population of the occupied country. We are, therefore, morally bound to apply this principle to those countries which we or our associates have been forced to occupy as well as to the territories occupied by the enemy. (2) This Government, and all of the United Nations, are vitally interested in the maintenance of the supply route to Russia through Iran and in the possible future use of Iran as a base for defensive or offensive operations against the enemy in the Middle East. It has seemed to this Department, and officers of the War Department have concurred, that the achievement of these objectives would be immensely complicated, if not entirely defeated, if our technical and combat forces in Iran should be confronted with a starving and rebellious population. This consideration, in our view, gains added force from the fact that about one-fourth of the population of Iran is composed of nomadic tribes whose preferred occupation until a few years ago consisted of preying upon transport routes and settled communities. Many of these tribes have recently resumed these activities, with the result that already some highways have become unsafe, or even temporarily closed from time to time. (3) It is highly probable that a real failure of the bread supply would result in the collapse of the Iranian Government, and that the United Nations would then be forced to proceed to military occupation of the entire country and establishment of a puppet government at Tehran. It is superfluous to point out that this would necessitate diversion of troops from the fighting fronts. It would also have unfortunate repercussions in the other Moslem nations and territories. Very truly yours, Cordell Hull.

Also on November 19, 1942, the Persian Gulf Service Command had expressed anxiety (Memorandum, 891.24/416):

Colonel Graham, who is a member of the Staff of the Persian Gulf Service Command, and Lieutenant Snyder (Iranian desk, G-2), called to discuss the food situation in Iran. Colonel Graham said that G-2 and General Connolly, head of PGSC, were very much concerned about this matter. One palliative which they had in mind was to pay in food part of the wages of the Iranian laborers whom they planned to employ. Ultimately these employees would probably total some 25,000, but for the present their number would be much smaller. The food required would be stowed on vessels carrying other supplies for the PGSC. I agreed that this measure seemed sound, but that it only scratched the surface of the problem. Colonel Graham and Lieutenant

> Snyder said that they entirely understood this. I showed them a copy of the communication which we were addressing to the Joint Chiefs of Staff and the War Shipping Administration regarding shipment of wheat to Iran, and Lieutenant Snyder said that the point of view and reasoning set forth in that letter were completely in accord with the views of G-2. He and Colonel Graham felt, however, that further concrete action should be taken at an early date in order to ensure that whatever wheat shipments might be necessary would arrive in time. . . . I pointed out that a cardinal factor in getting the desired action would be War Department support, and I hoped that G-2 would be able to convince Operations Division and General Somervell's S.O.S. of the soundness of our views. Lieutenant Snyder said that he would discuss the matter in the War Department and would let me know how things developed. . . . Colonel Graham made the suggestion that one way to get wheat to Iran might be to have a Presidential directive issued requiring that every ship leaving for the Persian Gulf should carry a certain minimum quantity of wheat in bags, say 300 tons. He believed that bagged wheat could easily be stowed in the spaces between other cargo. He recognized that this would mean a certain reduction in other types of shipments, including Lend-Lease goods to Russia and even materials for the PGSC itself, but he felt we must accept this.

Elements in the War Department opposed the plan to ship wheat to Iran. Alling's memorandum of November 24, 1942, to Murray, Acheson, and Welles (Memorandum, 891.24/304-½):

> As you will recall, an officer of the War Department recently urged that immediate steps be taken to prepare for wheat shipments to Iran, in fulfillment of the wheat commitment which the American and British Governments have agreed to make. We have, of course, addressed letters on this subject to the Joint Chiefs of Staff and the War Shipping Administration, but the officer in question, Colonel Graham of the Persian Gulf Service Command, felt that further concrete action should be initiated at once and suggested that a meeting of all interested agencies in Washington be arranged. It was understood that Colonel Graham would take the matter up at the War Department. This Division has now been informed that General McNarney, Deputy Chief of Staff, has ruled that the question is not one in which the War Department should take the initiative, even to the extent of giving an advance expression of its views. However, we have reason to believe that at least some of the appropriate divisions of the War Department do, in fact, take the same view as Colonel Graham, and it would undoubtedly be

of great assistance to the Department in getting action if we could be definitely assured of War Department support, or at least acquiescence, in our efforts to arrange whatever wheat shipment may prove to be necessary. Accordingly, I should like to suggest that Mr. Welles take the first convenient opportunity to broach the matter to General McNarney and ask whether the War Department would be willing to participate in a meeting such as that suggested. An officer of the War Department, who prefers that his name not be used, has expressed the personal opinion that a favorable reply would be forthcoming. General McNarney could be informed that we regard the question as one directly concerning the War Department, since it affects both the security of the Persian Gulf Service Command operations and the quantity and timing of shipments to Russia and to British and American armed forces in the Persian Gulf supply area. Barring an unexpected improvement in the shipping situation, wheat shipments to Iran can only be made at the expense of some other type of cargo, which in practice will probably mean that military shipments of some kind (American British or Russian) will have to be reduced. This Division feels that the War Department should understand this from the outset, and that it should also understand that failure to provide necessary wheat for the Iranian people might very well produce a disastrous situation which would be much worse in its result than a temporary reduction in certain military shipments. If it should seem desirable to elaborate on this, General McNarney could be shown the attached copy of the Department's letter to the Joint Chiefs of Staff.

The reply from Admiral William D. Leahy, Chairman, Joint Chiefs of Staff, to Secretary Hull, December 8, 1942, was not encouraging (Letter, 891.24/349):

Your letters of November 19th, inviting the attention of the Joint Chiefs of Staff to the critical economic and political situation in Iran, and requesting a monthly estimate of US military expenditures in Iran, are acknowledged. United States troops are in Iran, which is a sphere of British strategic responsibility, for the purpose of insuring an uninterrupted and increased flow of supplies to Russia. This they are doing by developing and operating transportation facilities. The grain shortage in Iran is inopportune because of the scarcity of water transportation. Diversion of United States shipping to meet the critical Iranian requirements can only be accomplished at the expense of sustaining US military operations throughout the world. Our present military commitments require more shipping than is available. The Joint Chiefs of

> Staff fully recognize the importance of Iran as a supply route to Russia. The presence, however, of US noncombatant units in this British area of strategic responsibility does not justify diverting US shipping to provide food for the local population. Security of the Iranian railway is a direct responsibility of the British, and if the feeding of the Iranian population is the condition upon which security of this transportation routes depend, such provision of food, including its shipment, is a British responsibility. It is noted that the British Government has informed the Russian Government that shipments to Russia will be reduced through Iran by the amount of grain supplied to that country. The Joint Chiefs of Staff are most anxious that our Russian commitments are not reduced. It would be helpful if such negotiations as your Department has recently concluded with the United Kingdom and Iran be coordinated with the Joint Chiefs of Staff in advance. This applies to all cases where obligations are to be imposed on this country requiring shipping and strategic materials which may already be committed and counted upon in the furtherance of the efforts of our armed forces in combat areas.

The letter adds that 25,000 American troops were expected to operate the Iranian transportation system. The projected cost for 1943 was $27.6 million, or $2.3 million per month.

On December 10, 1942, Murray had written to Assistant Secretary Berle (Memorandum, 891.00/2001):

> With reference to our telephone conversation last night, I am attaching copies of telegrams which we have gotten off to London and Tehran regarding the highly alarming situation in Iran. We are also drafting a message with specific reference to the arrest by the British of the Governor General of Isfahan, which seems to have come at a most inopportune moment, not to mention the apparently unwarranted and drastic manner in which it was carried out. It is our feeling, however, that no rearrangements of the Government or other political maneuvers will have any real effect upon the situation. The only remedy, so far as we can see, lies in the immediate provision of food supplies which will reassure the Iranian people. As you will recall, we have previously expressed this view and have urged the British Government to take all possible steps in this direction. We were given to understand that the Foreign Office was in agreement and, in consequence, on November 19 the Department addressed a letter to the Joint Chiefs of Staff setting forth the importance of action and requesting that body to take such measures as might be necessary to meet the anticipated deficit in the

Iranian wheat supply. (A copy of that letter is attached.) We have now received a reply, likewise attached, to the effect that the Joint chiefs of Staff are unwilling to take any action and consider that the entire question is a matter for the British authorities to handle. At the same time, it is stated that, whatever may be done, shipments to Russia via Iran must not be reduced. I should like to point out that this last statement in fact means that nothing at all should be done, even by the British, since, according to our information, the capacity of Iranian ports and internal transport will not permit an increase in future grain shipments without a corresponding reduction in other types of cargo handled. In view of the extreme urgency indicated by the latest telegrams from Mr. Dreyfus, I wonder if you would not feel justified in raising the question once more, possibly at the meeting of the Joint Intelligence Committee which it is understood you plan to attend this afternoon? Perhaps it would be well to request that the matter be taken up immediately with the Combined Chiefs of Staff and that they be urged to reallocate to Iranian civilian needs some part of the Allied military grain stocks in the Middle East. It could be pointed out that shipments from this country or from Australia will not arrive in time to meet the present needs, even if agreement is reached on the allocation of the necessary shipping space. I think we would be justified in making this move both because of the importance of the question and because Admiral Leahy's letter specifically states that action is up to the British. The appropriate British agency here would appear to be their representatives on the Combined Chiefs of Staff.

WSA was equally discouraging. L.W. Douglas, Deputy Administrator, to Acheson, December 17, 1942 (Letter, 891.24/348):

I have your letter of November 19 on the shortage of food in Iran and the necessity of supplying wheat for civilian consumption in that country. It is my understanding that the British Government is making arrangements to procure the 20,000 tons of wheat to be moved in replacement for Iranian grain purchased by the Soviet Government and to furnish shipping space for it. You are aware that the limiting factor on shipping to Iran is at the present time and will be for some time to come the capacity of Persian ports and of the inland transportation system, with the result that these and any other shipments to Iran will be at the expense of urgently needed military cargo destined for Russia. I infer from your letter that the Iranian wheat must nevertheless have priority, that the British Government has agreed that it should, and that the Russian Government has been informed of the program. I note your statement that further shipments of wheat will probably be necessary during the forthcoming year in addition to the 20,000 tons referred to above. In view of the essentiality of the Russian cargoes that will be displaced, I trust that the analysis of the Iranian requirements will be severe and that they will be held to a truly irreducible minimum. I know you will understand when I express my hope that in accordance with your usual practice you will consult with us before formulating any firm statement of Iranian requirements for next year. Without this consultation a commitment may be made that cannot be fulfilled easily, if at all.

On January 5, 1943, Alling had written to Dreyfus (Letter, 891.24/325):

Dear Louis: I refer to your various reports on the grain situation in Iran and to the American-British-Iranian agreement signed December 4 by which the British and ourselves are obligated to make up by imports any deficit in Iranian grain supplies which may be ascertained to exist. As you are aware, the Department has supported you throughout in your recommendations that this agreement be concluded and that an initial lot of 25,000 tons of wheat be sent forward as soon as possible. Although things did not go so rapidly as we had hoped, we have at least made the agreement, and shipment of the 25,000 tons of wheat is expected to be completed during January and February. There remains, however, the question of possible further shipments which it may be necessary to make in fulfillment of our undertaking of December 4. The Division feels that this Government must make every effort to live up to its obligations in this respect, and we are prepared to back you to the limit if you and Sheridan determine that the Iranian food supply can only be maintained through additional imports of grain. However, we are faced with no easy task in convincing the various agencies concerned of the importance of the matter. Those who are primarily concerned with the use of shipping space for the supply of our fighting forces, or the transportation of material to Russia, quite naturally feel reluctant to divert ships to feed a noncombatant country such as Iran. To show you what we are up against, I am enclosing a copy of a letter sent by the Department to the Joint Chiefs of Staff and the War Shipping Administration, and copies of replies which we have received. In view of this situation, I hope that it will be possible for you to give us considerable advance warning if further grain shipments become necessary. You should take into consideration not only the time lapse between the departure of a cargo ship from this country and its arrival

> at a Persian Gulf port, but also the probable time consumed in obtaining agreement of the competent agencies to the allocation of the necessary shipping space and priority of movement of the supplies inland upon their arrival at the port of destination. Please also bear in mind the importance of giving us all the information you can which would substantiate your recommendations. From the enclosed letters, you will see that it is not always enough to convince the Department of the desirability of a course of action. It is also necessary that other agencies, with other points of view, should be convinced, and to do this we need plenty of ammunition.

The OSS was convinced of the need to send wheat to Iran. Its report of February 11, 1943, entitled "Food in Iran," states (Research and Analysis, 891.5018/22):

> The situation is still critical. The December 4th agreement now commits the United States and United Kingdom to supplying the cereal deficit. Of the 25,000 tons of wheat promised by the Allies, 5,055 tons went forward from the US in November, another 5,000 in December. It is not clear when they may arrive. Sheridan urges that the remaining 15,000 be sent as soon as possible, saying that 20,000 tons beyond that will doubtless be needed to tide over the country until the 1943 harvest. This is not surprising in view of the considerable amounts used within the country by the Allies and the Polish refugees during the last year. Whether the Allies like it or not—whether they deem it just or unjust—the fact remains that the Iranians believe the Allies have pillaged their land and brought upon them this distress and near famine. The USA, as one of the Allies, inevitably has to share this resentment. It behooves us, therefore, to do everything in our power to counteract it by just, and even generous action. It is impossible to emphasize too much this point. In the first place, no little security and effectiveness of our own task force in the area depends upon the proper solution of this food problem. It is good to hear that this force is to be maintained entirely by shipments from outside Iran. It would contribute to the reception and efficiency of the force if they could at least supply wheat to the Iranian labor they shall need. There is no question but that backing the American Adviser in his efforts to solve this problem of food would help materially in winning the war in this area. The sending of wheat and a small supply of other essential civilian goods with each shipment to American forces would bring them the good-will and cooperation of the populace, free them from any necessity of policing, indirectly aid their own morale, and contribute much to their early

success. Moreover, this is an instance where immediate and long-range policies coincide. Such a policy of feeding Iran and meeting some of her most essential civilian needs would bring dividends later in Iranian good-will and friendliness toward the United States. At the present our prestige is high, and the Iranian government is turning to us for advice and aid in a variety of fields of endeavor. We must make every effort to conserve this position and extend it by assuring the conspicuous success of our advisers.

Iranian Request for Additional Wheat

Dreyfus on December 17, 1942 (Telegram 447, 891.24/326):

> Department's 371, December 14. Sheridan urges in view of seriousness of food situation that the balance come forward as promptly as possible in 5,000 tons lots. A factor not usually taken into consideration is that there is a shortage of seed wheat for spring sowing. As much as possible of the 25,000 tons should, therefore, arrive before spring in order that Iranian wheat can be released for planting. . . . Sheridan states that not a ton of this year's wheat crop has yet come out of Azerbaijan."

On December 23, 1942, Alling had written to Thorold (Letter, 891.24/325):

> I refer to our meeting at the Department on November 17, 1942 and to your recent conversations with Mr. Jernegan regarding the Iranian wheat situation. The Department has now received a telegram, dated December 17, 1942, in which the American Minister at Tehran reports that Mr. J.P. Sheridan, the American Food and Supply Adviser, urges that as yet unshipped balance of the 25,000 tons of wheat being forwarded by your Government be shipped at the earliest possible moment in 5,000 tons lots. . . . You may recall that at our meeting on November 17, 1942, you read us a telegram from Tehran or London indicating that the Soviet Government had agreed to release immediately 7,500 tons of wheat from Azerbaijan for the supply of the city of Tehran. In the telegram we have just received, our Minister advises that, according to Mr. Sheridan, not one ton of this year's wheat crop has as yet left Azerbaijan. It would be appreciated if you would transmit this information to your Government for such consideration and action as may seem appropriate. I need not repeat that the Department is very anxious to see wheat supplies for Iran go forward with minimum possible delay.

On January 6, 1943, Dreyfus had forwarded a cable from Sheridan informing that wheat imports were being "pooled" and consequently the quantity supplied to the Iranian government was only a fraction of the imported wheat (Telegram 12, 891.50A/13):

> I wish to inform you on behalf of Iranian Ministry of Food that I was told yesterday by British Legation and MESC that they intend to pool all wheat imports to Persian Gulf on behalf of (one) Iranian labor employed by Anglo-Iranian Oil Company, (two) workers hired by American and British armies, (three) Iranian civilians. It was intimated to me that all arrivals of the 25,000 tons wheat imported under the Tripartite Agreement will have to be used as well as other British imports for this pooling since Iran Government has been unable to feed Iranian labor and oil company employees. . . . I must point out that present abnormal situation with 70,000 workers taken off the farms creates a burden in furnishing food on works locations. British state arrivals of wheat for military and oil company up to January 15 will amount to 5,685 tons and that stocks at Abadan as of January 1 are 2,074 tons. They estimate total arrivals by March 31 under 25,000 ton program including the above amounts will be only 19,000 tons. British monthly requirements for army and oil company personnel of 3,450 tons will leave only 8,650 tons for Iranian civilian use up to March 31. It is impossible for me to carry on these three months with this amount even with maximum local purchases possible due to total failure of supplies from Azerbaijan caused by bad local organization. I am sending an American Rex Vivian, there as provincial manager to reorganize. For the present (wheat) is either hoarded or sold over the frontier. I have a supply in Tehran today of 60 tons. Against a need tomorrow of 250 tons. Local Iranian army garrison has not been fed since January 1. This week I am opening soup kitchens with an estimated maximum capacity of 50,000 persons daily. 300,000 people in Tehran eat bread alone. I am providing rice and potatoes at same price as bread but fear there may be internal disorders in next few days. . . . I urge immediate shipment of remainder of 25,000 agreed on as well as an emergency shipment from India of 5,000 tons. In addition we presented requests December 28 to both British and American Legations, complete with statistics, for an additional 20,000 tons from the United States.

Dreyfus on January 6, 1943 (Telegram 14, 891.24/371-1/2):

My 12, January 6, 11 a.m. Wheat situation critical. Result of the pooling arrangement described by Sheridan will be that Iranians will obtain for famine areas of Tehran and Southern Iran less than half of the 25,000 tons anticipated. Sheridan has presented to me convincing figures showing that he will have a deficit up to next harvest of 20,000 tons, assuming that all of the 25,000 ton program arrives. I therefore support his request that the 25,000 ton program be expedited and that an additional 20,000 tons be shipped to Iran as soon as possible. It is hoped that this amount will tide country over until next harvest.

State Department reply on January 8, 1943 (Telegram 12, 891.24/371-1/2):

Your 13 and 14, January 6. Please advise whether you have discussed Sheridan's request for additional 20,000 tons wheat with British Minister and whether your recommendation is based upon decision contemplated by Article I of food agreement signed December 4. Does British Minister concur? In order to save shipping space, would be possible to substitute flour for wheat?

Dreyfus replied on January 13, 1943 (Telegram 44, 891.24/352-1/2):

Department's 12, January 8. At wheat meeting last night attended by Sheridan, British Minister and myself following unanimous decision was reached. (1) Iran's shortage of cereals for human consumption up to next harvest will be approximately 23,500 tons. This is in addition to the 25,000 en route of which 2,500 tons must be repaid British army for advances during present period. (2) It was agreed that British and American Governments be requested to make up this deficiency under article one of Tripartite Food Agreement. (3) To save shipping space it was decided to recommend shipment of 7,100 tons of wheat (or flour if additional shipping space be saved) from United States or Canada and 16,400 tons of barley from Iraq, latter to be used as bread adulterant. Iran will also use 10,000 tons of own rice as bread adulterant. Bread henceforth will contain 60% wheat and 40% adulterants. (4) In case part or all of barley is not for any reason forthcoming from Iraq the shortage will be made up by wheat or flour from United States or Canada. Above represents in my opinion careful and conservative estimate of Iran's cereal needs and I recommend Department's approval. British Minister is recommending his government's approval and is taking steps to endeavor to obtain the barley from Iraq. Since matter is urgent I shall press British for early shipment of barley from Iraq, failing which I will be compelled to recommend to Department shipment of equivalent amount of wheat from United States or Canada. Repeated to Cairo for Winant.

On January 16, 1943, Acheson had written to Lewis Douglas of WSA (Letter, 891.24/280):

I refer to my letter of November 19, 1942 regarding the food shortage and generally unsatisfactory economic situation in Iran, with which there was enclosed a copy of a proposed agreement whereby the American and British Governments would undertake, under certain conditions, to make up any deficit in Iranian grain supplies which might be found to exist prior to the gathering of the 1943 harvest. The agreement in question was signed in Tehran on December 4, 1942, and the Iranian Ministry of Food and the American and British Ministers on January 12, 1943 unanimously decided that a deficit of approximately 23,500 tons of cereals was to be expected. This deficit was calculated after including in available supplies a total of 25,000 tons of wheat which has been in process of shipment from North American ports since the month of November 1942 and the last of which is expected to go forward during February 1943. In accordance with Article 1 of the agreement signed December 4, the American and British Ministers and the Iranian Ministry of Food have recommended that 16,400 tons of barley be obtained from Iraq and that 7,100 tons of wheat (or its equivalent in flour if shipping space would be saved thereby) be shipped from the United States or Canada. The British Minister at Tehran is transmitting this recommendation to his Government, and the Department of State is likewise informing the Foreign Office at London of its approval of the recommendations made. It is assumed that the proposed shipments from the United States or Canada will be handled by the British Ministry of Food and Ministry of War Transport by the same procedure as that adopted in previous shipments of grain to Iran. I shall be glad to inform you whenever word in this respect is received from the British Government.

Cable to London on January 18, 1943 (Telegram 397, 891.24/346A):

Tehran reports that British Minister, American Minister and Iranian Ministry of Food have unanimously decided that over and above 25,000 tons wheat now being shipped from North America, Iran will have a deficit of approximately 23,500 tons cereals during current crop year. This decision was taken in accordance with provisions of Article One of Tripartite Food Agreement signed December 4, 1942. The parties to this decision recommend shipment 7,100 tons wheat from North America and 16,400 tons barley from Iraq to make up anticipated deficit, in accordance with obligations established by food agreement. It is understood British Minister Tehran is transmitting above recommendation to his Government and is taking steps to obtain barley from Iraq. Department entirely approves recommendations made. Please transmit substance of foregoing to the Foreign Office and urge that action be taken as soon as possible. We assume British Ministry of Food will arrange wheat shipment from North America. Upon receipt of confirmation, Department will notify appropriate agencies in order that shipping programs may be adjusted. Please inquire whether a saving in shipping space could not be effected through shipment of flour equivalent to 7,100 tons of wheat instead of wheat itself.

London replied on January 20, 1943 (Telegram 508, 891.24/347):

Substance of Department's 397, January 18, 4 p.m. has been given Foreign Office and prompt action with reference to recommendations regarding wheat and barley for Iran has been urged. When doing so, we were told that as soon as British Minister at Tehran had informed Foreign Office of these recommendations, Foreign Office took up with the Ministry of War Transport the question of transporting this additional wheat from North America. While no definite reply has been received from the War Transport Ministry, Foreign Office says that limited shipping facilities will most likely make it difficult to arrange for the shipment of this wheat. In this connection, Foreign Office added that it has been found necessary to cut Middle East shipping program by fifty percent and that while this cut will probably not affect January shipping plans, it will become effective in February. Foreign Office will promptly inquire of shipping experts whether space could be saved by shipping flour instead of wheat. We were also told at the Foreign Office that the Soviet Ambassador in London is being requested to urge his government to take steps to induce Soviet authorities in Iran to facilitate transportation of wheat from Soviet occupied Iran where according to Soviet statements there is a supply of 35,000 tons to points in Iran where it is most needed. It is being pointed out to Soviet authorities Foreign Office states that for every ton of wheat made available from that which is in Soviet occupied Iran just so much more shipping space for supplies for Russia will become available.

London followed up with another cable on January 26, 1943 (Telegram 662, 891.24/360):

> Department's 397, January 18, 4 p.m. and Embassy's 508, January 20, 11 a.m. Foreign Office now informs us that it agrees that recommendations regarding wheat from North America and barley from Iraq should be approved and that it has instructed British Embassy at Washington so to advise Department. Foreign Office adds that British shipping authorities in United States are being told to take up with appropriate American authorities the arrangements that have to be made, so that adjustments can be effected in the shipping programs. Experts who have been consulted have informed Foreign Office that only about ten percent of shipping space would be conserved if flour were substituted for wheat. This the experts explain is because of the high percentage of flour which is being extracted from wheat in Iran.

Soon after, the British had again withdrawn their "consent" to send the additional wheat to Iran. Schnare from Tehran on February 1, 1943 (Telegram 121, 891.24/367):

> Legation's 44, January 13; and Department's 35, January 18. British Legation has withdrawn its approval for import of 7,100 tons wheat although its commitment thereto was formal and was communicated to London. This action was result of trip to Cairo of Squire, British Legation Counsellor handling food matters. Squire convinced Middle East Supply Center that decision to import 7,100 tons should be cancelled and that any additional cereals needed be made up by barley from Iraq because of shipping shortage. This they agreed would necessitate increasing adulteration rate for bread to 47%. British Legation refuses accept Sheridan's firm estimate that 16,000 tons wheat are needed up to next harvest for southern famine areas and gives own estimate as 11,000. Question of whether Iranians have taken all practicable steps to carry out their undertakings must be decided as provided in article 1 of Tripartite Food Agreement before Allied pledge to furnish wheat becomes operative. The British contend that they have not (repeat not) done so; this Legation is of opinion that they have, taking into consideration their limited resources, impotence and broken morale. I cannot admit that Middle East Supply Center has full jurisdiction in this matter which is based on special international agreement. Sheridan and this Legation are in full accord as to Iran's wheat needs and further agree that adulteration of bread beyond 40% is not fair in this country

where the masses are exclusively (repeat exclusively) bread eaters. My studied opinion is that the 7,100 tons of wheat should be shipped. This proposal should be binding since it has support of two of three parties mentioned in article 1 of food agreement. I recommend, however, that final decision be deferred until return from leave of Minister. Copy to Cairo for Winant's confidential information.

Cable to Tehran on February 5, 1943 (Telegram 67, 891.24/328):

Your 121, February 1. For your confidential information, Department is continuing with plans for shipment of balance of original 25,000 tons promised and additional 7,100 tons agreed upon January 12. Program being worked out here in collaboration with British shipping authorities calls for despatch of approximately 10,000 tons monthly in February and March and a somewhat smaller amount in April. Total will include some supplies for British forces and for Arab states on Persian Gulf. About two-thirds will probably go forward on American vessels, as Ministry of War Transport advises it can handle only some 3,000 tons monthly. We have not repeat not as yet received any indication from London or British authorities here that they propose to withdraw approval of the 7,100 tons. If necessary, however, Department is prepared to support your position in this matter.

The "withdrawal" of consent was a successful British ploy to reduce shipments. Schnare on February 8, 1943 (Telegram 144, 891.24/370):

Department's 67, February 5. Another wheat meeting attended by Sheridan and representatives of Britain-American Legations held February 6. Sheridan at meeting formally agreed to reduce his additional request from 7,100 tons wheat or flour to 5,000 tons. British agreed to provide additional millet and barley from Iraq which will more than make up the difference. Sheridan believes this change will not seriously affect his adulteration rate for bread. In view of Sheridan's agreement to above change it is now recommended that only 5,000 tons be shipped in addition to the 25,000 tons already agreed.

Dreyfus on March 6, 1943 (Telegram 242, 891.24/395):

Bread situation in Tehran remains critical. Internal stocks are nearing exhaustion and wheat from United States has not yet begun to flow into Tehran in sufficient volume. Several thousand tons have arrived or are about to arrive at southern ports destined for wheat pool to feed

Tehran, AIOC and Allied labor. In view of great and inexplicable delays in bringing wheat to Tehran over the railway I have sent Byron MacDonald of Lend-Lease office southward to investigate and endeavor to institute a system which will insure rapid and regular deliveries. It seems apparent to me that present agreed allocation of 200 tons a day northward for Iranian civil use is woefully insufficient and that revision upward should be made as soon as Americans take over remainder of this line and increase capacity of railway. British allocation officer agrees that for present 160 tons of wheat will be moved northward daily which item alone will almost exhaust the 200 ton allocation. Since there was such great delay in shipping the 25,000 tons of wheat I believe that bread situation here will show little improvement for several weeks.

Cable to Dreyfus on March 12, 1943 (Telegram 123, 891.24/370):

Please also report whether the grain situation in Azerbaijan, as described in Kuniholm's letters to you of February 1 and 10, will affect the wheat import program presented by Sheridan (your 44, January 13 and 144, February 9) and approved by British and American Governments. Does Sheridan still expect to get supplies for Tehran from Azerbaijan, and if not may we expect any request for additional imports? Present program, on which Department is working in collaboration with British and other agencies of this Government, contemplates total deliveries to Iran of about 30,000 tons wheat, plus some 25,000 tons additional for civilian employees of Anglo-Iranian Oil Company, Persian Gulf Service Command and Persia and Iraq Command. This may require some reduction in shipments to Soviet Union. We can give no repeat no assurance that quantity for Iran could be increased, but in this connection with possible reply to Soviet complaint, we should like to have as accurate a picture as possible of the present grain situation. Any increase in Iranian wheat imports would almost certainly be at the expense of planned shipments to Russia, and we may wish to point this out to Soviet Government as an argument against its purchases of Azerbaijan grain.

Dreyfus on March 15, 1943 (Telegram 273, 891.24/401):

My 272 today. I am convinced after consulting Sheridan and Middle East Supply Center representative that the wheat program of 30,000 tons for Iranian civil needs is adequate if it arrives. The program was based on assumption that almost no wheat will be obtained from

> Azerbaijan. I recommend no (repeat no) increase in the contemplated shipment of 55,000 tons of wheat to Iran to cover all needs up to next crop.

Dreyfus on March 31, 1943 (Telegram 332, 891.24/411):

> Department's 147, March 26. All wheat arriving in Iran is pooled by Middle East Supply Center. Distribution is made by Ministry of War Transport, in keeping with prearranged Middle East Supply Center program under supervision of the PAI (Persia and Iraq) force (and) Middle East Supply Center liaison officer. Total Iranian demands for imported wheat are about 13,000 tons monthly divided as follows: Iranian civil 9,500 AIOC 1,500 and army labor 2,000. Last figure includes American army labor but General Connolly does not wish to submit to Middle East Supply Center pooling arrangement and intends to import own wheat. A possible bottleneck in shipment of wheat is railway. The program now calls for movement from ports to Tehran of 160 tons wheat plus 100 tons other goods daily. Minister State is being asked to approve increase of wheat figure to 300 daily without reducing the 100 ton figure. Confidential. Much will depend on attitude to be adopted by American Army when they assume in near future full responsibility for movements control. General Connolly and staff in their desire to move maximum possible goods to Russia have so far shown little appreciation for necessity of moving Iran's essential requirements. I am hopeful, however, they will adopt a more liberal interpretation of term "Iran's minimum needs." I do not, therefore, recommend any immediate action and will keep Department informed of developments.

Wheat Shipments to Iran, November 1942 to June 1943

Of the agreed 30,000 tons for civilian needs, 10,000 were to be shipped during November and December 1942, and the remaining 20,000 tons were to reach Iran prior to the harvest in June 1943. Actual outcome turned out to be very different. On December 11, 1942, Thorold had telephoned Jernegan (Memorandum, 891.24/327):

> Mr. Thorold stated he had been advised as follows regarding progress on the shipment of the 25,000 tons of wheat to Iran: 3,905 tons had been shipped from American ports during November; 1,150 tons had

> been shipped during the first week of December; 3,350 tons additional were definitely scheduled for shipment during the balance of December. Efforts were being made to schedule a further 1,595 tons for December shipment. If this additional quantity were gotten off, it would complete the quota of 10,000 tons for November-December shipment which had been set by the British authorities in London.

Cable to Dreyfus on December 14, 1942 (Telegram 371, 891.24/325A): "British Embassy states 5,055 tons wheat for Iran shipped from American ports during November and first week December. It is planned to ship additional 5,000 tons during balance of December." These figures turned out to be exaggerated.

On February 5, 1943, Armstrong of Lend-Lease had telephoned Jernegan (Memorandum, 891.24/394-1/7):

> Mr. Armstrong said that War Department officials had raised the question of consignment of the wheat which was to be shipped to Iran in American vessels. They felt that at least part of it should be American wheat and should be sent to General Connolly, in order that he might have a supply under his control with which to feed his native employees. I said it had been my understanding that all the wheat would be furnished by the British Ministry of Food and would, presumably, be consigned to the UKCC for delivery to the Iranian Government. However, I thought the Department would have no objection to consigning our part to General Connolly, provided arrangements were made to see that our obligations to deliver wheat to the Iranian Government were strictly fulfilled. . . . It was my recollection that the British in Iran, in agreement with the Iranian authorities, had laid out a plan for pooling imported grain to take care of the needs of native employees of the British and American forces, Anglo-Iranian Oil Company, and the general run of Iranian civilians. Mr. Armstrong said that the War Department appeared to feel that General Connolly was being "pushed around," presumably by the British, and that his position would be strengthened if he had a supply of grain under his own control. If he had to go to the UKCC for his supplies, it might weaken his prestige vis-à-vis the Iranians. I agreed that it would be desirable to assist General Connolly if possible. Mr. Armstrong asked me to advise the appropriate officers of the Department of this development.

On March 5, 1943, General Robert Wylie, War Department, had telephoned Jernegan (Memorandum, 891.24/394-4/7):

> General Wylie said that the War Department had agreed to provide 1,500 tons of space for wheat shipments to Iran on each of five ships scheduled to sail during the month of March with supplies for the Persian Gulf Service Command. However, at the urgent request of PGSC, it had been decided that the first of these ships should carry 2,000 tons of wheat for the use of General Connolly's civilian employees in Iran, instead of the 1,500 tons originally allocated for general distribution under the MESC program. Consequently, the maximum to be carried on Army supply ships this month for general use would be 6,000 tons. I said that the Department could not object to the provision of wheat for General Connolly's people, but that we very much hoped the general program would also be met. We had heard that the five Army supply ships would not all sail in March, and that in reality only about 2,000 tons of wheat would be gotten off by that means this month. General Wylie said that it would depend upon the ability of the War Shipping Administration to provide the promised ships, but that his present information indicated they would be available in time and that from 4,500 to 6,000 tons of wheat, in addition to that for General Connolly, would be sent forward before April. (If General Wylie's estimate is correct, it would seem that the picture for March shipments, June arrivals, should turn out as follows: United States Army supply ships: 4,500-6,000 tons; British ships: 3,000 tons (estimated); Tankers from Australia: 1,500-2,000 tons. This leaves a balance of from 2,000 to 4,000 tons to be made up, presumably by shipments on Russian-aid vessels from the United States. If shipments on Army supply vessels fall below Wylie's estimate, as is quite likely, this balance will have to be increased.)

As below reported, the US Army had only shipped 2,000 tons in March 1943 "instead of the 7,500 tons as promised." The Army had subsequently shipped 7,500 tons in April.

On March 5, 1943, Thorold had written to Jernegan (Letter, 891.24/398):

> With reference to our discussion yesterday on the subject of the provision of wheat for Iran, recent telegrams which we have received from London emphasize that in the view of His Majesty's Government the only solution to this problem lies in the loading of the wheat on Russian aid vessels. It is pointed out that His Majesty's Government from

the first, fully recognized that the provision of wheat for Iran would have to be at the expense of Russian supplies, and it was because they realized all the grave disadvantages attendant on any curtailment of supplies to Russia, that they were reluctant to come to the decision to provide wheat for Iran until it was proved absolutely essential to do so. Once this decision had been come to and the commitment to Iran entered into, the consequences as far as regards Russian supplies were fully recognized and His Majesty's Government have repeatedly warned the Soviet Government that Russian supplies would have to suffer. In the first place it has to be appreciated that even if wheat for Iran could be shipped without encroaching on tonnage earmarked for Russia, it must displace Russian supplies on Persian inland clearance. It is for this reason that provision of a vessel from Australia is not altogether a solution. It will help, in that it will make the wheat available on the spot, but it will only displace Russian supplies in Iran and thereby involve a waste of shipping space in respect to Russian aid vessels which will be unable to discharge. Secondly, apart from our obligations to Iran under the food agreement, the situation has now become such that failure to send wheat to Iran *immediately* (original emphasis) will endanger the security of the trans-Iranian routes and consequently the transit of Russian supplies.

Dreyfus on March 19, 1943 (Telegram 285, 891.24/403):

My 273, March 15. British Ministry is informed that March loadings in United States of wheat destined for Iran will be very small. This is disturbing since Tehran is still living from day to day and because it now appears that considerable part of the 30,000 tons for Iranian civil use will not arrive much before next harvest. To ease the situation in June could not Department arrange for tankers returning from Australia to bring back larger cargoes of wheat? I should appreciate receiving from Department by telegraph a statement of wheat loadings from United States and Canadian ports for Iran monthly since November. This is needed to check the conflicting statistics received locally from various sources.

In response to the inquiry, Thorold had telephoned Jernegan on March 24, 1943 (Memorandum, 891.24/394-5/7):

In response to my request for figures on wheat shipments from the United States to Iran, Mr. Thorold said he had obtained two conflicting sets of statistics, as follows (tons):

1)	November	2,854	2)	November	854
	December	6,200		December	6,887
	January	4,700		January	5,714
	February	800		February	800
	Total	14,554			14,255

> Mr. Thorold said he was trying to ascertain the correct amounts, but he pointed out that the totals of the two sets were substantially the same. He went on to say that British shipments from this country during March were going to fall far below the anticipated 4,400 tons. Some of the ships scheduled had been taken away entirely and others were going to be delayed until April in getting away. The probable amount to clear in March would be 1,400 tons, and the maximum possible 1,900 tons. Adding 2,500 tons by tanker from Australia, this would mean only 4,000 tons probable arrival in the Persian Gulf in June. Consequently, Mr. Thorold felt we must endeavor to obtain a second dry cargo vessel to load in Australia in April in order to bring June arrivals up to at least the agreed minimum of 10,000 tons. Mr. Thorold went on to say that he had been informed scheduled loadings on United States Army supply ships in April would not come up to the anticipated amount of 6,000 tons. (It may be noted that these ships were originally announced as loading at the end of February, later as definitely for March, and then for April.) Mr. Thorold mentioned that up to February 18 the British Government had delivered to Iran for civilian requirements, in one way or another, 7,993 tons of wheat. This figure included advances made by the British Army in the Middle East. It did not, of course, include shipments now at sea.

According to Thorold, of the 14,554 tons imported, 7,993 tons were for civilian use and by implication 6,561 tons for British use. As below reported, of the latter amount, 5,024 tons consisted of Australian wheat shipped on returning oil tankers. Thus by the end of February 1943, the Allies had only met 27% of their commitment to Iran, and the wheat they had imported for Allied labor, AIOC employees, other British labor and the British military did not even cover Russian purchases in Azerbaijan.

To justify the failure to deliver, the British had again claimed that there was ample wheat in Iran. Thorold who on March 5, 1943, had urged immediate wheat shipments to Iran, was now taking the opposite tack. On March 22, 1943, he wrote to Jernegan (Letter, 891.61311/7):

We have just received a rather interesting repeat of a telegram from the British Minister in Teheran to the Minister of State in Cairo regarding Persian wheat supplies. From this it appears that a certain contractor (who had evidently been referred to in a telegram which we have not seen), armed with a government permit, has been making enquiries as to wheat and barley available on the open market. He has purchased or contracted for some 200 tons at the current local price of approximately £110 a ton and has just reported that the following further purchases could be made at about £130 a ton (i) within an 80 mile radius of Tehran - 15,000 tons (ii) around Qum—1,000 tons. The prices are of course, absolutely fantastic, but it is certainly a revealing fact that such large quantities, the provision of which would obviously very greatly ease our troubles in shipping wheat to Persia, are actually available if the owners could be induced to part with them. It seems certainly as if something more energetic on the part of the Persian Government is urgently needed.

Cable to Dreyfus on March 26, 1943 (Telegram 147, 891.24/403):

Your 285, March 19. British agencies here, which have handled details of all wheat shipments to date, furnish following loading figures from North American ports: November, 2,854 tons; December, 6,200; January, 4,700; February, 800 (repeat 800); total to February 28: 14,554. To make up for the small February shipments, War Shipping Administration is arranging to provide a Liberty ship to load about 8,000 tons at an Australian port in late March or early April for arrival Persian Gulf in early May. British further advise that tanker shipments from Australia have been as follows: October, 803 tons; November, 878; December, 1,417; January, 797; February, (incomplete) 1,129; Total: 5,024. Shipping authorities are understood now to have ordered complete utilization of all available tanker space, which averages about 500 tons per vessel, and it is hoped that average monthly shipments for March and succeeding months will be about 2,500 tons by this means. We are informed, however, that wheat brought by tanker is allocated first to AIOC and PAIC for their civilian employees and cannot, therefore, be counted as part of the 30,000 ton commitment to Iran. In this connection, we should appreciate information regarding arrangements in Iran for the division of wheat arriving on British and American vessels from North America or elsewhere. March loadings from United States are still uncertain, but Department is actively working on this problem and will make every effort to see that total June arrivals in Persian Gulf are adequate. For your information, War Department

> plans to send 2,000 tons wheat for General Connolly's civilian labor on a ship scheduled to clear from this country in near future. This is in addition to supplies promised Iranian Government, AIOC and PAIC.

By the end of March 1943, according to Thorold, wheat shipment to Iran was 8,000 tons behind schedule. On April 13, 1943, Thorold had written to Jernegan (Letter, 891.24/429-1/2):

> We have heard that the Government of India have agreed to continue supplies of flour for the PAIC (Persia and Iraq Command) rations, which you will remember were put at 1,700 tons a month. This therefore reduced the total requirements figure for the months of June, July, and August by 5,000 tons, but on the other hand, we are informed that no wheat was loaded in tankers during March. This means that 1,600 tons for Abadan and Caltex will have to be drawn from the pool so that we are at the moment some 3,400 tons nett to the good, so reducing the deficit to something under 8,000 tons.

From the paraphrase of a telegram dated "Middle of May" from the British Legation in Tehran to the Foreign Office and repeated to the British Embassy, Washington, one is able to get a measure of wheat shipments to Iran for civilian use during November 1942 to May 1943 (Memorandum, 891.24/440-3/4). It is stated that of the 25,000 ton commitment to Iran (not the agreed 30,000 tons), 9,000 tons remained to be met. By implication, 16,000 tons of wheat for civilian use had been shipped to Iran during November to May, of which, as above noted, 7,993 tons consisted of wheat shipped up to the end of February 1943, and as below described, 8,800 tons consisted of Australian wheat shipped on an American vessel. As the commitment to the Iranian government consisted of 30,000 tons, by May 1943, the two powers had only met 53% of their undertaking, and had it not been for the 25,000 tons of Russian wheat sent to Tehran during May to July, Tehran would have been without bread, claim to the contrary notwithstanding.

Dreyfus on June 9, 1943 (Telegram 597, 891.24/452):

> Department's 249, May 21 (800.24/896). After consultation with British Legation and MESC it appears that deviation of ship to Ceylon will not seriously affect our wheat commitments to Iran. It would seem unnecessary for Department to take steps to arrange for additional wheat shipments from India. MESC is programming for arrival of full 30,000 tons of wheat at Persian Gulf ports. 18,761 tons have already

> arrived and 6,422 tons are definitely known to be discharging or afloat. In addition wheat is being received from Russia, 8,000 tons having already arrived. Tehran silo has cereals reserve of more than 7,000 tons. It appears reasonably certain that our commitment to furnish Iran 25,000 tons of wheat will be fully met. The additional 5,000 tons will be placed in the MESC Persian Gulf wheat pool and furnished to Iran only if required. Repeated to Cairo and New Delhi.

Attempts to Obtain Indian and Australian Wheat

Numerous references to Indian and Australian wheat were noted. As India was facing famine, attempts to get Indian wheat for Iran were doomed. Following Dreyfus' suggestion in telegram 375 of November 14, 1942 (chapter 14), the State Department had cabled Winant in London on November 18, 1942 (Telegram 5788, 891.24/284):

> Your 6340, November 11 and previous. Tehran telegram 375 November 14 reads, in part, as follows: "Wheat situation in Tehran has taken even more critical turn. Sheridan has only half day supply in silo and wheat is coming in from provinces very slowly. Famine may come at any time and Sheridan is preparing to open soup kitchens if necessary. In view of the dangerous situation I feel we should take positive and immediate steps. I recommend that Department arrange urgently shipment of wheat to Iran from India at rate of 5,000 tons a month. Shipment from India is recommended because wheat from more distant places might not arrive in time to meet the crisis should it arise. While Sheridan may possibly be able to obtain sufficient wheat to tide country over for several months, my opinion is that we cannot afford to gamble while the lives of several thousand people are at stake." Please ask Foreign Office to give urgent consideration to possible immediate shipment of wheat from India or Middle East, rather than North America. Quantity furnished to meet Iranian emergency could, of course, be replaced later by shipments from this loading area. We are asking New Delhi to make inquiry in this of the Government of India.

Winant replied on November 19, 1942 (Telegram 6518, 891.24/296):

> When wheat situation in Tehran, as described in Department's 5788 of November 18, 6 p.m., was brought to attention of Foreign Office, Foreign Office informed us that it had received a telegram from the British Minister at Tehran, also dated November 14, in which he too

stressed the critical trend in the wheat situation. Consequently the Foreign Office telegraphed Minister of State Casey on November 16 to do whatever he could to secure in Iraq or India 3000 tons of wheat for immediate shipment to Iran, on the understanding that this 3000 tons would be replaced from shipment of 5000 tons previously scheduled for Iran for this month. . . . No reports have been received as yet from Minister Casey and the British Minister at Tehran regarding the results of their efforts to get wheat and barley to Iran from the sources mentioned above. Foreign Office, in giving us the foregoing information, added that unfortunately British authorities were not at present in a position to do anything further.

On November 18, 1942, prior to receiving Winant's reply, the State Department cabled the American Mission in New Delhi (Telegram 662, 891.24/296A):

Food situation in Iran has become a source of great concern to American and British Governments. . . . Our Minister reports as of November 14 that wheat shortage in Tehran has become acute and that immediate shipments of about 5,000 tons monthly are urgently needed. He suggests shipment from India, since wheat from more distant sources might not arrive in time. Foreign Office London has already agreed to ship 20,000 tons as follows: 5,000 tons November, 5,000 December and the remainder as soon as possible thereafter. However, it is believed these shipments are to be made from North America. We are asking Foreign Office to give urgent consideration to suggested shipments from India in order to save shipping time. Please take this up with Government of India and ask whether it would be possible to send wheat in quantities indicated. You may say that this Government attaches utmost importance to maintenance of Iranian food supply because of serious difficulties which would be encountered in moving supplies to Russia if there should be any breakdown of internal order in Iran. It would be understood that wheat made available in India for this purpose would be replaced by later shipments from other sources.

New Delhi replied on November 20, 1942 (Telegram 897, 891.24/297):

Question of wheat supplies for Iran was discussed this morning with Foreign Secretary (reference Department's 662, November 18, 7 p.m.) From his statements, made prior to consultation with Supply and Commerce Departments, it does not appear that favorable reply to this office's strong representations is likely. India's own wheat situation is

> critical. . . . Definitive reply will be cabled as soon as received. Repeated to Tehran.

Follow up on November 27, 1942 (Telegram 917, 891.24/303):

> In a note received this morning Government of India states it regrets that cereal shortage here is so severe that wheat cannot be loaned to Persia from either civil or military stocks in India. Note adds that Government has been watching Persian food crisis for many months with increasing anxiety but all assistance possible in the circumstances has already been rendered. Large quantities of seed wheat, in addition to personnel and materials, have already been sent to Persia. Strictly Confidential. A highly responsible official not directly concerned with foodstuffs but in a position to follow All-India food situation and military stocks, indicated informally today that shipping will very probably have to be found for imports into India of a minimum of 25,000 tons of wheat per month for six months. This for Indian needs alone and not including Persia. He estimates this amount, plus stocks which would consequently be released from hoarding, will be needed to carry India through until next crop (March-April 1943) which should be bumper. Repeated to Tehran, sent to Department.

State Department had next looked to Australia. On February 17, 1943, Armstrong of OLLA had written to Alling (Letter, 891.24/394-2/7):

> This will acknowledge receipt of your memorandum of recent date with respect to the shipment of wheat to Iran . . . and it is understood from recent conversations with Mr. Jernegan that the State Department will take up the matter with the War Shipping Administration with the objective of having a ship assigned to carry the necessary wheat from Australia to the Persian Gulf. . . . From the point of view of the Russian supply program, it proved impossible to make any space available during the current month. . . . If the wheat for Iran can be made available in Australia, it would seem that the assignment of vessels for this purpose should be definitely urged upon the War Shipping Administration.

Cable from London on February 21, 1943 (Telegram 1334, 891.24/387):

> To Acheson, Stettinius and Douglas from Harriman. . . . I understand total Persian civil requirements which has been agreed to by the United States and British Ministers in Persia is 30,000 tons. . . . I understand that it has been suggested in Washington that War Shipping Administration put on additional ship from Australia to carry wheat to Persian Gulf for arrival in May. I do not believe this proposal will help matters any unless one less Russian aid ship is dispatched. The bottleneck is, as you know, the capacity of Persian Gulf ports and railroad to Tehran. . . . The arrival of an additional shipload of wheat will therefore merely delay another ship unloading Russian aid cargo. Furthermore the transportation of wheat for Persian civil use from Persian Gulf to Tehran will also displace an equivalent amount of Russian aid. No matter how the wheat may be shipped its delivery to the Persians must be at the expense of Russian aid. It therefore seems that a definite decision of high policy must be made between carrying out our commitment to the Persians or to the Russians. We must evidently either face the consequences of further bread riots in Persia or of further straining the Russian supplies. If the decision is to supply the Persians, the most economical method of carrying the wheat would be to take it on Russian aid ships. There is some doubt whether, at this late date, wheat loaded in the United States would arrive during May. If this is the case it may be feasible for War Shipping Administration to put on ship in Australia and deduct one ship from Russian aid program. The balance could be loaded in Russian aid ships between now and the end of April if there is no additional space in Army vessels. I understand the Russians were told some months ago when they took wheat out of North Persia for their own requirements that it would be necessary to deduct wheat shipments from Russian aid shipping program. Leathers advises me that the British War cabinet after full consideration recommend that the joint decision should be to fulfill the Persian commitment even at the expense of Russian aid, and I am cabling you at his request.

On February 25, 1943, there was a meeting which included Stettinius (OLLA), Douglas (WSA), Generals Burns and Spalding (War Department), and Jernegan (Memorandum, 891.24/394-3/7):

> Mr. Douglas stated the problem as being that of ensuring the arrival of a minimum of 10,000 tons of wheat in the Persian Gulf in the month of May. It was brought out that the British have scheduled 2,400 tons for February shipment from the United States, leaving a total of about 7,500 tons to be taken care of otherwise. It was further brought out

that it is now too late to make any additional shipments from this country, for May arrival, even if space should be made on Russian-aid or other ships. Mr. Douglas said that the unknown factor in the problem was the possibility of shipments by tankers returning from Australia to the Gulf. Although the British Embassy had estimated that 2,500 tons monthly could be carried on British tankers. . . . He believed that some 3,500 tons could, in reality, be handled. In any case, a telegram had been sent to London to clear up this point. . . . Mr. Stettinius asked whether we had definite information on the urgency of the need for wheat in Iran. Mr. Jernegan replied that we had had repeated reports on the subject from our Legation at Tehran and had just received a letter from the Consul at Tabriz to the effect that Azerbaijan faced the prospect of famine within three months. He emphasized that Azerbaijan was the great wheat-producing region of Iran, and that this report, therefore, was indicative of the critical nature of the situation. Mr. Jernegan expressed concern lest the proposed tanker shipments might be delayed is some way, as had happened with wheat shipments originally scheduled from the United States during February, and actually arrive in June rather than May. . . . The meeting decided that no action could be taken pending receipt of definite word on the possibility of tanker shipment from Australia.

In a memorandum of March 5, 1943, to Rostow and Acheson, Alling writes (Memorandum, 891.5018/16):

To keep the record straight, I should like to summarize the Iranian wheat situation as I understand it at the present moment: 1) London's telegram 1487, February 28 shows, and Mr. McPherson of WSA agrees, that tanker shipments from Australia cannot be counted on to cover more than a very small part of our commitment. 2) Mr. McPherson has recommended, and Mr. Douglas is believed to have agreed, that a dry cargo ship must be put on from Australia, to sail around the end of March or early April. This ship could, presumably, carry 8,000 to 9,000 tons of cargo. This, of course, presupposes the availability of bags in Australia, but Harriman's telegram says MWT has encountered no difficulty in this respect. 3) It may or may not be necessary to subtract a Russian aid ship to make room for this wheat ship from Australia. Mr. McPherson proposes to take this up with General Burns et al., but he has given me his personal opinion (subject, I imagine, to change on notice from Mr. Douglas) that the wheat ship will get through somehow. 4) It now appears that only about 2,000 tons of wheat for Iran will be shipped on US Army vessels from this country instead of

> the 7,500 tons as promised. Mr. McPherson is aware of this and has promised to keep the question of March shipments from the US (for June arrival in Iran) in mind. I have also called this to the attention of Willis Armstrong (OLLA) and have asked him to consider the possibility of getting some tonnage on Russian-aid ships. He has promised to discuss it with General Burns. Unless WSA is willing to put on a second ship from Australia, or another ship from the United States for March sailing, it would appear that about 5,000 tons of space must be gouged out of Russian-aid vessels if we are to meet the program for June arrivals. 5) Our recent reports from Tehran and Tabriz, and those received by the British, indicate that the political and economic situation is getting worse and worse and that failure to meet our present wheat program would disastrous. The British War Cabinet has agreed that Iranian shipments must go through even at the sacrifice of Russian supplies, and they have warned the Russians of this. Consequently, we do not have to take all of the onus for any reduction in Russian shipments on this account.

A postscript dated March 16, 1943, adds: "Jernegan is getting the British to provide the wheat in Australia and to inform WSA as to where it will be. He will inform our rep. in Sydney when he hears."

Cable to Harriman on March 18, 1943 (Telegram 1676, 891.24/391):

> Your 1487, February 28 to Douglas. As Douglas has advised you, War Shipping Administration has agreed to put on a Liberty ship at an Australian port end of March or early April to carry approximately 8,000 tons bagged wheat to Iran for May delivery. Taken together with tanker shipments and such small quantities from the United States as may arrive during the month, it is believed this will meet the minimum Persian Gulf requirements for May. However, June, July, and August arrivals are still unprogrammed and uncertain. . . . Department is informed that Indian wheat situation has improved recently and that the next wheat crop, which will begin to reach market first of May, is expected to be largest in history. It is also understood that 68,000 tons Australian wheat is scheduled to load for India in March and April and that most of this will arrive after new domestic crop has begun to be available. We feel strongly that immediate consideration should be given to diversion of at least a substantial portion of this to meet Persian Gulf and Red Sea requirements. It would seem that this would effect a great saving both in time and shipping and might prove essential in any case to make up possible deficiencies in loadings from

North America. While Department has every reason to believe that diversion of this wheat would of itself have no repeat no adverse effect on Indian situation, it is desired to emphasize that any steps which may be taken should be kept secret to prevent speculators in India from taking advantage of them to create an artificial shortage. Please take this matter up with appropriate authorities.

Harriman replied on March 27, 1943 (Telegram 2195, 891.24/410):

Reference your 1676 of March 19 regarding the possibility of diverting Australian wheat from India to the Persian Gulf. I have put this matter to Lord Leathers but have as yet received no reply. I agree wholeheartedly that, if your reports are true, this diversion should be made and will press the matter. The decision to supply wheat to India was made by the War Cabinet and it will probably require similar decision to change it. It would be very helpful therefore if you could advise me the source of your reports and provide full details.

State Department reply of April 5, 1943 (Telegram 2126, 891.24/410):

For Harriman. Confidential. Our information was provided by American Mission New Delhi, which requests that it not repeat not be cited as source, in telegram 127, March 15 to Department. Mission states Government of India has succeeded in buying large quantities domestic wheat since beginning of February and has forced prices down 30 percent, thus indicating that artificial scarcity of wheat in Indian market has been at least partially overcome. Believes actual effect on local markets of balance of Australian wheat scheduled for shipment will be relatively unimportant in view of improved domestic situation and imminence of new harvest.

On May 11, 1943, Thorold had given Jernegan some supposedly good news (Letter, 891.24/431-1/2):

The British Merchant Shipping Mission have now had a telegram from the Ministry of War Transport confirming the release by the Government of India of two cargoes of wheat totaling 19,000 tons, now in Karachi, for on-shipment to the Persian Gulf. Although it is not altogether clear whether the provision for PAIC rations is included in this 19,000 tons, the cargoes in question will in any case undoubtedly relieve the wheat position in Persia and the Ministry of War Transport say that it will not be necessary to arrange for any further shipments of

> cereals in WSA vessels for Persian civilian needs; nor will it be necessary to arrange further shipments of cereals in British controlled vessels in May. I understand from Mr. Hart that arrangements had already been made for a further 2,000 tons to be loaded in US Army vessels, and 2,000 tons in BMWT vessels, and no doubt these arrangements will stand. In these circumstances there should be an opportunity of building up in Teheran some small reserve of cereals.

But the wheat ended up in Ceylon. Thorold to Jernegan on May 25, 1943 (Letter, 891.24/447-4/7): "We now understand that the ships carrying 19,000 tons of wheat which were to have been diverted from India to the Persian Gulf were in fact discharged in India, but the Indian Government has undertaken to supply 15,000 tons of wheat in their place." On May 31, 1943, Christelow of the British Civil Secretariat had written to Jernegan (Letter and enclosure, 891.24/447-5/7): "I attach a copy of a cable from MESC to Teheran concerning Persian Government wheat requirements. If you have any comments I shall be glad to hear from you." The telegram reads:

> We have been informed that "SS John Sedgwick" which was carrying wheat from Australia to the Persian Gulf has now been sent to Ceylon to meet the crisis there. We understand that the authorities concerned in Washington and London were in agreement on the necessity for this. However, we understand that there is a possibility that other supplies will be shipped to the Persians in replacement of the cargo on the "SS John Sedgwick." In order that we may decide on the urgency for replacement will you please take immediate action along the following lines: (a) Please consult the US Minister at once and cable us the actual quantity of cereals and flour which must be imported for provision to the Persian Government under the terms of the Food Agreement. It seems clear that 25,000 tons must be supplied in any circumstances. However, there is considerable confusion as to the amount to be provided above and beyond the 25,000 tons. Moreover, we would like to know whether there is any possibility of reducing the amount to be provided to the Persian Government by the quantities now coming forward from the USSR. (b) Please inform us earliest possible quantities of Russian wheat received in Teheran by June 1st together with information you may have on further quantities arriving at Caspian ports and awaiting movement.

The cable adds:

> We re-affirm that MESC will do its utmost to make available whatever quantities may be indicated by the signatories to the Food Agreement as essential for the supply to the Persian Government. As soon as we have your reply to the questions above we shall put the necessary recommendations to London and Washington.

Russian Wheat for Tehran

Reference was made in the above telegrams to Soviet wheat arriving in Tehran. As noted in chapter 19, Bullard had been greatly exercised by the dispatch of Russian wheat and had fired a "pin-prick" note to the Russian Ambassador. Dreyfus on April 13, 1943 (Telegram 382, 891.24/433):

> Russians out of a clear sky have announced they are shipping 25,000 tons wheat for consumption of people of Tehran. This will be transported by Russians down Volga via Caspian ports to Tehran and delivered at rate of 7,500 tons a month have been promised. The gesture is beautifully timed to embarrass the British and ourselves who despite the fact that deliveries are now being made, are felt by great many Iranians to have failed to live up to our agreement. The political motives behind this move are shown by fact that wheat from America is arriving and it would appear that no further supplies for Tehran are necessary. If as is being suggested Russian wheat be used for Tehran and American wheat to be used in south Iran, the Iranians in the capital will be left with impression that Russians fed them with grain and Americans and British with promises. Iranians while highly suspicious of this sudden generosity have accepted with an expression of gratitude. Iranian official reaction is typified by Shah who in conversation with me on Monday stated frankly he wonders what the Russians will now ask in return. Both British Minister and I had conversations with Soviet Ambassador immediately previous to this announcement but neither was given any indication that such a step was contemplated. British Minister feels move is designed primarily to influence Majlis elections referred to in my airgram No. 9, March 20. I would appreciate an indication from Department of the amount of cereals shipped to the USSR by either the United States or Great Britain under Lend-Lease or other arrangements. Repeated to Moscow.

On April 19, 1943, there was a meeting on the Soviet wheat offer, attended by Armstrong (OLLA), and Colonel Luscomb (PGSC), Murray, Alling, Jernegan and Loy Henderson (Memorandum, 891.24/440-1/4):

> Mr. Armstrong reported that between 200,000 and 250,000 tons of wheat and flour have been shipped to the Soviet Union by the United States and Canada since October 1941. Although the bulk of these shipments have been sent by way of Siberia, 13,000 tons were sent by way of the Persian Gulf in the period January-March 1943, some of which has probably now arrived in Iran. It was agreed that an absurd situation would be created by the movement of Lend-Lease flour north through Iran to Russia while, at the same moment, Russian wheat moved south into Iran. It was further agreed that this particular situation could best be adjusted by direct conversations with the Soviet Commissariat of Foreign Trade, keeping discussions on purely practical supply basis and avoiding any political issues. . . .

Cable to Dreyfus on April 22, 1943 (Telegram 193, 891.24/335):

> Your 382, April 13. Total Lend-Lease shipments wheat and flour to Soviet Union from October 1941 (repeat 1941) to April 1943 have been about 185,000 tons. In addition, Canada is understood to have shipped some 50,000 tons flour. Rate of shipment is increasing, as Soviet authorities have recently given foodstuffs relatively high priority in their requests. Most of American and Canadian shipments have been by other routes, but at least 20,970 tons flour are now afloat for delivery via Iran. Department is suggesting to Lend-Lease Administration that it take up with Soviets, through General Burns in Moscow, question of apparent waste of transport which would result from a two-way movement of cereals through Iran. . . . Department is considering possible approach to Soviets along following lines: 1. Ambassador Standley would be instructed to inform appropriate authorities that this Government is delighted to have the collaboration of the Soviet Government in meeting the urgent food problem in Iran. As we have previously stated, we regard the maintenance of the Iranian food supply as vitally important to the security of the United Nations position in Iran and, consequently, to the unimpeded movement of supplies to the Soviet Union by that route. 2. As the Soviet Government knows, the United States and Great Britain signed an agreement with Iran on December 4, 1942, whereby we undertook to make up any ascertained deficiency in the Iranian grain supply during the current crop year, which ends in August 1943. In pursuance of this agreement, the Ameri-

can and British Governments have made considerable shipments of wheat to Iran, and further shipments are now en route or scheduled to be made in the near future. 3. Since it now appears that the Soviet Union is in a position to join in meeting Iran's needs, we suggest that it might well be for the Soviet, British and American authorities in Moscow or Tehran to consult together regarding the total amount of grain required and the best sources of supply, having in mind the general supply and transportation picture. We would also suggest, if only to demonstrate the solidarity and common purpose of the United Nations, that the Soviet Union might wish to become a party to the Anglo-American-Iranian food agreement of December 4, 1942. Department would appreciate your comments, and those of Ambassador Standley, on foregoing. It is our thought that an approach along these lines might serve as a further step to bring about real cooperation among all three major powers in Iran, cooperation which seems to us to be more and more vitally necessary. We have not (repeat not) as yet consulted British on this matter. Although we may do so in near future, we do not (repeat not) contemplate a joint approach to Soviets, since we wish to avoid the appearance of presenting a concerted American-British front. Repeated to Moscow as Department's 248 April 22.

Dreyfus on April 26, 1943 (Telegram 430, 891.24/432):

Department's 193, April 22. Am in full accord with Department's suggested approach to Soviet Government. The proposed line appears to be positive and constructive whereas an approach based on a strong protest might well defeat its purpose. This might be good occasion to suggest to Russians that their full collaboration in matters of mutual interest to Allies in Iran will be beneficial and that consultation with the British and Americans before taking steps of this kind would undoubtedly be in the common interest. British Legation here has published articles in press taking substantially the line given in paragraphs one and two of Department's suggested American approach except that the articles were so exaggerated as to give impression of sarcasm. British are being strongly criticized for these articles. For Department's information in this connection present wheat position in Tehran is the best in the past year. The silo contains wheat to cover several days needs and wheat from Ahwaz and barley from Khanaqin are flowing into the capital at rates which permit the building up of a small reserve. For the moment there appears to be no cause to worry as to Tehran's supply and the Soviet wheat would seem to be surplus to Tehran's needs. Repeated to Moscow.

Dreyfus discusses the British press articles in a report of April 28, 1943 (Dispatch 536 and enclosure, 891.24/438):

> I have the honor to enclose a copy of an article printed in the April 21, 1943, edition of *Daily News*, which is published by the Public Relations Bureau of the British Legation, on the subject of the Soviet offer to furnish 25,000 tons of Russian wheat for the consumption of the population of Tehran. As indicated in my telegram No. 430, April 26, this article is rather sarcastic in its reference to the Soviet offer as an illustration of the economic unity of the United Nations. It declares, perhaps too pointedly, that the allies are furnishing far greater amounts of wheat to Russia, a fact which permits the Russians to make this generous offer. It points somewhat unkindly, too, to the fact that the best way to provide Tehran with wheat would have been to permit Iranian wheat to come down from Azerbaijan, where there have been three good successive crops. The Russians have not, to say the least, appreciated this British press release and there is considerable criticism of it in Soviet circles. The British points, omitting the sarcasm, are well taken but one doubts the wisdom of taking an ally to task in the public press. The Russians are proceeding with their plan to deliver wheat to Tehran in spite of the fact that the wheat being delivered under the British-American engagement is reaching Tehran in sufficient flow to take care of Tehran's daily needs and permit the building up of a modest reserve. The Soviet plan calls for the delivery of 7,500 tons monthly, beginning in May, at Caspian Sea ports. The wheat will be moved thence by the Iranians but the Russians have agreed to give all possible help in arranging transport facilities. The agreed price is 3,200 rials a ton, or about $100 cif Caspian Sea ports. This is understood to be about the same as the cif Persian Gulf price being charged by the UKCC for American wheat and the price was undoubtedly arrived at with the charge for American wheat in mind.

The *Daily News* article is entitled, "Unity of United Nations: Soviet Government's offer of 25,000 tons of Wheat for Tehran." It reads:

> The offer of 25,000 tons of wheat to the Iranian Government by the Soviet Government affords a good illustration of the economic unity of the Allied and United Nations in the present world struggle. In order to compensate the Soviet Government as far as possible for the loss of some of the Russian wheat lands, the British and American governments have sent to the northern ports of Russia, besides large quantities of other foodstuffs, huge quantities of wheat—many times 25,000

> tons. These are the figures up to January, 1943. The result is that in spite of their difficulties the Soviet Government are able to spare 25,000 tons for Tehran and some of the wheat which is being provided by Great Britain and America and which otherwise would have been brought to Tehran can help to make up for any shortage there may be in Shiraz, Isfahan and other places in the south. Of course, the best way to provide Tehran would be to bring wheat from Azerbaijan, where there have been three good harvests in succession and the stocks are large; but as the landowners of Azerbaijan have not been delivering even enough to feed the town of Tabriz properly, let alone the unfortunate people of Tehran, it is most gratifying that the Soviet Government, whose own needs are being met in part by British and American help, should now come forward to help Tehran.

On April 27, 1943, John S. Dent, Second Secretary of the British Embassy had written to Livingstone T. Merchants with copy to Jernegan (Letter, 891.61311/4 ½):

> You will recollect that at a recent MESC meeting a telegram from your Legation in Teheran was mentioned which reported that the Soviets had offered to supply Teheran with 25,000 tons of wheat from Russia at the rate of 7,500 tons a month. We telegraphed the Foreign Office in London asking for their comments. We have now received a reply from London saying that according to their information the report is quite correct. The Foreign Office continue however by remarking that previous Russian promises of assistance in regard to the Persian wheat problem have led to very little and it remains to be seen whether or not the present offer is an exception. It is therefore felt in London that this report offers no reason for interrupting our own programme for the supply of wheat to Persia. In any case the United States and British Governments are committed to supply wheat to Persia and this commitment was not conditional on the absence of supplies from other sources. In the opinion of the Foreign Office the effect upon Anglo-American prestige in Persia would be disastrous if we were to make this Russian offer an excuse for not fulfilling our own undertakings. Moreover since it is many months since the Persian Government had more than a few days' supply on hand, and since political stability in Teheran cannot be expected so long as the food supply of the people is not assured, it is urgently necessary to create a small reserve of wheat in Teheran. In addition the Foreign Office point out that South Persia has hitherto had to go very short because of the demands of the capital and relief of the scarcity in the South is also becoming more and more

> imperative. In the circumstance the Foreign Office urge most strongly that despite this recent Russian offer every possible effort should be made to implement our joint undertaking to supply wheat to Persia at the earliest possible moment and that the Agencies concerned should be urged to continue their efforts to find the necessary shipping space.

Merchant replied on May 4, 1943 (Letter, 891.61311/4 ½):

> Thank you for your letter of April 27, your reference WT 212/143/43, with reference to the supply of wheat to Iran. The Department is in complete agreement with the opinion of the Foreign Office that despite the recent Russian offer, every effort should be made to execute the joint undertakings of our two Governments to supply wheat to Iran in the quantity promised. I am glad to inform you that the Department was informed by the War Shipping Administration during the past few days that the wheat ship from Australia is sailing as previously arranged and will carry to the Persian Gulf 8,800 tons of wheat and flour. In addition, the Department has been recently informed by the US Army that five Army supply ships began to load 1,500 tons of wheat apiece in the first ten days of April. This wheat is also destined for Iran. The Army stated further that it was expected two more Army ships would load similar quantities by the end of April.

The letter concludes:

> I can assure you that no relaxation has occurred in the efforts of the Department to press for a full discharge of the obligations assumed. I think you will agree that the figures given above indicate gratifying progress in the loading of wheat on Army ships and the special arrangement whereby a ship was put on the run from Australia.

On May 3, 1943, Thorold had called on Jernegan (Memorandum, 891.24/450):

> Mr. Thorold called at my suggestion. I said that I had wanted to tell him about a new development in connection with the Soviet Government's announcement that it would send 25,000 tons of wheat to Iran. The Office of Lend-Lease Administration had found that some 20,000 tons of American and Canadian flour was at sea en route to the Persian Gulf for delivery to the Soviet Union. The American flour had been shipped under Lend-Lease and the Canadian flour had been purchased in Canada by the Russian Government. Both classes had been

> shipped from the United States on American vessels. Since it would seem a little absurd to have flour from this country moving north through Iran to Russia while wheat from Russia moved south to Iran, OLLA had cabled its representative at Moscow to take the matter up with the Soviet Foreign Trade Commissariat and suggest that the Soviet authorities divert the American and Canadian flour to Iran, for Iranian civilian use, thus conserving domestic Russian wheat and at the same time avoiding a waste of transportation. . . . Mr. Thorold remarked that the proposed action seemed eminently sensible. He wondered what excuse the Russians would find to answer it, since their offer of wheat was obviously political in its object. A diversion of our flour to feed Iran, instead of shipment of Russian wheat, would considerably reduce Soviet "kudos" and, therefore, might be expected to be unacceptable. I went on to say that there had been some discussion in the Department of the advisability of asking the Soviets since it appeared they might become a source of supply for Iran, to join with the British and American authorities in working out the supply program. It was thought that we might try, gradually, to get the Soviets more and more into the picture, possibly starting with this wheat question. It seemed to us that greater Soviet cooperation would be generally desirable. . . . Mr. Thorold expressed agreement with this point of view and said the he would report it to London and ask for the comments of the Foreign Office.

Thorold had again visited Jernegan on May 17, 1943 (Memorandum, 891.24/440-2/4):

> I told Mr. Thorold that Lend-Lease had received a reply to its suggestion that the Soviet Government conserve transportation by diverting to Iranian use the American and Canadian flour en route to the USSR via Iran, instead of shipping Russian wheat south to Iran. The reply had said that the Iranian Government needed 25,000 tons of wheat, the Soviet Government needed 30,000 tons of rice, and an exchange had therefore been arranged. The Soviet authorities asserted that this did not involve any waste of transportation. Mr. Thorold asked whether the Department had taken any further steps in this matter. I said that we had not yet had time to consider the Soviet reply carefully.

The memorandum adds:

> Mr. Thorold referred to our conversation of May 3, during which I had told him of the Department's thought that the Russians might be invited to adhere to the Anglo-American-Iranian wheat declaration of

> December 4, 1942 and otherwise join us in solving Iran's food supply problems. The British Embassy had referred this to London and had received a reply saying that the Foreign Office would welcome such Soviet action; the Russians had, of course, been invited to join in the wheat declaration even before it was signed, and the Foreign Office considered that the way had always been left open for their adherence. However, Mr. Thorold remarked, the tone of the Foreign Office cable indicated that the British Government did not believe there was much chance that the Soviets would act favorably on a suggestion of this kind.

The next day, May 18, 1943, Christelow had telephoned Jernegan (Memorandum, 891.24/440-3/4):

> Mr. Christelow said that he had received yesterday a cable stating that the first nine railroad carloads of Russian wheat had arrived in Tehran and that an additional 30 truckloads were expected momentarily. The cable went on to say that if this rate were maintained, Russian deliveries to Tehran would average about 7,500 tons a month and would be sufficient to keep the city going until the new harvest without other assistance from outside sources. (According to a report made last month by Mr. Jackson, Director of MESC, the Russian shipments were scheduled to begin May 1, with the first wheat arrivals in Tehran expected on May 15. It appears, therefore, that they are right on schedule.) I told Mr. Christelow that we had just received a cable indicating that the Soviets regarded their wheat shipments as being in exchange for 30,000 tons of Iranian rice. He remarked that this would not, in fact, detract from the benefit to be expected from the wheat supplies, since the rice in the Russian occupied zone would not have been available for other parts of the country in any case. I agreed that this was true, so far as the immediate situation was concerned. I pointed out, however, that if the Russian zone were to continue indefinitely segregated from the rest of Iran with respect to food supplies, we should have a permanent grain shortage in the deficit areas which normally draw upon the northern provinces for wheat, barley and rice. Mr. Christelow agreed but seemed to doubt anything could be done to change this state of affairs.

The British cable reads:

> On May 10th and May 11th 9 wagon loads of Russian wheat arrived in Tehran and 30 military truck loads are due on the 14th. Tehran should

be able to subsist until harvest time without further assistance from us if deliveries continue at the promised rate of 7,500 tons a month, especially as we have already built up a reserve of some 4,500 tons of wheat and Iraqi barley and millet. I do not however recommend any modification of our own programme for the present as it is too early to be sure of this. In any case we must deliver the balance of 9,000 tons still outstanding on our 25,000 tons of wheat. The question of disposing of any portion of this balance not eventually required for Tehran can be discussed with Sheridan on his return from Cairo. It might be our best policy to allow a substantial reserve to accumulate in Tehran. Assurance of adequate food supplies for Tehran during the remaining months before the harvest is not only an essential factor in political stability, but will have great psychological value in discouraging hoarding and speculation when the new harvest is gathered and preventing a repetition of last year's difficulties.

Departure of Sheridan and Assignment of Food Matters to Millspaugh

With so little wheat coming in, Sheridan's tenure was an unhappy one. Following Farrokh's resignation due to disagreement with Sheridan, Taddayon was named Minister of Food (Dreyfus, Telegram 240, 891.002/381, March 6, 1943). Dreyfus on March 8, 1943 (Dispatch 479 and enclosures, 891.01A/224):

> Mr. Sheridan is having a stormy passage. Before going into the reasons therefore it will be useful to record what the Iranians are saying about him. The following reports and comments in the Majlis are typical: *Dad* February 14. "The people expected that with advisers the wheels of the country would move better. Unfortunately, they saw nothing but serious differences of opinion between Mr. Sheridan and Mr. Farrokh (Minister of Food) which usually led to rows in the Ministry. . . . Thus the people are less benefited by the services of the adviser than they had expected. The people have no bread and no clothes and are waiting for reforms. Who is the man to remove these difficulties?" *Eqdam* February 17. "This black bread contains everything but wheat. It is better to take poison than such bread. To eat this bread means to take one's life, especially children who develop dysentery. The promises of the Food Adviser were all devoid of truth. This bread contains date pits. We will all develop diseases if this condition continues." *Mehr-i-Iran* February 18. "This bread they are feeding the

people is harder than granite. The people eat it and die. Then they are sent to the morgues and piled there without shroud. . . . Put aside lengthy programs and do something." Speech in Majlis by Deputy Amir-Teimur on February 20. "We created a Ministry of Food. It did not remedy our pains. We brought a Food Adviser. It became worse. We enacted an Anti-Hoarding Law. It caused trouble to the people. We took the people's food, without which they die. We gave the Ministry of Food 500,000,000 rials. It is gone. The adviser of the Ministry of Food is no expert at all. He may be an economist but no Adviser. They say he was a druggist in Egypt. . . . I request Mr. Soheily to give Mr. Sheridan another job for he is not worthy of this work. Let them give him five times his salary but remove him from this work. The bread they are giving to the people is not bread. They are mixing it with a thousand things, but one thing you will not find in this bread is wheat. . . . Put out Mr. Sheridan. Go, Sir, to the morgue and see how many people are dying (this was said in an inflammatory tone)." *Dad* February 22. "Instead of bread they are feeding the people a mixture of plaster of Paris, date pits and other things. If plaster of Paris is white, this bread is black; you can get the former easily but to get the latter one has to break his neck." *Dad* February 24. Leading editorial entitled "Mr. Sheridan is in Error"—"The Iranians are starving and they know the reason for it. They do not expect their Food Adviser to call the bread problem a historical problem. They expect him to find a remedy, not pour salt on the people's sores. Why does Mr. Sheridan speak of 2,500 tons of wheat and 3,300 tons of barley the British are giving? We exported wheat in former years. Were we in need of their help? Why do you speak of flour loaned us by the American Red Cross and Polish Red Cross? Are we beggars? We are suffering from the results of the allied invasion. They took away our wheat and took hold of our transport. We are not responsible. The responsibility for the death of innocent Iranians rests on those who took away our wheat." *Rahbar* February 28. "The mud brick bats produced in the silo do not require such pomp and circumstance as one finds in the Ministry of Food, especially when that organization is unable to distribute these mud brick bats in a more suitable manner among the poor." *Keihan* February 28. "We do not have the least doubt of Mr. Sheridan's good will. But we do not expect him to proceed with words, arguments and propaganda instead of action. . . . If the allies have not been withholding assistance in food supplies, why then is it that rice which sold for 300 rials a kharvar now sells for 13,000 rials in spite of the fact that the crop was the best in years? The people believe, and perhaps their view is sound, that the existence of the Ministry of Food is responsible for these high prices. This is the superhuman power which has been shown by the Ministry of Food. The Ministry of Food fixed the price of sugar. As soon as the price was announced the price of sugar went up from 110 to 400 rials a "man" (measure of weight, about 3 kilos). . . . In a later article we shall tell the Food Adviser what the people think of the miracles performed by the Ministry of Food." *Eqdam* March 1. "Oh, God Almighty, to show that thou hast the power to do anything, take this burden of the Ministry of Food off our shoulders regardless of the allies. . . . Do not place the people any longer in the hands of the executioners. . . . No bread, no kerosene, widows crying in the silence of the night over their dead husbands. . . . Hungry children are moaning. . . . Everything in this country has a high price except human lives." Majlis Proceedings March 11. Deputy Teimur again demanded that Sheridan be given another job. He stated that half of Iran's troubles are due to the thoughtlessness and misdirected work of the Ministry of Food. In any case, he said, a handful of imposters had devoured the 500,000,000 rials allotted to the Food Ministry and a thorough investigation should be made. As to Mr. Sheridan, Deputy Teimur said he would say nothing further, in accordance with his promise, except that Mr. Sheridan should be removed.

The above quotations will give the Department a good idea of Mr. Sheridan's present status. What are the causes of these violent attacks? It should be explained at the outset of fairness to Mr. Sheridan that he faced a thankless and almost impossible task. The people demanded results but how was he to produce wheat where none existed? There is growing evidence that Iran's wheat production in recent years has been declining. Some of the causes of this decline are: the low price paid for wheat by the Government; trend toward planting opium and other uncontrolled crops in preference to wheat; Shah Reza's well-known policy of cheap bread for the people; the policy of settlement of the tribes strangely enough reduced the tillage of the soil; and finally the industrialization of the country brought large numbers of peasants to the cities in search of high wages. Add to this the disruption of road transport due to the taking over of most of Iran's trucks by UKCC, the disappearance under Shah Reza of the former great herds of camels and donkeys, the exploitation of the Iranian railways by the British and Russians, and superimpose on the whole the breakdown in Government morale and efficiency because of the invasion and it will be seen that Sheridan was confronted with a difficult situation. All might still have been well had the British not stubbornly clung to their contention that there was wheat in hoarding in the country which could be brought to light if only sufficient pressure were put on the Iranians to disgorge. For this reason the British delayed so long in approving shipment of wheat to Iran that it has not arrived in time to save the people from hunger during the winter. Had wheat been shipped by the British and Americans when this Legation first requested it, it would have begun to arrive in January and Sheridan's position would today be entirely different. He would perhaps now be considered a great hero. Sheridan has had to give undue attention to the problem of feeding Tehran from day to day, which has prevented him from as much time as he would have liked to the more important question of organizing governmental machinery for the collection of next year's harvest. That is the paramount problem – to make sure that the crops are collected at harvest time, from May to August, on the threshing floor so that the country's wheat supply for next year is assured.

There is no doubt that Sheridan is sincere, honest, courageous and a hard worker. No one, I believe, denies him these attributes. However, on the demerit side of his report card, we have much to note. He has been rash in putting quickly-conceived ideas into practice without mature consideration. He took a "know-it-all" attitude with his Minister of Food with the result that there was very bad feeling between him and Farrokh. He has been much too sure of himself. For example, he won the dislike of an important young Iranian, Habib Naficy, by pretending to know all about Iran immediately after his arrival. He has been careless in making rash promises to the people. His press and verbal statements have usually promised that all would soon be well, when a child could see that all would not be well. He has changed like a weather vane from day to day. In his disputes with Farrokh, he would sometimes threaten, sometimes state he was resigning and sometimes ride rough shod over the Minister. . . . Sheridan's greatest fault is his inability to keep a leash on his tongue. The surest way to launch a report or rumor in Tehran is to tell Sheridan. I could give dozens of examples of this. For example, he told me and other persons that Dr. Millspaugh brought his son to Iran in order to escape the draft. One of the worst examples of Sheridan's wagging tongue is the following, to which I was witness. At a luncheon at the Danish Legation, attended by important persons, Hossein Ala, apparently deliberately baiting Sheridan, asked whether Sheridan had yet chosen a new Minister of Food (the incident occurred just after Farrokh had resigned because of Sheridan). Sheridan, taking the hook, line, and sinker, replied to the effect that he had not made up his mind as yet, but he was grooming Mostafa Adl, whom he considered a gentleman of ability, for the post.

Sheridan ran afoul of Dr. Millspaugh and came out second best. He apparently saw, soon after Dr. Millspaugh's arrival, that the Millspaugh Mission would probably invade his sphere and exert considerable influence in the policies of the Ministry of Food, particularly in financial aspects. He succeeded temporarily in winning to his side Dr. Atkins, one of Dr. Millspaugh's assistants, and both took the view that Millspaugh was not capable of running food matters and therefore Sheridan should be made supreme in these questions. Both came to me with insinuations that Dr. Millspaugh was "getting old and losing his grip." Dr. Millspaugh, in his quiet and competent way, took the swift action for which he is noted and proposed directly to Sheridan the following solution. Realizing that proper action in food matters should be based on greater powers, Sheridan should go to the Majlis to request such powers. If he were unable to get them, Dr. Millspaugh would obtain the powers for himself and take over responsibility for Sheridan's food mission. Sheridan, knowing full well that he could obtain nothing from an unfriendly Majlis, appears to have decided to terminate his mission after a few months and permit Dr. Millspaugh to take over. He is already telling about town that he will leave Tehran as soon as Colonel Bonneville of the Millspaugh Mission arrives, or at most after a few months. Dr. Atkins, as I am reporting by separate despatch devoted to the Millspaugh Mission, has apparently seen the light and has returned to the Millspaugh fold wiser and somewhat chastened.

In conclusion, it is a regrettable fact that Sheridan has reflected little credit on our adviser program. The reasons are, to a great extent, beyond his control; no one else could have succeeded in feeding Tehran with non-existent wheat, with wheat the Russians never permitted to leave the Russian zone, with wheat consumed already by the allied forces in Iran, or with wheat which refused to arrive from the United States. Nevertheless, he could, in my opinion, have saved himself somewhat by not "barging about like a bull in a china shop." Let us, however, give him full credit for his energetic action, particularly for setting the stage for the collection of next year's crop. He has engaged a number of Americans to take charge of this important task and it is hoped they are already on their way to Iran. It would be a mistake to say categorically that Sheridan is finished. The Iranians, as I have often remarked, are very fickle and they will perhaps love him when they are well fed as much as they hate him in their hunger. He has to "take the rap" temporarily. Dr. Millspaugh, moreover, has no desire to assume responsibility for food matters and would take it reluctantly.

Consequently, if Sheridan can hold on and wishes to do so he may still weather the storm. Certainly his position will improve as soon as wheat begins to arrive in volume from the United States, as I am hopeful it will do in the very near future, for then Tehran would be assured of bread until the next harvest. A hopeful sign is that the new Minister of Food, Mr. Tadayyon, is cooperating well with Sheridan and has defended him nobly in the Majlis. . . . The Department may be assured that I have given, and will continue to give, my full support to Mr. Sheridan, with whom I remain on the best of terms. It is, in my opinion, much to be preferred that he continue on at least until such time as the results of his efforts become apparent to the Iranians. I have, I may add, impressed upon Sheridan and all of our advisers the necessity of coordinated action and a united front on the part of our American advisers.

Dreyfus on June 29, 1943 (Telegram 673, 891.01A/231):

Sheridan, acting under terms of his contract, has given Iranian Government three months notice of intention to terminate contract at end of one year. He intends to leave Tehran in September at latest. Prime Minister, being very much dissatisfied with operation of Food Ministry under Sheridan and Tadayyon, is most anxious to dissolve this Ministry and have its functions taken over by Ministry of Finance. Millspaugh, in view of unsatisfactory work of Food Ministry, has agreed to accept responsibility for food matters and a decree making the transfer is now being prepared. Millspaugh is accepting this responsibility notwithstanding fact that he does not have personnel to deal with problem. He urges that War Department be requested to detail Colonel Bonnevalle and Major Speaks to Tehran temporarily to assume these functions under his supervision until such time as permanent personnel can be obtained. . . . I agree as to necessity of placing food matters under jurisdiction of Millspaugh and urge that Department endeavor without delay to arrange detail of Bonnevalle and Speaks.

Dreyfus on September 1, 1943 (Dispatch 659 and enclosures, 891.01A/238):

Mr. Sheridan departed from Tehran for the United States by airplane on August 28, 1943. While he will be missed socially by the many who came to appreciate his buoyant spirit and personally attractive qualities, all circles have heaved a sigh of relief at his departure. The Iranians have been so anxious to get rid of him that they have given

> him leave of absence of a month to permit his departure a month before the termination of the first full year of his contract. . . . Sheridan's work in Iran cannot be described as a success. His main failings were rash action without mature thought, a tendency towards political intrigue and absolute inability to keep his mouth shut. However, in fairness to him it must be said that his sincerity, honesty, and devotion to duty have never been questioned in any quarter. This is important because, while Sheridan failed in Iran, the affair has left no great stain on the almost unbroken favorable record of our advisers in Iran. . . . The functions of the Ministry of Food have been transferred to the Ministry of Finance and are under the supervision of Dr. Millspaugh. Mr. J. Forrest Crawford, who has been loaned by the Foreign Service Auxiliary Service, is temporarily in charge of these activities pending the arrival of Colonel Speaks, who is to head the Ministry of Finance Food Department.

The situation looked more promising at the onset of the 1943 harvest. Thorold to Jernegan on June 3, 1943 (Letter, 891.24/447-6/7):

> We are informed from Tehran that by June 1st 3,279 tons of Soviet wheat had arrived at Tehran and a further 2,000 tons were reported to have arrived at Caspian ports. The total stock of grain in the Tehran silo on the same date was 7,112 tons. I think we can feel therefore that the wheat position is decidedly more hopeful, but a new appreciation is now being got out by MESC and from past experience I do not think we can afford to sit back and regard our problem as solved!

Dreyfus on June 5, 1943 (Telegram 583, 891.24/449):

> Iranian wheat crop prospects are excellent. While plantings were perhaps 10% below the average higher yields will probably produce a crop above normal. Barring unforeseen circumstances I do not believe that it will be necessary to import wheat into Iran during crop year which begins in July.

Millspaugh's takeover of food matters added to the optimism. On July 20, 1943, the Executive Director of MESC, accompanied by Hayter of the British Embassy, met with Murray, Alling, Merriam, and Jernegan (Memorandum, 891.24/472):

> Commander Jackson, who had very recently arrived from Cairo and expected to return within a few days, said that the general supply posi-

tion in the Middle East had improved somewhat. Arrangements to meet the basic needs of most of the territories were pretty well in hand. . . . Iran, Commander Jackson said, was considered the prime problem of the entire area and was being given the most earnest consideration by the MESC. Its immediate importance was twofold, as a supply route to Russia and as the source of the petroleum products needed for the Allied forces in India and elsewhere. Both were vital and both could be safeguarded only by preventing collapse in Iran. During the past year, Iran's economy had been maintained and starvation avoided only by the narrowest of margins. At one point the situation had been saved only by the diversion to the Persian Gulf of 20,000 tons of grain destined for the Red Sea. In the end, partially thanks to the Russian shipment of 25,000 tons to Tehran, the food needs of the country had been barely met, but Commander Jackson felt that it was most unwise to operate so close to the borderline. He felt that it was short-sighted to take risks of this kind merely for the sake of saving two or three ships for other uses, and he intended to press this point in London on his way back to Cairo. For the coming year, he hoped the Ministry of War Transport and the War Shipping Administration would take a more liberal view, especially since the general shipping position was improving.

The new harvest in Iran was promising to be very large, more than 2,000,000 tons, Commander Jackson explained. Of this, the Iranian Government must gain control of 350,000 tons, in order to assure the supply of the cities until the next harvest. This could not be done, MESC felt, by any rigid, elaborate plan of organization and the promulgation of decrees; the administrative machine in Iran was too weak. The only possibility was to send out as many good men, as soon as possible, into the countryside to buy grain before it disappeared into hoards or was smuggled across into neighboring countries. Mr. Sheridan was not following this policy as yet, but Dr. Millspaugh agreed that it was the proper one. It might appear economically and commercially an unsound procedure, but it was the only practical one MESC could visualize under the circumstances. If it were adopted energetically, Commander Jackson believed, Iran could be self-sufficient in food during the coming year, even if no large quantities of grain should be obtained from the Soviet-occupied areas.

Commander Jackson spoke repeatedly of Dr. Millspaugh as the key man and the main hope of stability in Iran. He said that MESC was in close touch with him and was prepared to give him everything he asked for in the way of supplies and believed it would be possible to provide as much as Millspaugh could receive and distribute under his new economic powers. Mr. Murray said that the Department was very glad to hear this, that we agreed as to the vital importance of Dr. Millspaugh in the Iranian picture. We ourselves were doing everything to assist him and welcomed the interest and support of the British. Together, we should be able to carry the day, whereas alone we might not. In this connection, Commander Jackson emphasized the importance of solving the immediate financial difficulty of the Iranian Government. He said he had had a conversation with Mr. Bernstein of the Treasury on this subject and was glad to learn that the problem was receiving attention. He was also glad to hear that additional American assistants for Dr. Millspaugh were being sent out, including a man (Lieutenant Colonel Speaks) to replace Sheridan in charge of the food administration.

With respect to supplies other than food in Iran, Commander Jackson said that the oil shortage at Tehran had been relieved, he thought cotton piece goods and sugar would come forward satisfactorily, and with the end of the grain shortage, railroad shipping space would become available to move other miscellaneous non-food articles. . . . Mr. Murray and Mr. Jernegan asked whether he could give any explanation of the reiterated Iranian complaints against MESC, especially the charges that Iran was not given equal treatment with other territories. Commander Jackson said that this complaint was common to all the territories, each one being convinced that its neighbors were better treated, and he could state positively that there was no discrimination against Iran.

Commander Jackson spoke of the attitude of General Connolly, head of the Persian Gulf Service Command, whose policy in general seemed to ignore the civilian situation in Iran. Commander Jackson felt that MESC and British and American Legations at Tehran should make a determined effort to enlist the interest of General Connolly in Iranian problems, through a gradual process of education in the relationship of those problems to the unimpeded movement of supplies to Russia. He cited one case in which diversion of civilian oil supplies to military movements had resulted in a stoppage of power and industrial plants in Tehran and had ultimately forced an equal diversion of military transport to replenish civilian stocks, thus nullifying the original gain to the military movements. He also spoke of the danger to the whole Allied position, military as well as political, if there should be a real internal collapse in Iran.

> Mr. Murray spoke of the Russian attitude, which was not only uncooperative but indicated possible ambitions in the country. Speaking personally, Commander Jackson expressed the opinion that the Soviets were much interested in the demonstration being provided of the utility to them of a warm-water port on the Persian Gulf, where supplies could be received the year round. He made no suggestions, however, regarding British or American policy toward the Soviets in Iran. The relations between the British and American authorities in Iran, Commander Jackson said, appeared to have improved, although he felt that there was still room for greater understanding and cooperation. Mr. Murray closed the conversation by asking Commander Jackson to keep the Department fully informed of problems as they developed, in order that we might be in a position to lend our support and have data upon which to base our representations to other agencies.

In the above conversation, Commander Jackson of the MESC claims that there had been no famine and that "starvation had been avoided" in Iran. In chapter 8 it was noted that in the consideration of Iran's request for the typhus vaccine, American and British officials had claimed that there had been no unusual incidence of typhus in the country. The next two chapters provide a documentary account of the famine and the typhus epidemic, thereby debunking these claims.

Chapter 22

The Famine of 1942-1943: A Documentary Account

Economic conditions deteriorated due to the disruption of foreign trade after the outbreak of war in September 1939, and the food situation was already precarious even before the Anglo-Russian occupation of Iran in August 1941.[1] At the time, the British had announced with much fanfare that they were bringing food to the people. An Associated Press report dated August 25, 1941, is entitled, "British Carrying Food for the People of Iran." It reads in part: "Simla, India, Aug. 25 (AP)—The British troops entering Iran are carrying food supplies for the populace, British sources said today, because the country is reported in a state of near-famine from heavy German food requisitioning, presumably for storage." "Britain sending Iran Wheat, Sugar," is the title of a piece in the *Montreal Star* issue of December 4, 1941 (MID-Iran, 4220):

> Tehran, Iran, Dec.2—Delayed—(U.P.)—Great Britain expects to send Iran (Persia) 40,000 tons of wheat and 20,000 tons of sugar this year, a British Legation spokesman said today. He said Britain had already sent 13,000 tons of wheat, and that Iran's supplies were expected to be "adequate." Although Iran is normally a wheat producer, the current shortage was blamed on exports to Germany under a barter agreement and general hoarding arising from a lack of confidence in the former government.

Reports in *Journal de Tehran*

A 1942 Office of Strategic Services (OSS) report contains translated excerpts from *Journal de Tehran* from December 1941 to the summer of

1942. Although the paper attempts to reassure a nervous public, the reports paint a picture of rising scarcity and anxiety. On the "Problem of Provisions" the issues of December 2-26, 1941:

> Hitherto Iran has been free to trade with all countries. Commercial and economic relations with the West were maintained even during World War I. Today she can no longer trade with belligerent countries. . . . During the last ten years we have very stupidly exchanged our wheat, wool, leather, cereals and fruits for machinery and implements which are of no help to the country. The whole country is suffering from urbanization. Agriculture is not only the real source of our wealth but also the source of our food.

It adds:

> In order to insure the sale of food at reasonable prices in Tehran the municipality has decided to establish the following temporary markets. . . . In order to diminish the sales prices of food and to fix a standard rate the municipality has also decided to open in various sections of Tehran twenty stores for the retail sale of food. These stores will put at the disposal of the public food which has been purchased at a slightly higher price.

Contagious diseases were on the rise:

> In order to prevent the spreading of smallpox and other contagious diseases the Minister of Health has installed sixteen dispensaries for free vaccination in Tehran. Vaccines have also been distributed in the hospitals and dispensaries. Parents are invited to bring their children to one of these institutions. Each child must possess a certificate proving that he has been vaccinated. The parents of an unvaccinated child will be held responsible and be prosecuted.

A British army telegraphic "Situation Report," dated October 28, 1941, reads (MID-Iran, 6910):

> Kermanshah. Serious food riot morning 27th October due to Tehran Govt order raising prices wheat; consequent rise price of bread. Persian troops fired and used armoured cars believed 6 dead. Proclamation issued by General Sharbakte that price of bread would not be raised and no wheat transferred until need of own district assured.

The *Journal* writes:

> Recently the population of Kermanshah and Hamadan have been very anxious about the transportation of wheat from these regions to other towns, and certain rumors have been circulating to the effect that the British authorities have been buying this wheat for their armed forces. According to the Minister of Finance this suspicion is unjustified since the British received during November 14,174 tons of wheat from India and in the course of the next few months 90,000 tons are expected. During 1939 the Department of Kermanshah sent to other regions 28,100 tons and in 1940, 28,800 tons, and in 1941, 6,600 tons and in the same year Hamadan sent to various regions 11,800 tons of wheat.

The paper also claims that "Several tons of sugar have been distributed among the population of Bandar-Gaz," and that "During last week 3,000 bags of sugar have been received at Bandar Abbas from India. This sugar was sent to Yezd and Kermanshah."

The issues of December 27, 1941 to January 9, 1942, indicate that the situation was fast deteriorating, attempts to reassure the people notwithstanding:

> The Tehran silo has a capacity of 65,000 tons and when it was constructed they hoped to have sufficient supplies for one year; actually it only provides for ten months on account of the increase in Tehran's population. There should be no further anxiety about the bread supply. Especially as wheat is brought regularly from India and there is bread enough in Tehran until the next harvest. It has been suggested that the Minister of Finance, who is concerned with the problem of wheat supply, should also organize an association of bakers in order to insure a superior quality of bread. During the last few years, seven silos were built. Unfortunately on account of the war only three were completed and contain the following (capacities): Tehran, 65,000 tons; Tabriz, 16,000 tons; and Isfahan, 16,000 tons. The most important silo is at Tehran. There are three threshing machines and 202 cylinders each 22 meters high with a capacity of 65,000 tons. The mill began to function as soon as the silo was completed. At the beginning the consumption was only 100 tons in 24 hours. Thanks to recent technical improvements the capacity was raised to 640 tons and today assures bread for the whole of Tehran. (Dec. 10, '41). . . . The municipality has also ordered several head of cattle and believe that Tehran will have sufficient supply of butcher meat for the coming winter. . . . In regard to

> the question of food supply energetic steps have been taken and there is now plenty of bread. News from Bushire states that 12,000 tons of sugar ordered from India have just arrived at Bushire. The sugar will be for sale at 4 rials per kilo. Further news states that three merchant ships laden with sugar and wheat have arrived at Bushire and unloaded 30,120 bags of sugar and 16,000 bags of wheat. It was announced that two or three more boatloads of wheat will arrive shortly.

It soon became clear that the cited import figures had no foundation in facts.

The issues of January 10-23, 1942, had continued with the optimistic tone while announcing sugar rationing:

> It was proposed by the Minister of Economics and approved by the Council of Ministers that rice should be imported for the needs of the population of the south and the necessary authorization will be given to persons to carry out the distribution. It is reported from Bandar Abbas that a ship has arrived with a cargo of 20,820 bags of sugar which arrived on the 16th of January. It is now being unloaded. Another ship brought 200 bags of wheat. From tomorrow, January 12 until January 26, sugar coupons will be given to the heads of families in each district. . . . From today the sale of Indian prints and white linen and of shirt material will be undertaken under certain conditions. Each person will receive a coupon for the purchase of linen amounting to a sufficient quantity for three months.

From the issues of February 1-16, 1942:

> A ban on the export of cattle was proposed by the Ministry of Agriculture and approved by the Council of Ministers. Between December 22, 1941 and January 5, 1942, Iran ordered approximately 35,000 cases of tea from India. The prices were said to have remained quite reasonable. In view of the lack of paper for newspapers and other paper material in current use, the economic section of the Ministry of Finance sent an order to Canada for 2,000 tons of paper of different qualities.

The paper adds:

> After extensive discussions, the Ministry of Public Health has approved the decision to distribute medicine free for the poor and the needy, the costs to be taken from the "Imperial Gift." Distribution will begin in

Tehran on February 21 and in the Districts on March 21. It was proposed by the Ministries of Industry, Mines and Commerce, and decreed by the Council of Ministers, that the sum for imports of pharmaceutical products should be increased by four million rials for the current year.

From the issues of February 17-23, 1942:

It was announced that a ship has arrived with a cargo of 45,000 bags of sugar. It has already been unloaded and placed in the warehouse. At the request of the Ministries of Commerce, Industry and Mines and the Council of Ministers it has been decreed that dates may be imported free of duty and that an added sum of 80,000,000 rials will be placed on the importation of tea (the total import for the year will be 200,000,000 rials). It has also been decreed that threads of all sort may be imported with the exception of that of natural silk (authorization will be given to those interested on request).

From the issues of February 28 - March 13, 1942:

It is noted that all kinds of vegetables are being planted in peoples' private gardens in order to help the general shortage. . . . It is announced that recently 35,000 sacks of wheat and 10,000 sacks of sugar arrived in Bushire and have been unloaded. In addition, the *Baharestan* landed 2,028 cases of various merchandise, particularly cloth. A ship has unloaded 5,624 bags of powdered sugar in Bandar Abbas. The Iranians, according to tradition, will celebrate No-Ruz again this year. . . . The Minister of Finance is engaged in talks with USSR commercial representatives for the sale of certain amount of rice to Russia in exchange for the purchase of Soviet wheat. These talks are going through the Soviet commercial attaché, and an agreement has already been reached. . . . The price of imported pharmaceutical products has become so high that the Minister of Health decided to facilitate the preparation of certain of these products from supplies existing in Iran.

In the issues of July 1- 24, 1942, the optimistic pretense had vanished:

Rationing in the suburbs. In the suburbs of Ghar and Fechavoyeh until July 13, 15,261 coupons had been distributed to 3,134 families; at Varamine 43,992 coupons had been given out among 10,087 families. Distribution of coupons is almost completed in the suburbs. The population can help the municipality by refusing to buy any foodstuff at a higher rate than the fixed price and by notifying the Municipality by telephone when this occurs. This is the duty incumbent on every citizen of Iran to help regulate the cost of living. . . . The Ministry of Public Health has appointed Dr. Taghi Majlessi as supervisor of a committee appointed to prevent people from hoarding pharmaceutical products in their homes as there is a general shortage. . . . Dr. Nasser Akhtarnejat, specialist in children's diseases will give free care and necessary treatment to poor children.

On the food situation in the provinces:

Bread situation in Ahwaz. News from Ahwaz states that the bread situation is still very bad since July 7, (a week ago) no baker has received any flour and the population finds itself in a very difficult situation. Many people have left the town and taken refuge elsewhere. . . . Bread at Shiraz. Bakers are now working regularly. The quantity of bread has improved and there is plenty of it; the price of sale has been fixed at two rials per kilogram. A telegram has been received from Shiraz saying that a group of proprietors gathered at the house of Mr. Mohammad Hassan Behbahani to discuss relief for the poor. As a result they decided to give three hundred tons of wheat to insure food for the poor and needy. . . . Bread in Arak. Thanks to financial aid by generous persons four new bakeries have been opened in the crowded sections of Arak. 4,000 special coupons have been distributed to the poor who will receive daily three kilos of bread priced at two rials. . . . Situation in Semnan. In view of the difficulties entailed in obtaining bread and the delay in the delivery of rationed goods the population has ceased work and installed itself at the Post Office in protest of its treatment. The store houses (silos) are almost empty and the situation in Semnan and the surrounding country is not very good. . . . Resht. Lately discontent has been growing in Resht over the rise in cost of living. This has been due to hoarding by the tradesmen. The exorbitant price of rice has particularly incited the population to raid certain store houses. Many persons were wounded. The Department of Finance of Resht has proceeded to distribute rice among the population and the authorities have quieted the people. . . . Amul. The people will buy rice at four rials for three kilos whereas on the free market it costs ten rials. Coupons for sugar, cloth, cigarettes and matches have been distributed.

Reports by Military Attachés and Intelligence Agencies

In October 1942, Colonel H. Norman Schwarzkopf, the American Adviser to the Iranian Gendarmerie, had traveled from Tehran to Khuzestan. His report, forwarded by US Military Attaché, Major John G. Ondrick, is dated October 20, 1942 (MID-Iran, 4540). Ondrick writes: "Herewith report of Colonel Schwarzkopf's observations during a trip south of Tehran. I consider the report factual." Excerpts from this informative report follow:

> Along the northern portion of the route there is rather expansive irrigation and relatively good crops of wheat, melons and alfalfa. Grazing is pretty good and there are reasonably sized flocks of sheep and goats. One hundred kilometers south of Tehran the country is quite arid, no wheat is to be found, but some barley is grown. The price of bread is very high. . . . Around Mashkabad crops have been good but there is much hoarding; the same applies in the vicinity of Shahzand. In Arak crops have been good but again there is considerable hoarding and no movement of produce out of the area. South of there crops have been reported to have been poor and prices are very high. Many villages have barely food enough for the natives and gendarmes report that it is not possible to buy any food locally. The natives in the south are in a state of existence rather than living. . . . In the southern areas the Arabs appear to be struggling for existence alone. The people are dirty, half starved, ragged, lazy and diseased. Many blind people and more evidence of trachoma, infantile paralysis, club feet and "solak" were seen than in any part of the country visited so far. In conference with local sheiks it developed that the Arab tribes are suffering from a lack of food supplies and a lack of water and that many depredations that occur are caused by hunger rather than by maliciousness or avarice. In this area women were often seen in the desert gathering tufts of grass and carrying them to villages beyond the horizon. . . . An impression of general underfeeding was obtained all along the route and particularly in the south, and the availability and distribution of potable water is quite a problem. Much of the personal uncleanliness and much lack of sanitation is directly traceable to the meagerness of the water supply. There is a general lack of fuel, coal being very scarce, wood hard to obtain and small and infrequent in quantity. Many sections were seen where no wheat was available and where barley was being used for baking bread. Where wheat was available the price of bread was

> around 15 rials a kilo. The price a year ago was from 2 to 2½ rials per kilo. This situation is particularly aggravating because of the low wages paid. A gendarme normally eats from one to two kilos of bread a day but his entire ration allowance for a day is only 4 rials. The effects of such prices and such shortage is evident in the condition of the people.

Not surprisingly, the memory of the Great Famine of 1917-1919 had weighed heavily on the minds of the people. An OSS report dated November 28, 1942, reads (891.00/1975½):

> From a confidential source in Tehran this agency has received reports, dated November 18 to 26, 1942, reading as follows: "The spectre of famine as remembered in the last war alarmed the public which has no confidence in the current cabinet. The latter is popularly believed to be subject to Allied dictation. . . . There exists declining desire to hold banknotes and there are daily rises in prices of all types of goods. Believe there is limited hoarding of foodstuffs general among all but preponderant among the poor. The British seem determined to coddle the Poles at all costs in order to use Poland as a buffer state after the war. It has been reported that there have been large purchases of foodstuffs for the Poles here and British Army at Qum against the wishes of the Iranians and American food adviser."

Another OSS report dated December 11, 1942 (MID-Iran, 3110):

> From a confidential source in Cairo this agency has received a report, dated December 10, 1942, reading as follows: "On the Iran black market prices are almost fantastic. Loaves of bread (sell at) four times the price of last week. The price of butter is 10 shillings per pound. Restaurants sell white bread and fancy cream cakes in the meantime. . . . From 3:00 a.m. crowds form bread lines and women are trampled and beaten around the shops by disorganized mobs. Soldiers and police have neither the ability nor the will to establish orderly lines."

An OSS report entitled, "Southern Supply Route to USSR," dated November 23, 1943 (MID-Iran, 4810):

> The large majority of Iranians are ill-clothed and ill-fed. Their diet of bread, cheese, sour milk and fruit, with an occasional rice dish containing mutton or fowl, is basically healthy but for the poor there is never enough of it. . . . During 1942 the food conditions in many

> districts in Iran were lamentable due to the heavy demands made upon food supplies by the occupying armies and hoarding of cereals by the Iranians themselves. In some districts, especially Kerman, Lur and Teheran itself, many people died of starvation and during that winter deaths from typhus were at the rate of 4,000 per month, a direct result of lowered vitality on account of malnutrition.

A Naval Attaché report on "Political and Economic Trends in Iran," dated February 22, 1943 (MID-Iran, 4220):

> The prices of foodstuffs have steadily been rising, and the people are becoming desperate which state may result in riots. At Shiraz and Isfahan minor riots have already broken out. The shortage and the quality of the bread in Tehran is causing great discontent. Often bread queues of 300 impatient people are seen, and many have been seen waiting at 0330 hours. Before the end of January 2,500 tons were delivered to the Persian Government out of 25,000 tons of cereals originally promised to meet their needs for the first eight months of 1943. . . . The prosperity of the Russian-occupied zone evidenced by plentiful food at low prices is the result of Russian restrictions on exports to other parts of Persia, but less favored provinces which normally rely on certain supplies from that area suffer therefrom.

A Persian Gulf Service Command (PGSC) report of February 26, 1943 (MID-Iran, 3115): "The Tehran silo has been running with no margin at all most of the time and some days has had to borrow wheat from other stores in order to issue the allotted 250 tons per day. The situation in Kerman is particularly bad." PGSC report of March 3, 1943 (MID-Iran, 4220):

> The total food situation continues unrelieved. Bahrain Island is facing genuine starvation. The Island produces less than half of its cereal supply and transport from India has ceased. Stocks of rice are about exhausted. In Iran prices of foodstuffs are rising in the provinces to equal those of Tehran. In spite of excellent rains, there is no sign of relief until the fall harvest.

A Naval Attaché report dated March 5, 1943 (MID-Iran, 5940):

> Tehran is still on the verge of starvation and the daily death rate has trebled. A complete breakdown of bread supply has been averted by

> good luck than by management and the bread issued is almost uneatable. At Sultanabad wheat supplies are at the point of exhaustion. In Meshed there has been an influx to the town of hungry villagers, causing a shortage of Government bread supplies and demonstrations against the authorities for having failed to issue tea, sugar and cloth rations for the past month. In Maragheh (Azerbaijan) there have been disorders.

A Middle East Intelligence Center (MEIC, a British agency) report for March 13-20, 1943 (MID-Iran, 4220):

> Owing to unprecedented frosts and snow, grain supplies from the south and Iraq have been held up en route and, as a result, the expected improvement in the food situation has not come about, or at any rate not to anything like the extent hoped for. In Tehran, it is true, there has been a "slight improvement," but deaths from starvation are not uncommon in other parts of the country. The Tehran improvement appears to be attributable to the Russians who, most unexpectedly, sent many wagons of wheat down from Gurgan. This may have been a last-minute attempt to save the Qavam Government, but unfortunately it had already fallen the day before the supplies started to arrive.

Naval Attaché in Cairo on "Political and Economic Trends in Iran," March 21, 1943 (MID-Iran, 2810): "The anti-Allied feeling in the press has not changed. It is apparent that by 'Allies' is meant 'Great Britain,' and some papers even go to the limit of stating that the Iranians should have resisted Britain to the last man as death in battle is believed to be preferable to slow starvation." MID report, March 27, 1943 (File 5970):

> The food situation in Northern Iran continues to deteriorate. Much suffering and death by starvation have been reported. The attitude of the population is now passive, as compared to a former riotous tendency, but such passivity may well be physical, as a result of starvation. The situation has dangerous elements.

PGSC report, April 10, 1943 (MID-Iran, 5940):

> The food situation in Northern Iran continues to deteriorate, with indications of far more serious results. There have been a number of deaths from starvation and some serious rioting. Indications are that rioting may increase substantially. Under these conditions subversive elements may be expected to take every opportunity to foster trouble.

An interview with Phillip Connor Kidd, April 23, 1943 (MID-Iran, 9900):

> Mr. Kidd represented Lend-Lease, State Dept., and the US Commercial Co., which implements Lend-Lease. He was in control of commercial road transport. 1. Iran has a population of 15,000,000. The Iranian Government has no authority outside of Teheran, and damned little inside it; the only security is in the zone occupied by the Russians. British armed guards are necessary along much of transportation route. The second famine of the war is imminent; there is always hunger and people dying of hunger, but this wide spread famine is of far wider and greater scope. Both the Russians and the US are supplying wheat but not in sufficient extent. There are between 17,000-23,000 Poles in Iran. . . . The diet of the Poles is higher than the diet of civilians in Britain, and includes white bread. This is a source from which serious trouble will inescapably develop unless the Poles are sent out of the country; the removal of refugees however, at a time when transportation facilities—never good—are over-strained with the movement of military supplies, presents a tremendous problem. 2. There are 8,000 trucks per month transporting materials across Iran; this is expected to expand to 12,000 per month, all of course, transporting to Russia.

An OSS report for July 1943 (Report 42416):

> Prices still show no signs of normal and expected seasonal decline. Rice has actually advanced considerably in price—four times the price of last summer. Free sugar is still two dollars a pound and cooking fat unchanged. Fruit is ten times the price of last summer. The general public has serious doubts as to the ability of the government to collect the current harvest of grain and rice and people believe that the coming winter will be more difficult than last year.

A Combined Intelligence Center Iraq (CICI, British agency) report, August 30, 1943 (MID-Iran, 4220):

> A reliable observer has expressed the opinion that there may be a grave deterioration in the food situation by October, possibly reaching famine level. There is little indication that the Government scheme of buying wheat will achieve its purpose; so far, of the excellent crop harvested this year only about 16,000 tons have reached Government

> granaries and of this 8,000 tons were collected in Khuzistan. It is reported in the Press that 320,000 tons would suffice for the year.

An OSS report, September 18, 1943 (MID-Iran, 4220): "It is reliably reported that British authorities are this week 9/18 buying two hundred thousand (200,000) tons of barley at I.D. 25,000 per ton and storing it in Iraq." An OSS report dated September 28, 1943 (Report A 12083, 891.00/2066-1/2):

> Most Iranians lay the chief blame for soaring prices on the advent of the Allied armies, with their buying of materials and supplies. An exception: the American command is credited with bringing in 90% of its food supplies. The greatest present hardship in the country is the high price of food and necessities, as against the (still) low scale of pay of government and other employees.

An OSS report by Lowe and Grant dated November 25, 1943 (report 79, 891.00/2075):

> It is reported that the value of real estate in Teheran has dropped 30%. The explanation given by the bankers is said to be that the Iranians anticipate the end of the war and believe at that time the present enormously swollen values will collapse. It is said that the cost of foodstuffs has dropped but our own experience has not borne that out. Eggs increased in price last week, now costing 6 cents. I was offered a fair sized cauliflower for 90 cents. A kilo of lamb costs 1.50 dollars. A 12-15 lb. turkey costs 12 dollars. White bread remains 30 cents for a half pound loaf. The very high cost of charcoal, largely used by the poorer people for heating in the winter, has made its use prohibitive. It is likely that this winter will see intense suffering among the poor (most of the population) and an increase in sickness.

"Suffering of the Masses"

The terrible conditions are further captured in Dreyfus' cable of April 21, 1943 (Telegram 409, 891.00/2009):

> Iran appears to be on the verge of another political crisis. Large part of bazaars closed yesterday afternoon and there is some uneasiness in city although no riots have occurred. Closing of bazaars is widely regarded as protest of merchants and politicians against passage of Millspaugh

> powers bill (my 385, April 14) which was to be considered yesterday by Majlis and which had already been approved by Majlis Finance Committee. It protests the passage of legislation which represents only hope of country in order that vested interests of merchant profiteers and corrupt political elements may prevail over common welfare. Suffering of the masses because of high prices has reached an unbearable pitch. Meat if it can be found costs several dollars a pound; pound sugar in black market costs $2. This suffering is a result a result of unbridled greed and cannot be corrected until government takes strongest of measures. General Ahmadi, who by decree of Council of Ministers of April 17 became military governor, has published proclamation asking commerce to reopen, calling attention to provision of existing law, ordering curfew at nine and warning public that strong measures to protect public interest will be taken. I am convinced Iran is headed for disaster unless a government strong enough to cope with entrenched classes can be instituted. Such a government might consist of a trinity of power—Millspaugh to make necessary regulations—a strong Prime Minister to put them into effect and a War Minister like General Ahmadi to enforce them on pain of summary and capital punishment.

The situation of the under paid government employees is described by Dreyfus in a report of June 30, 1943 (Dispatch 594 and Enclosure, 891.5018/27):

> I have the honor to enclose for the information of the Department a translation furnished to the Legation by Dr. A.C. Millspaugh, Administrator General of the Finances for the Iranian Government, of a petition presented to the Shah and other important Iranian Government Officials, including the Administrator General of the Finances himself, as well as to four of the local newspapers. Even in the poor translation given the petition presents a deeply moving picture of the bitter hardships still being undergone by these lower-paid employees in spite of the solemn undertaking of the United Nations to provide "minimum essential needs" for Iran. There is no reason to think that the picture is in the slightest degree overpainted. With the cost of living, recently increased more than 1,000%, in large measure owing to the inroads on food and necessities of life by Allied armed forces, Poles and others for whom Iran cannot properly be held responsible, as well as the rigid control by the Allies of Foreign imports to replace these necessities of which the country has been denuded, conditions for the poor have become indeed tragic.

The petition addressed to "H.M. Pahlevi, the Majless, the Minister of Finance, the Administrator General of the Finances, and newspapers *Hour*, *Towfigh*, *Baba Shemal*, and *Ettelaat*," provides an excellent example of the use of famine by the British to gain legitimacy for the Pahlavi regime. After the downfall of Reza Shah Iranians were given a "New Deal" of which punishment for Reza Shah's collaborators and restitution to his victims were integral parts.[2] With famine and the struggle for survival, the New Deal was forgotten and the Reza Shah era came to be remembered by many as a "golden age" in which the people had ample bread. This, of course, brought added legitimacy to his son and successor. As soon as economic conditions had improved in 1944, there was a resumption of demand for punishing Reza Shah's henchmen, and his prison executioner, the notorious "Physician" Ahmadi, was promptly hanged and others were given prison terms.[3] The petition reads:

> We employees that are receiving between Rls. 1000 and 1500 monthly salary have to pay about Rls. 400 for rent and with the rest we have to maintain a large family. For two years we have stand all the pressure of life and due to ever increasing of the cost of living we have sold whatever we could, and now nothing is left. Up to now we have not said anything, but now we like to inform you that we cannot continue any longer. Our children do not get proper food, they are weak and pale because they do not get butter and milk. We cannot feed them with 200 grams bread, they crying out day and night for food, and for fruit we have to show them the picture of it. What is this tragic and disastrous life that we and our children are having, and what is the fault of these children? Why no one cares for us? The 5% children's allowance is not even sufficient for one sickness case of a child. Since three months we do not get even that little rice which we used to get, why do we not get rice? Why should we and our family be hungry? We are not belonging to this country? We are fed up, and we cannot stand the present miserable life. Unexperienced young men are drawing good salaries, and also those who are having grade six and upwards. These fortunate employees are getting everything, but we have to do the heavy duties and at the same time die of hunger. You statesmen must know that the groan of our children will vanish you and your families as well. You must understand that we are not asking luxury, radio and automobile from you, whatever we want from you is but food and clothing. You have withheld these two things from us! God may grant you same miserable life so that you may know too the taste of it. We will vanish ourselves and family, because it is better to die

> sooner and not gradually. It is no justice that you should have everything, and we should have nothing and at the same time be hungry. We want bread from you and cheap living and not radio, etc. Almighty God may send back Reza Shah Pahlavi for us. This is our petition No. 1 and if you do not consider our case, we and our family are to die, and the whole world will know that we vanish because of being hungry. On behalf of 286 employees of Tehran.

Letters from Tehran

Under the provisions of the Tripartite Treaty of Alliance of January 29, 1942, the British and the Russians had imposed mail censorship. Fortunately, the British Censor in Tehran had provided the US Military Intelligence Division (MID) periodic reports of its actions and excerpts from the seized mail. These letters provide a telling account of conditions in Iran in World War II. An Iranian in Tehran writing to his son in America on May 27, 1942, writes (MID-Iran, 5970):

> The British authorities . . . import wheat from India, but this is sufficient for Teheran only, whereas the other regions are in dire need of bread. A good crop is expected this year, but our Government is much too weak to seize it, and to distribute it evenly among the whole population. The Persian people are utterly helpless, there are no capable men to manage for them. In the last 20 years all capable politicians have been killed, poisoned or have rotted away in prison. We have no people to turn to. . . .

From an Iranian writer in Tehran, on July 7, 1942 (MID-Iran, 5970): "It (the war) brought us nothing but misery and is going to bring us hunger that I hope not. We have still sufficient food stuff but I am afraid it won't be long that we will have the shortage of many things."

Arthur C. Boyce of the American Mission, Tehran, had written numerous letters to his friends, all of which had apparently been intercepted by the British Censor in Tehran (MID-Iran, 5970). Several letters are addressed to friends in Collinsville, Illinois, dated July 14, 1942. To Mrs. Charles Leech he writes:

> Everyone is worried over the bad prospects for food and fuel in the fall. . . . In some sections there was little rain and there is shortage of wheat for that and other reasons. . . . The Government seems helpless to control prices. Teheran is overcrowded, people think it is safer to be

here if anything happens. . . . There might be more chance of order in the capital than other small places, but the food situation would be worse here.

To Mr. A. Baghamian:

We are having a time of high prices the like of which Iran has never known. The prices are due to a variety of things—war conditions, presence of foreign troops and refugees and more than anything else I believe, profiteering. The Government seems powerless to control any prices.

To Miss Potter:

We fear food shortages in the fall and winter for the wheat crop is less than usual. For a year prices have been constantly rising until the situation is really impossible for the poor even though a day laborer who got two krans in your days gets 12-15 a day now. . . . I think the biggest reason for the prices is profiteering and the Government seems helpless, but of course war conditions, influx of people from outside etc. all have a bearing on the matter. In the Spring, 12,000 Polish refugees from Russia were moved here. They are in a camp out Doshan Tappe way.

To Mr. and Mrs. Kermani:

There is a curfew which keeps people off the streets after 11 p.m. There is a terrible shortage of tires and it is getting more and more difficult and expensive to travel. . . . There are no troops in Teheran itself, but one sees many British officers, mechanics, drivers etc. connected with transportation—Indian drivers and many Poles in uniform. . . .

Boyce on July 16, 1942, to Dr. and Mrs. S.M. Jordan, c/o Dr. J.L. Dodds, 156 Fifth Avenue, New York (MID-Iran, 5970):

Iran is surely between two claws which may pinch us any time but there seems nothing to do but hold on. In any case, indications point to something like famine conditions the coming winter. There was very little rain in some places, and the wheat crop is less than usual. Transportation is getting more and more difficult and profiteering is apparently utterly uncontrolled. We have just bought coal at 22 tomans a kharvar, wood at 18, rice at 19 a man, charcoal 42 tomans a kharvar (300 kilos). Roghan (ghee) is actually 14 tomans a man. Fruit is plentiful and beautiful, but grapes, apples, cherries, (over now) keep at 4 to 5 rials a cherek and vegetables at absurd prices. A carriage driver said yesterday that barley is 11 rials a man (3 kilos).

Boyce to Mrs. W.A. Manchee, 108 North Maple Avenue, East Orange, New Jersey, on July 17, 1942 (MID-Iran, 4630):

Everyone is worried over the prospects of food and fuel shortage this fall. Transportation is getting worse and worse because of shortage of tires, that and profiteering seem to be the chief factors in the situation which is very bad indeed. At present we can get almost everything in the food line for sky-high prices, fuel is more difficult. We have just bought coal (soft) at about $25 per ton. . . .

Letter from Tehran on July 19, 1942 (MID-Iran, 5970):

Living in Teheran is becoming impossible with the prices of everything soaring sky high. The barest necessities of life cost a fortune and prices are 3 to 4 times higher than they were a few months ago. Bread is difficult to obtain and unless you go at a certain time you get no bread at all.

Letter from Rasht, July 12 and 19, 1942:

The sugar situation is rather acute in Resht now. I had none in the home this morning but am hoping to secure some today. . . . There was a bit of trouble in Resht on Thursday afternoon over rice. This has gone up to an absurd price and supplies are short in the Bazaar. A crowd raided some warehouses and helped themselves. Some shops were also looted and at night the Bazaar was all shut up. . . .

G. Lynn Browning, American Mission, Rasht, to George Browning, Park College, Parkville, Kentucky, on August 26, 1943 (MID-Iran, 4220):

Prices, instead of dropping a bit when the new (rice) crop comes in, have actually gone up and now are twice what they were five months ago. Since rice is almost the sole food of this region, I don't see how people are going to live through the winter.

Imperial Bank of Iran, Rasht, to the London office, September 20, 1943 (MID-Iran, 5060):

> Little rice has been moved from Guilan except by the government owing to various restrictions, but the total crops of tobacco, silk and tea have been bought up by the Government Monopolies and dispatched. . . . The lower classes appear to be extremely poor and there are hundreds of beggars on the streets. Discontent with the present cost of foodstuffs and commodities is voiced by all sections of the community. Prices of goods are fantastic and bear little relations to the cost of production.

A.E. Perigal, Tehran, on November 15, 1942, to Mrs. A.E. Perigal, 24 Church Street, Hatfield, England:

> Teheran is a very good shopping centre from what I have seen of it but prices are terribly high. . . . Yesterday, Friday, we all had to stay put in our houses all day as the authorities were taking a census of the town and taking the opportunity at the same time of issuing coupons for bread, sugar and tea.

Paraphrase (by the British Censor) of a letter dated December 7, 1942 (MID-Iran, 4000):

> A minister in Tehran writing to another minister in London states: "Prices don't stop rising; they rise daily. The money is depreciating rapidly. The silver rial which used to be in circulation can now be turned to nine paper rials in the market. In the third place certain articles of vital need are scarce. For bread, for instance, one has to line at the bread shops for two or three hours, and what bread we get in this way is full of grits and very unhealthy to eat. . . . An ordinary loaf of bread for which we used to pay Rls. 3 last year is now being sold for as much as 30 rials and strong measures have not been taken against this black markets and things are daily going from bad to worse."

Letter from Tehran to New York, February 14, 1943 (MID-Iran, 5970):

> The cost of living in Teheran and in other cities of Iran has reached to an incredible point. A pair of lady's shoes costs $187.50, and a pair of men's shoes costs $93.75. One suit of clothes costs about $300. This

will give you an idea about other prices. Bread and other things are rare and are sold at very strange prices.

O. Hempel, 1779 Khiaban Pahlevi, Tehran, to Hedwig Nelson, 1121 N. Tejon Street, Colorado Spring, Colorado, April 9, 1943 (MID-Iran, 5970):

We here do not see or feel the war but for the exorbitant prices. The poor are actually starving, their only food is bread, rationed of course, and for that hundreds are waiting for hours, clamoring, shouting. Whenever I see one of these emaciated figures, I buy him a bread—for people who are willing to pay 4 or 5 times the price, can get as much as they like. On top of this famine, typhus (Flecktyphus) pervades all the town, especially of course the dirty quarters of the poor. Even here, where there is no war, no Hitler, no Jew-baiting I see so much misery that my heart is bleeding for unfortunate people. Prices have risen so high and their earnings, if they can work, are so low, there is nothing for them but to beg and starve and die.

J.D. Payne, American Mission, Tehran, to Lt. Joseph T. Payne, MD, Strong Memorial Hospital, Rochester, New York, August 7, 1943 (MID-Iran, 5970):

Dr. Millspaugh and his staff are trying valiantly to hold prices to the present level and to bring down bread, charcoal and staples. We hope they succeed. The big problem is of course transport because products are not so much more expensive in the provinces and villages than they were a year ago. Cucumbers are rials 1.50 to 2 here in Tehran; they are rials 15 a hundred in Semnan. Typewriter ribbons are quoted in the bazaar at from rials 170 to 200 each, hence the need to use the red side of the ribbon as long as it will give any color. Rajab Ali Khan told us yesterday that he had paid rials 735 for two pairs of shoes for his little boys; they are 7 and 6 years old respectively. Akhtar told me she had to pay rials 1500 to get a good pair. The people are saying that a toman now will barely do what a rial used to do. This is a bit of an exaggeration, as a general statement, but it isn't so far off. It is the exact proportion when applied to the cost of coal and charcoal; people are going over to kerosene which has not been raised but 30%. This is a small increase really, because the cost of transport enters so largely into its price. If Iran did not produce its own kerosene and gasoline I don't know what the country would do.

Alinaghi Mortazi, Tehran, to Mohammad Fakhr Rejai Gilani, c/o Mohammad Ali Farokh Tootoonchi, Karbala, Iraq, September 18, 1943, translated by the British Censor (MID-Iran, 5970):

> It is now so difficult to live that one is never in a mood to write letters to one's friends. I say "difficult" but I do not mean what we used to when we said "difficult" in former days. I do not wish you may understand what it means now. Although this year the harvest was wonderfully rich as it has not been for the last 30 years, and although it is the beginning of the year there are so many people crowded in front of the bakers shops every day that it is impossible to buy any bread. Those who have a big family of ten can obtain bread for four members after hours of waiting and shouting and can take their bitter tears for the rest of the family. And the winter has not come yet. There are still fruits to satisfy the people's hunger. Typhus has not started yet. Still the poor people can live without any fuel. But imagine the winter. Everybody has prepared for death and such a death as last winter to be buried without any wrapping and campher. Never think of coming here. Stay where you are and be happy. I will write some prices of materials for your information and surprise. . . .

Imperial Bank of Iran, Tehran, to Baghdad office, September 26, 1943 (MID-Iran, 5060):

> The transport situation has been temporarily eased by the progressive arrival during the last three months or so, of 900 Lease-Lend trucks for the Iran Government. These trucks, together with many others contracted for locally, are under the control of the Edareh Barbari Rah. Many of the available trucks of this administration have been held in readiness for the transport of cereals from this year's harvest. Unfortunately delivery of cereals have not come forward as readily as was hoped, and this has caused trucks to be withheld from other uses longer than anticipated. The last available figures show that growers have contracted to deliver 200,000 tons of cereals of which so far 40,000 tons have come in.

It adds: "Iran's declaration of a state of war with Germany had been under discussion for some time with the Allies and it was purely fortuitous that the actual notification coincided with news of Italy's surrender."

Famine in Areas under British Occupation

Azerbaijan, Gilan, Mazanderan and northern Khorassan were occupied by Russia and the remaining part, called the "southern zone," was under British occupation. The southern zone was often called "the famine zone." Letter from Sherkat Ghalibafi Kerman (Kerman Rug Weaving Company), Kerman, to Kerman Rug Weavers, Inc., 261 Fifth Avenue, New York, May 9, 1942 (MID-Iran, 5970):

> There is first the food question which makes all contracts illusory. When I wrote you 4 months ago the wheat price was 8 rials a batman, today the poor wretches have to pay almost anything to get a little bread. Even at 14 and 15 rials per batman they cannot get it, and more and more is asked. It is strange, Iran could be one of the happiest countries in the world. Plenty of space, a small frugal population, fertile soil, great mineral riches, etc. and all the same everything is upside down. Well let us hope that this state of affairs will pass! Conditions in this country have gone from bad to worse, and we have to face nothing but difficulties and troubles. To work with a crowd of underfed and hungry weavers is no pleasure. . . . Somehow one has the impression, that in certain quarters one does not care a hang about the working class here, the sooner they die of hunger the better. . . .[4]

Letter from a British resident of Shiraz, June 8, 1942 (MID-Iran, 5970):

> Things have gone up by leaps and bounds and we are having a pretty thin time of it. . . . A lb. packet of tea is now 12/S, so we scarcely have any. Butter is a fabulous price. The British Government does nothing to interfere, but we think eventually they'll have to step in and control prices. The poor folk around us are seen starving. Our trouble is that we haven't the money to buy a fair quantity of stores.

Miss Nightingale, C.M.S. Hospital, Yezd, to Olive Nightingale, Parkside, Henley on Thames, England, June 26, 1942 (MID-Iran, 5970):

> We are quite well aware of a war being on, the prices of everything soaring high. Robbers are out again on all the lonely roads, and stealing flocks from the villages; in Taft which we passed on the way up that week 2,000 sheep had been stolen, the poor people are suffering a great deal. . . .

Letter from an Armenian writer in Isfahan, dated July 1, 1942 (MID-Iran, 5970):

> Here conditions are bad. The Government is going to move from Teheran to Isfahan. The Bakhtiaris have again rebelled and a big army has gone to suppress them. The Bakhtiaris have already made several attacks and a great number of their men were killed. A few soldiers were also killed. Anyhow, the roads are very unsafe for they attack motor cars and steal whatever they find.

Letter from Shiraz, July 7, 1942 (MID-Iran, 5970): "The feeling against Britain is strong, as it is felt that we let the Russians in, who are not likely to leave their section of the country again, despite their promises." From Shiraz on July 19, 1942 (MID-Iran, 5970):

> We are having a very stiff time, dear, financially, and it daily becomes more difficult to manage. We live in a country entirely uncontrolled economically and profiteering, hoarding etc. is quite unchecked. Things are definitely worse since the Russian and British occupation. I feel ashamed to mention it but really it is getting impossible to buy food.

From Isfahan on July 20, 1942:

> Even out of the way mountain villages are suffering indirectly from the war, prices of food and everything else are fabulous. Since the abdication of the previous Shah the robber tribes are out again, they swoop down on the helpless villages and carry off all the flocks, the poor people are suffering a good deal.

From Kerman on July 27, 1942:

> The situation in the grain market is thus, that the Government takes 40% of the harvest from the growers, at prices which are still the same as last year, although the cost of living has in the meantime doubled and tripled. . . . What remains besides what he needs for his own people he of course tries to sell at highest prices. The quantities thus at the disposal are hidden away and only sold slowly, in continually raising prices. . . . The prices they (the village weavers) have to pay are exorbitant. . . . If we do not do anything in this matter, or cannot do anything, we consider the future to be very black. Owners of grain will not stop at present high prices and we should not be surprised if

> we get later on serious troubles. . . . Work will suffer and stop altogether, and we may even have to face riots.

Letter from a British missionary in Shiraz, August 6, 1942 (MID-Iran, 5970):

> The situation in Iran is very difficult now. The entry of foreign troops into the country has occasioned a feeling of resentment and insecurity. Hoarding of food-stuff is on a prodigious scale with the result that cost of living more than twice as much as a year ago, and there is acute scarcity and much economic distress. The British are extremely unpopular because they let the Russians into the country, and also because of the misdeeds and incredible rapacity and aggression of the late Shah are put down to us, who are supposed to have favoured the coup d'état he made.

Mrs. L.G. Griffiths, Isfahan, to Joan and Wendy Griffiths, Victoria, Australia, August 24, 1942 (MID-Iran, 4220):

> Excuse this paper but paper like everything else is getting an awful price. Prices are going up and up every week. Butter is now about 3/6d a pound. I have just made a little jam, but sugar is scarce and awfully expensive so I can't make much. Tea is a terrible price and we very seldom make cakes now because sugar and butter are so expensive.

The censorship files contain numerous letters written by the staff of the Anglo-Iranian Oil Company (AIOC). Letter, June 18, 1942: "Abadan judged by the general standards of English colonies in tropical climes is well catered for. Only an oil company could manage to do so well by its employees." Letter, June 21, 1942: "The Americans in Abadan are giving such colossal wages that we company people simply cannot compete unless the AIOC give us a grant or something to meet the increased cost of living." Letter, July 14, 1942: "These Americans will just pay any price the boys ask and in that they feed them too and the bazaar prices since they arrived here have risen over 200% . . ." AIOC's Iranian Press Summary of June 17-25, 1942:

> It is commented that lack of means of transport is one of the greatest difficulties in regard to Iranian food supply conditions. A number of vehicles are worn out by long usage, and many disappeared in the first days when the Allies entered the country, and the position is that if one

> locality has sufficient foodstuffs available there is no way of transporting this to another locality in need of it. As the Allies promised economic help, and as they themselves have brought this state affairs about, they are requested to see to adequate provision of automobiles, buses and accessories.

An AIOC official in a letter of June 25, 1942:

> I have got a most interesting and difficult job on hand at the moment, namely collection of the local harvest, which the cultivators are very loathe to part with. It is really being done under the aegis of the Consul, but I expect that most of the work will fall on my two British assistants. I have spent the last few days trying to cope with uncooperative Government departments, but am at last getting some sense into them. . . .

This official had subsequently gone to Ahwaz, whence he flew to Agha Jari, and proceeded to the hill country to meet with a tribal leader. On July 22, 1942, he writes:

> The big shot himself proved to be well educated and intelligent, and I had a most interesting time with him, he told me frankly that his men were hungry, and that they would be obliged to take what they could in the way of food by force, but he alleged that the Company would be left in peace—kind of him. I cannot help sympathizing with many of these people, for their lot is hard, and the Government do nothing to help them. I am working on a scheme of my own for getting tea, sugar, and piece goods to the tribes, and am very keen to get into action as I believe that it will make a great contribution to the stability of the province, but it is going to be uphill work persuading others that this is so.

Letter, July 7, 1942:

> We are being denied food as the Company refuses to comply with the Ministry of Food regulations, inasmuch as they refuse to bring food in here unless it can be supplied to the Persians as well as us. . . . I would rather do without than see these, pro-axis, ungrateful cast-offs have it, when my own mother has to go short.

Letter, July 13, 1942:

> We can also only have 1 lb. of tea, 5 lbs. of sugar, 500 cigs and 10 tins of milk per month. I expect this really sounds a lot to you, but the thing that annoys most of us is the fact that the Iranians can have the same, even a coolie can get a bag of tea and sugar and is also supplied with bread. It is a shame that our sailors have to risk their lives for these people who do not in the least appreciate anything that is done for them.

An AIOC official refers to the arrival of the staff of the Burma Oil Company in Abadan in a letter of July 13, 1942:

> The Burmese have arrived. We call them the Burmese and they don't like it or the place. They complain of the heat and the un-Sahib like way in which we work. All kinds of jobs here have to be done by whites because the other breeds are not capable thereof and the Burmese are consequently amazed.

Conditions in Kerman are described by a member of the C.M.S. Hospital, Shiraz, in a letter to Tasmania dated October 30, 1942:

> There is no middle class in Kerman. They are all very well off (land owners or carpet factory owners) or very poor (weavers etc.), and now they say two of the carpet factories are closing because the American market is closed, so the winter ahead is terrible to think of, unemployment, inadequate food, and bitter cold.

A missionary in Shiraz, writing to England on November 14, 1942:

> We are having a pretty bad time. The cost of living for most articles of food has gone up 400%. Our sugar ration is about a quarter what it is in England so I am obliged to buy outside in the bazaar to add to the children's allowance. It is 3 shillings a pound. The British Government is doing a lot in the way of relief work for the starving poor in many parts of Shiraz. The consul here has sent maize and millet grain stores and clothings to the worst parts. The difficulty is to get anything honestly administered in the way of public funds with so many scally wags about. We are all much alarmed at the prospect of any American troops in these parts. They have got nearly as far as Isfahan. Life would be intolerable for ordinary folk. Do you know that the private

> American soldier is paid 25 Sh. a day in these parts, which is more than our junior officers get. The price of everything would be fabulous.

Another missionary in Shiraz writes to a missionary in Uganda:

> It was very kind of you to say you would send us a parcel of coffee and other things, but I think it is likely to be snatched in the Persian post office which is very corrupt. . . . The cost of living has risen by much over 200%, partly through the depredation of armed tribes and partly through hoarding on a terrific scale. Wood for fire is six times the price it was last winter, and great distress is prevalent.

C.W. Mast, Isfahan, to Mrs. H. Raves, 1 Northdown Road, Romford, Essex, England, November 15, 1942 (MID-Iran, 2200): "I wish they could get a fair system of rationing going here—prices are fantastic—bread, eggs, rice and charcoal are 7 (seven) times their old price."

Manager, Imperial Bank of Iran, Isfahan, to Tehran Branch, November 15, 1942, intercepted by the British Censor: "The food situation continues to deteriorate. Prices are rising daily. Supplies of bread have been insufficient. The position appears to be aggravated by the Iranian troops who are commandeering supplies both outside and in the town." An Englishman in Hamadan to England, November 24, 1942:

> Conditions are getting more and more difficult. If something is not done soon I am afraid there will be trouble. Prices continue to go up and up, there seems no limit. The bread situation gets worse instead of better. The poor people wait for hours to get their bread, pushing and fighting. They can not afford to buy other food. Only solution is for us to take over this country. The Persians are in such a hopeless muddle that they will never straighten themselves out without help. It is so wrong that one class of persons should be making thousands and thousands, building themselves big houses, driving about in new and expensive cars. The other class are going short of food.

English resident of Kerman to England, December 5, 1942 (MID-Iran, 2200):

> The poverty in this town is pitiful and appalling. Food is scarce and often literally 10 times as expensive as 18 months ago. We ourselves have found it very difficult to live. . . . There is no sort of control of prices here and so merchants and shopkeepers sell goods for what they

> can get, the prices go up almost hour by hour. . . . Here the worst effect of the war is the awful shortage and fantastic price of foodstuffs. Kerman is poor enough at the best of times, but now there is sheer, stark tragedy in the shape of starvation wherever you go. Bread is either unobtainable or a wicked price and meat, milk, butter, eggs etc. are an awful price—not to mention firing.

A.T. Howden, Kerman, to Mr. and Mrs. E.A. Wilson, St. Albans, England, February 15, 1943 (MID-Iran, 5970):

> This has been a very hard winter in Kerman. Everything has been five, six and even ten times more expensive than it used to be. There has been very little wheat indeed, and the poor people have had to eat dates or potatoes, and not even them sometimes, in place of bread which is such an important item in the Persian diet. There have been many deaths due to cold and starvation, and the wretchedness and poverty and misery around us have been very hard to bear; there is so little we can do to help.

British woman in Hamadan to her parents in London, February 28, 1943 (MID-Iran, 5970):

> Prices are still going up. Most things are six or seven times their cost of a year ago. The sugar ration does not always work. There has been none for this month. It costs about 3/6 (3.5 shillings) a pound. And a pound does not last long. . . . Butter is about 5/- a lb. All very difficult for us but a thousand times worse for the poor people.

Letter from Ahwaz to New York, March 1, 1943:

> The cost of living here now is very high, the bazaar prices go up every week; for one kilo of sugar it is 70 rials . . . for a packet of tea, about 19/- . . . 1/- each for razor blades. The Abadan people are worse off, there are so many people there now, the army, Americans, Poles, etc., that meat, chickens and eggs are very scarce, and dear; they have to have two meatless days per week; of course they get fish. . . .

Norman and Barbara Sharp, Shiraz, to E.S. Sharp, The White Cottage, Shanklin, Isle of Wight, England, March 19, 1943 (MID-Iran, 2400): "There is much distress generally and even starvation. It is dreadful to see the general underfed condition of the poorer classes. We are now beginning to get the inevitable pestilences associated with famine and war. Typhoid is very prevalent and typhus has now begun."

L.M. Norris, AIOC, Abadan, to Mr. and Mrs. Norris of Birmingham, England, March 14, 1943 (MID-Iran, 5940):

> Prices here are soaring by leaps and bounds and really it is time some control was introduced, but as usual the British government seem incapable of doing any job properly. Do you remember our propaganda of just over a year ago when British forces entered Iran? How Britain would feed the starving Persians and only came into Iran as a friend of the people. Yet last week we had to give out over the BBC, that there were food riots in Tehran and that wheat would have to be supplied from the Middle East Forces stores to make bread for the people. A regiment of troops too had to be sent to Tehran to quell the rioting. Talk about German propaganda back firing, I think ours must be just as bad.

Combined Intelligence Centre Iraq (CICI) report for March 13-20, 1943, on conditions in Kermanshah (MID-Iran, 5910):

> The big landowners wish to see acute shortage and famine conditions in order to keep up the black market price of wheat. This policy also suits the holders of alternative foodstuffs such as rice, beans, peas and ghee of which thousands of tons are known to be hoarded in Kermanshah itself. The streets of the town during February have been full of hungry and half-naked beggars of whom about 15 die each day of starvation and typhus cases among the people have been numerous.

Middle East Intelligence Centre (MEIC), Cairo, report for March 27 to April 3, 1943 (MID-Iran, 4220):

> Tehran was almost faced with another crisis owing to a breakdown on the line from Ahwaz which disorganized traffic, and consequently the grain supplies from the Persian Gulf, on which the capital is to a large extent dependent, were held up for some days. On March 14th Tabriz had only four tons of wheat in hand, the daily issue being 60 tons. In Kermanshah bread is bad and scarce although local charity is doing something to alleviate the lot of the very poor. In Hamadan living conditions are worse but the bread situation is slightly better owing to the efforts of the C.L.O. In Sultanabad the position is also worse, and between Andimeshk and Khurramabad the peasants are said to be so

> badly off that they are having to eat grass. Rice, barley and lentils were distributed to 500 poor people by the Anglo-Iranian Relief Committee in Yezd in sufficient quantities to provide them with five meals per week for a period of six weeks. In Kerman, the food kitchen opened by the local Anglo-Iranian Relief Committee some six months ago now serves as many as 1,500 poor persons every day. The food provided consists of rice, potatoes and dates.

Report by an American ship captain, dated March 29, 1943, on port conditions in Abadan (OSS Report 39371). The ship carrying supplies for Russia had sailed from New York on July 13, 1942:

> Arrived at Abadan September 7. Waited here for four days to get to the dock. The discharging was done by natives who receive nine rials per day and have to "kick back" part of that to the contractor... Native winch drivers were used, some of whom are only twelve and fourteen years old. The natives . . . are all dirty and ragged and underfed and receive no medical attention unless the ship's crew takes care of them. Most of them go around with dirty bandages on their legs, arms, or other parts of their bodies. There were several deaths among the men while this ship was in port. The natives bring their own cooking gear along, including a charcoal burner to cook what little rice they have. They are not allowed to drink water on the ship, so they have to get their water from the river. The river water is covered with scum and is an outlet for sewage, but the natives have no choice, but to drink it. Americans seem to be better liked here than the British since the Americans treat the natives better; however they don't have much love for any white man.

British GHQ, India, April 2, 1943 (MID-Iran, 2700):

> There has been a slight improvement in the bread situation in Tehran thanks to the arrival of wheat from the Persian Gulf and barley from Iraq. There is still, however, no reserve, and Tehran continues to live from day to day. In the provincial towns also the positions remain precarious. A fairly serious bread riot broke out in Khorramabad during the week ending 15th March which had to be quelled by military action, and economic conditions in parts of Kermanshah and in Luristan are reported to be so bad as likely to lead to disorder.

CICI, April 26, 1943, on Hamadan (MID-Iran, 5970):

> There has been a slight deterioration in the local situation due to the continuing rise in the cost of living, though bread improved slightly in quality. Officials of the Finance Department have stated they will go on strike if their salaries are not raised. As a result of this threat, a ration of rice was issued to all Government officials to allay discontent which is not confined to the Finance Department. So strong is the belief, as a result of hostile propaganda, that the British are deliberately creating a state of misery among the Persians that it was seriously proposed among the common people to march in a body under a white flag to the British Vice-Consulate to "submit" unconditionally and to beg the British to take over the administration and prevent them from starving. It is said that this demonstration was not intended to be a gesture of friendliness but was the outcome of hopelessness. However, local notables dissuaded the people from realizing their project. Typhus in Hamadan is on the increase due in part to the weather being abnormally cold. In Sultanabad there continues to be much discontent (and) among the Lur tribesmen in the Burujird area. It is reported that wages of an unskilled laborer in Hamadan which were about 7 rials a day prior to August, 1941, are now about 35 rials a day and have risen markedly during the last fortnight, an inevitable change if the laborers are to attempt to live on their earnings.

On Isfahan, the same report states:

> There is little news from this (Isfahan) area. The factory workers continue to be dissatisfied and the cost of living continues to increase. Bread prices are rising and the Government granary is empty but the bakers say they can obtain wheat for the next 30 days; on this reckoning there will be a breadless month before the harvest is gathered.

A woman in Abadan calling herself "Mother of Ishmael," writing to Haji Kandar Ali Ansari, Karachi, on April 25, 1943, says that those in India cannot begin to imagine the pitiable conditions in Iran (MID-Iran, 5970): "Disease, misery and famine stare in the face everywhere." She says that in Abadan the number of death is 80-90 a day, mostly due to hunger. Typhus and typhoid were also exacting a heavy toll. Abdul Rahim Sawal from Zahedan writes to a friend in Dera Ghazi Khan that due to the epidemic business had ceased, and shops and factories were closing.

Armenian in Isfahan to Garegin Johannes, Calcutta, India, April 28, 1943 (MID-Iran, 2020):

> We see plenty of Polish immigrants; their arrival has caused a typhus epidemic and has created a crisis. Since their arrival in Isfahan we are deprived of eggs, milk and butter. They have much money and can afford to buy everything at any price. We see them always in shops, eating with greediness.

J.B. Gibson, AIOC, to his wife, 303 Bilbington road, Rock Ferry, Birkenhead, England, on conditions in Abadan, April 30, 1943:

> The servants are very troublesome and trying. The Americans have ruined the whole area paying fabulous sums, £300 for a carpet, and Rials 800-1000 a month for a cook and Rials 35 per day and food for coolies. The day is not far distant when the whole place should be taken over by the military; that will be the only safeguard Europeans will have; plenty of married people in Abadan are living without cooks and house servants and probably it is only a matter of time when the same trouble will come to Fields.

Dr. Ali Dehghan, Shiraz, to Mrs. M.G. Naqi, 16 Glenloch Road, Belsize Park, London N.W.3, May 19, 1943 (MID-Iran, 5970):

> There is not much to write about the general conditions. Times are very bad and hard. On the one hand the cost of living is so high that it can easily be said that Shiraz is even more expensive than New York. Everything is scarce and disease is raging furiously in most places. In our city typhoid is in full swing inflicting heavy casualty on the population.

OSS report "A Review of the Economic Situation in the Frontier Districts of Kurdistan, May-June 1943" (MID-Iran, 5970):

> Two officers have recently made independent tours of the outlying districts in Kurdistan on the Iraqi-Persian frontier. In their reports they stress the bad economic situation, both past and present, and are not optimistic about the future. Last winter was disastrous for the villagers and many people died of starvation. Some idea of their sufferings may be gained when it is realized that even under normal conditions there are several permanent factors which mitigate against a state of well-being and the poor find it extremely difficult to eke out an adequate existence. . . . Their plight last winter was further aggravated by the effects of: (d) An exceptionally cold winter in 1941/42 which caused the death of a large number of livestock. (e) Considerable damage to

> the 1942 grain crop in this region by the Sunn pest. (f) The inadequate provision by the Government of grain to see the populace through the winter. (g) The sale, during the winter of 1942/43, of further large numbers of livestock in order to purchase at exorbitant prices what little grain was on sale on the free marker. (h) The progressive decline in the quantity of motor transport available in the region. The main characteristic of this fertile region is that it is not self-sufficient in foodstuffs and relies on the sale of the main crop, tobacco, for the purchase of staples. Wheat and barley are grown in small quantities as is rice, which, though fairly plentiful, is of secondary importance in this bread-eating community. . . . It is estimated that only about half the population is in a position to make adequate provision for food supplies, the other half, whose condition is said to range from extreme poverty to complete destitution, is dependent on such measures as the Government may put into force. Last year's efforts give no grounds for optimism in this respect.

CICI, July 17, 1943 (MID-Iran, 3410):

> On July 5th there was a minor demonstration in Ahwaz at the quality and quantity of bread; the Governor General, Mispah Fatemi, as a result has deported to Burujird four leading merchants who are believed to have engineered the affair in their own interests and in an endeavor to obstruct Government control of the price of bread.

US Military attaché's report on the condition of Iranian dock workers at Bandar Shahpur, August 3, 1943, based on his interview in New York with A.C. Newberry who had been in Iran as assistant field engineer with Foley Bros., Spencer, White and Prentice, New York, from March 1942 to May 1943 (MID-Iran, File 5940): "The natives do not have the strength to lift fifty-pound loads and are prey to many diseases: smallpox, typhoid, digestive troubles, eye and skin diseases, and syphilis. The native diet of bread and tea is inadequate." While the dock workers starved, "Source saw large stocks of food (destined for Russia) piled up at this port and estimated that foodstuffs accumulated for six or seven months."

G.Z. Zoeckler, American Mission, Hamadan, to Mrs. Funk, Londerdale, USA, August 22, 1943 (MID-Iran, 5060):

> Our greatest problem has arisen from the rapid increase in the cost of living. This has hit us in several directions, the high cost of food and

> fuel and the problem of workers' salaries. We have increased some salaries and given bonuses to employees several times in the course of the year in the endeavor to ease the situation, but at best all salaries are woefully inadequate to meet the cost of living. At one time one of the highest paid workers was getting just enough to buy 4 lbs. of bread a day to feed a family of seven, the ordinary ration being 2 lbs. a day per person in this bread eating country. Naturally there has been a good deal of unrest and discontent at this state of affairs. . . . The food problem has been a knotty one. Not only has the cost of food steadily advanced but hours and hours of time and quantities of paper and ink have gone into the attempt to obtain sugar, tea, rice and potatoes from the food administration. We were not included in any rationing system and it has been a constant struggle to obtain the supplies we were supposed to have. In one day when bread rationing went into effect the price of one day's supply of bread for the hospital rose from 84 rials to 220 rials, near which figure it has remained ever since. . . .

Robert Brandly, Kerman, to Annie Brandly, Lindenberg St. 10, Kuesnacht, Zurich, Switzerland, August 27, 1943 (MID-Iran, 5970):

> Sometimes we hear that a lorry of the post has been pillaged between Kerman and Isfahan. I do not know whether that is true but I only know that nothing is coming in. . . . It is really a shame that now I am spending more than Swiss Francs 500 a month here (1 rial = about 0.14 Swiss Francs) and that only for the most necessary things. . . . And unfortunately you cannot see the end. The speculation is still very active. There are people making a fortune, whilst the largest part of the population is condemned to vegetate miserably.

OSS report, October 5, 1943, on conditions in the Iran-Iraq frontier region in Kurdistan (MID-Iran, 5940):

> There is a great scarcity of wheat and barley and the Kurds are in a bad way. Scarcity is due to crop failure, due to Sunn pest, primarily. Contributing factors are purchase of Persian wheat by Russians; lack of pack animals (these have been gradually used less and less over the past few years due to use of motor transport. Numbers have further diminished in past two years due to buying by the British and lately by Russian army.). . . There is a great deal of sickness. Among grown people malaria is quite common, among children, whooping cough, malaria, mumps, measles, diphtheria. . . . Medical supplies are also very inadequate.

Imperial Bank of Iran, Isfahan, to London head office, October 9, 1943 (MID-Iran, 5000):

> The living conditions of the people have become worse. Efforts to collect the bumper harvest into the Government ambars have not been very successful and requirements for the coming year are by no means assured. Bread has been reduced in price but the quality varies and supplies are often unobtainable. Adequate supplies of fats, sugar, tea and many other necessities are beyond the reach of all but the well-to-do.

F.M. Stead, Kermanshah, to Clement P. Heydenburk, 1043 Curtis Avenue, Petoskey, Michigan, October 14, 1943 (MID-Iran, 2200):

> Stealing, highway robbery and even the looting of villages are becoming more common. A large village only 10 miles away was looted last week and two men were killed. Two families that possessed Government rifles succeeded in defending themselves. A number of Kakavend tribesmen have banded together for looting and robbery and have not yet been captured. Deserters from the Army and police have joined them, as well as others, who think it is easier and pleasanter to earn their living by looting and robbing than by honest labor. . . . It is reported that there is a plan to raid our compound in daytime for the sake of the Government rifles that have been lent us for our protection. . . .

A British resident of Kerman on December 30, 1943, to a friend in Bombay, states there is more freedom since Reza Shah left (MID-Iran, 5070):

> On the other hand living conditions have grown extremely bad. The population is fast decreasing owing to famine and epidemics. In every community a few got richer at the expense of the mass of the population. This, in particular, coupled with the unsafety of the roads, villages and countryside which seems to be the characteristic feature of the South, is furnishing an extremely fertile ground for Russian propaganda.

Another Britisher in Kerman to a friend in Karachi (MID-Iran, 5070): "Dearness still prevails. The price of wheat per kharvar is 300 tomans; barley per kharvar, 200 tomans; sugar per maun, 40 tomans; a packet of tea costs 10-11 tomans; ghee per maun, 20 tomans; rice of good quality per maun, 15 tomans. Every article of food is dear but thank God it is available." As below described, by the end of 1943, conditions were slowly improving.

In contrast to the general misery, the oil company had taken good care of its own. G.M. Shaw, AIOC, Abadan, to E.L. Colston, 'St. Bernard,' Gerrards Cross, Bucks., England, September 6, 1943 (MID-Iran, 5070):

> I am Food Controller! I wonder if you can have any idea what that means in a place like this? I didn't actually start the job off but I took it over when it was a tender stripling about two months old, when its original parent had to go home. None of us knew anything about rationing, we had no basis, no population figures and, incidentally no food—that is almost literally true. . . . Although food has not any time been scarce here, it has mostly been unprocurable or obtainable only at famine prices—bread, for example, last year could be bought but only at 1,200% of its pre-war price; meat was deliberately held in short supply, even when there was lashings of it, and retailed at something like 5,000% of its pre-war cost; sugar was—and still is—about 4,000%, tea about 400%. Increases in pay merely resulted in the bazaar prices going up in proportion, the Government were apparently powerless to stop it and finally the Company had to take the drastic (and reluctant) step of supplying the basic commodities in order to keep this vital industry going, and we had to start, if you please, by taking a census of the whole of the Company's various theatres of operation. The result is that today I am feeding 110,000 people on Abadan island and about 50,000 more in other centres; we have ration cards, coupons, ration days and meatless days; in Abadan alone I have built seven shops and am now building five more for the supply of our labourers alone; I have created a meat shop, a fish shop and a vegetable shop in each of our two residential (staff) areas; I have built a fish market in the town and am now finishing a vegetable market there as well; I have 600 fishermen fishing for me down below the bar, launches plying up and down with ice bringing the catches in and a contractor retailing the fish to the staff and the public at rigorously controlled prices; I am importing wheat from Australia, Canada and the States, barley from Iraq and millet from Egypt; frozen meat from Australia and South Africa; dehydrated meat and dried milk from Australia—all in our own returning tankers, thus avoiding any call on shipping space; vegetable seeds from South Africa and the Argentine; I am now trying to get a trawler complete with crew and nets from home and combing India, South Africa and the Gulf area for supplies of smoked or salted fish; I have imported drill and printed cotton from

India and bought more in this country; I bring sheep from 1,000 miles away by train and ship; I have bought a whole dairy farm in Abadan and am negotiating for another up-country, have engaged a professional farmer from Europe and am buying cattle of good stock as I can get them; at present I have to buy fodder for them but am putting 400 acres under cultivation to provide my own next year; have built a piggery and am trying to get good breeds from South Africa; have bought incubators from Palestine and will start a hen farm this autumn; I provide barley and other foods for private poultry-keepers to eek out supplies; I send a cart round with the milk; I have a 15 acre vegetable garden of my own and have installed four contractors in a big way for additional supplies of vegetables—we put in pumps to bring them a water supply from the Shatt, lend them agricultural implements, give them lime, manure and allied things, give them seed and feed their cultivators; I bring cigarettes, ghee, dried vegetables, shoes, etc. from North Persia, rice and dates from Iraq; tea from India and sugar from East Africa and I actually got some ghee from Kenya before export was frozen. I dare say I am doing others as well, but these are the main ones and will give you an idea of the scope of the scheme. I might have mentioned also that I am making about 200,000 chupatties a day in Abadan and issuing them to labour and dependents, three a time—nice little job that!

Notes

1. Majd, Mohammad Gholi. *August 1941: The Anglo-Russian Occupation of Iran & Change of Shah*. Lanham: University Press of America, 2012. 34-42.

2. Ibid, 371-400.

3. Ibid, 400-406.

4. The reports on conditions in Kerman are particularly interesting because this was the second time in 25 years that the rug weaving industry was ravaged by famine. In a report on "Trade Conditions in Persia," dated March 30, 1920, US Consul Ralph H. Bader, writes: "Prices for this commodity remain high, due to the fact that rugs, and especially the finer makes, are getting scarce on account of the death from starvation in 1918 of many of the best weavers. Production is, therefore, greatly limited." Commerce Reports, Part 1. Bureau of Foreign and Domestic Commerce, Department of Commerce, 1920—Consular Reports, page 1787.

Chapter 23

The Typhus Epidemic: A Documentary Account

Typhus was widespread in the spring of 1942. For instance, during the six-week span of March 13 to April 17, 1942, there were 86 reported cases and 34 fatalities in Tehran, 28 cases and 2 fatalities in Tabriz, 42 cases in Rasht and 24 cases in Isfahan. (Dreyfus, Telegram 155, 158.919/23, May 14, 1942) Of course, the actual prevalence was far worse than the reported cases. With the advent of summer, typhus had ceased. Dreyfus on June 17, 1942 (Dispatch 288, 891.20/155):

> I have the honor to enclose a copy of a speech made in English by the Iranian Minister of Public Health at a banquet given by him at the Hotel Darband on June 11, 1942, in honor of Dr. Abraham Neuwirth, Colonel, United States Army Medical Corps. The occasion of the banquet was to pay homage to Dr. Neuwirth, who was decorated by the Iranian Government on June 11 with the Scientific Order, first class, for the part he played in dealing with the threatened typhus epidemic and the treatment of Polish refugees in Iran. The Minister, a graduate of the American School, pays warm tribute to Dr. Neuwirth and to American activities in Iran. Dr. Neuwirth well deserves his decoration and the homage being paid to him by the Iranians. He worked voluntarily, untiringly, and with great buoyancy of spirit to see that adequate medical attention was given to the Polish refugees. He inoculated many persons against typhus as long as his serum held out, then assisted the Pasteur Institute in the manufacture of typhus serum here in Tehran. He completely won over the hearts of the Iranians, who are presently carrying on a campaign to have him assigned to the Iranian Government as a medical adviser. Here is yet another example of the

> friendly and unselfish services which have won Americans so high a regard in the hearts of Iranians. Iranians, generally speaking of sentimental nature, are touched by these manifestations of friendly interest in them and their problems, where they would be largely unaffected by volumes of propaganda.

Neuwirth's subsequent request that a large quantity of vaccine be sent to Iran was based on his experience in the spring of 1942. Subsequently, the MESC had sent its own "expert," Colonel Sams, to Iran in the fall of 1942 when typhus was rare. For instance, A.E. Chapman of AIOC, Abadan to Mrs. Chapman, Cambo, Morpeth, Northumberland, England, October 6, 1942 (MID-Iran, 2400): "There seems to be much more typhoid this year, even the boy has had it and has been off work over a month." Dr. Frank Marsh of the AIOC, Abadan, to Mrs. A.H. Marsh, 68 Evelegh Road, Portsmouth, England, December 12, 1942 (MID-Iran, 2400): "Our latest event is an epidemic of smallpox . . . we have beginning of an epidemic of Diphtheria as well." No mention of typhus. Not surprisingly, Sams had reported that there was no typhus in Iran and the vaccine had been held at Cairo for the "MESC pool."

An OSS report of March 16, 1943 (MID-Iran, 2400):

> From a reliable source in the Near East, this Agency has received the following report, dated March 5, 1943: "Reports, unconfirmed, of yellow fever on northeastern Iraq-Persia frontier. Typhus cases are occurring in the Kurdish hills. There are sporadic cases in the Rowanduz district. The Sulamania district has been closed. There have been two fatal cases in Mosul. Cases of smallpox among civilians and soldiers, but not yet numerous enough to be serious."

The Persian Gulf Service Command (PGSC) Weekly Intelligence Bulletin No. 6, April 2, 1943 (MID-Iran, 2400):

> Added to other fears, there has been an "epidemic" of typhus, greatly exaggerated by rumors. There are no statistics available since many poor people (where the disease spreads most rapidly) do not report to physicians. On the floor of Parliament a statement was made that there were estimates of from 5-20,000 cases in Tehran alone. There is talk of closing down schools for a month. Actually there were about 30 deaths in Tehran the week of March 14-20. Miss Nightingale, a nurse in Isfahan died last week. A few US troops have developed the disease. The serum apparently does not guarantee immunity but it does

> seem to blunt the attack and make cases lighter. Typhus is carried by the body louse. US soldiers should avoid public places such as cafes, cinemas, or anywhere that contact with the local population might expose them. The epidemic is now at its height and will disappear in May, when people wear less clothes and bathe more frequently.

Charles E. Bailey, Assistant Director in Charge of Civilian Relief, ARC, Tehran, to Ralph Bain, Director of Middle East Operation, ARC, Cairo, April 5, 1943 (MID-Iran, 2400):

> Of immediate importance is the fact that there is a Typhus epidemic in town which is increasing in magnitude daily. There are 11,000 known cases at the moment and in the "Caves" are many unknown cases. I went through the hovels and mud dug-outs yesterday and witnessed scores of cases of Typhus, lying around on the ground without care or without sufficient food. In one small enclosure not over ten feet square were three cases of Typhus, one active case of Small-pox, two cases of advanced Malaria and one case of starvation—all living together and sharing each others rags that were being used for blankets.

The Tehran press had tried to reassure a terrified public. An OSS report on the Iranian press, April 8, 1943 (MID-Iran, 2400):

> On Friday next the British Indian hospital at Doshan Tappeh will be thrown open for the reception of Iranian typhus patients. This hospital can provide for 1,000 patients. . . . Typhus serums have been distributed recently among the hospitals with typhus patients for the inoculation of the physicians and the hospital staffs. A meeting of the physicians, deputies, Ministers of Health and Agriculture, presided over by the Prime Minister, has taken place to discuss methods of combating typhus.

PGSC Bulletin No. 7, April 9, 1943 (MID-Iran, 2400):

> A baffling problem is faced in an effort to get facts about the typhus epidemic now existing in Iran. Reliable doctors vary greatly in their estimates. In Tehran, an average of several "guesses" would indicate a death rate of about 70 a day during the week with a total of about 7500 cases. The British have opened the Doshan Tapeh Hospital of 1000 beds for civilian cases, which is still inadequate. If these figures represent the approximate proportion throughout the larger cities, it would

seem that 1% of the city population is affected. Qum and Kashan report no epidemics. Kermanshah and Rezayeh report severe epidemics.

A British report, April 9, 1943, (MID-Iran, 2400):

> An epidemic of typhus has broken out in Tehran with several thousand cases. The G.O.C. in C., Paiforce (Persia and Iraq Force) has recommended that the tented hospital, provided originally by India for the use of Polish refugees, should be used complete with doctors and orderlies for civilian typhus cases.

Translation (by the British censor) of an extract from a letter, April 13, 1943, from Alireza Sobhani, Tehran, to Ahmad Sobhani, c/o Iranian Legation, Baghdad (MID-Iran, 5970): "As regards typhus, Teheran's average deaths were 5 a day, now they have increased to 1000 a day. The corpses are bound with rope into bundles of 100 corpses, then carried by trucks and emptied into pits. Every day several persons die of hunger in the streets." PGSC report, April 16, 1943 (MID-Iran, 5940):

> We are in the midst of the worst typhus epidemic that has ever been known here. Figures are hard to find that is accurate, but in the last Intelligence Bulletin I reported that there were probably 8,000 cases with a daily death rate of about 80. Some swear that my figures are too low. This is partly the result of some bungling. Last spring Lt. Colonel Neuwirth anticipated an epidemic this winter. He persuaded the Iranian Government to order typhus serum for this expected attack from the USA. It was ordered but by some strange misuse of authority, was held at Cairo for a "pool" for the Middle East and not forwarded here. Cairo had a few cases in the hospitals with only a few deaths per week. In Iran the epidemic is violent all over the country. Yet the typhus serum has not been sent here and Lt. Colonel Neuwirth was sent back to the USA, probably not to return. Farnsworth wrote this up in a dispatch for AP. He left out the story about the "pool" of serum in Cairo.

Mohammad Ali Ehsani, Tehran, to Hadji Mohammad Hossein Ehsani, Kerbela, Iraq, translated by the British Censor, April 18, 1943 (MID-Iran, 5970):

> The situation in Persia is critical. Prices of all foodstuffs, provisions, clothing etc. have increased; typhoid and typhus reign in Tehran and

the people fall victim to these diseases. The microbes of the epidemic spread in buses, cars and carriages. People die from hunger and typhoid by thousands every day. What a misery will come forth if the war extends into Persia. . . . May God bless the poor people who suffer and die from this famine.

Iraj Pirnazar, Ave. Pahlevi, Kucheh Soheily, Tehran, to Fereidun Saleh (son of Allah Yar Saleh), Mount Hermon Agricultural School, Massachusetts, April 20, 1943 (MID-Iran, 2400):

> Listen to a few words about typhus. Have you, heard the word typhus? No doubt you have heard it. Before the Polish refugees came here, I had not heard of such a strange and serious word. Life gives men new experiences. Typhus is a very dangerous disease which the Polish refugees brought into Persia. The disease has spread in most of the provinces of Persia. Thirty per cent of the population of Tehran die of this dreadful disease. Every day a number of people fall victim to it. . . . The disease has spread to such an extent that the schools have commenced their final annual examinations before time. As soon as the examinations are completed they will close the schools so that in case of emergency the school premises may be converted into hospitals and on the other hand the number of victims may be reduced.

An OSS report on the Tehran Press during the period March 22 to April 21, 1943 (MID-Iran, 2400):

> Apparently no official figures on the number of (typhus) cases in Tehran and in other parts of the country have appeared, but, beyond question, the epidemic is serious. A reasonable estimate made a week ago by the head of the Pasteur Institute was some 14,000 cases in Tehran. The fact that the vaccine was held up in Cairo by the MESC is entirely inexplicable: had it been available here the situation could have been put under some control at an earlier stage. Typhus is always dormant in Iran and Persians explain its current prevalence in part to the severe and rainy winter which kept people cramped up inside of their crowded shelters. The shortage of fuel had increased the price of the public baths to the point where the poor could not make their normal use of these facilities. Examinations are now being held in the Tehran schools and they will close more than a month earlier than usual. Persians state that the present warm weather will cause a great decline in the number of new cases.

The British, not surprisingly, played down the gravity of the epidemic. The *New York Times* of April 22, 1943, has a brief piece entitled, "Typhus Epidemic in Iran." It reads (MID-Iran, 2400):

> Cairo, April 21—A typhus epidemic of a limited nature is now prevailing in Iran, Richard G. Casey, British Minister of State, reported today on his return from a trip to Teheran. The number of cases runs into the hundreds and not thousands, he added. The British authorities have turned over thousands of hospital beds to the Iranian Government for typhus cases only and serum is being shipped in.

S.V. Pill, AIOC, Masjid-i-Sulaiman, Khuzestan, to Mrs. K. Todd, Naharia, Palestine, May 4, 1943:

> My hands are full with all my stock and the feeding problem is acute. Contractors are buying the barley and the wheat crop as it stands in the field so as to corner the market. . . . The hospital is quiet except for the typhus cases which number to-day 28. The epidemic seems to be slowly on the wane but Aschot Daulatatian arrived back from Abadan with fever and is warded as a suspected case.

An OSS report of May 6, 1943, entitled, "Typhus in Iran," (MID-Iran, 2400):

> The following report is classified as secret, can be employed for background purposes only, and if digested must be carefully paraphrased and also classified as secret. Mention has been made in a previous roundup of a developing epidemic of typhus in Iran. Recent news has added numerous details which add up to a disturbing picture. Although typhus is found in most of the principal cities, Tehran has been the hardest hit. There by mid-March there were thirty deaths a week, the cases estimated variously from five to twenty thousand. By the middle of April the daily death rate in the capital had risen to eighty. The press has called for the closing of all schools, cafes and cinemas. All US troops have been warned to avoid public gatherings. . . . Blame for the situation is placed naturally on the Allies and their war effort, which allegedly has brought famine and malnutrition, and the overcrowding of Tehran under squalid conditions. In this blame the US must share. We also share in the blame put upon the local government, because until lately US Lt. Col. Abraham Neuwirth has been adviser to the Ministry of Health. Actually, however, this is misplaced blame,

> since Lt. Col. Neuwirth many months ago foresaw this possible outbreak, persuaded the Iran Government to order large quantities of typhus serum from the USA. This serum does not completely immunize against the disease but does lighten the case once it is contracted. By some unexplained short-circuiting in authority, the serum was held in Cairo in a "pool" for the Middle East. The story of this mishap, although reflecting somewhat on the British administration in Cairo, was passed by the British censor in Tehran but suppressed by the Russians. The latter recently denied access to Russia to a US naval officer who wished to study their methods of combating the disease. In Tehran they claimed that typhus did not exist in Russia. The Iran Government has responded to the situation by pushing through the Majlis, or Parliament, a bill authorizing the Ministry of Health to order large amounts of pharmaceutical supplies from the USA. The Iranian Minister in Washington has been instructed to employ an American to administer this pharmaceutical company.

A British intelligence report for the period May 9-22, 1943 (MID-Iran, 2400): "Typhus is still very prevalent in Khorramshahr and Abadan. Occasional cases of sandfly fever occurring here in Basra as well as Khorramshahr." S.M. Stead, American missionary in Kermanshah, to Mr. and Mrs. G.G. Crosier, Assam, India, May 25, 1943 (MID-Iran, 2400):

> By the way, they are having a bad epidemic of typhus in Kermanshah. Blanche Bussdieker had it. Was free from fever 2 or 3 days and came down with phlebitis and then pneumonia. There is an epidemic of typhoid or para typhoid in villages nearby and they say there is much smallpox in nearby villages, but we have been spared.

An OSS report on the Iranian press dated May 28, 1943 (MID-Iran, 2400): "In the past five weeks 1388 typhus cases were treated at the Thousand Bed Hospital."

A censor report on a letter of June 4, 1943, from the ARC, Cairo, to the head office, Washington, DC (MID-Iran, 2400):

> Sender encloses a copy of a letter of May 24, 1943, from C.E. Bailey, Assistant Director, Middle East Operations, to Mr. Hassan Adhan, Assistant Director, Persian Red Lion and Sun, Teheran, Iran. In this letter Mr. Bailey writes that the American Red Cross has given substantial assistance during the typhus epidemic in Teheran. In a conver-

> sation with His Excellency Ala, Mr. Bailey states that they both agreed that the best preventive of a typhus epidemic next winter is not importation of typhus serum, but an organized program for cleaning up the slums. Last year many people left other districts for Teheran because bread was sold there at a cheaper price. Since Iran has had an abundant wheat harvest, many of the poorer people will now be able to return to their former homes.

Dr. H. Jamieson, AIOC, Abadan, to Major E. Jamieson, Carrow Villa, Nairn, Scotland, June 11, 1943 (MID-Iran, 2400): "We have had two very bad epidemics this year, first small-pox, and lately typhus, which was of course practically unknown here before. We have had about a thousand cases in Abadan in the last two months, but thanks to all concerned we have the outbreak well in hand. . . ."

CICI report for the week ending June 14, 1943 (MID-Iran, 2710):

> On May 20th the Commissioner of Police stated that he had received no funds for feeding prisoners since March. (This callous inefficiency compares with the conditions in the lunatic asylum in Hamadan where the feeding of the inmates is still paid on the pre-war scale which was fixed prior to the enormous rise in the cost of living; the lunatics are therefore on the verge of starvation since the allowance is heartlessly inadequate).

W. Stocken, UKCC, Mashad, to M.J. Stocken, 1263 Prospect Street, Pretoria, South Africa, June 16, 1943 (MID-Iran, 2400): "Even in Meshed they had plenty of typhus this year amongst the poor people. But strangely enough only 17 to 20% are fatal."

In the OSS report entitled "The Southern Supply Route to Russia," discussed in the previous chapter, it was stated that the monthly death from typhus during the 1943 epidemic was 4,000. The report did not specify whether this was for the country or for Tehran. Since other reports give the daily typhus deaths in Tehran at 80, it clear that the 4,000 was just for Tehran. Of course, given that actual typhus fatalities were considerably greater than reported fatalities, even the 4,000 figure understates the actual number. It can be confidently stated that conservatively 15-20,000 died of typhus in Tehran during January to May of 1943. Given that the population of Tehran was reported at 700,000, it follows that 2-3% were lost to typhus. The pre-war population of Iran was reported to be 15 million, consequently, in the typhus epidemic of

1943, 300-400,000 Iranians died of the disease, of whom many would have been spared if vaccinated.

Typhus and the Kerosene Shortage

The shortage of kerosene was briefly mentioned in chapter 16. While Iran oil was fueling Allied forces and Iranian roads, railways and trucks were used to deliver war goods to Russia, very little space was allocated to Iranian needs, including the transport of vital fuel and kerosene from the south to the north of the country. Dreyfus on March 10, 1943 (Telegram 253, 891.6363/796):

> Department's 118, March 6. Several days ago at request of Iranian Government I requested General Connolly to take all possible steps to bring adequate stocks of fuel oil and kerosene to Tehran. His reply was that British movements control, which alone is responsible under present arrangement for allocation of space on southern section of railway, is doing all possible to insure adequate stocks and create safe reserve. Situation is showing signs of improvement and will I believe soon be under control. The severe shortage is attributed by British to delays on railways caused by (1) freezing weather in mountains and (2) inevitable confusion attending taking over of railways by Americans from British. Americans attribute it to British allocation officers. In my opinion primary cause is insufficient allotment on railway for Iranian civil use (see my 242, March 6). Whatever the cause of the block long queues in front of kerosene shops, together with bread shortage have had damaging effect on Allied Iranian relations. Matter of allotment of tonnage on railway for Iranian civil use is now under study and I hope the present figure of 200 tons daily will be increased sharply upwards. In my opinion some 500 tons daily will be required to move wheat and other goods and to retire part of the estimated 20,000 tons of civil goods backed up in customs houses in the south. British railway officials show keener appreciation of need for meeting Iranian essential civil requirements than do American officials who seem to feel their only responsibility is to move goods to Russia. Since I am hopeful that General Connolly will soon come to appreciate political and practical necessity of taking care of Iranian needs I do not for the moment suggest any action by Department.

Having deprived Iran of the typhus vaccine, the Allies had further aggravated the epidemic by their failure to transport fuel. Dreyfus on

March 11, 1943, in a classic report entitled, "Kerosene Shortage in Tehran" (Dispatch 486, 891.6363/796):

> With reference to my telegram No. 253 of March 10, 1943, I have the honor to offer the following observations on the present shortage of kerosene and fuel oil in Tehran. In other places, this would not appear to be a serious matter nor one worthy of notice. Here, however, it is a matter vital especially to the poorer people of Tehran who are dependent on kerosene alone for heating and lighting their houses and for cooking. To have this occur during the middle of the winter and at a time when a great number of people in Tehran are getting very little or nothing to eat is doubly unfortunate. The present prices of charcoal, wood and coal makes the substitution of these for kerosene completely out of the question. The shortage was caused by the failure of the railroad to make the necessary deliveries and the blame for this must rest largely on the shoulders of the British authorities controlling movements of the Iranian railroad system. The Iranian press has been quick to accuse the "Allies" of failing to live up to that part of the Tripartite Pact which assures the maintenance of the economic life of the country and the Legation has been formally requested by the Foreign Office to take steps to remedy the situation. Insufficient stocks stored in Tehran, freezing weather in the mountains, and a certain amount of confusion in turning over parts of the railroad to the American Army all helped cause the shortage. In answer to an inquiry by the Legation, however, the Commanding Officer of the American forces in Iran stated that the movement of petroleum supplies was so far solely the responsibility of the British. The head of the Tehran office of the Anglo-Iranian Oil Company points out that the safeguarding of the essential oil needs of this area can only be achieved by the maintenance of reserve stocks sufficient for at least two weeks.
>
> This incident is an extremely good example of the difficulties encountered in using the Iranian railroad system as a supply line to Russia and at the same time trying to meet the essential needs of the Iranian population. It is possible that, in order to keep the flow of supplies moving at a steady pace, the Soviets may be willing to bring in some oil supplies from the Baku region and a suggestion to this effect has been made to them by the British Minister. They have already shipped some 800 tons of fuel oil for the railroad, and the British Minister has expressed to the Soviet Ambassador his hope that it may be possible to increase the supply of oil products in general from the Soviet Union. The queues in front of the kerosene shops have been enormous and

> there has been a certain amount of disorder. One disagreeable phase of the shortage from the point of view of the civil population has been the closing of the public baths on which Iranians rely exclusively for bathing. Lack of cleanliness in turn encourages typhus. All in all it has had a markedly bad effect on allied prestige in Iran, and public opinion, inflamed by the irresponsible press both on this issue and on the food situation, has become increasingly ugly. As indicated in my telegram No. 242 dated March 6 it has become apparent to me that the allotment of 200 tons a day for Iranian civilian use on the Trans-Iranian Railway is woefully insufficient, especially now that 160 tons of wheat are to come forward daily. Conversations in regard to raising this figure are now taking place and I will inform the Department promptly of their progress.

Typhus in Azerbaijan

On July 6, 1943, the Iraqi consul in Tabriz had sent to Baghdad a report entitled "Typhus in Azerbaijan," which was intercepted by the Anglo-Russian censor. Its text is given in an OSS report dated October 15, 1943 (MID-Iran, 2400):

> The symptoms of Typhoid and Typhus appeared during the end of summer 1942. Typhus alone has remained, growing in intensity as winter approached, the disease reaching its utmost seriousness in the intense cold weather during the end of February and all the month of March. The poverty of the inhabitants, negligence of cleanliness, and carelessness of health in general have helped the prevalence of the disease in this area, as well as the scarcity and high cost of medicines. All this has caused the past mortality. The number of cases increased to where the Government Hospital was over-congested by patients. The Health Authorities were therefore compelled to use the Municipal Hospital also, although this institution had been for non-infectious diseases only up to this time. That Hospital likewise became full of patients. The focal point of this dangerous disease was the jail with its filth, lice, and malnutrition. Early in March, three judicial officers visited the jail on inspection—i.e. the Public Prosecutor, the Medical Officer, and a Magistrate. All three of them were quickly infected with typhus. The Prosecutor and the Medical Officer recovered after long treatment, but the third official died. The transmission of this disease and circulation to the public is effected principally by means of carriages on which patients are transported to the hospitals. In this way the lice are left in the carriages, and infect healthy people when next

used. . . . Some of the Tabriz doctors had small supplies of old stock ampoules of anti-typhus serum, which they injected on request on payment of fabulous fees. The local authorities did practically nothing to combat the epidemic. . . .

After being concentrated largely in the poorer class quarters, especially in the northern areas of the city, the disease declined in intensity during April and May, and the number of cases decreased substantially. Unfortunately we could not obtain any accurate or reliable statistics on cases, for all the doctors we asked who were employed in the hospitals, etc., replied only with vague figures which were merely guesses on their part. The control of the typhus was due to two facts: the passing of winter and the approach of spring and warm weather in which there is much less lice activity, and the improved conditions of cleanliness within the home when the average family comes out from under the huge quilt under which they have been sleeping all together in one kursee (bedding) during the months of cold and snow. However, with the appearance of warm weather there also again came typhoid—from fruits and vegetables, as well as the greater consumption of drinking water. All Tabriz water is brought in from points outside the city where streams flow to a ford. Poor peasants are often washing their clothing and rags in it, it becomes contaminated, and is then brought through the city to the homes and confined in cisterns, which exist in every house.

The second reason for the decrease in typhus in the area, is in the fact that during the latter part of April the Russians imported large quantities of anti-typhus and anti-typhoid serum to inoculate the inhabitants, in their various categories, free of charge and on as large a scale as possible. The local authorities at first opened four centers for the doctors and health officials of the Russians and Persians to inoculate therefrom. The number of city centers was later increased and traveling centers established to permit transfer between workshop, schools, factories and institutions in charge of the Russian and Persian physicians working in cooperation. Twenty thousand persons were inoculated up to the end of May, and this is a small number in view of the popularity which the local regimes succeeded in exciting the people for the treatment, as a help to the doctors. In June the numbers were still higher. The Russian serum is being injected into the back under the shoulder, three series a week apart, for typhus, typhoid, and paratyphoid. Some of the weaker persons have fainted and the Fifth Column is taking this and the fever which follows the serum, as a pretext for many Axis rumors. The first rumor was that the Russians were intending to kill the local population, that a number had already died, and the public became terrified. This later disappeared, and then another report that it was illegal for Russians to inoculate Moslems of the Faith. The Russians then immediately increased the number of Moslem doctors working for them in the inoculation clinics. The next rumor had it that the Russians were marking the back of each victim with a sign which they would later recognize and call that person a subject of the Soviet. And finally, in the serum there is a special chemical which "affects the blood and changes the patient into a Bolshevist."

The report ends:

The result of all this has been that the Russian officials have had a real fight to combat rumor as well as fear among the ignorant lower classes who have eagerly passed on each new story. Everything possible has been done to bring them in. Newspaper notices, and even the opening of clinics in the market places where many pass, with policemen there to stop and force the uninoculated in to the doctors. In this connection it may be noted that two groups have sprung up among the lower classes: One, those who go through with the inoculation in order to get the certificate so that they can sell it to others who are afraid of the ordeal, and the other, those who are willing to pay the sum for the paper which says they have had the serum—rather than take the needle—and remain exposed to the epidemic. There are some responsible people who believe that the number of inoculated persons in the city of Tabriz itself is not large, due to above conditions. But this does not obtain in other parts of Azerbaijan. Outside the city the inoculation attendance is very high. Advantage is taken by the authorities in the outside areas of the example set by the prompt inoculations of the Sheikhs and Religious Chiefs of the Tribes. This influences the subjects to follow. In many villages practically 100% of the people have had the serum, and Azerbaijan is now largely immune against a recurrence of an epidemic next year.

An OSS report for September 14-18, 1943 (MID-Iran, 2400):

In Tabriz and outlying areas, the Russians are inoculating all military personnel with a new single all-inclusive serum which they have developed, whereby one ampoule immunizes against typhus, typhoid, plague, and dysentery. Large scale civilian inoculation is publicized, but because of the size of the population, is actually limited largely to war workers in the factories (and for them not the new, but the old typhus serum is being used.

Renewed Outbreak

Military attaché report, October 28, 1943 (OSS Report 49320): "The first of the fall typhus cases have appeared in Tehran (see MA report No. 184, Section III). The outlook for the coming winter is not good. . . . Conditions causing last winter's cases remain, such as undernourishment, crowded bread and kerosene lines, and inadequate clothing." OSS report of December 3, 1943 (MID-Iran, 5060):

> According to the American Mission doctors in Meshed, there is a large increase this year in the number of sick people and several cases of typhus have already appeared. The explanation is general under-nourishment and exposure last winter to the cold. The doctors anticipate a large number of deaths in the area this winter due to the fact that the large majority of the people cannot afford to buy either adequate food or clothing; nor can they buy fuel. The result will be overcrowding and the spread of disease. The explanation for the high price of fuel is lack of transportation and heavy Russian purchases of wood for cooking and heating purposes of their troops in the area. The high prices of food is partly attributed to large Russian purchases, though the country-wide increase of prices also plays a large part.

CICI report for the week ending February 8, 1944 (MID-Iran, 2400): "Typhus has been on the increase in Tabriz and the local centre has been the prison; the Director of Public Health's telegram for money and drugs have been ignored; there is no hospital accommodation available." CICI report for the week ending February 15, 1944 (MID-Iran, 2400):

> The situation in Hamadan remains quiet. As a result of the gross overcrowding of the prison, there was a serious outbreak of typhus among the prisoners. Most of them have therefore been transferred to another prison but it would seem that the lot of these unfortunates is now worse than before since the new gaol is stated to be most unsatisfactory owing to damp and lack of ventilation.

American Military Attaché, Tehran, March 7, 1944 (MID-Iran, 2400):

> Statistics published by the Iranian Ministry of Public Health have shown a sharp rise in the number of typhus cases over the past few weeks. In

> Tabriz, there is little typhus, but appeals for medical assistance have come from Isfahan, Damghan, Semnan, and Saveh. Nevertheless, the number of cases is small in comparison with the number at this time last year, and it is felt that the unusually mild winter, better economic conditions, and preventive measures will combine to make the attack much less serious than last year's.

Ford in a dispatch of April 29, 1944, entitled, "The Typhus Situation in Iran." (Dispatch 925 and enclosures, 158.919/40):

> I have the honor to submit the following information with respect to the typhus situation in Iran, and concerning the disposition made of the supplies of anti-typhus vaccine delivered to Iran late last year from Lend-Lease stocks in Cairo. . . . While the number of cases reported during the winter just passed was not as large as the number reported during the preceding winter, there was still a considerable incidence of typhus, and outbreaks of moderate severity occurred in Tehran, Semnan, Damghan, Kashan, Resht, Pahlevi, Shiraz, Abadan, Sari, and in the area around Kerman. Although there was still a disturbingly large number of cases, Dr. Bennett F. Avery, the new American Director of Public Health, has given it as his opinion that the situation this year will not reach epidemic proportions, or approach that of last year. Dr. Avery's reasons for his conclusion are: (1) the unseasonably warm weather so far this year, coupled with an unusually warm spring; (2) the fact that the "epidemic" is in its second year; and (3) the fact that a considerable amount of control has already been accomplished. A total of 413,180 cubic centimeters of anti-typhus vaccine was received in Iran last fall from Lend-Lease stocks in Cairo. It was planned to use this vaccine in inoculating certain groups of persons, and a list of the groups agreed upon, together with the estimated number of persons in each group, will be found annexed to this despatch as enclosure No. 2. The records of the Ministry of Health indicate that 345,960 cubic centimeters of vaccine have been distributed so far to the groups mentioned. . . .

A total of 225,500 persons were designated to receive the vaccine: 100,000 factory and silo workers; 50,000 railway workers and transport drivers, including droshky drivers; 38,500 policemen, gendarmes, prison employees and prisoners; 14,000 public bath attendants and hairdressers; 13,000 bakery and flour mill workers; and 10,000 medical workers consisting of doctors, nurses and midwives. City slum dwellers most susceptible to the disease were not included.

Chapter 24

Tribal Uprisings and the Spreading Chaos

In the summer of 1943, widespread chaos in the country and the tribal uprisings in the south had led to fears of government collapse. Ever since August 1941, the Iranian government had faced conflict with the Kashkai tribes. Dreyfus on October 14, 1942 (Airgram-2, 891.00/1931):

> There have been serious clashes between migrating Kashkais and Government forces south of Shiraz and it is reported that the Shiraz-Bushire road is closed. The fighting, according to reliable sources, began when Government forces endeavored to disarm a tribe which was migrating to the lowlands. First clash was won by Government forces but second by Kashkais who took three machine guns and 30 rifles.

Nine months later, turmoil and renewed conflict had created a crisis. Dreyfus on July 16, 1943 (Dispatch 616, 891.00/2034):

> Iranian Government forces, I have the honor to inform the Department, suffered an important and humiliating defeat at the hands of Kashkai and Boir Ahmadi tribesmen at Samirun, Fars, between the 28 and 30 of June, 1943, a reverse which has radically altered the security picture in southern Iran. The facts are briefly as follows. A large band of Kashkais, under Khosro Khan (brother the great Kashkai leaders Naser Khan), and Boir Ahmadis, under Abdollah Khan Zarghampur, on June 28 successfully attacked a convoy of seven Iranian trucks and one armored car about seven miles north of the garrison town of Samirun, in Fars not far south of Isfahan. The trucks were burned and

their contents consisting of uniforms, money and supplies were taken by the tribesmen. The following night the tribesmen, wearing the uniforms they had seized, attacked the Iranian garrison at Samirun, which consisted of two infantry battalions and two troops of cavalry, a total of about 1,100 men. The garrison was well armed, possessing in addition to small arms two machine gun companies, four mortars and two 75 mm mountain guns. In spite of the size of the garrison and its superior equipment, the tribesmen after almost three days of assault subdued the defenders and captured the post. Casualties among the defenders were heavy, including the commanding officer killed. Some of the survivors were stripped and released while others were held prisoner. It is difficult to understand, in spite of the treachery of the tribesmen in wearing army uniforms, how a band of irregulars was able to defeat a larger force of trained soldiers possessing prepared positions and superior equipment. It would certainly seem that there was treachery within the garrison as well as without. I have frequently called the Department's attention to the broken morale of the Iranian army, a condition deriving mainly from the soul shattering invasion of 1941 and the events which followed. However, the defeat cannot, in my opinion, be passed off with the glib statement that the morale of the army is bad. The question of subduing and disarming the Kashkais has, in fact, been made a political football in Tehran with the result that the officers in the field have hardly known how to proceed. General Shabakhti, certainly one of Iran's most able and hardened officers, was at wits end in Fars after his arrival there several months ago to know whether he would be backed up by the Government if he proceeded with vigor. Certain politicians, deputies and newspapermen in Tehran were preaching moderation in dealing with the tribes in order to win them over by calm persuasion instead of by force. Subtle propaganda was spread to the effect that the Allies wanted action taken against the tribes merely in order to turn brother against brother. Hence the individual soldier, already reduced in morale to a low ebb, had little official inspiration from Tehran to reinforce his determination to get on with a distasteful job. The Shah, too, played his part by sending emissaries to the south to deal in a friendly way with Naser Khan.

General Shabakhti, as I have said, did not know whether or not to move but, having finally obtained assurances from the Prime Minister that forceful action against the Kashkais would be supported by the Government, decided at last to strike. He marched against Firouzabad, the seat of the Kashkais, and took it about May 22. Naser Khan and his henchmen escaped to the hills. In the opinion of many it was "all over bar the shouting" and the Government then decided on a policy of friendly negotiations with Naser Khan. With the aces in the hands of the Government at long last, there seemed to be some hopes of bringing about a final settlement of the troublesome Kashkai problem. But while Government emissaries were trying to lure Naser Khan out of his mountain fastness with sweet words, the wily Kashkai leader was apparently preparing, in unholy alliance with Boir Ahmadis, a stroke of his own. In despatches 194 of February 2, 212 of February 19, 260 of May 6 and 337 of August 31, 1942, I developed the theme of deteriorating internal situation in Iran, how the tribes quickly rearmed themselves with weapons thrown down by the Iranian soldiers at the time of the invasion, how governmental authority in the tribal areas became precarious or was completely lost, how the broken and helpless Iranian Government was impotent to remedy the situation, how the allies failed in their primary obligation to see that internal security was maintained and how security, the greatest boon of Shah Reza, appeared well on the way to being lost at least for some years. While the Government has been unable for the last year or so to reassert its authority in the tribal areas, it has been able at least to hold the line and prevent further serious deterioration. The Kurds in northern Azerbaijan have been held somewhat in check since the Rezaieh incident by the Russians, although the Iranians themselves have not been permitted to take strong action. In southern Kurdistan the fighting north of Senna has died down and a period of relative calm, accompanied by canny and cautious negotiation by the Kurds, has set in. In Khuzistan, while there have been occasional raids, the Iranians with the help of the British, have been keeping the situation under fairly good control, the while trying to disarm the tribes by persuasion rather than by force. In Khorassan relative quiet has prevailed since the depredations and arrest of Yousof Hezarehi. The principal threat to security has come from Naser Khan Kashkai, whose defeat by Shabakhti a few weeks ago appeared to presage a happy improvement there. It was something of a shock, therefore, when the tribesmen destroyed the garrison at Samirun.

The Samirun disaster may, however, serve a useful purpose and be a blessing in disguise. It should not only force the Government to redouble its efforts but also should quiet those who have preached the false doctrine of winning the embittered tribesmen with soft words and empty promises. The tribesmen, especially the Kurds, hate the Government and all that it stands for. They hold the Government, as unfortunately does the average Iranian, to be their deadly enemy and consider Government officials instruments of exploitation and thievery.

They have not forgotten the period during the late 1920s when Shah Reza, using the unscrupulous Ahmadi as his tool, subdued the tribes with cruelty and then ground them under foot and left them in a hopelessly subordinate position. Instead of roads and schools, they received only blows and overlordship by corrupt officials, then finally suffered the crowning indignity of expropriation of large part of their lands. No, the tribes cannot be won by honeyed words and perhaps the politicians who have taken that line, mainly for their own political advantage, will come to realize that fact. Another element which is favorable to the present position of the Government is that the Allies, awakening from their slumbers of the past two years, are beginning to provide Iran with tools without which the tribes can never be subdued—trucks, tires, equipment and, almost as important, a certain degree of sympathetic encouragement. The Iranian army was, in fact, so immobile that they could not move a small force to Azerbaijan without outside help. Shahbakhti's force was actually moved to Fars only when the Allied-Iranian Transport Board agreed to lend him 50 civil trucks which were badly needed for other purposes. Small wonder indeed that the tribal situation did not get completely out of hand. The tribes must be subdued by force but they can be converted into peaceful and useful elements of the population only through an enlightened and kindly policy. That was the mistake of Shah Reza; it is to be hoped that a more intelligent course will be followed when the tribes come once more, as they eventually must, under control. Tribal complaints as to expropriation of their lands must he heard and settled; the tribes must have schools, roads, lands and water; they must have more voice in the Government; they must become useful units in a progressive society in which they participate and not mere objects of exploitation by corrupt officials. First, however, they must be brought under control.

The Samirun incident will probably have its political repercussions in Tehran, some of which are already becoming evident. The policy of certain politicians and the Shah of babying the tribes may give way to a stronger line. The Iranian financial position will suffer, since some 70,000,000 rials are now being requested by the army to fit out a sizable expedition to send to Fars. The wheat collection program, so essential to Iran and to allied shipping, may suffer in view of the insecurity prevailing in the Shiraz area at this time when some 32,000 tons of wheat are ready to move from the threshing floors. How futile for the Allies to help Iran with trucks to collect wheat and at the same time fail to encourage a return to security, the most fundamental element in the entire Iranian problem! I have often remarked to the Department

> that security was the cornerstone and sine qua non of the Iranian problem but for some reason the British and the Russians have failed to appreciate this fact. If they did, they certainly failed to take constructive action. Help is at last coming to the Iranian army but only as a result of the appearance of American influence in this country. General Ridley has been a God-send to the Iranians and through his efforts equipment, especially several hundred trucks, the tools to do an essential job, should soon be in the hands of the army.
>
> An interesting sidelight on the Kashkai problem is furnished by Turkish interest in this tribe. The Turkish Ambassador has gone so far as to suggest to the Prime Minister that instead of proceeding against the Kashkais with force the tribe be permitted to migrate to Turkey where they would be given permanent lands. Turkish interest in the Kashkais springs from the belief, generally accepted as fact, that this tribe was transplanted to Fars from Turkey by Nadir Shah (1736-1747). Ethnologically white, this Turki speaking and distinctly Aryan tribe is the most important, and the most troublesome, tribal unit in Fars. While the Turkish Ambassador probably does not anticipate compliance with his suggestion of the transplantation of the Kashkais to Turkey, the incident reveals the maternal interest the Turks continue to display in the Turki speaking minorities scattered through the Middle East.

The reference to Qavam's appointment as governor of Fars refers to Ibrahim Qavam (Qavam-ol-Molk), no relation of Ahmad Qavam. Dreyfus on August 4, 1943 (Telegram 801, 891.00/2035):

> An important and potentially dangerous situation in Kashkai situation is the appointment of Qavam-ol-Molk as Governor General of Fars. Qavam family has been for centuries leading family of Fars and the Khamseh tribes they control are traditional and bitter enemies of Kashkais. It is widely believed since Qavam has long been known as British tool that British engineered appointment for purpose of endeavoring to break Kashkai power in Fars by encouraging the Qavam tribes. It is reported that Qavam will distribute arms among his tribes for use in fighting Kashkais. Millspaugh informs me confidentially that he has been requested by Government to approve a large grant of money to Qavam but that he has not yet consented. There is strong opposition in press and Majlis to Qavam appointment on grounds that tribal situation can only be aggravated by arming one tribe to fight the other.

Dreyfus on August 13, 1943 (Telegram 831, 891.00/2049 ½):

In spite of denial of British envoys here and at Ankara there is not the slightest doubt that Qavam appointment was made on British insistence. Prime and Foreign Ministers inform me they wished to send a commission to Washington to seek solution to Kashkai problem, but were persuaded by British to make Qavam appointment instead. Qavam has departed for Shiraz, but exact nature of his orders are not clear. Although Prime Minister informs me Qavam is empowered only to seek peaceful solution, British Minister states Qavam will be permitted to distribute up to 1000 rifles. I will seek clarification on this point. . . . Turk Ambassador in conversations with Iranian officials has made it clear that he opposes appointment of a tribal partisan like Qavam and that he supports idea of impartial commission. He has told me in confidence that arrest of Nobakht will serve to destroy freedom of speech in Majlis. He is of firm opinion that constant and objectionable British interference in Iranian affairs has brought about condition under which no self-respecting Iranian would enter but which must necessarily be left to unscrupulous elements. Ambassador himself told British Minister of nature of his statement to Iran Foreign Office. Bullard was furious and ensuing heated argument ended in virtual break between the two.

Dreyfus on August 21, 1943 (Dispatch 647, 891.00/2043):

I have the honor to report the following developments in the Kashkai tribal problem, especially my interview on this subject with Khosrow Khan Kashkai. Khosrow Khan Kashkai, considered to be the second most important Kashkai leader, arrived in Tehran by air on August 16 accompanied by General Jehanbani, general officer commanding Fars area, who engineered the visit. The purpose of his visit was to discuss the Kashkai problem with the Iranian Government with a view to arriving at a satisfactory and peaceful solution of this now aggravated question. He apparently came under a firm guarantee of immunity since it must be recalled that he was one of the leaders in the tribal attack against Semirun, in which the Iranian garrison of more than 1,000 was destroyed (see despatch No. 616, July 16, 1943). In addition, Khosrow, as well as Kashqais in general, is in the bad graces of the British, who allege that the tribe has been consistently anti-British and has recently given refuge to German agents. Khosrow left Tehran by air on August 19, after having held conversations with the Prime Minister, the Shah, the British Minister and myself. Khosrow's visit to

Tehran, while described by the British as unsuccessful, seems to have cleared the atmosphere considerably and paved the way for future negotiations. At any rate, he and the Prime Minister and Shah agreed that a peaceful settlement of the Kashkai problem is essential and they pledged themselves to seek a means of bringing this about and to avoid armed clashes in the future. The Iranian Government is said to have agreed to a general amnesty for tribesmen but a formal agreement on this and other points has not yet been arrived at. Khosrow has promised to endeavor to persuade his brother, Naser, to come to Tehran for discussions in the near future. While General Jehanbani believes he and Khosrow can persuade Naser to make this visit, it is said that Naser will not come to Tehran until the Government appoints him a deputy from Firouzabad, summer headquarters of the tribe. Although the Prime Minister could do this by special by-election, he is reluctant to do so because he feels the Government would lose face by such action. Naser is wisely skeptical of promises of the Iranian Government and of the British and it is doubtful if he can be lured to Tehran without most convincing guarantees of immunity.

The British are not pleased with the activities of General Jehanbani in bringing Khosrow to Tehran for direct negotiations, preferring to proceed in settlement of through their tool, Qavam, recently appointed Governor General of Fars. They were pleased, however, at Khosrow's assurances that Germans in the Kashkai country will be told that their status as honored and protected guests, based on tribal custom, is at an end and that any Germans remaining in Kashkai territory will be handed over to the British. The British Minister continues to be intransigent in the question of the mission of Qavam, a matter discussed in my telegram No. 831, August 12, 1943. The British Minister told me yesterday that "an attack on Qavam is an attack on the British. We have evidence that Qavam is considered by the Germans as Iranian enemy No. 1 and that is enough excuse for us to support him." What the British fail to take into consideration is that the Iranians desire and peaceful and permanent solution of the Kashkai problem through conciliation, an end impossible of realization when the agent is a partisan with a history enmity for the Kashkais. In spite of the Iranian opposition, of the attitude of the Turkish Ambassador (see telegram No. 831, August 12, 1943) and of my frank statement to the British Minister that the appointment is unsound and unwise, the British insist on going ahead. Qavam has left for Shiraz, after having obtained a large sum of money from the Iranian Government to cover his mission and permission to distribute arms. The number of rifles he will take for distribution is said by the British to be 1,000, by the Turkish Ambassador to be 3,500 and by Khosrow Khan to number 5,000. Whatever the number of rifles, I am more than ever firmly convinced that the procedure of arming one tribe to fight another is basically unsound and not in conformity with the duties of the Government. Qavam's appointment itself is, in my opinion, a great mistake and must be described as an attempt to impose a settlement rather than an honest endeavor to arrive at a solution through mediation. General Jehanbani's approach in bringing tribal leaders to Tehran for discussion seems to have a great deal of merit and should be definitely encouraged. The Shah seems to be of the same opinion since it is said he will decorate General Jehanbani for his efforts.

Khosrow, of his own volition and without encouragement from me, called on me on August 18. His purpose on calling, he stated, was merely to pay his respects because he is an admirer of Americans and all things American. His professed affection for Americans and belief in us appear to be fully sincere and spring mainly from the fact that he attended the American missionary school at Tehran. To digress for a moment from the theme of this despatch, one cannot help but remark on the profound effect the missionary schools have had on the youth of Iran. As a typical example, here is a boy of about 23, of fine appearance, able to speak English, of education and character far above the average Iranian level, whose superior qualities can be traced in part directly to the American missionary school. This striking example of the lasting value to Iran and to our country of missionary education should not be lost sight of in considering the general question of reopening of the schools.

To return to Khosrow, he began the conversation, after his introductory remarks about his regard for America, by stating the Kashkai case against the Iranian Government. He related how his father had been imprisoned and later killed by Shah Reza, how the tribe had been harried, abused, disarmed and exploited by the Iranian Government and how their lands have been in many cases expropriated. His father, he said, and he seemed to feel this was the crowning abuse, in spite of having been a rich man was buried though the charity of a friend, who was in turn persecuted by the Iranian Government for his act of decency. Notwithstanding these bitter experiences, Khosrow declared that he and Naser wish ardently to arrive at a solution which will be just, peaceful and permanent. They wished to avoid, he averred, any more incidents such as that at Semirun and are willing to pledge their good conduct if the Iranian Government will grant amnesty and will honestly endeavor to give some degree of justice to the tribesmen.

Khosrow said he was absolutely confident of his ability personally to settle the problem and therefore regretted that his offers had not been taken advantage of by the Iranians or the British. He left not the slightest doubt that he considers the Qavam appointment an error. Without evident animus, he remarked that the Qavam family, through the Khamseh tribes they control, have been bitter enemies of the Kashkais for five centuries. He felt that Qavam, as an enemy of the tribe and a British agent, could not possibly bring about a solution. I must admit that I was impressed by Khosrow Khan, both by his personality and his evident ability as a tribal leader. I was pleased, too, at his evident sincere regard for our country, a fact which may prove of some importance in the future. Although he made it clear that he was merely calling to pay his respects, he asked during the course of the conversation for my support in obtaining justice for Kashkais. I replied to the effect that my Government would not approve of any overt interference on my part in purely internal Iranian affairs but that I would naturally wish to do all in my power to encourage a friendly and just settlement of the Kashkai problem. Khosrow's visit served at least to put the disputants at long last in direct contact with each other and to open the way for future conversations which may bear fruit.

Dreyfus on August 25, 1943 (Dispatch 648 and enclosure, 891.00/2044):

I have the honor to report the following developments which have occurred in the Qashqai tribal dispute and the internal security situation in southern Iran since my despatches No. 646 dated August 20 and No. 647 dated August 21. The Prime Minister told me yesterday that Khosrow Khan Qashqai, on the occasion of his visit to Tehran last week, agreed in writing to the following four points. The demands on which this agreement was based, the Prime Minister stresses, were dictated by the British Legation. (1) The Qashqais will surrender any German who may remain in their territory after he has been invited to leave and any Germans who may find their way into Qashqai country in the future. They will surrender documents and papers, but not gold, found in the possession of Germans. (2) The Qashqais will permit British officials to go into their territory and will facilitate their travel. (3) The Qashqais will inform the British as to the location of any airfields which have been laid out in their territory. (4) The Qashqais will endeavor to maintain security in their territory and will also offer protection to the Trans-Iranian Railway. While Khosrow was willing to agree to these four points, he refused to acknowledge Qavam-ol-Molk as the arbiter in the Qashqai dispute. The British are still intransigent on this question, taking the view that Qavam was appointed by the Iranian Government to carry out this task and must therefore be supported. Further, and final, evidence that Qavam is backed fully by the British was obtained in a letter addressed to the Prime Minister by the British Minister. The Prime Minister yesterday permitted me, in the strictest confidence, to copy the pertinent portion of the British Minister's letter, which is quoted herewith: "Paragraph 3. Finally may I remind Your Excellency of what I said about His Excellency Qavam-ol-Molk, against whom, Your Excellency admitted, there are many intrigues in Tehran and elsewhere. The opinion of His Majesty's Legation that Qavam is a faithful servant of the Iranian Government is fully borne out by incontrovertible evidence that the Germans hate and fear him as a redoubtable opponent. Consequently, His Majesty's Legation will be obliged to regard any persons who intrigue against the Qavam as intriguing against the allies. The Iranian Government has appointed him and I look to Your Excellency to see that he receives from the army and the civil servants concerned the support on which any high official ought to be able to count as a matter of course." The above language leaves no doubt that the British are squarely behind the Qavam appointment, especially when the Prime Minister admitted to me freely that he is being required to proceed in the Qashqai negotiations in conformity with British desires. I do not quite see how Sir Reader Bullard, in supporting Qavam in this manner, can pretend to speak for the Allies. If he means by "Allies," the nations allied against the Axis powers he certainly is not in a position to assume this attitude, since the United States was not consulted. If, on the other hand, he had in mind the nations to which Iran is allied by treaty, Great Britain and Russia, he still is not in a position to state the question thus, since I know that the Soviet Government has not yet taken a stand in the question of Qavam or the matter of the arrests.

Dreyfus on August 26, 1943 (Dispatch 653 and enclosure, 891.00/2045):

I have the honor to enclose a translation of a letter written to the Prime Minister by Khosrow Khan Qashqai outlining the Qashqai complaints against the Iranian Government and suggesting measures to settle the Qashqai tribal dispute. While the letter is not particularly important or profound, it is, to my knowledge, the first time a tribal leader has taken the trouble to reduce tribal complaints to writing in a restrained and constructive manner.

In his letter of August 18, 1943, Khosrow had made two demands: unconditional and full restitution of lands taken by Reza Shah and full compensation for lost income from these properties over the years. Subsequent events in Khorassan showed that the government had no intention of reaching a just settlement of these grievances. Information on government's insincerity is provided in an OSS report by Lowe on his trip to Mashad during October 26 to November 10, 1943 (Report 74, 891.00/2091):

> Yusuf Hezara (Solat as-Saltaneh) with his two brothers headed the tribe of the Hezaras who lived on the Afghan frontier. Riza Shah took some of their villages near Fariman, gave them to the Qashghais and gave to the Hezaras in exchange certain villages south of Shiraz. When Riza Shah left, the Qashghais took back their villages south of Shiraz. Using this as an excuse, the Hezaras rose in arms to take back their villages in Khurasan. The chiefs, in fact, seemed to think the time ripe to carve out for themselves an independent area in the Meshed region. They were defeated and dispersed by the Persian army. The leaders were arrested and brought to Teheran where negotiations concerning the property were supposed to be going on. Yusuf seems to have been allowed to move about freely in Teheran. About two months ago, I was told confidentially that he had been to call on an official of the British Legation to inquire whether he had better to remain here and continue the fruitless discussions or return to his home and again try force. He was not encouraged to use force. In any case, he left Teheran and returned to Meshed. From there he went to a village near the Afghan frontier. The Gendarmes were told to go and bring him back to Teheran. An officer went with about 20 men. The village was surrounded and the officer went unarmed to call on Yusuf. When the message was delivered, Yusuf shot the officer and then with twelve of his followers mounted horse and tried to escape. He and two of his followers were shot and killed by the gendarmes, two of whom were also killed. The above information about the shooting comes from an officer in the Gendarmerie in Meshed. The rumor that Solat was deliberately murdered does not seem to be true. The affair simply demonstrates again the government's continued unwillingness to reach and put into effect a fair settlement with the tribes.

British Desire to Recreate the South Persia Rifles

In their apparent panic, the British had sought to recreate the South Persia Rifles of World War I.[1] Dreyfus on July 20, 1943 (Telegram 751, 891.00/2031):

> Strictly Confidential. British here are alarmed at Iranian security situation and appear to be considering remedial action. British Minister is approaching me rather formally on subject stressed disastrous defeat in which the Iranian army garrison of more than a thousand men was eliminated as a military unit by tribesmen in Samirun in Fars at end of June (see despatch 616, July 16 which reported this incident and discussed general tribal situation). He alleged that German parachutists have been dropped near Qum and have not been apprehended. He summed up by expressing opinion that there is almost total lack of security in Iran and that country verges on anarchy. Since he attributes this condition to great extent to weakness and incompetence of Soheily Government he asked my support and that of Soviet Chargé in bringing about fall of present Government and installing Ali Mansur as Prime Minister. I replied that while I hold no brief for Soheily and rather incline to British view of him and while I consider Mansur to be one of the most suitable candidates for Prime Minister I could hardly go so far as to assist in engineering fall of Government in view of policy of my Government not to interfere in internal Iranian political affairs. Although Soviet Chargé has promised to consult Moscow it is very unlikely that Russians would offer their cooperation because they appear to be well satisfied with Soheily and in view of their reluctance to join other Allies in any action affecting their mutual interests. Russians appear to be getting on well with Mansur at Meshed although he has been criticized by some Russians as willing tool of ex-Shah.
>
> General Pownall's current visit to Iran is closely connected with this subject. Pownall takes serious view of situation and feels that some action must be taken to bring about improvement. He told Schwarzkopf in strictest confidence that he is considering recruiting a special Iranian force against tribes to maintain security supply lines. Force would apparently be similar to South Persia Rifles of last war. However in a conversation with General Ridley Pownall made no mention of this idea. British seem to be making conscious endeavor to build up picture of Iranian insecurity. Foreign Minister remarked to me yesterday with some bitterness that British are permitting or encouraging press in England to paint picture of Iran as insecure, chaotic and bordering on

> anarchy. I am not sure to what extent his British view of Iranian security situation is due (one) sincere belief that situation is getting out of hand and that British as Allied Government responsible for Iranian security must take effective action or (two) desire to use situation as excuse to get rid of Soheily Government. I shall report developments.

The suggestion on the South Persia Rifles was not well received in Washington. Cable to Dreyfus, July 29, 1943 (Telegram 377, 891.00/2031):

> Secret. Your 751, July 20. Department is inclined to feel that creation of a new force of British-officered Iranian troops, similar to the South Persia Rifles, would be a mistake at this time, since it would be an invitation to the Soviets to create a similar organization, a counterpart of the old Cossack Brigade. It seems to us that development of two new military groups, under foreign domination, would only lead to confusion worse confounded and that equipment and effort devoted to their organization could better be employed under the direction of Ridley and Schwarzkopf in building up the existing Iranian Army and Gendarmerie. If these latter forces are unable to cope with the tribal situation, do you not believe that from a political point of view it would be preferable to employ British troops to maintain security, rather than create a pseudo-Iranian force which would, we imagine, be regarded with suspicion by the Iranians themselves?

The British had dropped the idea. Dreyfus on August 4, 1943 (Telegram 801, 891.00/2035):

> Department's 377, July 29. After discussing with British Minister Ridley Schwarzkopf and Foreign Minister general question of recruitment of special Iranian force I do not believe British intend to develop this idea. Schwarzkopf's impression is that Pownall was only exploring the ground and had in mind perhaps a small force of levies for railway security to affect that British have sent troops to Southern Iran to take care of convoy security. Ridley told me in strictest confidence that the tribal situation will be met by calling upon additional ten thousand conscripts to create a special striking force. He stated that this force cannot for various reasons including lack of money and equipment be brought into being before winter or spring.

A "Flurry" of British Political Intervention

Dreyfus on July 23, 1943 (Telegram 761, 891.00/2032):

> My 751, July 20. British Minister informs me that on Monday at his own request and accompanied by his Military Attaché, he was received by the Shah. Purpose he declares was to bring to Shah's attention forcefully and frankly his dissatisfaction with conditions in Iran and with Shah's interference in Government affairs. He states he made following points: One, the weakness and incompetence of Soheily Government have been largely responsible for bringing about present condition of chaos and insecurity in Iran; two, Shah's constant interference in Government is improper and has tended to aggravate situation. Minister intimated to Shah that he and career army clique were responsible for riots last December. Three. Tribal situation is getting out of hand. Government has failed to act on British suggestion that tribal complaints be looked into with view to arriving at just and permanent settlement. He referred to defeat at Semirum and deprecated Shah's efforts to place blame on War Minister whereas responsibility lies with Shah and springs from mistaken tribal policy. Shah's reply to above was to effect that if he has in fact interfered it was because he cannot govern like another Ahmad Shah (last of Kajars who has won an unenviable reputation for weakness and incompetence). Strangely coincidental with Minister's visit to Shah, Iran press opened its first overt campaign against Shah since his advent two years ago. Briefly press accuses Shah of interfering with and endeavoring to direct Government affairs. One paper warns that if he follows in his father's footsteps he will suffer the same fate as his father. Shah in his conversation with British Minister attribute press attacks to vindictive action by certain papers he failed to subsidize and by those he actually aided financially because he withdrew his support. Despite explanation it seems unlikely that press would dare make such attacks under present conditions without blessing or actual connivance of a foreign power. Department will recall that at time of invasion I reported that British looked with disfavor on young Shah and decided to support him only because of absence of any alternative and then only on definite understanding that he was on trial. Since then I have frequently remarked on increasing British dissatisfaction with Shah's activities a trend culminating in present gesture of disapproval.
>
> Present flurry of activity by British is the more obvious since British Legation has been acting in a relatively restrained manner since the frank conversations between Department and British officials concern-

> ing arrests and interference in Iranian political affairs. It is not clear to me whether they intend merely to bring about fall of Soheily or whether they hunt bigger game and envisage departure of Shah and institution of new kind of Government. There is, of course, some justification in British interference. They can hardly be expected in view of their interest in Iran and considering their responsibility to Allies for maintenance of security on Russian supply route to sit by complacently while conditions degenerate to point where effective Government has almost ceased to exist. Nevertheless, open interference of this kind is fraught with dangerous implications and will bear careful watching.

The British had soon after resurrected another ghost of 1919. Dreyfus on August 8, 1943 (telegram 818, 891.00/2036):

> Department's 76, February 11. I am reliably informed that the return to Iran of Seyid Zia-ed-Din Tabatabai is imminent. British Minister confirms this fact but denies any complicity therein. To prove this point, he states that he has refused to assist Tabatabai to obtain seat in plane from Palestine. Notwithstanding this denial I have every reason to believe British have at least encouraged him; for example, British Minister admitted to me that there was correspondence between him and British Oriental Secretary Trott. Since both Shah and Russian Ambassador have told me they are very much opposed to Tabatabai, our wisest course for the moment may be to permit them to offer any resistance they desire and ourselves await developments.

In the same telegram, Dreyfus adds:

> With reference to my 761, July 23, British continue their political activity. British Minister informed me yesterday that he is now preparing a letter to Prime Minister demanding that deputy Nobakht have his immunity waived by Majlis and be arrested by Government. Nobakht is accused by British of working in German interests, a charge based mainly on the Mayer document (see despatch 495, March 25). In justification of this British demand, I must say that Nobakht has been not only generally obstructive, but has taken a consistent anti-Allied line. As far as I am aware, he is the only deputy who has made public statements against the United States (see despatch 192, March 30 1942).
>
> Political situation continues to drift hopelessly with virtual breakdown in government and daily threats of riots and strikes of woefully underpaid government employees. Soheily seems to feel that tenure of office

is an end in itself and hangs on for dear life despite weak position of his government and British desire to oust him. Millspaugh's recent regulation creating government monopoly in grains has further embarrassed government by subjecting it to violent attacks by speculators and war profiteers who prefer huge profits to common welfare. Millspaugh in matters of grain monopoly, income tax, and government salaries has reached critical and climatic point in his struggle with selfish and corrupt elements. Under attack now from all quarters, including Majlis, Cabinet, press and merchants, he sticks to his guns with equanimity, secure in knowledge that he is working for welfare of people. His test of strength is close at hand and outcome in the balance.

Dreyfus on August 13, 1943 (Telegram 831, 891.00/2049 ½):

Department's 398, August 7. One. Arrests. British Minister informs me he will shortly request Iranian Government to arrest some thirty Iranians alleged to have engaged in pro-German activities. He has delivered to Iranian Government the note requesting the arrest of Deputy Nobakht and is awaiting developments (see my 818, August 7. Copy of note being sent to Department airmail). After mature thought and based to large extent in considerations given in concluding section of this telegram I have come to conclusion that we should not (repeat not) oppose the arrests but should suggest to Iranians if they approach us the overriding military necessity of restraining persons who have obstructed or are potentially harmful to war effort. However, British should be required to support each request by obviously authentic documents of highly convincing nature. Since Mayer documents will form basis for arrests it is suggested Department have these documents carefully examined by experts. . . .

British activities. I must admit bewilderment as to possible motives behind present surge of British political activity in Iran. Turkish Ambassador who is fair, intelligent and well informed expresses opinion that British, viewing Russian ascendancy in Iran, feel it necessary to step in with forceful action to endeavor to salvage as much as possible of their position in this country. It is possible that British are by the arrests deliberately endeavoring to alienate Iranians to such an extent that they will refuse to join United Nations declaration, a step British have admittedly not favored.

> Conclusion. We have arrived at important crossroads in Anglo-American-Iranian relations. We must weigh on one side our desire to protect Iranians from British and Soviet domination and on the other side our obligation toward our British allies, and endeavor to find somewhere between the two extremes a workable solution. Certainly Iran has recently degenerated to state of confusion and virtual breakdown of government, a condition to which the British, who are charged with maintenance of allied security in Iran, cannot close their eyes. However, it must be remarked that Iran's present condition is due in great degree to allied failure to give country the kind of assistance, sympathy and constructive leadership which an occupied country has the right to expect. While I incline to view that British "pin prick" action in Iran has and continues to have harmful effect, I hardly see how we can take a firm stand unless we are prepared to have an almost open break with British here and forfeit the feeling of Anglo-American solidarity which we have been at pains to develop since the frank discussions of last year. Would not this be a good opportunity for discussions in Washington and London, without criticism and recrimination, as to allied aims in Iran in light of war effort and Atlantic Charter with view to determining best means of arriving at the desired ends? Department requested to repeat to London.

Dreyfus on August 12, 1943 (Dispatch 637 and enclosure, 891.00/2042):

> I have the honor to enclose a copy of a note of August 5, 1943, addressed by the British Minister in Tehran to the Iranian Prime Minister, in which the arrest of Deputy Habibullah Nobakht is requested. The Prime Minister has not yet replied to the British Legation note or taken any action to comply. He told the Turkish Ambassador, who passed the information along to me, that he is completely at a loss to know how to proceed. He fully realizes the consternation which will reign when he asks the Majlis to waive deputy Nobakht's immunity preparatory to his arrest and he feels certain the incident will provoke a wave of anti-British feeling. He is aware, also that the affair may well result in the fall of his Government. In spite of these adverse considerations, it is difficult to see how the Prime Minister will extricate himself from this predicament without endeavoring to comply with the British request. The British request for the arrest of deputy Nobakht is the first of a series of such demands which the British intend to make. The political implications of these arrests were discussed at some length in my telegram No. 831, August 12. The Department will be kept informed of developments.

Bullard's letter of August 5, 1943, to Soheily:

Your Excellency was so good as to inform me recently that, if I provided you with written evidence, you would be prepared to arrest any Iranians whose name I might think fit to bring to your notice in connection with pro-Axis activities prejudicial to Allied cause. 2. I now have the honor to inform Your Excellency that the evidence which has been accumulating against Nobakht, at present a member of the Majlis, is such that I can no longer refrain from bringing his case to your urgent and personal attention. As Your Excellency is aware, Iran has reached a danger point in her history and events are now justifying the foresight of those who concluded and ratified the Tripartite Treaty of January 1942. However, among those who opposed that treaty was Nobakht and eversince that date he and those like him have, in spite of the smashing blows which have been delivered against Germany, Italy and Japan on land, sea and in the air, been endeavoring to drag Iran into the Axis camp and transform what should be an allied country into the last bastion of the Axis Powers. All those who are helping him and his satellites in these nefarious activities and now attempt to shield and protect him can only be classed as traitors to their country and enemies of the United Nations.

3. Your Excellency knows as well as I do that a dangerous movement, supported by German agents in the tribal areas of the South, is at present on foot against the Iranian Government and is being instigated first and foremost by Nobakht. The latter is known to have been in close contact with Nasir Khan and his German advisers during the last year and he has spared no effort to stir up the Qashghais not only against the Allied Powers, but even against the Imperial Government with whom His Majesty's Government are in close and friendly relations. Documents which were seized by the British Security Authorities in the house of the German agent Franz Mayer, in Isfahan, in November last, conclusively show that Nobakht was closely implicated in a wide organization composed of Germans and Iranians, who were preparing a coup in Iran to be carried out at the most favorable moment. The coup, which provided for the reception of German agents in the country, preliminary to the overthrow of the existing Iranian Government and the establishment of a Military Government hostile to the Allied powers, failed to materialize owing to the fact that German campaigns in Russia and North Africa met with defeat.

4. According to documents in possession of His Majesty's Legation, of which I enclose a few extracts for Your Excellency's information,

Nobakht is beyond question deeply implicated in these treacherous activities which the conspirators hoped would expose the Allied position in this country to serious danger, particularly as regards the supply of Aid to Russia. I have refrained from taking the matter up earlier with the Imperial Government as the Government could not be unaware of the activities of Nobakht and I had assumed that the Imperial Government itself would take firm action against all those concerned without representations on my part. To my deep regret my assumption proved to be ill-founded and accordingly in view of the constant deterioration of the situation throughout the country I have no alternative but to request Your Excellency to arrange forthwith for the removal of Nobakht's parliamentary immunity and for his arrest and despatch to Sultanabad for detention and interrogation in accordance with the Agreement reached last year between the Iranian and British Governments.

5. During conversations which I have had with Your Excellency at various times about the suggestion that Iran should join the United Nations, I have said more than once that in my opinion His Majesty's Government and her Allies would judge Iran less by her signature to some formal document than by her acts.

I avail myself of this opportunity to renew to Your Excellency the assurance of my highest consideration. (Sgd.) R.W. Bullard

Dreyfus on August 25, 1943 (Dispatch 648 and enclosure, 891.00/2044):

There are as yet no important developments in the general question of British demands for arrests. The Iranian Government has advertised, at British request, an offer of a reward of 50,000 rials to any person giving information which will lead to the apprehension of a German who has no residence permit. The British Minister has handed me a copy of a draft of a letter he intends to send to the Iranian Government demanding the arrest of Iranians included in lists which he will attach. A copy of this draft is attached. Even if the charges are made in the draft before delivery, I feel it is significant as an indication of the severe line being taken by the British. While I do not for a moment suggest altering the course we have chosen of not opposing the British in these arrests, I must express amazement at the belligerent and unfriendly tone of the British in this entire question. Their action may be justified by their apparent belief that the fifth column danger in Iran menaces the Russian supply line and the position of the allies in this country. However, one is constrained to remark that it is strange the British have found it necessary to take such strong and vehement action against an allied power.

In Bullard's intended letter to Soheily, STBD stands for Sultanabad:

I have the honor to inform Your Excellency that for several months past the activities of pro-Axis Iranian agitators in this country, supported by German agents, have seriously increased without the Imperial Government having thought fit even in one single instance to take the initiative in instituting severe measures against those who are deeply implicated in such treacherous and nefarious designs. It was hoped that the Imperial Government, in their position as an ally, would have been ready to put an end to this dangerous state of affairs without constant representations by His Majesty's Legation, but unfortunately the Iranian police authorities have proved to be useless in this respect. In many cases the police appear to be condoning, if not actually supporting, the work of these agents against Allied interests in Iran, and it is therefore impossible for His Majesty's Government to have any more confidence in them. 2. It is hardly necessary for me to remind Your Excellency of the serious shortcomings of the Iranian Police Department in the past, since Your Excellency is well aware that Vaziri, Mehvandy & Akhbari, whose arrests I have been requesting for more than a year, are still at large—possibly with the connivance of members of the Iranian Police themselves. 3. It is certain that German agents in Iran are now making a desperate effort to delay the inevitable defeat of the Axis by trying to sabotage the Allied war effort in this country. It is essential to the interests of the Allies that the pro-Axis organization should be broken up completely, and I therefore have the honor to request Your Excellency to give immediate instructions for the arrest of the persons whose names figure on the attached lists, and for their despatch forthwith to STBD for detention and interrogation in accordance with the agreement concluded between the Imperial Government and the British Government last year. 4. I can assure Your Excellency that I should not be making this request unless my Government were fully convinced that it was essential to the interests of both our countries. All the evidence accumulated against these suspects will be forthcoming as soon as they are in safe custody in STBD. Past experience has shown that evidence communicated to the Imperial Government in advance has often been improperly used and has even reached those persons whose arrest the Imperial Government had been asked to effect.

Arrest of Iranian "Plotters"

Shortly after Bullard's latest letter to Soheily, many Iranians were arrested by the British and sent to Sultanabad for interrogation and detention. An OSS report dated September 28, 1943, contains the following (Report A 12083, 891.00/2066-1/2):

> Iranians although slow to speak of it, resented sudden arrests of Iranian officials by the British in the south, several months ago, as an infringement of their sovereignty. Recent arrests by the British (August 30, 31, September 1) on a wide scale (including the commander of the Gendarmerie, an ex-Prime Minister, Mullah from Koum) may have been made directly, instead of through Iranians authorities in some cases. The British have not as yet revealed the evidence on which they acted.

Two of the "plotters," Deputy Nobakht and Molla Kashani, whom the British were very anxious to catch, had remained at large for nearly a year. Nobakht was arrested in May 1944, while Kashani was caught a month later. Ford on June 26, 1944, in a dispatch entitled, "Arrest of Molla Kashani" (Dispatch 1005, 800.20291/6-2644):

> I have the honor to refer to my despatch No. 956 of May 23, 1944 and to previous despatches regarding the arrest and interrogation of suspected Axis agents in Iran, and to report that on June 17 British security agents, accompanied by an Iranian police officer, arrested the fugitive Molla Abol Ghassem Kashani, last of important suspects to escape detention. The arrest was made at a shrine (imamzadeh) near Tehran. Kashani has been taken to Arak (Sultanabad) for interrogation by British authorities. The arrest brought about a certain amount of public protest, as was to be expected in view of Kashani's political and religious influence. The Tehran bazaar closed briefly on June 18 and there was a slight disturbance which was quickly quelled. The same day Deputy Firuzabadi spoke in the Majlis, calling Kashani "a member of the Majlis" and declaring that his detention was contrary to the principles of freedom upheld by Great Britain. A group of mollas also met and sent messages to the Shah and Prime Minister requesting his release. However, there seem to have been no further developments along this line.

Ford on August 10, 1944 (Dispatch 1064 and enclosure, 800.20291/8-1044):

I have the honor to refer to my despatches No. 956 of May 23 and No. 1005 of June 26, 1944, reporting the arrest of Hassan Nobakht and Molla Abolghassem Kashani, and to transmit herewith a translation of a communiqué which has been issued by the Iranian Ministry of Interior outlining evidence against these two Axis agents. An Anglo-Iranian board has been interrogating Kashani and Nobakht at Arak, and this communiqué was issued at British insistence in order to counteract the assertions made by certain newspapers that both of the accused were innocent patriots who had been "railroaded." Between June 23 and July 26, a total of 25 more of the internees being held in Tehran were released, somewhat to the annoyance of the British security authorities, who felt that sufficient care had not been taken to obtain adequate guarantees of good behavior from them before release. In addition, ten of the so-called Russian prisoners who were taken to Resht for interrogation have been set free on condition that they promised to refrain from all activity hostile to the Allies and to keep the authorities informed of their whereabouts. Among these was Dr. Matin Daftary, brother of the Counselor of the Iranian Legation at Washington. The press report mentioned in my despatch No. 956, to the effect that the Resht internees were to be brought back to Tehran, has proved inaccurate, and the balance of the group held for Russian questioning is apparently still in Resht.

Note

1. For a history of the establishment of the South Persia Rifles in 1916 and its successful imposition of "law and order" in southern Iran, see Majd, Mohammad Gholi. *Persia in World War I & Its Conquest by Great Britain.* Lanham: University Press of America, 2003. 101-139.

Chapter 25

British-American Exchanges and Memoranda on Iran and the Tehran Declaration

On July 31, 1943, W.G. Hayter, First Secretary of the British Embassy, had called on Alling (Memorandum, 891.00/2035):

> Mr. Hayter called at his request to inform the Department of certain developments in connection with the situation in Iran. He stated that General Pownall, commanding British troops in Iran, had become greatly disturbed by recent attacks upon Iranian forces by tribesmen. Mr. Hayter pointed that, as we knew, tribesmen had recently annihilated an Iranian garrison. General Pownall proceeded to Tehran a few days ago to discuss with the British Minister recommendations which might be made to the Foreign Office regarding steps to be taken to improve the situation. The British Minister and General Pownall both agreed that it would be unwise to use British troops against the tribesmen. After lengthy discussion they submitted the following proposals to the Foreign Office: (1) 550 trucks carrying Lend-Lease supplies to Russia would be sent north convoyed by British troops; (2) it would be suggested to the Shah that, in view of the weakness of Prime Minister Soheily, it would seem desirable to replace him by appointing Ali Mansur; (3) it would be desirable to appoint Qavam-ol-Molk as Governor-General of Fars. The Foreign Office replied that it had no objection to using British troops to convoy the trucks as far as Isfahan but it desired that the Russians authorities be informed; (2) the Foreign Office would be glad to see Mr. Soheily replaced by Ali Mansur if that could be done without too much difficulty; (3) the Foreign Office ap-

proved of the proposal regarding the appointment of Qavam-ol-Molk as Governor General of Fars but pointed out that the Shah might disapprove.

The Foreign Office had instructed the British Embassy in Washington to bring the foregoing to the attention of the Department of State and to point out that the Foreign Office regarded interference in the internal affairs of Iran "with reluctance and repugnance." However, the British Government had responsibilities regarding the transport of supplies to Russia and could not allow the disturbed situation in Iran to interfere in the supply program. I said that I was sure that all of the interested officials in the Department would be glad to learn that the Foreign Office regarded interference in the internal affairs of Iran "with reluctance and repugnance," and that we certainly all hoped that a solution could be found without such interference. Mr. Hayter said that he had one further communication to make. German parachutists had recently landed in Iraq near the borders of Iran and the British authorities had some reason to believe that German agents were operating in Iran with the connivance of Iranian officials and nationals. It was possible therefore that it would be necessary to arrest some of the Persian officials who were alleged to be in contact with Axis agents. I told Mr. Hayter that as he doubtless knew it had been the general feeling in the Department that it was better, when Iranian officials came under suspicion, to request their arrest by the Iranian authorities rather than having them arrested by British or Russians. Mr. Hayter indicated that he would recall this point of view to the attention of the authorities.

Alling on August 5, 1943 (Memorandum, 891.00/2035):

Today Mr. Hayter called at his request. He said that the British Government was still disturbed regarding the activities of certain Iranian nationals who, they had reason to believe, were in contact with Axis agents in Iran. Therefore the Foreign Office had telegraphed to Moscow to lay the situation before the Soviet authorities and request that the Soviet Chargé d'Affaires in Tehran be instructed to concert with his British colleague in drawing up a list of alleged offenders, together with a statement of their offenses. It was then proposed that the British Minister and the Soviet Chargé d'Affaires should present this list to the Iranian Foreign Office with the request that the persons in question should be arrested. Mr. Hayter said that he had been directed to bring the foregoing to the attention of the Department and point out that

> while the United States Government was not directly interested in this problem, the British Government would welcome American support in the step proposed. In any case, the British Government hoped that the American Minister in Tehran might be authorized if he was approached on the matter by the Iranian authorities to say that he concurred in the desirability of the arrests. I asked Mr. Hayter whether he had any information to the effect that Mr. Dreyfus had been informed of the foregoing. He said that he had no such information. I told him in the first instance we would probably confine ourselves to informing Mr. Dreyfus of the proposed steps in asking his views in the matter.

Dissatisfied with State Department response, on August 25, 1943, at a conference in Quebec, Canada, Sir Ronald Campbell, the British Chargé d'Affaires in Washington, handed a memorandum to the Secretary of State entitled "Situation in Persia." It reads (Memorandum, 891.00/2055):

> Our views on Persia are as follows: The most pressing problem is security. Tribes near Shiraz have been largely out of hand since their recent success against a Persian army detachment and although the Shiraz road is no longer used for aid to Russia disorders may spread. The Germans, who are planning a sabotage campaign in all Middle Eastern countries, are naturally exploiting the situation and have dropped parachutists with the immediate object of increasing disorder and diverting our troops, and with probable ultimate object of damaging the oil installations and the railway. Both HM Minister in Tehran and we wished to see British troops stationed at Shiraz as the best means of keeping the situation under control, but with the forces at his disposal the Commander-in-Chief cannot agree to this. We must therefore concentrate on (a) efforts to improve local Persian administration and (b) drastic measures against Persian pro-Axis plotters.
>
> As regards (a) HM Minister has with difficulty induced the Persian Government to appoint as Governor-General of Shiraz a reliable Persian of local tribal origin. His appointment will encourage the tribes which have not yet joined the rebels to remain loyal. As to (b) we are naturally anxious to act jointly with the Russians if possible and we have done all we can to get them into line. But time presses and we can not wait indefinitely for the Soviet representative to receive instructions from Moscow. HM Minister was recently authorized to present to the Persian Government our demands for the arrests of Persian suspects if necessary without waiting for Russian support and in the last resort to have the arrests effected by British security authorities. Since

then one particularly dangerous German who has organized a widespread plot with the assistance of prominent Persians and two newly-arrived German parachutists have been captured by our security authorities, and a mass of new evidence against Persian suspects has come into our hands. It is now a fortnight since HM Minister gave the Persian Prime Minister our evidence against the most dangerous of Persian Axis sympathizers but the Persian Government have still taken no action. It is therefore likely that HM Minister may soon have to have recourse to direct arrests by British forces.

Meanwhile the political situation is unsatisfactory and continues to deteriorate. Soheily, the Persian Prime Minister, is ineffective. The Persian Government command no confidence and have little authority in the country as a whole. The financial situation is also bad and likely to get worse. In spite of a large harvest administrative inefficiency may again result in shortages.

We should certainly welcome closer cooperation with the United States Government in Persian affairs. The most important thing at present is to have United States support for our action on security questions. We have not asked the United States Government to act jointly with us, as security is not their responsibility, though we have kept them generally informed of our intentions except as regards possible direct arrests by ourselves. But we are entitled to hope that the United States Government will present a common front with us to the Persians and in case of need make it clear to all concerned that they are at one with us as regards the vital importance of checking the activities of hostile Persians which would assist the German threat to supply routes. If the United States Government for their part, in the light of the experience gained by the American adviser, have any suggestions for improving Persian administration we shall of course gladly do our best to help. It has been suggested that the situation might be eased if reasonable quantities of consumer goods could be imported into Iran. Probably two shiploads would suffice, and this would cause only a small retardation of the increase of supplies to Russia. It is hoped that the United States Government will give this question their benevolent consideration.

In forwarding the full text of the Quebec memorandum to the Embassy in London on September 22, 1943, the instruction adds (Telegram 1271, 891.00/2053A):

Please send the Foreign Office a memorandum in reply reading in substance as follows: The Department is, of course, fully aware of the importance of the security problem in Iran. On August 20 the American Minister at Tehran was instructed to support British action leading to the arrest of the persons believed to be engaged in pro-Axis activities by explaining to the Iranians, if approached by them on the subject, the overriding military necessity of restraining persons who have obstructed or are potentially harmful to the war effort. This course of action had been suggested by Mr. Dreyfus. It is to be hoped that the recent Iranian declaration of war will strengthen, at least to some extent, the hand of the Iranian Government in dealing with security matters. The Department has also discussed security questions with the War Department, which, we understand, is engaged in conversations with the British military authorities on the subject. We shall be glad to bear in mind the Foreign Office's assurance that it will do its best to help if we have any suggestions for improving the Persian administration in the light of experience gained by the American adviser. The Department has under active consideration the Foreign Office's suggestion that the situation might be eased if reasonable quantities of consumer goods could be imported into Iran. For a variety of reasons, it would be very difficult to provide the shipping space for consumer goods for Iran at the expense of military supplies for Russia. In any case, this problem appears to lie primarily within the sphere of the Middle East Supply Center, and we have telegraphed Cairo for an expression of their views.

London replied on October 22, 1943 (Airgram A-1207, 891.00/2061):

Reference Department's Airgram A-1271, dated September 22, 1943. Following is text of informal note from the Foreign Office in reply to the Embassy's presentation of the Department's views on the security problem in Iran: "Many thanks for your letter of the 30th September, about Anglo-American co-operation in Persia. We are happy to have this confirmation that the State Department are particularly aware of the importance of the security problem in Persia. The support of the United States authorities in connection with the recent action by the British and Soviet representatives to ensure the arrest of Axis agents and suspects in Persia contributed in no small measure to the satisfactory results obtained. We are aware of the difficulties entailed in the proposal to increase the supply of consumer goods to Persia, and agree with the State Department's view that this is a question which must be referred to the Middle East Supply Centre." Winant

Memorandum to the President

Greatly alarmed at the situation in Iran, on August 16, 1943, Secretary of State Cordell Hull had addressed a letter to President Roosevelt (Letter and memorandum, 891.00/2042A):

> My dear Mr. President: I enclose herewith, for your consideration, a summary statement of policy which has, in general, served as the basis of the Department's attitude towards Iran during the past eight or nine months. I believe that you will agree with the fundamental principles expressed therein. During recent months, it has become apparent that political and economic situation in Iran is critical and may dissolve into chaos at any moment. I feel, therefore, that the Department's policy should be implemented more actively than heretofore, but before taking measures along this line, I should like to have assurance that you are in accord. It is clear that this policy can be implemented effectively only if it is followed by all interested agencies of this Government. In particular, it is important to have the support of the War Department authorities in Washington and of the American military commander in Iran. At the present time, the instructions of the commander in Iran are understood to confine him strictly to the transportation of supplies to the Soviet Union. In consequence, he does not feel free to cooperate, even informally, with the efforts of the American civilian representatives and agencies to solve the numerous, pressing, internal problems of Iran. Accordingly, if you approve the course of action proposed in the enclosed memorandum, I would like to suggest that it be presented to the Joint Chiefs of Staff for their consideration. If they perceive no insuperable military objection, I believe it would be well to have instructions issued to the commander in Iran to lend such assistance as may be practicable to the carrying out of the policy in question. I hope, also, that following such consideration by the Joint Chiefs of Staff the War Department will feel free to lend its assistance in other ways, perhaps, if need arises, through the provision of certain personnel and supplies to assist the American advisers now in Iran.

The memorandum is entitled "American Policy in Iran":

> The historic ambitions of Great Britain and Russia in Iran have made that country a diplomatic battleground for more than a century. The geographical, political and economic bases of these ambitions remain unchanged, and the present attitude of the British and Soviet Governments and their representatives in Iran give strong reason to fear that

their rivalry will break out again as soon as the military situation permits. This danger is greatly increased by the existing economic and political weakness of the Iranian Government and the presence on Iranian soil of British and Soviet armed forces. If events are allowed to run their course unchecked, it seems likely that either Russia or Great Britain, or both, will be led to take action which will seriously abridge, if not destroy, effective Iranian independence. That such action would be contrary to the principles of the Atlantic Charter is obvious. Its effect upon other peoples of the Near East, and elsewhere, might well be disastrous to our hopes for an equitable and lasting post-war settlement.

The best hope of avoiding such action lies in strengthening Iran to a point at which she will be able to stand on her own feet, without foreign control or "protection," and in calling upon our associates, when necessary, to respect their general commitments under the Atlantic Charter and their specific commitments to Iran under the Treaty of Alliance of 1942, the provisions of which were noted by the President in a communication to the Shah of Iran. The United States is the only nation in a position to render effective aid to Iran, specifically through providing American advisers and technicians and financial and other material support. We are also the only nation in a position to exercise a restraining influence upon the two great powers directly concerned. Since this country has a vital interest in the fulfillment of the Principles of the Atlantic Charter and the establishment of foundations for a lasting peace throughout the world, it is to the advantage of the United States to exert itself to see that Iran's integrity and independence are maintained and that she becomes prosperous and stable. Likewise, from a more directly selfish point of view, it is to our interest that no great power be established on the Persian Gulf opposite the important American petroleum developments in Saudi Arabia.

Therefore, the United States should adopt a policy of positive action in Iran, with a view to facilitating not only the war operations of the United Nations in that country but also a sound post-war development. We should take the lead, whenever possible, in remedying internal difficulties, working as much as possible through American administrators freely employed by the Iranian Government. We should further endeavor to lend timely diplomatic support to Iran, to prevent the development of a situation in which an open threat to Iranian integrity might be presented. In carrying out this policy, we should enlist the support of all branches of the American Government. The success of the proposed course of action is favored by the exceptionally high regard in which this country is held by the Iranian people. There is also reason to believe that the British Government would acquiesce, or even lend its active support. The attitude of the Soviet Government is doubtful, but this Government should be in a position to exert considerable influence if occasion should arise. It goes without saying that the safeguarding of legitimate British and Soviet economic interests in Iran should be a basic principle of American action.

On September 30, 1943, Murray wrote to Assistant Secretary Berle (Memorandum and enclosure, 891.00/2048 - 5/8):

> Mr. Berle: As far as we have been able to learn, no reply has ever been received to the attached letter of August 16 last which the Secretary addressed to the President regarding the political and economic situation in Iran, which is described as so critical that "it may dissolve into chaos at any moment." Very pertinent in this connection is the still unresolved question of whether the War Department can be induced to furnish General Connolly, who heads the Persian Gulf Service Command, with the necessary instructions to interest himself forthwith and without delay in the common problem facing all of our people in Iran to prevent a collapse. . . . Colonel Schwarzkopf, who is, as you know, in charge of the Iranian gendarmerie and is a thoroughly first-rate person, is back in Washington on a flying trip to try to induce the War Department to instruct General Connolly to cease his vigorous efforts to block the flow of vital supplies for the functioning of the Iranian gendarmerie under Colonel Schwarzkopf. While Colonel Schwarzkopf furnished us with still further information regarding the manner in which General Connolly's outfit is functioning in Iran, he obviously will convey none of that information to the War Department since military discipline would prevent him from any such action. Such being the case, the question arises whether any means might be found to bring about an investigation of the activities of General Connolly's command in Iran by the competent authorities of the War Department; in other words, is it not possible to suggest in proper quarters that the Inspector General might send out at once a competent officer to look into the matter and furnish him with a completely unbiased report on the situation?

Assignment of General Hurley to Iran

On October 5, 1943, Brigadier General Patrick J. Hurley, adviser to the President, who had recently returned from Iran, had called on Berle

(Memorandum, 123 Hurley, Patrick J. /109 ½):

> General Patrick Hurley came to see me today by reference from the Secretary's Office. He gave me orally the substance of a report he had made to the President on conditions in Iran. He said that he had been over the ground thoroughly, had seen and talked to the people, British and Russian and American, and his conclusions were considered. General Hurley said that the British policy towards Iran was "cruel and avaricious." They had first entered the country; then commandeered its railroad without compensation; then seized all of the Iranian trucks; then commandeered what food they could get hold of; then insisted on the Iranian Government's printing currency to be used for the pay of the British troops, causing inflation. The result of all this had been literal starvation in a number of areas. This was not, General Hurley said, hyperbole. He had seen the corpses in the streets and had heard the women and children crying over their dead. Worse, he said, this was a considered policy of the British representatives. He had seen and obtained a copy of Bullard's report, who had stated that hunger was an excellent way of controlling the country.
>
> The situation had finally blown up, he said, because having first rendered the Iranian Government impotent so that it could neither control its people, meet the emergency forced upon it, or maintain its authority, the British had then insisted that the resulting situation was the fault of the Iranian Government. Finally, he said, while this was going on the Anglo-Persian Oil Company had extended its operations and had declared a dividend of 20 percent in London. The United Kingdom Commercial Corporation, he said, had obtained lend-lease goods and likewise controlled imports and had used this to force independent Iranian merchants out of business to a point where it or selected British companies were obtaining an important and airtight monopoly on the entire commerce and resources of the country. The phrase "lend-lease millionaires" was current in the Middle East, based on the fact that lend-lease goods (he mentioned specifically an item of 26,000 tires) were sold by the UKCC or some similar agency; only after protest was made did they put the money obtained back to the credit of the United States Government. He spoke rather bitterly about the entire situation, and said that he had very bluntly and frankly explained it in this sense to Minister Richard Casey after he returned.
>
> He knew of the difficulties between Dreyfus, Connolly, and the British. He believed that Dreyfus had been right from the beginning; that he had endeavored to uphold the prestige and honor of the United

> States and assist the Persian Government in keeping its head above water. Connolly, he said, had been so interested in cooperation with the Russians that he had ceased really to maintain any other point of view. He felt that a first-rate two-fisted man, preferably in uniform, ought to go to Iran and sit on the situation. Also a man who could assure the cooperation of Connolly or an appropriate replacement, and could support Dreyfus since he would not be restricted by the protocol and diplomatic limitations attaching to a regularly constituted Minister. He suggested that the Legation at Tehran ought to be raised to an Embassy so as to give added rank to our representative there in view of the extreme importance of Iran as a cross-road.
>
> Finally, he said, publicity and the opinion of the world ought to be brought to bear on the situation. He considered that the Iranians were quite as able and entitled to govern themselves as most other peoples and they could do so if the powers allowed them. . . . He added that Iran would like to play with the United States if possible. If we were out of the situation, and they had to choose between the British and the Russians, they would choose the Russians by an overwhelming majority.
>
> His hope appeared to be that the Department would ask the White House to assign him to the Department, giving him some sort of a rank although he remained in uniform. His reason for this was that he was presently directly attached to the White House and of course reported to the President; but there was no secretariat at the White House which could back up or implement anything he did. The President was unwilling to have him report directly to the War Department because everything he reported found its way into the newspapers. He seemed to feel that the President would be sympathetic if the request came from this Department.

On October 6, 1943, Berle wrote to Under Secretary Stettinius (Memorandum, 891.00/2087):

> The attached memorandum, and particularly the last page of it, I think offers some possibilities. The War Department has from time to time assigned officers to the State Department for special missions and I see no reason why we could not ask the President to have the War Department assign General Hurley to us.
>
> I am perfectly clear that the Iranian situation is a terrible mess and that only a two-fisted hard-hitting man is likely to clear up. Unfortunately,

> our own reports bear out Pat's statement as to the results of the British-Russian policy in Iran. In the last war, 25 percent of the entire population of that unhappy country starved to death as the result of the German activity there. This time, it looks as though the Allied occupation might produce about the same results. This result ought to be avoided if there is any human possibility of doing so. I think Pat's assignment to the problem might be a good place to begin.

On October 7, 1943, Murray wrote to Stettinius (Memorandum, 891.00/2042 - 5/8):

> I should be glad to discuss with you at your convenience Mr. Berle's attached memorandum of his conversation with General Hurley on the critical situation in Iran. You may be interested to know that the Secretary addressed a letter to the President on the subject, dated August 16, a copy of which is attached. Only within the last few days, however, does it appear that consideration is being given to the matter, and both Admiral Leahy and Mr. Harry Hopkins have started to move. Mr. Hopkins has sent word to me that he would like to speak to me either today or tomorrow on the subject, and I am holding myself in readiness for such a discussion. It is not entirely clear from Mr. Berle's memorandum just what part General Hurley believes he might usefully play in the present situation in Iran, but if he in fact would be prepared to proceed there on a special mission to function at least during the time of the leave of absence of Mr. Dreyfus, who is expected to return to this country next month, we are, generally speaking, of the opinion that General Hurley might be in a position to bring a certain measure of order out of the present chaos, particularly with regard to the relations between General Connolly's Persian Gulf Service Command and our Legation, as well as the various other American agencies now functioning under desperate difficulties in that country.
>
> From all reports Mr. Dreyfus is not a well man and it may be that he will be in no condition to return to Iran. I doubt that General Hurley would wish to remain in Tehran for any length of time in the capacity of Chief of Mission, although if he desires such an appointment rather than the capacity of the head of a special mission or personal representative of the President, as the case might be, his services might be equally useful. In any case, I think it would be highly desirable for General Hurley, if he proceeds to Iran, to go there with his full military rank and even with two stars, rather than one, since there are already two American major generals carrying on in the country. The

situation there today is so predominantly military that an American military chief of mission would not be out of order. There is ample precedent for such an appointment in the case of Admiral Bristol who functioned for years in Istanbul as the American High Commissioner and retained his rank in the Navy during the entire time.

On October 15, 1943, Berle had written to Admiral Leahy (Letter, 891.24/604A):

Dear Admiral Leahy: The State Department is seriously concerned over a situation which has arisen in Iran and which appears to be due to lack of coordinated effort between the diplomatic, the military and the American-sponsored Missions. The situation is precarious, and plainly needs prompt attention. The Secretary sent a letter to the President on August 16, 1943, outlining the situation and I believe that it may have been referred to you for consideration. Since the letter was sent, conditions in Iran have continued to deteriorate. A summary of the difficulties purely from the point of view of the State Department would of course be one-sided, and it is believed you will wish to ascertain the facts through your own channels. But the salient points appear to be these: General Connolly considers his task to relate solely to the transport of supplies through Iran to the Soviet Government. Under this consideration, the considerable force which he has is not available to do even elementary service such as protecting the American Legation in Tehran; as a result of which (the Iranian police being disorganized) the Legation has been repeatedly robbed. In contrast the British Legation is continuously guarded by a considerable contingent of British troops. Security for the railway line is a British responsibility but it is claimed that our forces are partial to the Russians. In any case, little consideration is shown the Iranians. In this situation, difficult at best, General Connolly's command and the American Legation in Tehran appear to be so much at cross purposes that it is a matter of common knowledge in the Middle East. Naturally, we hear only the Legation side of this, but it is pretty impressive.

The American policy is to endeavor to hold Iran together if it can possibly be done. This task is difficult at best, and can only be performed if all American elements there work shoulder to shoulder supporting each other's hand in every possible way. The interest seems to the Department not merely diplomatic. Should Iran disintegrate into an anarchic mass of hostile population, warring tribes, and armed movements (a situation which has already begun in some parts of Iran),

> the task of transporting supplies to Russia through that country would be vastly more difficult. The long range results to American interests in the Middle East (among which may be noted the oil interests we have in Iraq and Saudi Arabia, and our relations with Turkey) might become extremely complicated. I know that you have had this in mind and have been looking into the matter. It would seem some pretty drastic remedial action is necessary. The Department's suggestion is that you review the facts independently, and thereafter, if you care to do so, confer with the Department as to possible reorganization of a dangerous situation.

On October 16, 1943, Murray had also written to Admiral Leahy (Memorandum and enclosures, 891.00/2042 - 5/8):

> Referring to Mr. Hull's letter of October 13, regarding the situation in Iran, there is attached a copy of Mr. Hull's letter to the President of August 13, 1943, mentioned in Mr. Hull's letter. There is also enclosed a copy of a memorandum of January 23, 1943, which explains the basis of the State Department's policy toward Iran. Department's actions in Iran have only confirmed our view that the policy outlined will best serve American interests in that area.

Berle on October 20, 1943, to Murray, Alling and Stettinius (Memorandum and enclosure, 891.00/2042 - 6/8):

> Admiral Leahy courteously came over to see me and stated: (1) That if the Department wrote a letter to the War Department asking them to provide a legation guard for Dreyfus, the War Department would be disposed to provide one. (2) Likewise, if we can specify what we want, Admiral Leahy believes that we can have men assigned to us from the Charlottesville crowd to assist us. (3) He is considering whether we cannot assign a two-fisted general to Iran and wonders whether Iran could request us to send a military mission in view of their recent declaration of war. He foresees some opposition from the British; we should have to overcome it. (4) This would solve the Connolly angle, since Connolly, properly speaking, is there to do railroading and nothing else. (5) He has a general feeling that Dreyfus, while he may have been right, is probably personally inadequate to swing a very wild situation. I told him in this regard that part of it, I thought, represented a campaign against him by British sources, and perhaps also Russian sources, but that we would take his comment into consideration. Attached, his letter.

Admiral Leahy's letter to Berle is dated October 20, 1943:

> Upon the receipt of your letters PA/M and NE 891.24 of October 15th, I at once took up with the American Chiefs of Staff the difficulties that your Department is encountering in Iran as enumerated in the above-noted letters. Some of these difficulties together with others affecting the US Army had already come to the attention of the Chiefs of Staff. The situation in Iran which controls action by the American Chiefs of Staff is briefly as follows: Iran has been accepted for war purposes as a British responsibility. By agreement with the Combined Chiefs of Staff, the US Army is charged with developing and operating transportation and port facilities in the Persian Corridor. The US Army has no other military function. The British military force in Iran has agreed to provide the necessary protection. The American Commander in Iran, General Connolly, has complained of inadequate protection and his complaint was on 17 September brought to the attention of the British Chiefs of Staff. We have as yet received no reply from the British Chiefs of Staff. It is my understanding that the Commander of British Forces in Iran has full authority to decide upon what material shall be transported by General Connolly's transportation facilities. Reports have come to us that this authority has at times interfered with shipment of war material to Russia and has restricted shipments by and to the native inhabitants. In view of the fact that Iran has definitely been designated a military sphere of British responsibility by the highest political authority, action by the American Chiefs of Staff appears to be precluded, and political complications in that Area would seem to be a problem for diplomatic solution. . . . I am informed by officers of the War Department that past experience indicates that cooperation with the United States Minister has been difficult.

On October 22, 1943, Murray had written to Berle and Stettinius (Memorandum, 891.00/2042 - 6/8):

> With regard to Admiral Leahy's thought that it might be desirable to assign "a two-fisted general" to Iran and his speculation as to whether Iran might not request us to send as military mission, in view of their recent declaration of war (September 7, 1943), the following observations are in order: a) Such a request was received from the Iranian Government many months ago and was enthusiastically supported by the British Government. As a result Major General Ridley was sent to Iran as head of a military mission and is now operating with eight or nine American officers under him. Recently the Iranian Government

> requested us to send additional officers to strengthen that mission. . . . I am strongly of the view that the existing mission should be strengthened with a view to reorganizing the Iranian army as soon as possible, for the purpose of preserving law and order in the country which appears to be disintegrating rather seriously. b) After discussion with Mr. Berle yesterday of the Iranian situation it was agreed that we might draft a memorandum to the President for Mr. Stettinius' initials, if he approves, suggesting the temporary assignment of General Hurley to Iran in the capacity of Personal Representative of the President with the rank of Ambassador, and with two stars on his shoulders. We are in agreement that after the forthcoming departure of Mr. Dreyfus on leave of absence, General Hurley might do a very useful job for us in bringing about a much needed collaboration between the Persian Gulf Service Command and the Legation, as well as with the numerous other American advisers functioning in the country. The memorandum in question will come along shortly for your approval.

In early November 1943, General Hurley was requested to go from Cairo to Tehran as Special Representative of the President with rank of Ambassador and given the temporary rank of Major General. He arrived in Tehran shortly before the summit meeting of the three Allied heads of state, and played a big role in arranging and getting approval of the Tehran Declaration.

The Tehran Declaration

The Tehran Conference was held during November 28 to December 1, 1943, and was used by Roosevelt to get Stalin and Churchill to sign the Tehran Declaration committing the three powers to respect and preserve the independence and territorial integrity of Iran. The occasion was also used to demonstrate support for the Iranian government. An unfortunate outcome was Roosevelt's removal of Dreyfus at the instigation of the American military authorities and, possibly, the British. Dreyfus on December 3, 1943 (Telegram 1086, 891.00/2070):

> December 1 a declaration was signed here in which United States, Union of Soviet Socialist Republics and Great Britain stated mutual agreement regarding policy toward Iran containing following points. One. Three powers recognize Iranian contribution to war effort against common enemy. Two. They realize war has caused special economic difficulties in Iran. Three powers express their intent to continue to

> provide such economic assistance as they are able. Three. Three powers agree that Iranian postwar economic problems should receive full consideration by international agencies and conferences which may be created or held to deal with such matters. Four. They reaffirm their desire for maintenance of sovereignty, independence and territorial integrity of Iran according to Atlantic Charter. Text has been submitted to Iran Government which has declared it acceptable. It is understood publicity will be withheld until December 6 when full text will be released. Issuance of declaration along these lines was requested by Iranian Prime Minister November 29. The President approved and directed General Hurley to obtain consent of other parties, which he and the Legation working together were able to do. Hurley and I feel that this has strengthened United States position in Iran and should have beneficent effect.

The Declaration was bound to strengthen the Iranian government. Dreyfus on December 6, 1943 (Telegram 1091, 891.00/2069):

> Declaration as to Iran was enthusiastically received by group of Cabinet members, deputies, Army leaders, and press representatives to whom Prime Minister announced it yesterday. . . . Deputy Taheri made fullsome speech in praise of Allied chiefs, thanking them for this demonstration of friendship and respect for Iran. Today's Tehran papers unanimously echo this enthusiasm.

Dreyfus on December 9, 1943 (Dispatch 750 and enclosure, 891.00/2078):

> I have the honor to report, for the Department's background information, the circumstances of the drawing up of the joint declaration regarding Iran signed at Tehran on December 1, 1943, by the President, Prime Minister Churchill and Premier Stalin, and on the same day declared acceptable by the Iranian Government through its Minister of Foreign Affairs. During a visit by General Hurley and myself to Prime Minister Soheily and Foreign Minister Saed on November 25, 1943, the Iranian officials spoke of the proposed declaration on Iran which was discussed, but not approved, at the Moscow meeting of foreign secretaries October 10 to 30. (See Mr. George V. Allen's despatch of November 4 from this Legation. I do not know how the Iranian Government learned of this Moscow proposal but assume they were informed by the British.) General Hurley informed me that on November 28 he discussed with the President the possibility of securing from

the conference of the chiefs of governments a declaration pertaining to the status of Iran. The President had authorized him to see Foreign Ministers Eden and Molotov and endeavor to work something out. On the morning of the 29, when I called at the Foreign Office regarding another matter, Prime Minister Soheily told me he had just seen Mr. Eden and had put forward the request that the conference should issue a joint communiqué regarding Iran, to cover the following points: 1) Allied recognition that Iran had given every possible help in the prosecution of the war. 2) Confirmation of the pledgees given in the Anglo-Soviet-Iranian treaty of alliance with respect to the independence, sovereignty and territorial integrity of Iran. 3) Assurance that the economic needs of Iran would be considered when the peace treaty should be negotiated. M. Soheily said that Mr. Eden had agreed in principle but had requested that he approach the Soviet representatives and the American Minister. General Hurley saw Mr. Eden on November 30 and advised me that he had reached agreement with the British Foreign Secretary on the desirability of a declaration such as that proposed. The Moscow draft declarations were considered, and General Hurley suggested that, in addition to the points which they covered, there should be a reaffirmation of the principles of the Atlantic Charter. Mr. Eden assented. It was further agreed that the provision of the Moscow draft calling for support for foreign advisers in Iran should be omitted. General Hurley advised me that, inasmuch as the Moscow draft had not been approved by the Russians, he and Mr. Eden had agreed it would be appropriate to have the Iranian Prime Minister present his request himself to M. Molotov and endeavor to obtain Soviet consent to the new proposal. Later that same day, the Iranian Foreign Minister told me that Premier Stalin and Foreign Commissar Molotov had expressed their willingness to meet the request for a declaration. However, from the information reaching General Hurley, it appeared that Soviet assurances was not certain, and the following day he requested the President to speak to Marshal Stalin on the matter. General Hurley tells me he was afterwards informed that the President had done so.

December 1 was the last day of the meeting at Tehran, and there was no time for joint discussions among the American Soviet and British representatives with respect to the text of the proposed communiqué. In consultation with General Hurley, this Legation had prepared a tentative draft, which was the first draft to include specific affirmation of the principles of the Atlantic Charter. It was approved by the American delegation to the conference and was submitted to Mr. Eden and M. Molotov late in the afternoon of December 1. With a few minor changes in wording, this draft was accepted by the final plenary session of the conference, held that evening. I understand time was so short that it was not possible to make three original copies, and that only one was signed, this original copy remaining in the possession of the American delegation. A copy of the final text is enclosed herewith.

I had previously given the Iranian Foreign Minister a copy of the Legation's first draft, which he had discussed with the Prime Minister. I had also informed him that the proposal would be discussed by the chiefs of government on December 1. Accordingly, when the conference session ended at about 11 o'clock in the evening, General Hurley and I took a copy of the final draft to the Foreign Minister and went over it word by word with M. Saed explaining the slight changes which had been made in the phraseology. The Foreign Minister called the Prime Minister on the phone and read him the altered phrases. He then informed us that the revised text was acceptable to the Government of Iran. He initialed a copy which we had brought for that purpose. The Foreign Minister agreed to give no publicity to the declaration until it should have been released by the three signatory governments. It was explained to him that this would probably be delayed for several days. In the course of the conversation with M. Saed, General Hurley emphasized that the American representatives had given special support to the proposed declaration, that certain objections had been encountered, but that he had, happily, been able to secure the agreement of the British and Soviets. Since the Foreign Minister could also see for himself that the Legation's draft declaration had been adopted almost in toto by the conference, I think there can be little doubt in his mind that the United States played a large part in the issuance of the declaration.

As the Department will recall, the Soviet delegation at the Moscow Conference resolutely opposed the issuance of any statement regarding policy toward Iran. I was, therefore, surprised at the readiness of Marshal Stalin and M. Molotov to agree to a substantially similar proposal when made at Tehran only a few weeks later. It may well be that the President's personal appeal, coming at the end of a successful conference, was the deciding factor, although I am inclined to think that some general shift in Soviet attitude toward Iran may also have taken place in recent weeks. (As I have previously reported, there are indications that Irano-Soviet relations have attained a more friendly basis.) Contributing or alternative reasons for Soviet acquiescence at Tehran may have been: 1) The opposition at Moscow may have originated with subordinates, such as former Ambassador Smirnov, who were not present here and so could not bring their views to the attention of the chiefs. 2) At Moscow, the proposal was made by the British and supported by the Americans, no Iranian representatives being present. At Tehran, the proposal came from the Iranians themselves, and the Soviets may have felt that they could not well oppose it without placing themselves in an unfavorable light vis-à-vis the Iranian Government, especially after both the American and British representatives had indicated agreement. 3) The Soviet leaders may have thought this a more appropriate occasion to make a gesture toward Iran, since the meeting was taking place on Iranian soil.

"Iranian Reaction to Declaration Regarding Iran. Significance of the Declaration" is the title of Dreyfus' report on December 10, 1943 (Dispatch 751 and enclosure, 891.00/2079):

I have the honor to refer to . . . the signing of the American-British-Soviet declaration regarding Iran and the initial Iranian reaction to its publication. Local reaction continues to be enthusiastic. There are enclosed excerpts from press comments, which provide a fair sample of the attitude taken by the Tehran newspapers. Some are almost rhapsodical in their tone, and no paper has expressed anything but pleasure at the honor shown Iran and the assurances given her. Perhaps more significant is the attitude of the Iranian Government. The Prime Minister and Foreign Minister have taken pains to express to me their great satisfaction at the success of their request that a communiqué on Iran be issued by the Tehran Conference. They assert that this feeling is shared by the whole people, and they obviously regard it as a triumph for the Government. Certainly, from all that the Legation has been able to learn, there is genuine rejoicing among the articulate, thinking portion of the population, even though the mass is probably almost unaware of the declaration and too much preoccupied with the quest for bread to give it much attention. As was to be expected, the press has been quick to seize upon, and perhaps overemphasize, the portions of the document dealing with Iran's contribution to the war and the promise of economic assistance from the Allies. The Department is familiar with Iran's just, and oft-repeated, plea for help, and it would be contrary to Iranian human nature not to take the declaration in a spirit of "now-all-our-troubles-are-over-because-the-Allies-will-take-care-of-us." However, this attitude is not universal, and the press has not failed to appreciate the general significance of the American participation nor the importance of the final paragraph supporting Iranian independence, sovereignty and territorial integrity.

My own feeling is that, from our point of view and that of Iran, the significance and potential utility of the document may be summed up in the following points: 1) The United States has declared itself for the first time, formally and publicly, as interested in the welfare of Iran and as supporting its free and independent existence. 2) The USSR and Great Britain have renewed their two-year-old pledges to respect Iranian independence, sovereignty and territorial integrity. Very many Iranians and others, as the Department is well aware, had begun to have grave doubts regarding those pledges, and this reassurance is most welcome. Further, if the great powers should be tempted in the future to disregard their promises, this public document, bearing the names of their highest leaders may well give them pause. 3) The reference to the principles of the Atlantic Charter again brings that document before the world, gives evidence that it is intended to apply to small nations as well as great, and may, therefore, have a heartening effect even beyond Iran's borders. I am told by General Hurley that the President regarded this as the most important part of the declaration. 4) It will be difficult to ignore Iran after the war, as she was ignored at the Versailles Conference, in the light of the statements in the declaration that Iranian economic problems should receive full consideration at post-war conferences and that the three powers count upon Iran's participation in the establishment of international peace, security and prosperity. The express recognition of Iran's contribution to the war effort should also count in this connection. I do not wish to appear to attach too much importance to the declaration. I realize that in many ways it is merely a pious wish and that the proof of the pudding will be in the concrete actions of the powers in the future. However, it does seem to me to be a step in the right direction, one more small stone in the foundation of international fair-dealing. It is encouraging that the British and Russians were willing to sign such a document, and, as I have already remarked, it should make it more difficult for them to have a change of heart later on.

Additional information is contained in an OSS report, "Notes on an interview with Honorable Louis G. Dreyfus, former US Minister to Iran, 28 February 1944." (MID-Iran, 3850):

This was managed largely by the army in co-operation with the immediate advisers of the President. Dreyfus was not allowed to go to the airport to meet the President. The Shah asked for the privilege of meeting him at the airport, as head of the state welcoming the head of a friendly power; but this was denied. The Shah then, seeing that the

President was apparently not coming to call on him, offered to go to see the President at the Soviet Embassy. He was kept waiting about ten minutes. He presented the President with a fine Isfahan rug, said to be worth between 15,000 and 20,000 dollars. For the President Mr. Dreyfus later took the Shah his autographed photograph framed in silver. As the Shah came from seeing the President, he was ushered into a side reception room where he received Mr. Churchill; and the British were able to say that the Prime Minister had done the proper thing, called upon the Shah. Stalin, however, went to the Shah's palace to call and stayed for two hours. The Iran Declaration was drawn up by Mr. Ferguson, Third Secretary of the Legation, approved by Mr. Dreyfus and sent to the President. The Iranian Prime Minister had previously spoken to Mr. Eden about such a declaration and secured his approval. Late the last night, Wednesday, the President raised the question of signing the document. Stalin at first demurred since it was only in English and he had not had a chance to study it. But the President insisted that it contained nothing that was not already in the Tripartite Treaty or previous commitments of the USSR, but that the US had never made any such declaration and wished to join the other Allies in such guarantees. The President said that since Mr. Molotov knew English and was acquainted with the matter, there was no reason why it could not be concluded then. To this Stalin agreed and with a change of but three or four minor words, including striking out of "proposed" in the title, the document was signed. The fact that this was initiated and concluded by the US helped to mollify the Shah and the Iranians over the Shah having to go to see the President who then did not return his call. The Shah was mollified further by the fact that the President sent a friendly letter on departure expressing gratitude for Iranian hospitality, on which, in his own handwriting, he expressed the desire that the Shah might come to the US for a visit before very long. This letter was also composed by the Third Secretary and delivered by Mr. Dreyfus, when he found it impossible to get to the President with his request that the President return the Shah's call.

Annex: "Declaration of Three Nations regarding Iran," December 1, 1943

The President of the United States, the Premier of the USSR, and the Prime Minister of the United Kingdom, having consulted with each other and with the Premier of Iran, desire to declare the mutual agreement of their three Governments regarding their relations with Iran.

The Governments of the United States, the USSR and the United Kingdom recognize the assistance which Iran has given in the prosecution of the war against the common enemy, particularly by facilitating the transportation of supplies from overseas to the Soviet Union.

The three Governments realize that the war has caused special economic difficulties for Iran, and they are agreed that they will continue to make available to the Government of Iran such economic assistance which may be possible, having regard to the heavy demands made upon them by their world-wide military operations and to the world-wide shortage of transport, raw materials, and supplies for civilian consumption.

With respect to the post-war period, the Governments of the United States, the USSR, and the United Kingdom are in accord with the Government of Iran that any economic problems confronting Iran at the close of hostilities should receive full consideration, along with those of other members of the United Nations, by conferences or international agencies held or created to deal with international economic matters.

The Governments of the United States, the USSR, and the United Kingdom are at one with the Government of Iran in their desire for the maintenance of the independence, sovereignty and territorial integrity of Iran. They count upon the participation of Iran, together with all other peace-loving nations, in the establishment of international peace, security and prosperity after the war, in accordance with the principles of the Atlantic Charter, to which all four Governments have subscribed. (Signed) Winston Churchill. J.V. Stalin. Franklin D. Roosevelt.

Chapter 26

Attempts at Revival of Dictatorship

British desire to bring back Seyid Zia Tabatabaii was reported in chapter 24. An act of great symbolic importance, the return of Seyid Zia was a clear indication that Great Britain desired to pursue its traditional policy. Dreyfus on October 2, 1943 (Telegram 976, 891.00/2057):

> My 818, August 7. Seyidzia Ed Din returned to Tehran on September 30. There is little doubt that his return was arranged, or at least encouraged, by the British, supported by a large group of prominent Iranians such as Ala, Ebtehaj and Ahmadi who profess to believe that Seyid is the only Iranian now capable of leading Iran out of wilderness. Shah was persuaded by the British not to oppose his return or his subsequent political activities. However, the Russian Chargé informs me his government still strongly objects to Seyid because of his alleged reactionary tendencies and his record in connection with coup d'état. While the next move of Seyid's supporters is not clear, it seems likely that he will be elected to the Majlis in the current elections. This will give him an opportunity to attain power gradually, to study the Iranian political scene and allow time for an effective buildup in the press and among the people. His eventual assumption of power as Prime Minister seems probable unless the Russians are willing openly to prevent it. In this connection, Seyid's bid for power combines all the elements for a more open and intensified struggle for ascendancy between the British and Russians in Iran. The Department is familiar with Seyid's record, how he supported the abortive 1919 treaty, how he attacked the United States violently in editorials in his newspaper *Raad* and how he engineered the coup d'état which led eventually to the disposition of Ahmad Shah and the advent of the Pahlavi dynasty (see, for example, despatch of October 1, 1919). In view of the far

reaching political implications involved, his activities will be carefully followed.

Dreyfus on November 1, 1943 (Telegram 1036, 891.00/2065):

The Government was interpellated yesterday on account of the food situation. After a long debate the Government was supported, the vote being 50 favorable, 5 against, 8 blank votes and 18 abstentions out of 81 deputies present. This Medjliss will expire on November 22 and, since the elections are proceeding very slowly and only some 35 deputies have been elected, it would appear that the next Medjliss cannot be inaugurated until at least December.

OSS report, November 25, 1943 (Report 79, 891.00/2075):

The 13th Legislature closed its two year term on November 23. Since the elections will not be finished for a month, the present Cabinet will apparently run the country within legal limits for the next four weeks. As has long been apparent, any great improvement in conditions in Iran is dependent on the results of the present elections. The returns in so far from the provinces show that about half of the Deputies elected are new men, but, as happened in the Meshed area, they often come from the same old group. Elections in Tehran began November 22 and will continue until December 22. Electioneering is active. One man was holding forth this afternoon in the main square to a crowd of about 100. The Election Committee in Teheran is composed of reputable people who are doing their best to run a free election. It will certainly be freer than any other in the last 20 years, but with the prevailing poverty, the large scale purchase of votes is almost inevitable.

Dreyfus on November 26, 1943 (Dispatch 743, 891.032/65):

I have the honor to report that the 13th Majlis came to an end on November 23. The final sessions was more in the nature of a farewell gathering, since no legislation was considered, and was devoted almost entirely to laudatory speeches delivered by the President of the Majlis, Hassan Esfandiari, and the Prime Minister, Ali Soheily. . . . With all its faults, however, it must be granted that the now-defunct legislature wound up its affairs in much more creditable fashion than any one expected. During its final two weeks of existence it met in full session almost every day, frequently twice a day, which in itself was an accomplishment for a body normally accustomed to only one short session three days a week, and it got through an astonishing number of bills. Among other items of interest to us, the past two weeks or so saw the passage of the vital income tax bill, the regular budget for 1322 (the current year ending March 21, 1944), most of the supplementary budget, the authorization of 400,000,000 rials for the Government wheat purchases, the authorization of the employment of Major General Reynolds as Director General of the Ministry of Health and the employment of an American director of the Pharmaceutical Institute, and the authorization of the minting of silver coins. No date has yet been set for the assembly of the new Majlis, elections for which are continuing in a desultory fashion. It is apparently impossible to obtain accurate figures, but something more than sixty deputies have now been elected, and, under the Constitution, a new Majlis may be inaugurated as soon as 69 of the 136 seats have been filled. It is theoretically possible, therefore, for the 14th Majlis to meet very soon. However, it is customary to await the election of the deputies from Tehran, and the elections in this city began only on November 22 and will not be completed until December 22. Consequently, the probabilities are that there will be a gap of at least a month between the old and the new sessions.

Rising Power of the Shah

The Tehran Conference and the departure of Dreyfus facilitated a power grab by the Shah. Richard Ford, chargé d'affaires, on December 15, 1943 (Telegram 1122, 891.01/93):

> Prime Minister Soheily resigned yesterday. It is thought this is merely a tactical move to enable him to eliminate certain members of Cabinet and that Shah will request him to form a new government in next few days. Soheily has been talking of a reorganization for months but has apparently been unable (to) persuade men concerned to resign.

Ford on December 16, 1943 (Telegram 1125, 891.002/391):

> Reference my 1122, December 15. Following is new Iranian Cabinet: Prime Minister Ali Soheily; Justice Seyid Mohsen Sadr; Foreign Affairs Mohammad Saed; Finance Amanollah Ardalan; Interior Abdol Hossein Hajir; Agriculture Mousa Noury Esfandiari; Education Issa Sadiq; Roads and Communications Nasrollah Entezam; Posts and Telegraphs Hamid Sayah; War Ibrahim Zand; Health Doctor Qasem Ghani; Without Portfolio Mostafa Adl.

Again on December 16, 1943 (Telegram 1126, 891.002/392):

> New Cabinet 1125, December 16 is regarded locally as clear victory for Shah who has been able to place his own candidates in a majority of Cabinet posts. Soheily has also gained his ends and strengthened his position by eliminating the opposing elements in the previous Cabinet including Tadayyon, Ahmadi, Bader and Etebar. Tadayyon was apparently dropped because of his summary dismissal of Mayor of Tehran without consulting Soheily who is close personal friend of deposed official. Ahmadi had incurred displeasure of Shah and was regarded in government circles as too ambitious to be left in a position of importance.

Ford on December 24, 1943 (Dispatch 770, 891.002/394):

> With reference to my telegram No. 1125 of December 16, 1943, reporting the formation of a new Iranian cabinet, I have the honor to offer the following comments on the personnel of the cabinet and on the developments surrounding the change. Prime Minister—Ali Soheily. It is now almost a year since Soheily returned to power succeeding the unhappy Qavam and in that time he has proved himself an expert at political tricks of every sort and a past master of the Iranian art of intrigue. Despite this, however, and despite his reputation among a good many Iranians for dishonesty, he has grown somewhat in stature during his present tenure of office and has proved to be satisfactory to most Iranians as Prime Minister. Although his power remains based on every known variety of political maneuvering, he can point to a large number of accomplishments during his Ministry, the most notable being the Tri-Partite Declaration of Tehran. He has moreover, been as cooperative with the American advisers as is possible for a man of his nature to be, and has supported Dr. Millspaugh in almost every issue, albeit a bit reluctantly in the case of the Income Tax Bill. . . . Minister of Foreign Affairs—Mohamed Saed. Saed appears to be a permanent fixture in the Foreign Office, a situation for which he may well be thankful. . . . The Foreign Minister is neither a vigorous personality nor an able politician and though his name is mentioned frequently, it is not probable that he would be able to muster enough support to remain Prime Minister for long should he eventually, as is not unlikely, to be given that post. . . . Minister of Finance—Amanollah Ardalan. The transfer of Ardalan to the Ministry of Finance from the Public Health Post has been expected for some time and was made, it is alleged because he worked well with Dr. Millspaugh. Dr. Millspaugh has expressed himself as being pleased with the ap-

pointment and by and large, it would appear to be a good one. . . . He is a close friend of Prime Minister Soheily and is one of the few members of the present cabinet of whom it cannot be said that he is a royal appointee. Minister of Commerce & Industry—Brigadier General Ismail Shafai. Shafai is a new face on the Iranian political scene. . . . He is an appointee of the Shah and concludes the rather long list of His Majesty's representatives on the new Council of Ministers. . . . Shafai was a personal aide to the Shah and a member of the latter's military clique.

Soheily has been anxious for some to time to be rid of the dissident elements in his official family as well as the Ministers he had originally been obliged to appoint to strengthen his position with the former Majlis. No political crisis precipitated the present turn-over which is important principally in its revelation of the greatly enhanced influence of the Shah. I took the occasion shortly after the formation of the new group to call on the Minister of the Court, Mr. Ala, who in the course of a more or less general conversation let fall the remark that Soheily when he had decided on the reorganization asked the Shah as a matter of courtesy whom he would like to see in power. The Shah replied that such matters were solely the concern of the Prime Minister but that he thought highly of certain men whom he named. The men named were all included in the new cabinet. Ala apparently realized that he possibly had said too much and a few moments later blandly denied that the Shah had any part in the formation of the cabinet.

The Shah's meddling has now come into the open and is causing a certain amount of uneasiness among those Iranians who cannot forget that the present ruler is the son of his father. The Shah is apparently unable to rule as a constitutional monarch especially as regards the army which he considers his private property and over which he has, at least temporarily, gained complete control. Soheily accepted the Shah's men in his new cabinet since it was the only way he could dispose of the hostile elements in the former cabinet and yet remain in power himself. It is not unlikely therefore that all of the Shah's men will be dropped if Soheily is assured of Majlis support. The most prevalent rumor in Tehran is that Soheily will do anything to stay in power until he has amassed a fortune sufficient to enable him to escape the country and take up permanent residence in the United States. Certainly he has an all-consuming desire to remain as Prime Minister and will hesitate at nothing to assure his continuity in office. Despite the political strategy involved and despite the possible impermanence of the new group, the fact that the Shah has been able to impose a cabinet of his own choosing on the Iranian people is an event of great importance to Iran regardless of the mechanics of the deal and regardless of the fact that none of his appointees may last long in the positions to which they have so suddenly been elevated.

Soheily is reported to have wished to postpone the formation of a new cabinet until the opening of the new Majlis, but this the Shah refused using his power to appoint the Prime Minister as a club over Soheily's head and forcing the issue at the time when he, the Shah, would be able to dictate the personnel of the new cabinet. While this report has not been confirmed, it seems unlikely that Soheily would risk losing his position by twice resigning with a period of few weeks unless it was the only means by which he could purge his official family of those persons whose presence had become embarrassing to him. The Prime Minister may encounter a certain amount of trouble in the Majlis over the interim cabinet since the formation of a new Council of Ministers when the Majlis is not in session is of questionable legality and some of the deposed officials are not without followers in parliamentary circles. Some day Soheily will go too far in his political twists and turns and find that by some brilliant piece of political "quarterbacking" he has maneuvered himself out of office. . . . There are no strong personalities in the cabinet and it is regarded by many Iranians as weak and composed of nonentities whose principal task will be to carry out orders sent from higher quarters. Soheily undoubtedly has a group that will cause him a few less official headaches as he no longer has to deal with such vigorous personalities as Ahmadi and Taddayon. I must confess relief at the departure of Taddayon from the Iranian political scene. The Department is thoroughly familiar with this character and his reputation of being a black reactionary and a politician with a strong antiforeign bias. Taddayon is not particularly anti-American as much as he is anti-foreign, and it has proved to be extremely difficult for any foreign diplomat to deal with him. The Department will recall the interminable delays in the signature of the Schwarzkopf contract caused by Taddayon's suspicion that the United States was trying to "put something over on him." He has recently fallen into political ill favor because of his practically open manipulation of the elections and an increasing reputation for being an expert at the art of graft. . . . Ahmadi's fall from grace has its disadvantages from our point of view in that he showed satisfactory cooperation toward General Ridley and the members of his mission while Minister of War. It has been widely reported that the Shah in his desire to control the army is opposed to the activities of the American military mission fearing it as a possible check on his ambitions. . . . The Shah's burning ambition to run the army in his own way is known to every one but in all fairness it must be said that he has officially supported the American adviser program from its start and was especially helpful in supporting Dr. Millspaugh at the time of the passage of the income tax bill. Ahmadi, ambitious and ruthless and undoubtedly competent, proved to be too strong a personality to remain in a cabinet position in Iran at a time when no acute national emergency existed. He and the Shah had been at loggerheads for some time over the administration of the War Ministry and his dismissal while not unexpected, shows that the Shah felt fairly sure of his position since Ahmadi is a man of considerable influence and has considerable backing in Iranian military and political circles. It may be said, however, that the Field Marshal is heartily detested by most Iranians, and his expulsion will probably prove to be one of Soheily's more popular acts. The dismissal of Minister Bader, Etebar, and Bayat is warmly approved locally. Bader although a rather able man, was widely accused of graft on a large scale, Etebar's reported dishonesty and lack of ability made him a liability to Soheily, and Bayat, though cooperative with Dr. Millspaugh, showed no noticeable ability as Minister of Finance. Etebar and Bayat moreover, were originally appointed to the cabinet to appease the now defunct thirteenth Majlis and with the passing of that body, the Prime Minister had no further need for their services.

In the Legation's Despatch No. 468, dated March 2, 1943, written when Soheily returned to office, it was stated that Soheily would probably "cash in" on certain improvements in the general internal situation of Iran. This has proved to be the case and Soheily is able to point to a number of accomplishments during his administration, many of which were effected in spite of rather than by him. The reforms of the Millspaugh Mission are beginning to be felt, and the general economic situation of the country has improved during the past year, Iran has declared war on the Axis and has been solemnly assured by the United States, Great Britain, and the Soviet Union that those powers have no intentions inimical to the territorial integrity and independence of Iran. The tribal situation is calm at the moment and the general security of the country has shown some improvement. Soheily, therefore, will probably be in a fairly strong position when the new Majlis assembles and may be able to reorganize his government again with parliamentary support according to his own rather than Shah's wishes. His vast store of political tricks may, however, as stated above carry him a little too far and both the Shah and the Majlis may turn on him and trust the Government to a man whose political policies are a little less

> devious. For the moment it is sufficient to say that Soheily will fall in with the Shah's wishes and whims just so long as the Shah is powerful enough to be able to dismiss him with impunity. The struggle for power between the Shah and the politicians is a fascinating development in the local scene and will be carefully watched. The Shah is playing a dangerous game which may eventually either make him another Reza Shah, or more likely, cost him his throne.

The Shah's boldness was unceasing. Ford on January 20, 1944 (Telegram 40, 891.00/3002):

> Shah yesterday summoned British Minister and told him he wants to cancel the Majlis elections now nearing completion, because of the widespread fraud, corruption and interference which has characterized them. This would involve, of course, suspending the opening of the new Majlis scheduled for January. British Minister says Shah also wishes to form new cabinet headed by Mohammed Mossadegh, who is now leading candidate for Deputy in Tehran election returns. Sir Reader states he pointed out to Shah difficulties which might result from cancellation of elections, but from a conversation this morning with Minister of Court he gathered that Shah intends to go ahead. He states Shah also consulted Soviet Ambassador, who confined himself to saying that the Soviet Union did not attempt to interfere in internal Iranian affairs, implying that there would be no (repeat no) Soviet objection to proposed action.

Ford on January 21, 1944 (Telegram 41, 891.00/3001):

> Prime Minister told me last night (reference my 40, January 20) that opening of Majlis will be postponed for fifteen or twenty days because so many deputies have left Tehran and also because there have been strong protests against the opening in the absence of Tehran deputies, whose election returns will not (repeat not) be complete for another two or three weeks. This postponement was confirmed this morning by the Foreign Office. Press this morning also states only fifty-eight deputies are presently in Tehran whereas sixty-nine are required for quorum.

Ford on January 22, 1944 (Telegram 43, 891.00/3005):

> British Minister has been told by Minister of Court that Shah has decided not (repeat not) to carry out his plan to cancel elections and form

new cabinet. (My 40, January 20). Reason for change of plan said to be that before proceeding with the elections Mossadegh wanted to hold a referendum to amend electoral law. There is no (repeat no) doubt that the proposed action would have created a great furor and it may well be that on reflection, the Shah and his advisers became apprehensive of possible consequences. It is also possible that Shah found Mossadegh too independent in his ideas, since he is regarded as a man of character.

Ford on February 2, 1944 (891.00/3008):

Political position of Soheily appears to be inexorably deteriorating and he continues being viciously attacked in Tehran press, latest campaign hinging on Prime Minister's failure to open Majlis as first scheduled (my telegram No. 41, dated January 21). Persistent rumor tends to widen alleged cleavage between Shah and his Prime Minister, and Ala, who is undeniably close to, if not especially influential with Shah, informed me yesterday that Soheily's power may well not (repeat not) survive opening of new Majlis now fixed for February 26. One factor favoring Soheily's position is the complete absence thus far of capable substitute. Mossadegh who denies ever having been offered Premiership by Shah (my telegram No. 40, dated January 20) and Qavam have both been mentioned as possibilities available to Shah as counter irritants to the allegedly British supported, Soviet despised, Seyidzia-ed-Din Tabatabai, who appears now completely discredited. The other British hope, Ali Mansur, has announced from Meshed that he will not consider Premiership at this time. Of possible successors now on horizon Saed, Foreign Minister, one figure acceptable to the Soviets, probably agreeable to the British, liked by Shah and generally popular in Iran, if not particularly strong personality, and definitely no politician. (Acceptability to Soviets is becoming something of criterion of success in Iran these latter days). However, none of these possesses Soheily's entrenched power or probably his politician's astuteness, and would undoubtedly have great difficulty in forming strong government unless personally aided by Shah whose accolade seems increasingly potent. Thus, while Soheily is losing ground and will almost certainly face hostile Majlis even if Shah lets him last long enough to ask that body for customary vote of confidence, the problem of a successor remains far from settled. Many observers believe Soheily will gracefully settle portion of problem himself immediately after the Ambassadorship in Washington becomes available.

Ford on February 10, 1944 (Telegram 82, 891.002/396):

> According to Minister of Court Ala Shah has been urging Taqizadeh Iranian Minister at London, to accept premiership (Reference my 59, February 2). Taqizadeh said to have declined on grounds of age and ill health but to have suggested Ala for the post. From a conversation with Foreign Minister Saed this morning I gather that he (Saed) would not (repeat not) refuse Premiership if offered, although he disclaimed any ambition in that direction. British Minister has informed Shah that Qavam-es-Sultaneh would not (repeat not) be acceptable as Prime Minister. Reason given is that British have discovered Qavam received German emissaries during his previous term of office.

The improving economic conditions had created additional space for political maneuvering. Ford on February 15, 1944 (Dispatch 845, 891.00/3014):

> I have the honor to refer to my despatch No. 789, January 17, 1944, and to submit herewith notes on various developments in Iran since that despatch was written: 1. A British milling expert temporarily on loan from Malta has taken charge of operations at the Tehran silo and has succeeded in increasing the amount of barley in the local bread to 27%. Largely as a result of this measure, the stocks of grain on hand in the city as of February 5 constituted 53.5 days supply. Better control has also reduced civilian consumption of flour to 180 tons daily from a former average of 200 tons. Complaints about quantity and quality of bread in the city have almost disappeared, although the quality of flour will not be really satisfactory until adequate cleaning equipment is obtained and installed at the silo and the local barley mill. 2. Stocks of petroleum products at Tehran have been satisfactory throughout the winter to date, in contrast to the scarcity which prevailed during part of last winter. 3. Attended by much fanfare, the Shah has been making a series of visits to local public schools, usually accompanied by the Minister of Education and other high officials. His remarks on these occasions stress the importance of improving educational facilities in Iran. He has also taken the leading role in recent ceremonies at the University of Tehran, the Military Academy, and the Normal School.

Majlis Attempts to Curb the Shah

Ford on February 28, 1944 (Dispatch 802 and enclosure, 891.032/67):

> I have the honor to report that the 14th Iranian National Consultative Assembly (Majlis) was formally inaugurated on February 26, 1944, at the Palace of the Majlis in Tehran. After listening to the Shah's speech from the throne, the deputies proceeded to the election of provisional officers and divided themselves into six committees for the scrutiny of each other's credentials. According to the press, 83 deputies, well over the quorum of 69, were present. No real business, of course, can be transacted until the credentials have been accepted and permanent officers elected. The next meeting has been set for March 5. Two of the deputies-elect from Tehran did not take their seats at the opening. Pirnia has declined to accept election, on the ground of ill-health, and Firuzabadi was disqualified by the electoral college because he is over the age prescribed by law. It is understood that these places are being filled by candidates who ran just below the first twelve in the Tehran elections.

Weeks after the opening of the 14th Majlis, elections in Azerbaijan were still underway. Ebling on March 16, 1944 (Dispatch 36, 891.00/3028):

> In view of conditions which prevailed in Iran just a few years ago during the Pahlevi regime, it is interesting to consider the present opportunities in Azerbaijan for the development of liberal ideas, as illustrated by the career of Mr. M. Beriyah. One of the best known liberal leaders in Tabriz is M. Beriyah who was formerly employed in a minor position in the municipality. At the time of the arrival of the Soviet occupying forces in 1941, Mr. Beriyah was practically unknown. To the conservatives Mr. Beriyah appears as a Soviet protégé, and it is alleged that he may receive a salary as a Soviet agent. In an election speech delivered on March 5th from a truck parked near the entrance of the Central Police Station, Mr. Beriyah directed the attention of a large crowd to the development of liberal ideas which has been possible since the Soviet occupation. The speaker described the conditions of suppression which prevailed for 22 years in Azerbaijan generally recognized in Persian history as the home of liberal thought. The speaker referred to the desire of the ex-Shah to suppress the people of Azerbaijan for their liberalism, and recalled words of a former Governor General who once stated that "wheat which is unsuitable for other Persians,

> can be sent to the people of Azerbaijan." Mr. Beriyah appealed to the laborers and underprivileged to seize the opportunity offered by the present election to elect liberal deputies and to defeat the candidates who stand for reaction. In a dramatic manner the speaker asked his listeners if the legislation of previous parliaments had ensured them any better food or security for the future. "This is the Iranian New Year and I see that you are all hungry" concluded Mr. Beriyah suggesting that this was time for people to get together and defeat the landlords and rich merchants who are only interested in adding to their personal fortunes. The speech ended with the words, "Long live liberals, workers, and free parties."

On March 7, 1944, Ford had conversed with Soheily whose predictions reported in a cable of the same date proved accurate (Telegram 165, 891.002/397):

> Urgent. Following is summary of statements made to me today by Prime Minister Soheily when I asked what he thought of the prospects for his cabinet: One. He regards his position as gloomy, with very little possibility that he can remain in power. Principal reason is that he is at odds with Shah over royal interference with army and also over policy toward American advisers. Two. Shah has turned against entire adviser group, even including Schwarzkopf, whom he had previously refrained from criticizing. In consequence, Soheily believes any cabinet which replaces his will have as one of its main policies the elimination of the American advisers. Three. Marshal Yazdanpanah, Shah's close adviser, is anti-American. Four. Russians have not (repeat not) concealed their dislike of American adviser program. Five. Shah is grooming Saed, who would be a yes man, as next Prime Minister. Six. Even if he (Soheily) remains as Prime Minister, the advisers will face a determined attack which he may not (repeat not) be able to hold off. I asked Prime Minister what measures he would suggest to save adviser program should he lose power. He replied that he thought the only possibility would be to present to the Shah a united American-British front. He said British have always supported advisers in their conversations with him. It is of course possible that Soheily has an ulterior motive in making these statements. Perhaps he hopes we will intervene to keep him in office. However Saed recently criticized Millspaugh Mission very severely in conversation with me (my 116 of February 21) and the last few weeks have seen an ever swelling volume of press criticism directed at almost all American advisers. There is talk of Majlis investigation of their work. I do not (repeat not) think

therefore that Soheily's remarks can be lightly dismissed. I plan to see British Minister this evening, tell him frankly substance of Prime Minister's statements regarding advisers and sound out his attitude toward a possible joint demarche, if such action should seem advisable. I also plan a more discreet approach to Soviet Embassy, and shall try to see Minister of Court with view to gauging court sentiment directly.

As predicted, Saed had replaced Soheily. Ford on March 17, 1944 (Telegram 196, 891.002/398): "Majlis having completed its organization cabinet resigned yesterday." March 18, 1944 (Telegram 199, 891.002/399): "Medjliss in secret mission today voted its confidence in Mohammed Saed as Prime Minister. Shah is now expected to request him to form a cabinet." The formation of a new cabinet, however, had not gone smoothly. Ford on March 22, 1944 (Telegram 204, 891.002/400):

> Saed informed Medjliss March 20 that he proposed to retain all members of previous Cabinet except Minister of Justice. Deputies objected strongly and insisted upon certain changes. Saed has agreed to make substantial changes but he insists he needs time to do so, is now generally concluded that formation of cabinet will await termination of new year holidays on March 26."

Ford on March 30, 1944 (Telegram 218, 891.002/402):

> Since Majlis and press have shown themselves completely dissatisfied with new Cabinet (my 204, March 22) that body will probably resign today or tomorrow without going through formality of asking for a vote of confidence. It is believed that Saed will be asked to try again and that he may include a number of deputies in Cabinet.

On March 31, 1944 (Telegram 222, 891.002/403):

> Leaders of majority groups of Majlis have conferred with Saed (my 218, March 30) and it was decided that Majlis would present a list of thirty men from whom he might select his Ministers. However, independent deputies, representing about one-third of total membership, are opposed to this procedure as creating undesirable precedent and likely to cause dissension and Majlis outcome remains uncertain. Saed told me last night he is endeavoring to work out a Cabinet which will

be acceptable to all groups but does not expect to complete task before April 4.

Ford on March 31, 1944 (Telegram 223, 891.00/3034):

There appears to be brewing a major constitutional conflict between the Shah and his supporters on the one hand and those who fear another royal dictatorship on the other. Indications are that majority of Majlis deputies resent influence Shah has wielded in recent Cabinets. They display strong opposition to Ministers, such as Zand, Entezam, and Nurie-Esfandiary, whom he is known to have nominated. At Nowruz Salam, Malek Madani, Vice President of Majlis, is said to have replied sharply to a remark by Shah critical of Majlis and to have stressed that (legislative) branch of government is responsible only to the nation. Seyid Zia Eddin is understood to be preparing measure whereby Majlis would define (and limit) constitutional powers of Shah, especially with respect to his authority over Army and in appointment and dismissal of Cabinet officers. This would bring conflict out into open, and it is possible issue will break as soon as new Cabinet is definitely installed and Majlis has finished discussion of election question.

Ford on April 5, 1944 (Telegram 231, 891.00/3024):

Although Saed yesterday told me it was definitely settled that Hossein Ala would go to Washington as Ambassador, Ala himself an hour earlier stated that he could not go unless the situation here improved and someone could be found to take his place as Minister of Court. (In this latter connection, he mentioned Pirnia as possibility). Ala expressed himself as gravely disturbed by public criticism of Shah and especially by attitude of British, who are, he says, definitely supporting Seid Ziawddin. (Reference my 223, March 31). He believes this can be interpreted only as evidence of desire to get rid of Shah. Ala also remarked there had been a distinct cooling of Irano-Soviet relations. Apropos of his dissatisfaction with and apparent uncertainty about present British policy in Iran, Ala asked me pointedly whether recent recall of Minister Dreyfus was indication that my government's policy in Iran was veering to a pro-British stand. His intimation was, of course, that British had been instrumental in having Dreyfus removed. (Rumors reflecting this local belief are indeed current in Tehran). I replied that so far as I knew there had been no (repeat no) change in American policy since Tehran conference. Saed is still trying to form Cabinet acceptable to Majlis. New group of Ministers will probably be presented tomorrow. During yesterday's conversation, Prime Minister again spoke of his dissatisfaction with Millspaugh and his hope someone could be provided to replace him.

Ford on April 10, 1944 (Telegram 246, 891.002/406):

> Majlis' debate on Saed's new cabinet began yesterday but no (repeat no) vote was taken. Deputies Mohammed Mossadegh and Seid Mahmud Tussi attacked American Economic Mission, criticizing especially the British-American work in connection with food supply, price control and distribution of monopoly goods it is likely Majlis criticism will continue and perhaps be intensified in subsequent sessions. Millspaugh, however, does not (repeat not) appear unduly perturbed.

Ford on April 17, 1944 (Telegram 260, 891.032/68): "Saed Government received vote of confidence from Majlis by a vote of 64 out of 85 deputies present."

Recall of Dreyfus

It turned that the recall of Dreyfus was a prelude to the removal of Millspaugh and the eventual reimposition of Pahlavi dictatorship. Dreyfus' replacement by Leland B. Morris as the first US Ambassador was unfortunate. While Dreyfus and his wife, Grace, were perceived as friends of Iran, Morris, the Minister to Iceland and the former chargé d'affaires in Berlin at the time of German declaration of war on the US, had little interest in and even less sympathy for Iran. As described in chapter 28, in September 1944, Morris had joined his British colleague in sending a note to the Iranian government in which it is stated that the relief of the newly liberated Europeans took precedence over aid to Iran, the Tehran Declaration by the Big Three notwithstanding. The note had so angered the Iranian government that it had not returned the favor of a reply. Unfortunately, only after approving the Morris appointment and after the submission of his name to the US Senate, the Soheily government had belatedly made some gestures to retain Dreyfus. Dreyfus departed on December 12, 1943. Ford on February 19, 1944 (Telegram 112, 123 D 82/585):

> Personal and Confidential for Alling. Press announcement of Bullard's promotion to Ambassador with continued uncertainty of status of her

> husband has deeply worried Mrs. Dreyfus who has asked that I send this personal inquiry. She does not (repeat not) wish Dreyfus to return to Iran unless he comes as Ambassador in view of possible embarrassment to both Legation and the British. If at all possible, I should greatly appreciate receiving an indication of the Department's intentions in this connection in order to relieve Mrs. Dreyfus' mind.

Ford on February 29, 1944 (Telegram 146, 123 D 82/589): "Confidential for Dreyfus from Mrs. 'Unnecessary to return here. Shall pack or dispose of equipment indicated (reference Department's telegram No. 110, February 26). Shall travel with household effects. Disgusted.'"

Murray on March 3, 1944 (Memorandum, 123 D 82/609):

> Acting under instruction from his Government the Iranian Minister called on me this afternoon to convey a most unusual message and request from the Foreign Minister of Iran. The Minister said that he had been instructed to see Mr. Hull personally, but in his absence had decided to talk the matter over with me in view of his feeling that I would better understand the Iranian reasoning in this matter. The Minister was instructed to state that while his Government had, as an act of courtesy and respect for the President, granted an agrément to the appointment of Mr. Leland B. Morris as the first American Ambassador to Iran, it is nevertheless so deeply appreciative of the great help and assistance which Mr. Dreyfus has rendered Iran in these times of trials and tribulations, and in view of the deep understanding which Mr. Dreyfus has come to have of the Iranian mind (which he said he knew was difficult to acquire) the Iranian Government desired to make a most earnest appeal to this Government to reconsider the transfer of Mr. Dreyfus from Iran and ardently hoped that he would be left there as the first American Ambassador to that country. I told the Minister that we were, of course, very grateful that the Iranian Government had such a high appreciation of Mr. Dreyfus, both officially and personally, and we could of course only be pleased that he had been able to render such assistance to Iran in these times as had called forth this high tribute to him. At the same time I felt that I knew him well enough to ask him to tell me frankly whether he thought the message from his Government was in fact more than an example of the traditional Iranian courtesy and politeness, or whether he thought his Government literally meant what he had been instructed to say to us on this subject. The Minister replied that he appreciated this question coming from me who, he felt, understood the Iranian mind, but that he could assure me from the exact context of the messages which he had received on the

subject of Mr. Dreyfus that his Government, and in fact even the Shah himself, felt deeply on this matter and would consider it a great courtesy if we could see our way clear to reconsider the present intention to withdraw Mr. Dreyfus. I then asked the Minister whether in his opinion the Shah felt so strongly on the subject that he might be inclined to send the President a direct communication making this request. The Minister replied that he had no doubt that the Shah would be so disposed *if he were assured that his request would not be turned down*. Immediately after my conversation with the Minister I took this matter up orally with Mr. Stettinius who felt that it was too late to suggest any change in the appointments involving Mr. Dreyfus and Mr. Morris, who has been appointed as our Ambassador to Iran and whose name has come to the Senate. Mr. Stettinius further pointed out that any reversal of our present decision would be very difficult to handle in view of the fact that it had already been cleared through the Secretary and the President, and finally that our relations with the War Department and our plans to bring about closer collaboration between General Connolly and our Embassy at Tehran would become hopelessly involved if we now reversed our position and announced that Mr. Dreyfus was to return to his former post. I subsequently explained to the Minister that the decisions in this matter had gone too far to permit reversal. As much as we would like to meet the wishes of the Iranian Government and of the Shah in this matter, I felt sure that he would understand and hoped that he would be able to make the situation clear to his Government. The Minister seemed much disappointed and told me he would keep me advised of any further communication that he might receive in this matter from his Government.

Schayesteh had been next instructed to continue his representations with Assistant Secretary Berle. Berle on March 9, 1944 (Memorandum, 123 D 82/613):

The Minister of Iran came to see me at his request. He wished to renew a request made earlier that our Government reconsider the recall of Mr. Louis G. Dreyfus, Jr., and to express the hope that we would appoint him as our Ambassador to Iran. He recited at considerable length the very great personal esteem in which Dreyfus and his wife were held in Iran; the fact that the Shah had given the agrément to Mr. Leland B. Morris' appointment, but coupled it with the request that Mr. Dreyfus might be considered for the ambassadorial post. Recognizing that representation was a matter for the President, and that there was nothing personal against Leland Morris, the Iranian Government and the Shah nevertheless ventured the hope that even at this late date the matter might be reconsidered. The Minister added that if it would assist matters the Shah would communicate directly and personally with President Roosevelt. The Minister gave at some length the reasons for this, including the fact that for two years Dreyfus had upheld the interests of Iran and of the United States at a time when the Middle East Supply Center was falling down badly on supplies and so forth. He said that these representations had been made by him pursuant to a cable dated February 26 and another one dated February 28; that the latter had directed him to take up the matter with Secretary Hull personally, but that Secretary Hull was out of town; he had subsequently received a cable from his Foreign Office directing him to take it up personally with me. I said I was gratified to know of the success which had attended Mr. Dreyfus, who was a personal friend of mine; that, as the Minister had stated, representation was, of course, a matter for the President; but that I would be glad to bring his representations to the attention of the appropriate authorities and he could be assured that they would be given every consideration.

Berle's letter to the President, March 9, 1944:

Attached, memorandum of conversation with the Minister of Iran, in which he transmitted a request from the Iranian Government for reconsideration of the recall of Dreyfus and expresses his Government's hope that Dreyfus will be appointed Ambassador to Iran. The Iranian Government asks that this message be conveyed to the White House and stated that if it will assist in the matter the Shah will be prepared to communicate personally with President Roosevelt.

Hull's note to the President, March 24, 1944 (Memorandum and enclosures, 123 D 82/612):

It does not seem to me that it would be feasible, in view of the announcements already made of the appointment of Mr. Morris to Tehran and of Mr. Dreyfus to Reykjavik, to attempt to do anything about the Iranian request. We have told the Iranian Minister that while we appreciate deeply the generous references to Mr. Dreyfus, appointments already made could not be reversed. I do not believe any further action necessary.

On March 17, 1944, Hugo A. Muller, Secretary of the Iran Mission of the Presbyterian Church in the USA, Hamadan, had written to Murray

(Letter and enclosure, 123 D 82/616): "The Executive Committee of the Iran Mission of the Presbyterian Church has instructed me to send you the enclosed copy of its minute of appreciation of Minister Louis Dreyfus and Mrs. Dreyfus, whose service in Iran has been very valuable and whose departure we regret." The minute of appreciation reads:

> The members of the Iran Mission wish to record their deep appreciation of the service rendered by the American Minister, Mr. Louis Dreyfus and his wife, during their stay in Iran. Since their arrival in Tehran in December, 1940, we have found Mr. Dreyfus ever ready to give sympathetic consideration to our problems and glad to assist us in every possible way. Especially in the perplexities and crises of recent years he has given us wise and helpful counsel, accompanied by a truly rare understanding of our viewpoint as missionaries and permanent residents of the country. By many kind expressions of their thought for us and by their gracious and delightful hospitality in the Legation on numerous occasions, Mr. and Mrs. Dreyfus have endeared themselves to all of us. Even more than for our happy personal relationships with the American Minister and Mrs. Dreyfus we are glad and grateful for their unremitting efforts to show the government and people of Iran the friendship and goodwill of the United States. With sincerity, tact and devotion they have improved every opportunity to strengthen the ties which bind our two countries together and in this effort they have been markedly successful. They are known and recognized as true friends of Iran. As a member of the Iran-America Relief Committee, for a year and a half, Mrs. Dreyfus has done outstanding work for the poor in a most neglected section of Teheran. She has given freely of her time and her own funds for this work and has carried a load which has severely taxed her physically. In her personal ministrations to the sick and destitute she has given to the people of the city a demonstration of the finest spirit of service which cannot be forgotten. At a time when Iran sorely needs loyal friends we deeply regret that Mr. and Mrs. Dreyfus are not to remain in our Embassy. Hundreds of Iranians who hold them in highest esteem are distressed by their going. As fine and worthy representatives of our great nation we know that wherever they are stationed they will increase American prestige. We are proud of their record in Iran.

Chapter 27

Another Looming Famine and Actions to Avert It

From the documentary evidence provided in the previous chapters, it is clear that Iran in the fall of 1943 was faced with another famine. The grim conditions in Azerbaijan and Khorassan in the fall of 1943 were described in chapter 20. As documented in chapter 22, similar conditions prevailed in Tehran and the southern regions, and General Hurley had reported seeing dead bodies in the streets (chapter 25). Consequently, the relative optimism expressed by Dreyfus and Jackson at the onset of the 1943 harvest (chapter 21) was short-lived. Concerned at the political situation and the spreading chaos in the summer of 1943, Dreyfus had conveyed Millspaugh's anxious request on July 20, 1943 (Telegram 752, 891.154A/5):

> My 737, July 18. Millspaugh strongly urges that May be granted leave to assume direction of transport services since present transport director is leaving in four weeks and there is no other suitable person available to assume charge of this important work. Millspaugh has become responsible for transport and food matters as result of transfer of functions of Food Ministry to Ministry of Finance. In view of extreme urgency of transport problem in Iran and the active cooperation we have given Iranians in providing trucks and keeping them moving I support Millspaugh's request for May's assignment. Department is requested to expedite selection of the transport men mentioned in my 577, June 3.

Dreyfus on July 31, 1943 (Telegram 792, 891.154A/6):

> My 752, July 20. Iranian road transport situation gives cause for alarm in view of departure next week of the present British director, illness of Granger, May, or other suitable person. Because road transport is the very cornerstone of Iran's wheat and other economic problems the British and American Legations have been instrumental in helping Iran build up a fleet of almost 2000 trucks which is capable of taking care of all needs. The organization cannot be maintained and in fact will disintegrate without adequate foreign personnel. Therefore I cannot stress too strongly the necessity of prompt selection and departure of transport experts mentioned in my 577, June 3.

Dreyfus in a report entitled, "Allied Responsibility for Grain for Iran," dated September 30, 1943 (Dispatch 686 and enclosure, 891.5018/30):

> I have the honor to enclose a copy of a letter from Dr. Millspaugh, chief of the American Financial Mission to Iran, addressed to Sir Reader Bullard, the British Minister, reporting that a serious situation seems about to occur in connection with the Allied undertaking to meet the essential food needs of Iran arising from the announced decision of the British and American forces in this country to cease the importation of grain for their Iranian employees. The situation is further complicated by the practice, which is well authenticated in the case of the Russian forces and suspected in the case of the British forces, of either actively collecting the grain for export or at least tacitly encouraging the export of the grain, so badly needed in this country, to such an extent that what should be a period of abundance, owing to ample crops, may actually develop into a period of scarcity. It may be necessary to import grain from abroad into this country to replace that taken from it by the Allies unless Iran keeps what it needs of the grain produced here and neighboring countries make their own imports. Dr. Millspaugh suggests, as a temporary palliative measure, that, for the present, the grain required to feed British troops be imported. Although not mentioned in this letter, it might be cited, as a precedent, that last winter, when the Russians were exporting grain from Northern Iran to the Soviet Union and actively preventing its distribution here, the British did, in fact, agree to Allied importation of grain for Iranian needs. The present situation in respect of wheat collection is roughly as follows: total commitments and landlords' undertakings amount to 204,000 tons as against the original target figure for this year of 350,000 tons. It

now seems that even the smaller revised figure of 300,000 tons could not be attained. The silo contains 5,000 tons of barley and other adulterants but only 3,000 tons of wheat, which makes the percentage of adulterants too high for the wheat stock. Wheat is coming into Tehran at the rate of only 250 tons a day, barely enough to feed the city currently. Unquestionably there seems to be enough transport and there is a good crop—the thing is to bring it out for use by the government and no solution has yet appeared to this problem.

Millspaugh's letter to Bullard, September 10, 1943, is a classic:

Dear Sir Reader: With further reference to your letter of 31 August, 1943, in which you state that after 30 November, 1943, you will no longer import grain to feed Iranian laborers employed by the British Forces, I wish to call your attention to an aspect of the food situation which appears to me extremely important. It is true that the harvest this year is ample to feed the Iranian population. Our problem, as you know, is one of collection and distribution. In addition, it is a problem of preventing exportation and consumption of grain by the Allied Governments in excess of the surplus. I feel assured from your letter that no Iranian grain will be purchased by British authorities either for export or for local use. I have the same assurance in the case of the American authorities. Unfortunately, we have no such assurance from or with respect to the Soviet authorities. On the contrary, we are certain that they expect to obtain in Iran a certain quantity of Iranian grain. The quantity is still undetermined and may remain so for some time. In addition, I need not remind you that the Soviet authorities, in effect, substantially control the collection, movement and distribution of grain of the northern provinces. None can be made available for the needs of Tehran without the permission of the Soviets or, at the least, without their active cooperation. As I have just said, we have no positive assurance at the present moment that any grain will be available from the northern provinces for Tehran and it is quite possible that, in any event, the grain from the north will not be available in Tehran.

It seems to me that, if a shortage should develop at Tehran due to nonavailability of northern grain, I am justified in assuming that such shortage would be due to the military needs of the Allies or to the virtual military occupation in the country by Allied forces; and, even in the presence of a bumper harvest, such a shortage would be beyond the control of the Iranian Government. Under the circumstances, therefore, if the Iranian Government is unable to obtain the needed quantity of grain from the north, I am forced to the conclusion that the Allied Governments are under an obligation to see that the people of Tehran are fed. In other words, it does not seem quite logical for one or two of the Allies to declare that they will import no grain into Iran this year while another Ally creates a shortage by consuming and exporting Iranian grain and interfering with its collection and distribution within the country. It appears to me that the policies and activities of the three Allied Governments and the Iranian Government are all parts of our problem and must be coordinated. Unless they are so treated and coordinated, Iran is likely to be left to suffer through no fault of its own. To put my view in still more definite terms, if Soviet Russia needs grain for its military forces or as a result of the war, the grain should be supplied directly by the other Allied Governments, leaving Iranian grain for Iranian needs, or, if Soviet Russia is supplied by Iran, Iran should be supplied by the other Allied Governments.

The quantity required to feed the Iranian laborers employed by the British and American forces does not appear to be large; but the administrative arrangements required for their feeding may involve some difficulties. I would suggest that, in view of the uncertainties of the situation, a final decision be deferred for a time and the grain required to feed these laborers continue to be imported. You may be assured that we are making every effort to the end that all of the needs of the Iranian population may be met. Yours very truly, A.C. Millspaugh

Dreyfus on "Grain Supplies in Iran," October 1, 1943 (Dispatch 688, 891.6131/2):

I have the honor to report that the Cereals and Bread Section of the Iranian Ministry of Finance, (the section which was taken over the functions of the former Ministry of Food), has furnished the Legation with a statement of the current and probable future situation in Iran with respect to domestic grain supplies during the present crop year. This statement may be summarized as follows: (1) To meet minimum requirements of the various cities, a total of 310,000 tons of grain will be needed. If possible, this figure should be exceeded in order to provide a reserve. (2) On the basis of reports received up to September 8, 1943, the Cereals and Bread Section believes that all provincial municipalities will either be able to draw their requirements from their own provinces or may be supplied without special difficulty from adjacent provinces. (3) The city of Tehran presents the most serious and most important problem. Its requirements for the year are estimated at

90,000 tons (of the 310,000 tons total). It is believed that 25,000 tons of this will be obtainable from the areas near the city and that an additional 35,000 tons can be brought in from other parts of the country outside the Soviet-occupied zone. This leaves 30,000 tons to be made up by shipments from the Soviet-controlled sections, and these shipments have been tentatively allocated, on the basis of the present information and estimates, as follows: 4,000 tons from Zenjan, 12,000 tons from Gorgan, 10,000 tons from Khorassan, and 8,000 tons from Azerbaijan. (4) The amounts to be furnished from the Soviet zone are far below the normal surpluses of the areas in question and have been scheduled with the idea that they do not represent what the provinces should furnish, but rather what, as a practical matter, they might reasonably be expected to provide under the circumstances. In making its calculations, the Cereals and Bread Section has taken into consideration the probable requirements of Soviet troops in Iran and has also tried to leave a margin for possible Soviet exports to the USSR. (5) If the requisite amount is not forthcoming from the Soviet zone, it may be barely possible to squeeze it out of the southern and central provinces, but this would be an extremely difficult and doubtful undertaking, necessitating drastic action which might well fail and would be likely to produce serious repercussions politically.

The foregoing statement was discussed fully on September 27 at a meeting called by Dr. Millspaugh, Administrator General of Finances, and attended by the British and American Ministers, other officers of the two Legations, representatives of the Middle East Supply Center, Tehran, the American Acting Director of the Road Transport Office, and American and British officials of the Cereals and Transport Section. It was brought out that the supply estimates were based upon the assumption that adequate truck transport would be available to move the grain from the producing areas to the consuming centers. It was believed that transport would, in fact, be provided, but it was emphasized that existing difficulties made this by no means certain. Apart from transport, it was recognized that the key to the success of the program would lie in the attitude adopted by the Soviet authorities toward the collection of grain in the northern provinces and its movement to Tehran. If their attitude should prove hostile, or merely passively obstructive, it would be almost impossible to collect the grain, even if they did not impose physical obstacles to its movement south, since local Iranian authorities would probably take their cue from the Soviets and do nothing to execute the orders of the Ministry of Finance.

Factors which might influence the Soviet authorities in this respect are: (a) The completion of the 1942-43 contract, calling for the delivery to them of 20,000 tons of grain other than rice. The Cereals and Bread Section reported that it had the required quantity on hand and had issued orders for its delivery. (b) The success of the Russians in purchasing, either direct or through the Iranian authorities, such quantities as they might want for their garrisons in Iran and for export to the Soviet Union. So far, they had made no demands in this connection, but it was to be expected that they would insist upon obtaining a more or less substantial amount from the provinces under their control. It is quite possible that the Soviets would find means to prevent any movement of grain south until after they had obtained their own requirements.

It was agreed that Dr. Millspaugh should give the Prime Minister a factual statement of the grain position, should point out the vital importance of Soviet attitude, and should request the Prime Minister to approach the Soviet authorities at once to enlist their cooperation. I believe that this is a necessary first step, and it seems quite possible that favorable assurances will be received from the Russians. However, such assurances were given last year, and, as the Department knows, were never translated into action. It is hoped that this season the understanding with the Soviets will be more specific and, therefore, more likely to produce results. In any case, the test will come within the next few weeks, when the Cereals and Bread Section plans to begin movement of grain to Tehran from certain of the provinces in the Russian zone. In laying emphasis upon the importance of the Soviet attitude, I do not wish to give the impression that there are no other factors which will influence the results or lack of results obtained. The landowners and Iranian officials in the northern provinces are notoriously selfish and corrupt, and, even if assured of Russian benevolence, the authorities at Tehran may find it extremely difficult to obtain the quantities of grain which they require. As indicated above, the provision of adequate transportation is also a doubtful matter. However, I think it is axiomatic that Soviet acquiescence, at least, is a sine qua non for any program of grain collection in the North. In my opinion, the United States and Great Britain should not sit idly by if the Russians should prove uncooperative, but should be prepared to make energetic representations, in Tehran and in Moscow, to obtain at least a minimum share of the surplus of the northern provinces for the consumption of the deficit areas of the south.

Dreyfus on October 16, 1943 (Dispatch 693, 891.6131/3):

I have the honor to refer to the Legation's despatch No. 688 of October 1, 1943 and to report below subsequent developments in the Iranian grain supply picture. As was reported in the despatch under reference, one of the requisites for assuring the grain supply of Tehran during the crop year ending September 1, 1944 is the procurement of minimum quantities of surplus grain from the Soviet-occupied provinces of northern Iran. During the past two weeks, Dr. Millspaugh and Mr. Crawford, (the American acting-director of the Cereals and Bread Section of the Ministry of Finance) have been in touch with the Soviet authorities in Tehran and have commenced negotiations for the division of the anticipated northern surplus stocks between the Soviets and the Iranians. At present, conversations are in progress regarding the rice crop, which is expected to be large and which the Soviets wished to discuss first. They have asked for 40,000 tons, and Mr. Crawford believes that this amount can be provided and still leave a roughly equivalent amount for the supply of the Tehran area. It is planned to have this crop bought up by a syndicate of Iranian merchants, formed through the Tehran Chamber of Commerce, which will buy and sell under the general direction of the Cereals and Bread Section and at prices agreed upon with that Section. The Soviet share will be provided by that syndicate, if plans work out, at a price only slightly above cost. The success of this plan with respect to rice will depend in part upon the price at which the syndicate is able to buy from the growers, which is expected to be ascertained within a few days, and in part upon agreement with respect to a barter arrangement proposed by the Soviets whereby they would pay for the rice in cotton piece-goods and other essential goods, rather than in cash. In principle, I understand, the Iranians would welcome payment in kind, since they are badly in need of goods of all kinds. It may be, however, that the Soviets will insist upon prohibitive valuations for the goods they would provide, or that they will demand that the price of rice be fixed at too low a level to make the scheme practicable.

To date, the Soviet authorities have made no specific requests with regard to wheat, nor have they been formally advised of the quantities of wheat which the Iranian Government feels it must have from the northern areas for the supply of Tehran. Mr. Crawford guesses that the Russians will want about 16,000 tons of wheat, and he believes that it would not be impossible to provide that amount. A specific Soviet request for 16,000 tons of barley has been received. This is only 1,000 tons more than was agreed upon for the 1942-43 crop year, and, in view of the much larger crop this year, it should be possible to meet this request. It remains to be seen, of course, whether the Soviets will insist upon receiving all the grain which they request before permitting, or assisting, the Iranian authorities to collect and ship the amounts needed for Tehran. If they do so, it will make things very difficult. Mr. Crawford reports, however, as an encouraging sign, that small quantities of wheat have begun to reach the capital by rail from Gorgan, in the Russian zone.

With regard to the general situation, throughout the country, the Cereals and Bread Section is cautiously optimistic. While admitting that the administrative machine is very unreliable, characterized by inefficiency and corruption, Mr. Crawford, nevertheless, points out that grain is being collected and that government-controlled stocks in Tehran are steadily, if not rapidly, rising. The latest figures available, (of several days ago), show that landlords have given undertakings to deliver approximately 250,000 tons of grain. This figure is expected to jump up to around 300,000 tons at the end of the current Iranian month of Mehr (October 23), at which time the Government is empowered to fix quotas for all landlords who have not already given undertakings for delivery of grain. To make up any remaining quantity needed to complete the estimated total requirements of 310,000 tons, the Cereals and Bread Section plans to attempt direct purchase from the peasants, possibly by bartering sugar or similar articles.

Apart from the continuing uncertainty with respect to the Soviet zone, the greatest potential danger faced by the grain administration is that of a breakdown of transport. Although there are probably sufficient trucks in Iran to handle grain and other essential movements, the Road Transport Department (Edareh Barbari Rah), is having great difficulty in controlling them in the face of the inflated freight rates offered by black market traders. Efforts are being made to meet this situation by seeking more widespread use of police and gendarmes and by stationing European employees of the Road Transport Department (mostly Scandinavians) in various key centers of the country. New road transport regulations are also to be prepared. This control program, however, is still in its infancy, and it may be that its results will develop too late to affect the grain movement. It has already been necessary for the Road Transport Department to confess its inability to move the sugar beet harvest, which is now ready for processing. In one sector, the Iranian Army, through General Ridley's mission, has offered much needed assistance by providing 100 army trucks to move from 8,000 to 12,000 tons of grain from Hamadan to the railroad at Arak. Half of this amount is to go to the Army for its own rations. The Iranian Army has also offered to assist the Cereals and Bread Section by using troops to enforce collection of grain. However, Mr. Crawford has, so far, preferred not to accept this aid, fearing that the Army's methods would antagonize the growers and, in the end, make the collection more difficult.

Allied Assistance in Grain Collection and Transport

The transport crisis had soon become apparent, but in contrast to 1942, the Allied armies had provided assistance. The changed response was undoubtedly due to developments discussed in chapters 24 and 25, and the forthcoming visit to Tehran of the three Allied heads of state. In addition, by late 1943, shipments to Russia were decreasing, thereby facilitating assistance to Iran. Dreyfus on October 28, 1943 (Telegram 1028, 891.24/601):

> Department will (have) now received paraphrase of telegram of British Minister addressed to PAI (Persia and Iraq) Force and repeated to British Embassy, Washington as No. 86 with instructions to transmit to Department. I agree fully with British Minister's statement and his conclusion that unless help from the Allies is forthcoming there may be another bread crisis this winter. The situation is urgent and desperate and unless PAI Force is able to furnish the necessary trucks without delay I shall ask the Department to approach the War Department for assistance from PGSC. In considering this matter it must be stressed that Iran's fleet of some 5,000 trucks has been decimated by old age, lack of parts and exploitation of large portion by UKCC and Iran-Soviet transport. Only 900 Lend-Lease trucks have been received and these are not fully suitable as load carriers for use in Iran; many of these vehicles are now laid up for repairs and lack of parts. We should therefore give serious consideration to a long range program of gradually replacing Iran's rapidly disappearing truck fleet or the situation next year will be even more desperate. A possible solution of the problem might be to turn over to Iran some of the PGSC trucks when haulage to Russia is reduced or stopped.

A note to Murray, November 4, 1943, reads in part (Memorandum, 891.6131/5):

> The grain situation in Iran is critical. . . . On October 25 the British Minister wired the PAI Command at Baghdad that a serious crisis existed and asked that it provide trucks to move 20,000 tons of grain from Hamadan and Kermanshah to Sultanabad. Dreyfus telegraphed (No. 1028, October 28) that if PAI could not supply the trucks he would ask us to ask the War Department for assistance from PGSC. (We sent War copies of both messages.) Dreyfus also asks for long-range replacement program of trucks for Iran. This is primarily a MESC problem. This program calls for distribution of 2,338 trucks in the Middle East in the nine months from August 1, 1943, of which Iran gets the lion's share, 922. The plan calls for shipments to Iran from Cairo of 50 in November, 120 in December, 221 in January, 150 in February, 190 in March and 80 in April.

On November 5, 1943, Hayter of the British Embassy had written to Gordon P. Merriam (Letter and enclosure, 891.6131/6):

> Mr. Pares of this Embassy gave you on October 28th a copy of a telegram from our Legation at Tehran to our Embassy at Baghdad about the provision of trucks for grain collecting in Persia. You may be interested to see the enclosed telegram from the Foreign Office to Baghdad of October 30th, which comments on the Tehran Legation's suggestion.

The Foreign Office telegram reads:

> We agree it is most desirable that we should assist on lines suggested by Sir R. Bullard. We understand that Russian cargo arriving in the Persian Gulf between mid-November and mid-January is unlikely fully to absorb capacity of Persian-Iraq L of C (Line of Communication) in which case it may be possible for Commander in Chief PAIC (Persia and Iraq Command) to arrange to release some UKCC vehicles without affecting aid to Russia. But if we can only assist with transport of grain at the expense of supplies to Russia we must (explain to the) Soviet Government that we should be prepared to do this on the basis that the only alternative, viz import of wheat into Persia, would have even more prejudicial effect on supplies to Russia. Fact that UKCC have many Persian contracted vehicles in their fleet makes it more important that we rather than the Americans (who do not use Persian vehicles) should assist. Every effort should of course be made to see that interference with supplies for Russia is kept to a minimum and

terminated as soon as possible. Above has been agreed with the War Office.

Ford on November 11, 1943 (Telegram 1054, 891.24/603):

British military have provided about 500 trucks and are expected to supply 150 or more again to move about 10,000 tons grain from Kermanshah to Hamadan Arak and Tehran. Movement expected to require about two months. Trucks taken from (aid) to Russia Transport Services. This will not only ensure delivery of part of stocks needed for Tehran but will release Iranian trucks to carry out in Soviet zone wheat program described in British Legation's telegram 86 to British Embassy Washington. Iranian Government continues grain negotiations with Soviet authorities who say they will arrange deliveries to Tehran of 40 to 50,000 tons if about 250 trucks are made available from Iranian fleet. This is not entirely worked out as yet but convoys of 46 and 40 trucks left Tehran last week for Azerbaijan and Khorrasan respectively. Cereals Director Crawford believes large part of balance of transport requested by Soviets can be made up from Iran trucks already working in north under road transport office. Soviets say they appointed Russians to supervise grain collection and delivery (in) their zone and to assist control Iranian contracted trucks, whose irresponsibility is one of the principal difficulties faced by Iran transport organization. Crawford says Soviet officials here have displayed generally reasonable attitude. It has been agreed they shall get 36,000 tons rice for export to USSR but they are confining their wheat and barley requests to amounts needed for Soviet garrisons in Iran about six and one six thousand tons respectively.

Despite these favorable developments situation as a whole is not encouraging. Total contracts for grain deliveries to government still about 30,000 tons below estimated requirements and it is unlikely that all contracts will be fulfilled. Furthermore, rate of consumption in Khorrasan has increased and at present rate will leave little or no surplus for Tehran. Crawford fears imports will be needed to cover requirements before next harvest and informal request has already been made through British Legation that a reserve British Army stock of 10,000 tons be created to be available for Iran civilian use if necessary. Later this month a formal request for imports may be submitted to MESC. Repeated to Cairo for Landis.

With the Big Three due to meet in Tehran at the end of November, matters had taken greater urgency. Dreyfus on November 17, 1943 (Telegram 1060, 891.5018/32):

> Commander Jackson Director General of MESC here for a week studying Iran grain civil transport situation in close consultation with this Legation, British Legation, Millspaugh Mission and MESC Tehran. Unanimously agreed outlook is doubtful and urgent steps are required to improve grain collection and transport if a crisis like last winter's is to be avoided. Efficient and reliable personnel is most critical need and Millspaugh and I feel this must be obtained where it can be found at the moment. Accordingly we have agreed to following to be effected as fast as possible: One. MESC to try to provide 16 officers and 9 noncommissioned officers from British army in Mid-East to assist in control and operation of Iranian civil transfers. These men must be stationed at various provincial centers outside Soviet zone. They will be attached technically to MESC Tehran but will act under Millspaugh and his United States aides. They will not receive pay or allowances from Iran Government and will have no titles. Their services will be temporary and will not affect purely American character of Millspaugh Mission nor its control of economic matters. Two. MESC will also provide 14 British officers to assist cereal collection and distribution in provinces outside Soviet zone. They will operate under same conditions as transport men. Three. Unless Soviets object the eight available Americans and non British Europeans now employed by Iran Road Transport Office will go to Soviet zone to control transport there. Four. British Minister and I will ask Soviet Chargé to arrange for Soviet officers to assist collections in northern zone in same way as it is proposed for British officers in the South. If Soviets are willing to provide transport control officers also, that will be welcomed. Five. MESC will seek milling technician to increase capacity of Tehran flour mill which is now well below city's daily consumption. MESC also to seek competent accountant forward transport office to fill in pending arrival of American staff. Six. Factual reporting on grain and transport situation will be centralized thru MESC Tehran to MESC Cairo but American and British Legations will continue to report direct to their governments on policy aspects. Seven. With approval of both Legations MESC Tehran is asking MESC Cairo to prepare reserve of 10,000 tons wheat to be available for Iranian civilian consumption six weeks notice. This would be called upon only as a last resort. General Connolly has been asked to assist by lending a few trucking experts on same basis proposed for British Army officers. He has declined on

ground that he has none to spare and that responsibility for conditions in Iran rests primarily with British and not at all on American forces. Repeated to Cairo for Landis.

Landis to Acheson on November 20, 1943 (Telegram 2143, 891.24/605):

Reference Tehran's No. seventy, ten six zero November 17, 2 p.m. to Department repeated Cairo. Grateful if you bring General Clay's attention to last paragraph. Cereals and transport situation in Iran as per reports extremely serious and unless difficulties surmounted will react on lift to Russia. Gesture of (US) Army Iran will in my judgment do much to further American prestige and promote more cooperative concern on part of United States, British and Soviet. Cooperation now good on civil and diplomatic side Tehran. To implement our Minister Tehran seems sound policy as well as making possible success of Millspaugh. Other aspects of cable working here Cairo to help feel Millspaugh's needs. But War Department help necessary to broaden Connolly's directive if aim of last paragraph to be achieved. General Clay is familiar with and understands situation.

Dreyfus on November 19, 1943 (Dispatch 736 and enclosure, 891.5018/33):

I have the honor to refer to my telegram No. 1060 of November 17, 1943 reporting the arrangement worked out by the Middle East Supply Center with the American and British Legations at Tehran and with the Millspaugh Mission for the provision of special, temporary British Army personnel to assist in the collection and transportation of the domestic Iranian grain crop. There is enclosed herewith, for the Department's information and records, a copy of a letter of November 17, 1943 from Dr. Millspaugh to Commander R.G.A. Jackson, Director General of MESC, in which Dr. Millspaugh confirmed his approval of the plan and defined his understanding of its terms. The letter is entirely in accord with my understanding of the arrangement.

Millspaugh's November 17, 1943, letter to Jackson reads:

Dear Mr. Jackson: It is with much pleasure that I write a letter confirmatory of our conversations and with particular reference to the Minutes of a Meeting at the MESC held on 15 November, 1943. No doubt can be entertained that assistance is needed in the work of grain-collection and transport, and the temporary assistance offered by MESC is accepted with much appreciation. I took the liberty of suggesting that the arrangements for assistance be understood as extending to about March 21, 1944, at which time the situation will be reviewed and a fresh decision arrived at after mutual consultation. In the interim, MESC will, of course, be entirely free to withdraw personnel, if such action should appear necessary, and, on my part, I would like to feel that no misunderstanding would arise if I should have reason to request the withdrawal of one or more individuals. It is our common feeling also, I take it, that the British personnel will be withdrawn if and when Americans arrive to do the work done by the British, or when Iranians are available to do that work, or in case of change of conditions which would make British assistance in any branch of the organization or in any locality no longer necessary. It is my belief that we have a full understanding that the British personnel can not be considered members of my Mission, and that they can not be given official titles, position or legal authority. . . . Let me say, in conclusion, how much I have been heartened by your generous cooperation. I am sending a copy of this letter to Mr. Landis, the British Legation, and the American Legation. Yours very truly, A.C. Millspaugh

Landis on November 24, 1943 (Airgram-292, 891.24/608):

I am quoting below a savingram dispatched from R.G.A. Jackson, Director General of MESC, from Tehran on November 17, 1943 to MESC, Cairo. . . . The savingram represents conclusions reached by Jackson after his recent visit to Tehran. It supports earlier reports made to the Department of the seriousness of the impending situation in Tehran. The potential flexible use of all British resources in Iran as contrasted with the inflexible character of American resources in Iran should be noted. It should also be noted that due to the presence of the Millspaugh Mission in Iran the primary responsibility for assisting in the solution of these internal problems in Iran is likely to be deemed by the Iranian population to rest with the United States more than with anyone else. United States nationals under Dr. Millspaugh head up administrative responsibility for both cereals and road transport. Please note also especially paragraphs 16 and 17, pointing to the key to cereal collection resting on getting grain from the Russian zone which depends on cooperation with Russian officials. The savingram follows:

"Immediate. Following from Jackson. Detailed discussions have taken place in Tehran with United States Legation, British Legation and

Millspaugh Mission, in connection with road transport and cereals situation in Iran. Generally agreed locally that organization of road transport is key to majority of economic problems in Iran. Effective control can only be achieved when sufficient reliable personnel is available to Dr. Millspaugh. Latter has now telegraphed to Washington asking that Mr. Shields, who is to take charge of road transport department, and two assistants, should be sent here as quickly as possible. In meantime Mr. Vivian is continuing to take charge of the Department, but is badly in need of personnel both to assist in administration and in controlling transport throughout the southern zone. Dr. Millspaugh states that there is no early possibility of sufficient American personnel being provided at short notice to carry out these duties. He immediately accepted an offer that we should try to find personnel from alternative sources as a temporary measure. Sixteen officers and nine technicians of NCO standing are required. If any personnel can be provided, they would be attached to MESC, Tehran, and then seconded to assist the Transport Department of the Millspaugh Mission. British and United States Legations would be kept informed of the manner in which they were employed.

"3. It is clear that a major crisis has only been averted by the prompt assistance of PAIC in providing several hundred trucks to move grain and oil. In addition, the Indian Army is also being asked to release UKCC transport to assist with oil distribution in eastern Iran. There can be no guarantee that this assistance can be given for a long period, and it is therefore imperative that some steps be taken immediately to strengthen the road transport organization.

"4. Mr. Ozzard, a United States member of MESC, who has been lent by the State Department to the Millspaugh Mission until the end of the year, has already made good progress in setting up a repair organization. Much more could be done if the additional personnel referred to above can be provided.

"5. Backloading in UKCC vehicles under control of PAIC is being followed separately with PAIC who have already indicated their willingness to try to help in this.

"6. An essential part of transport organization is that the movement of all civil supplies, both by rail and by road, should be planned in advance. Dr. Millspaugh has recently proposed a Transport Advisory Committee with a working sub-Committee with the primary duty of planning movements. (This will probably supercede the Road Transport Board eventually). He agreed to bring both the Committee and the working sub-Committee into operation with the least possible delay.

"7. In connection with the movement problem, the appointment of a Movement Officer at Ahwaz (as suggested in May by MESC, Tehran) has already been very effective in increasing to Tehran the flow of civil supplies held in the Gulf Ports. This experience encourages the belief that additional personnel should have some effect both on the road transport and movements problem.

"8. The road transport situation is obviously of vital importance in the movement of grain. It is true to say that if PAIC had not responded promptly to the request for assistance in moving wheat from Hamadan and Kermanshah Tehran would have been without bread in a few days' time.

"9. Mr. Crawford, a United States agricultural production official attached to MESC, has been lent to the Millspaugh Mission since the departure of Mr. Sheridan to take charge of the grain collection scheme. He is badly in need of assistance, especially in the provinces. As in the case of the road transport organization, there is no immediate possibility of American personnel being provided by the Millspaugh Mission. A first-class administrative assistant is required to help Mr. Crawford in the Food Department and another thirteen officers are required for work primarily in the provinces. If we can also assist in this respect, personnel would be appointed in the same way as transport personnel referred to in paragraph 2. . . .

"10. It has been emphasized that if any British assistance can be given, it must be of temporary nature only. No official titles should be given to any personnel seconded through MESC and the American character of the Millspaugh Mission must be maintained. It is apparent, however, that unless some assistance with personnel can be provided, the transport and cereals situation in Persia must continue to remain critical. A disastrous situation would result if PAIC were to withdraw its present assistance with trucks.

"11. Dr. Millspaugh would replace any personnel provided under the above arrangements immediately he is able to recruit suitable personnel himself. Again, he recommends that the personnel situation should be generally reviewed again at the end of the Iranian year, 21st March, 1944, when it will be possible to forecast the new harvest.

"12. Any military personnel would require plain clothes. Cars would be necessary for officials working in provinces. They cannot be provided locally.

"13. General Connolly has been interviewed to see whether any transport personnel can be lent from USPGSC. He is sympathetic and recognizes that if the transport and grain situation were to deteriorate still further, it would be necessary to import grain to prevent starvation on his line of communications. Nevertheless, he is unable to help for any personnel whom he can free from this theatre are being sent, under instructions from the United States War Department, to other theatres.

"14. Strongly recommend we should do our best to help. As to transport personnel; I shall discuss with PAIC when I am in Baghdad next week-end. Again, Civil Affairs Branch and MEF might be able to assist. I feel assistance with personnel at this stage would be a cheaper investment in the long run in so far as it would provide an opportunity for getting some sort of organization into Iranian road transport, thus lessening the existing burden on PAIC and also reducing the danger of having to import cereals early next year.

"15. I hope that assistance in cereals collection can be provided by transferring British OCP officers from the Levant States for the winter months. If this is agreed, I shall discuss with General Spears early next week.

"16. The United States and British Ministers intend to consult the Soviet Chargé d'Affaires in Tehran and to inform him of the proposed plan of assistance. The Russians have already been asked to appoint Russian Liaison Officers to assist with transport and cereals collection in the northern zone. In addition, it is hoped that a Russian official might be appointed to assist in the Road Transport Department and also in the Food Department so that coordination of road transport and cereals collection in both zones may be improved.

"17. Separate telegram is being sent about existing grain situation. Present stock of wheat and flour in Tehran is only about ten days. Situation should improve if PAIC continue to transport grain from the south. Position would then seem moderately secure until about mid-January. After that, everything depends on getting grain from the northern zone and this is as yet by no means certain.

"18. What is far more important at the present time is that milling capacity in Tehran is only about 200 tons of flour daily, while 215 tons are being issued. Immediate deficiency is being covered through use of final shipments of flour sent here under the Food Agreement. Milling problem is also being dealt with separately.

"19. Many of the factors which contributed to the Food crisis of 1942 are again developing in Iran. If we assist with personnel now, we shall reduce the chances of repetition. I do not suggest assistance proposed above can solve transport and food problems, but dangers should to some extent be reduced. The alternative of taking no action would most probably lead to emergency calls for assistance early in 1944 and with the existing world grain and truck situation, it might be impossible to meet such demands. Again, if an effective grain collection scheme is to come into operation in 1944, the plans and organizations for that scheme must begin now.

"20. In this telegram I have concentrated only on transport and cereals for, in my opinion, they are the fundamental problems in this country at the present time and everything else is secondary to them in importance.

"21. United States and British Ministers will telegraph separately any observations which they wish to make on the political aspects of these proposals.

"22. This telegram is agreed by the United States and British Ministers and is based on a memorandum agreed with Dr. Millspaugh. Please pass copy to Minister of State Resident in the Middle East. It is assumed that the Minister of State and London will comment immediately if it is not desired to proceed on above lines.

"23. MESC Cairo please pass this telegram by fast bag to London and Washington. Signed: RGA Jackson."

The use of British army trucks to move wheat had created the impression among Iranians that the British were taking their wheat. Ford on January 17, 1944 (Dispatch 799, 891.24/622):

I have the honor to inform the Department that the British Ministry of Information has recently completed the filming of certain scenes at Hamadan, Sultanabad and Tehran, depicting American-British-Iranian

> cooperation in the collecting and transporting of the Iranian wheat harvest. It is hoped, by the showing of these films in Iran, to counteract the rumors which have been circulating here recently to the effect that the British were stealing Iran's wheat. These rumors no doubt had their origin in the fact that the British Army, through the loan of trucks and drivers, has been assisting the Iranian Government in its wheat collection program. The films, which were taken during the period from December 3 to January 8, show the following scenes: wheat being loaded on British Army trucks at Hamadan for transport to the railroad; wheat being unloaded from British Army trucks at Sultanabad for forwarding by rail; the unloading of wheat from railway cars at Tehran; Mr. Crawford, an American and, at present, Acting Director of the Cereals Section of the Iranian Ministry of Finance, greeting a party of British experts arriving in Tehran from Syria to assist in the wheat collection program; various processing operations in the Tehran silo; and, finally, the distribution of bread in Tehran. The films, which have just been sent to Cairo for developing, are expected back in Tehran shortly. Upon their return here, they will be viewed, a decision reached as to the film to be retained, and a suitable Persian script prepared. It is planned to exhibit the completed film, as part of a newsreel, throughout the Middle East, and to accompany the showings in Iran with a complementary campaign in the Persian press. As the Russians have been assisting in the wheat collection drive in facilitating shipments from the Northern Zone, the suggestion was made by a member of this Legation's staff to the attaché of the British Legation charged with the handling of the film that suitable mention of this fact ought to be made in any of the articles prepared for publication in the Persian press. It is understood that such a mention will be made. An officer attached to this Legation has arranged to be present at the private showing of the films to be held upon their return from Cairo, and to follow up, and report upon, any subsequent developments of interest, and particularly, so far as possible, upon the Persian reaction to the film.

The Russians, as above noted, had actively assisted in the collection and transport of wheat from Azerbaijan to Tehran and points south. Ford on November 11, 1943 (Telegram 1054, 891.24/603): "Iranian Government continues grain negotiations with Soviet authorities who say they will arrange deliveries to Tehran of 40 to 50,000 tons if about 250 trucks are made available from Iranian fleet." Dreyfus on November 17, 1943 (Telegram 1060, 891.5018/32): "British Minister and I will ask Soviet Chargé to arrange for Soviet officers to assist collections in northern zone in same way as it is proposed for British officers in the South. If

Soviets are willing to provide transport control officers also, that will be welcomed." Russian assistance in grain collection and transport to Tehran had created tension in Azerbaijan. Ebling on November 27, 1943 (Dispatch 5, 891.00/2084):

> With reference to the food supply it is reported that the request of the Soviets to buy wheat was disapproved by local Iranian officials. The Soviets have been requested to defer their purchases of wheat to a later date, after the landowners have completed their obligations to the local Iranian authorities. The Soviets can then buy in the open market. . . . As a further illustration of the distrustful attitude of the Azerbaijan population to the Tehran Government may be mentioned the agitation which was aroused by the recent announcement that the Ministry of Finance was sending trucks to Tabriz for the purpose of importing wheat from Azerbaijan to increase the supply of wheat in the silo at Tehran. It is feared that such action would result in an increase in the local price of wheat for sale to the Government.

Landis to Dreyfus on December 7, 1943 (Telegram 2256, 891.24/609):

> Would suggest for your consideration implementation of Tehran declaration by following steps. One. Representation by you and Bullard to Russians of necessity of getting 40,000 tons of grain from Russian zone of necessary Russian personnel for purpose. Two. Introduction of Russians on those Anglo-American-Iranian committees now participating in various angles of distribution and transport. Three. Consideration with Bullard of desirability of introduction some Russian representation on MESC particularly on Iranian requirements so as to inculcate habit of Russian responsibility for economic assistance to Iran. This Russian representation need not go to all activities, for example supply cut can be limited to consideration of essential Iranian requirements. Sent Tehran, repeated to Department.

Dreyfus responded on December 10, 1943 (Telegram 1104, 891.24/610):

> I agree with your suggestions which are in line with general policy being followed by Legation under Department's instructions. As you know Bullard and I several weeks ago approached Soviet Chargé about need for grain from Russian zone for Tehran and he expressed willingness of Soviets to furnish transport for 40,000 tons if that quantity were delivered main loading areas such as Tabriz. We also suggested

that Russian personnel be provided to help in collection and control of transport. Soviets are nominally represented on Road Transport Board but never attend. They have been invited to sit on new Transport Advisory Committee. Legation will consult Bullard about Soviet representation on MESC and I think he will agree but I think it doubtful that Russians will accept invitation to participate. . . . In general Legation plans to intensify its efforts to obtain closer participation in Allied efforts to relieve Iran's economic difficulties and I hope Tehran Declaration will prove useful talking points in this connection. However, we may not be able to accomplish much until new Soviet Ambassador arrives. Sent Cairo as No. 92.

Kirk from Cairo on December 18, 1943 (Telegram 2323, 891.24/612):

For George Washington from Short. Repeated to Landis care Atchinson Washington. "Foreign Office London has just cabled British Minister Tehran suggesting that he discuss with US Legation progress made by Russians on delivery of surplus cereals from Russian zone or desirability of publicizing Russian offer of 40,000 tons together with figures at regular intervals showing deliveries. Understand Landis initiated or participated in arrangements for such deliveries during his last visit Tehran. Imperative no publicity be given out without permission of Russians and would appreciate your so advising US Legation immediately." Sent to Tehran. Repeated to Department as our 2323.

Publicity on Russian assistance, as noted, was delicate. Ford on December 22, 1943 (Telegram 1133, 891.24/613):

For Short. Your December 18 to George Washington regarding cereals from Russian zone. We assume you have seen British Legation's telegram of December 19 to Foreign Office, repeated to Minister of State, Cairo as No. 337. British here agree with us that it would be unwise at this time to single out cereals situation in Russian zone for special publicity; Andrive asked Crawford to avoid distinguishing between zones in proposed publication of progress reports. There is no (repeat no) intention to publicize any Soviet undertaking regarding delivery of grain, especially since their agreement is only to transport grain from Tabriz to railhead in Mianeh, and from railhead at Bandarshah, Shahrud and Mianeh to Tehran. They have made no (repeat no) commitment regarding local collection or transportation of grain to main shipping centers, which appears to be the greatest difficulty at the moment. We have discussed foregoing with George Washington who concurs and suggests you refer to his latest mail report. Sent to Cairo as No. 101.

Improving Conditions

Tentative signs of improvement had first appeared in Azerbaijan. Ebling on November 27, 1943 (Dispatch 5, 891.00/2084):

> With reference to the food supply attention is invited to the lower prices registered for certain commodities. Stocks of provisions formerly hoarded are now being displayed in the bazaar. Such products include rice, raisins, wheat, and peas. The lower prices are attributed to: (a) Approval by the parliament of Dr. Millspaugh's income tax bill. (b) Successes of the Soviet Army. (c) Prospective entry of Turkey into the war.

Ebling on January 4, 1944 (Dispatch 15, 891.00/3006):

> The year 1943 came to a close with all classes of people in Azerbaijan manifesting gratitude and contentment at a slight improvement in local living conditions. There has been a noticeable decline in the cost of certain staple products. The price of fuel wood, alone, has decreased from $21.00 to $15.00 per metric ton during the past few days. Vegetable and food shops are displaying large stocks of products. It is the general opinion that the hoarders desire to dispose of accumulated stocks. Further price reductions are anticipated. It is rumored in the bazaar that the American Adviser in charge of price stabilization has recently announced that arrangements will soon be perfected for an increasing number of products to be imported from the United States.

Conditions in Tehran were also improving. As reported in Ford's dispatch 845 of February 15, 1944, given in chapter 27, complaints about quantity and quality of bread in Tehran had almost disappeared. This was mostly due to the arrival of northern wheat. V.G. Danielian, 7 Ave. Pahlevi, Kouche Bidi, Tehran to Habib Sabet, R.C.A. Building, New York (MID-Iran, 2200):

> Now let me tell you something about Tehran. Business is slack and there are no more contracts given out by the Allied Armies. Life in Tehran is alright. Food, clothes and other indispensables are plenty

> but terribly expensive. For example, wheat costs 9,000 rials per ton, rice 20 rials per kilo, butter 100 rials per kilo, and sugar 120 rials per kilo. A 1941 Buick costs 600,000 rials, and a single tire 35,000 rials. A suit of clothes costs 6000 rials, a pair of ladies shoes 1500 rials, men's shoes 1,000 rials and so on ($1 = 35 rials). Otherwise it is alright and much better than Irak, Syria or Palestine.

Imported products, however, showed no sign of decline. The improvements were not yet evident in the British zone. An OSS report on Kermanshah, February 2, 1944 (MID-Iran, 5070): "Local prices have taken another sharp rise, particularly cloth and tea. Two weeks ago tea was 400 rials per mann (3 kilos). Today the market price is 600 rials. No reason is advanced for this jump."

Ford on January 24, 1944 (Dispatch 814 and enclosure, 891.24/ 626):

> I have the honor to refer to previous communications regarding the Iranian domestic grain supply and to transmit herewith, to show the present situation, a copy of the weekly cereals collection report for January 15, 1944, prepared by the Tehran office of the Middle East Supply Center. As will be seen from this table, the estimate of local consumption for the country as a whole during the current crop year has been revised and now stands at 318,500 tons of bread grains. Against this, the cereals authorities hold contracts and undertakings from landlords and others to deliver to the Iranian Government 328,811 tons. They do not expect, however, that all undertakings will be fulfilled, and on the basis of the present information they estimate ultimate deliveries at 317,700 tons, or a trifle short of the estimated consumption. Stocks in Tehran on January 15 amounted to 17,000 tons, more than half of which was barley and other adulterants, equivalent to 32 days supply for the city at the present rate of adulteration of wheat flour. During the past month daily receipts of grain in the capital from all parts of the country have averaged from 300 to 600 tons, which is well above the daily consumption and has permitted the building up of reserves. The general picture is fairly satisfactory, taking into consideration the many difficulties and the desperate situation which prevailed last winter. Contracts and undertakings have not reached the 350,000 ton target originally set last summer, but they exceed minimum estimated requirements and have surpassed the gloomy expectations of a few months ago. Collections in most parts of the country

have been going fairly well, remarkably well in the Tehran and Khuzistan areas. There has been no evidence of foreign interference, such as was feared on the part of the Soviet authorities. On the contrary, the Russians are substantially living up to their offer to move grain to Tehran whenever it is delivered to a proper point on one of the road or rail routes over which they operate. For five or six weeks, grain from the Soviet zone has made up roughly one-third of Tehran's daily receipts, coming at first only from Gorgan but later also from the Zenjan area and, in small quantities, from Khorassan. The enclosed report shows that first deliveries from Azerbaijan have just been received.

The greatest difficulty continues to be transport. The Iranian Transport Department has not been able to handle the volume of essential goods which must be moved within the country, and only the assistance of British Army trucks and the UKCC on the main routes, has enabled deliveries to Tehran to be maintained. According to the Acting Director of the Cereals Section, Mr. Crawford, the transport weakness has been the main reason for delay in receiving grain from Azerbaijan. He is sending an additional 30 Iranian Government Pool (Lend-Lease) trucks to that province. The Road Transport Department is also sending a Danish employee to Tabriz to try to bring about more efficient use of trucks in the area. Other difficulties still confronting the cereals section include: a) Reluctance of local governors and other officials to allow grain shipments to Tehran until they have collected and stored away sufficient grain to cover the whole year's requirements for their own localities; b) The perennial desire of landlords to hold back their grain for higher prices, or other inducements in the form of sugar, cotton piece goods, etc. Mr. Crawford says that this is especially marked in the western part of Azerbaijan, where the landlords made fortunes out of the sugar and piece goods paid them last year as part of the price of their grain. In consequence of this attitude, he has given orders that no payment in kind shall be made for grain in the northern zone this year, hoping thus to establish the Government's position for next year, even though it may make things more difficult at present. Mr. Crawford feels that the country can be pulled through until the next harvest, although he anticipates a rather tight period in the spring. To meet possible unfavorable developments, MESC Tehran is keeping current its request to MESC Cairo for the maintenance of a reserve stock of 10,000 tons of imported grain or flour, to be available for Iranian civil consumption on six weeks notice.

One problem which loomed very large on the horizon last fall, but which seems to have been settled fairly well, is that of Soviet requests for grain from Iran. As has been reported previously, a contract has been signed for the delivery of 36,000 tons of rice to the USSR. The financial terms of that contract are unfavorable to Iran, but the quantity of rice involved is not excessive in view of normal Soviet imports from Iran and the large rice harvest last year. There has been no Russian request for Iranian wheat, and the barley request was for only 16,000 tons, just 1,000 tons higher than last year, when the harvest was very much smaller. The barley delivery contract was signed December 2, 1943. A copy is enclosed, from which it will be seen that deliveries are to be made at various points within Iran during the period December-April. The price, 2,750 rials per metric ton (gross) seems reasonable, since the official price which the Iranian Government pays to growers for barley is 2,250 rials per ton. (It remains to be seen, of course, whether the Government will be able to obtain sufficient quantities of barley at that price.) Another notable feature of the contract, in contrast to the rice agreement, is that the penalties for non-performance on either side are comparatively small, only 2½ per thousand per day of delay in delivery or acceptance. Since it is understood that the Cereals Section put up a fairly stiff fight to obtain these relatively favorable terms, it may be justified to venture the tentative conclusion that the Iranian authorities would be well advised to adopt a stronger bargaining attitude in their financial dealings with the Soviets.

Getting wheat from Azerbaijan remained difficult. Ebling on April 4, 1944 (Dispatch 42, 891.00/3033):

Merchants in the bazaar report an advance in the cost of all commodities. The increased prices are attributed to the general impression that the war will be of long duration and stocks cannot be replenished. Much opposition has been manifested by leading citizens concerning the desire of the Food Department to purchase wheat in Azerbaijan. The new policy has been put into effect of offering 12 kilos of sugar for one ton of wheat or 9 kilos of sugar for one ton of barley. Dealers announce an increase of 600 rials (US $18.75) per ton in the price of wheat following the concerted efforts of the Government to purchase wheat in this district. Wheat is now quoted at 3600 to 3700 rials (US $113 to $115) per ton.

Ford on April 4, 1944 (Dispatch 903, 891.5018/37):

I have the honor to refer to my despatch No. 814 of January 24, 1944 regarding the developments in the Iranian grain collection program and to submit a summary of the present situation:

Progress of Collections. Latest available figures for March 20, 1944 show that the Government has received delivery of a total of 301,692 tons of wheat and barley, only 17,000 tons short of the estimated consumption through the month of August. There appears to be no question that the minimum requirements for the crop year September 1943 to August 1944 will be covered without importation of grain. In fact, officials of the Cereals and Bread Section of the Iranian Ministry of Finance believe that they will have a carry-over amounting to one month to six weeks' supply for the cities of the country. Receipts in Tehran of grain from the northern zone, under Soviet control, have not been satisfactory, except from the province of Gorgan. On March 15 the total from the north stood at 17,237 tons, as against a program for the crop year calling for 40,000 tons. However, a small but steady flow is coming from Khorassan, and an American is being sent to Azerbaijan to expedite shipments from that area. It does not appear that the blame for slow deliveries can be attributed to the Soviet authorities.

Soviet Purchases. Although they had not previously indicated a desire to buy Iranian wheat this year, the Russian authorities some weeks ago asked the Cereals and Bread Section to sell them 2,500 tons of wheat for consumption by Soviet troops in Iran. Mr. Crawford, head of the Section, has agreed, and deliveries are being made. No formal contract was signed to cover this transaction, as Mr. Crawford insisted that the Russians should deal with the Section on the same basis as other agencies which buy limited quantities from it from time to time. He was also successful in obtaining what he considers a reasonable price.

Exchange of Zabul Wheat for Flour. The Iranian organization has been negotiating for some time with the Government of India to barter 3,000 tons of wheat at Zabul, in southeastern Iran, against 3,000 tons of wheat flour under British control in the Basra area. Arrangements have been virtually completed, although Mr. Crawford has recently heard that there may be some difficulty because the Zabul wheat is not up to specifications. The transaction would be advantageous to Iran, since it would eliminate the long, wasteful haul by motor transport necessary to bring the grain from Zabul to Tehran.

Coming Crop Year. The Iranian crop year is from September through August, but in the southern areas harvesting begins as early as the end of April. Accordingly, the Cereals and Bread Section and the Middle East Supply Center are already making plan and calculations for the coming year. Rain and snow fall during the past winter has been disappointing in a large part of the country, especially in the south, and considerable alarm is being expressed with respect to grain prospects. It is said that the yield in Fars, Khuzistan, and other extreme southern regions will undoubtedly be very poor, with the result that the northern provinces, Azerbaijan, Gorgan and Khorassan, will have to supply a much higher percentage of the country's needs. Mr. Crawford is, of course, unable to estimate collections for the 1944-45 year beyond saying that there will be no need for importations for consumption during the calendar year 1944. He anticipates, however, that it will be necessary to import an indeterminate quantity of grain for distribution during 1945. In this connection, he and his provincial assistant, Colonel Ata-Ullah, have made the informal suggestion that it would be well, if shipping permits, to begin shipments from abroad at an early date. Their thought is that this would give them a much stronger position in collecting the coming crop, since they would have a reserve on hand to reassure consumers against shortage and discourage growers from withholding their produce in the hope of higher prices. They feel that psychological factors involved are very important. Furthermore, if given an assurance of foreign supplies, they would feel able to reduce the domestic price of grain, with a corresponding deflationary effect on the general price structure. No definite request along this line has as yet been presented, and I do not know whether Dr. Millspaugh has given the matter thought, but I should like to suggest it for the Department's consideration. There can be no doubt that early shipments of grain, at the rate of 5,000 to 10,000 tons monthly, would be helpful to the general situation here and might well prevent a crisis during the winter and spring of 1945, but I assume that the shipping situation must necessarily be the first factor to be studied. The Legation has no information on this, or on the availability of grain supplies for shipment to Iran.

Renewed Anxiety on Grain Supply

Inadequate precipitation in the central and southern parts in the spring of 1944, as noted, had caused anxiety. CICI report, March 21, 1944 (MID-

Iran, 4220): "The widespread lack of rain this spring means that poor crops in most of the districts around Sultanabad may be expected. Wheat is therefore being hoarded and prices are rising, although stocks held in the municipal granary are considered sufficient to last Sultanabad until the end of August." CICI, April 4, 1944 (MID-Iran, 4220):

> The absence of spring rains in large areas of the country is arousing anxiety regarding the next harvest with the inevitable result of the rise in prices in the wholesale and free retail markets and an increase of hoarding and speculation. The immediate grain situation is satisfactory, some 300,000 tons of the estimated 310,000 required to feed the towns until the next harvest having been collected. But the latter figure includes no reserve, and the Government should have a reserve of at least 50,000 tons. The prospects of collecting this amount are not good, although there are still stacks of grain in the country. Of 18,000 tons expected from Azerbaijan only 700 tons have as yet reached the capital.

CICI, April 11, 1944 (MID-Iran, 4220): "Retail prices in Tehran have risen and reports of developments on the frontier of Burma have given rise in the price of tea. In spite of the relatively dry season so far, it is believed that crops in Kermanshah, Hamadan and in the north of Persia may be good enough to prevent a grain shortage." CICI, April 18, 1944 (MID-Iran, 4220): "In Bushire lack of rainfall is causing apprehension of famine conditions."

Ford on April 15, 1944 (Telegram 266, 891.5018/36):

> We have recently discussed grain collection prospects (for) 1944-45 harvest year with Millspaugh, MESC and British Embassy. Situation seems to be as follows: (One). Despite excellent harvest in 1943, Iranian Government will have only small reserve of perhaps 25,000 tons on hand as it enters new crop year; (Two). If northern provinces of Azerbaijan and Zenjan, and to some extent Khorassan, which are under Soviet occupation, had contributed even their minimum expected share, this reserve would have been larger by at least another 18,000 tons; (Three). Joint Anglo-American efforts have produced results 25% above original target in southern areas of Iran; (Four). At most an average harvest for country as a whole is expected for the coming crop year, but good harvest is again anticipated in Zenjan and Azerbaijan as well as other northern provinces. Because of expected smaller harvest, Millspaugh fears large scale hoarding may make collections difficult unless something is done quickly to establish public confidence. He

therefore wishes to have at an early date a guarantee from the Allies, including Soviets, along lines of 1942 grain agreement. Along with guarantee, Millspaugh feels Allies should make early shipment to Iran of about 10,000 tons grain. In addition to assisting in establishing of confidence and so helping collections, such an actual delivery would enable Iranian Government further to reduce prices paid for grain, with wholesome effect upon economy of country as whole. (It is proposed in any case to reduce grain prices by about 10%). Amount delivered if not ultimately needed by Iran, could be returned later to Allied Armies or other agencies in this area. Although British Embassy, MESC, Tehran and ourselves agree that guarantee would be desirable, Dr. Murray of MESC, Cairo tells us that Allied Governments would probably find difficulty in assuming an obligation of this kind in light of present world grain supply and transport situation, increasing Allied commitments, and shortage of shipping. It is therefore doubly necessary that complete Soviet cooperation with Iranian authorities be obtained in order to ensure collection and delivery to Tehran, from next harvest, of at least 25,000 tons from Zenjan and Azerbaijan, as well as normal amounts from other northern provinces. (25,000 tons is well within capacity of two provinces cited). Important reason for unsatisfactory results during present harvest year in north has been refusal of Soviet authorities to allow foreign advisers to Iranian Government free access to and freedom of movement in Soviet zone. Such freedom of action is essential for adequate organization and coordination of Iranian Government's transport and grain collection operations in the area. Although Soviet authorities have recently issued three month permit for Azerbaijan to an American employee of Cereals and Bread Section, there is no (repeat no) assurance that they will continue this slightly more liberal attitude. The fact that three month limit was imposed is not (repeat not) good augury for future grain operations in the region. In summary, if times were normal it would appear that Iran could be self-sufficient in grain for 1944-45. Under present conditions, however, and in view of anticipated serious deficit in extreme southern districts, it seems that Allied Governments must choose between three alternatives: (one) making sure that maximum possible surplus of grain from northern provinces is moved to Tehran; (two) bringing in grain from outside Iran; (three) risking famine conditions in certain districts of the south. British Embassy is sending similar telegram to London. I would appreciate an indication of Department's views. Paraphrase by air mail to Cairo for Landis.

Ford's cable had elicited a memorandum from Harold B. Minor, dated April 18, 1944, and entitled, "Grain Situation in Iran":

The problem presented herein is not an easy one and the responsibility entailed is great. The situation is similar in many respects to that two years ago. . . . The present situation, however, is different in four respects. First, there is this year a rather good carry-over of grain, some 25,000 tons, which, together with the harvest will be collected in the period June to September, even if it is poor, should carry Iran over adequately until mid-winter. Second, there are as yet no indications of a crop failure in Iran. Third, the Russians this year gave slightly better cooperation in allowing, or encouraging, crop collection and transport southward. Whereas two years ago no wheat came out of Azerbaijan, this year at least several thousand tons were obtained and it is to be hoped that much more will be forthcoming next year. This does not mean the complaint that the Russians are not allowing Iranian grain to flow to Tehran is unfounded. It is very real and presents a problem which will cry for solution in case the crops this year are poor or bad. The north of the country is the chief grain-producing region and must, as it always has, provide to a considerable extent for Tehran's needs. The point of better Russian cooperation was made above only to show a more encouraging trend. Fourth, the shipping situation is slightly better and the transit time to Iran has been cut considerably, which allows us more time to reach a decision. My opinion is that we should not be precipitated into any action at the moment. It appears unreasonable to expect a guarantee of this sort from a country which is normally self-sufficient in grain, especially in the absence of indications of crop failure and considering the tight grain supply situation of the world. . . . Dr. Millspaugh must be told that we will not turn a deaf ear to Iran's plea for grain if the need is clearly established. In the meantime, we should, it seems to me, do what we can to bring about a condition of Allied-Iranian cooperation in Iran which will insure that the Russians in the next crop year will allow the surplus grain from Azerbaijan, Zenjan and Khorrassan to flow to the south. The fact that bread shortage has not developed in Tehran this year is due not to Russian cooperation but rather to the happy condition of a bumper crop and to magnificent British-American cooperation with the Iranians in wheat collection and transport in southern Iran.

Cable to Ford on April 22, 1944 (Telegram 244, 891.5018/36):

You may inform Millspaugh and any other Iranian officials that this Government will give, as it has in past instances, its earnest and sympathetic consideration to Iranian requests for grain should a serious shortage develop. (Your 266, April 15.) However Department does not feel justified, on the basis of evidence at hand, in supporting Millspaugh's suggestion for immediate shipment of 10,000 tons of grain or for an allied guarantee along lines of 1942 Anglo-American-Iranian wheat agreement. This view is based on probability of a sizeable carryover of Iranian grain into next crop year, lack of indications of a crop failure in mid-1944, heavy demands on allies for cereals for other areas, and continuing tight shipping situation. Please follow grain situation closely in consultation with MESC and your British colleague, reporting especially on prospects for coming crop and on deliveries of this year's harvest surplus from northern provinces. Department agrees that it is essential, in order to avoid necessity for importation of foreign grain into Iran during next crop year, to obtain Soviet cooperation in collection and transportation of surplus cereals from northern Iran. A paraphrase of your telegram has been sent to Mr. Murray in London for use in discussing this phase of the problem with the British. Repeated to Cairo for Landis, and to Moscow.

Ford on May 31, 1944 (Dispatch 968 and enclosures, 891.5018/41):

I have the honor to refer to my telegram No. 255 (266) of April 15, 1944 reporting conversations with MESC (Tehran), British Embassy and American officials of the Iranian Government regarding anticipated grain supply situation in Iran during the new crops year, and to the Department's telegram in reply, No. 244 of April 22. The substance of the Department's telegram has been conveyed orally to Dr. Albert G. Black, new American head of the Cereals and Bread Section of the Iranian Ministry of Finance, and to the British Embassy. As the Department will recall, a telegram similar to my 255 (266) was sent by the British Embassy to the Foreign Office at London, but no reply to the message has been received. There is enclosed herewith a copy of a letter which Dr. Black sent to Dr. A.C. Millspaugh, Administrator General of Finances, under date of May 16, 1944. This letter sums up prospects for Iranian Government grain collections during the period of the new harvest, now getting under way in some area, as they appear at present to the Cereals and Bread Section. It will be noted that the table attached to Dr. Black's letter sets forth an estimated minimum total collection at 301,500 tons, as against an estimated urban consumption of 305,200 tons leaving an estimated deficit of roughly 4,000 tons. However, it will also be noted that the Cereals and Bread Section expects a carry-over from the 1943 harvest amounting to perhaps 40,000 tons. (Both collection and consumption from the 1943 harvest is still going on, and it is as yet impossible to say definitely what the carry-over will be.) On the basis of these calculations, therefore, it would seem that Iran should be self-sufficient in grain during the coming year, that is, from about mid-1944 to about mid-1945. (The crop year is ordinarily stated as from the first of September to the end of the following August, but in reality the harvest in different parts of the country is in progress from late April to September). However, as Dr. Black indicates in his letter, there are certain unknown factors which might tip the balance unfavorably. These are: 1) The fact that weather conditions in the next few months can still affect the harvest in the northern regions. 2) Uncertainty regarding quantity of surplus from the northern zone which it will be practicable to move south to deficit areas. 3) The fact that all the estimates are unreliable, in the absence of adequate machinery for gathering statistics. 4) The possibility of almost total crop failure in some of the southern districts, which might mean that even the rural sections of those districts, in addition to the cities, would have to be fed by grain brought in from other areas. Some rather alarming reports in this regard have been received from Khuzistan, but full investigation has not yet been completed. In previous years, as this year, consumption schedules have been taken into consideration only the needs of cities, it being assumed that rural areas would at least be able to feed themselves. If this should prove not to be the case, it will necessitate a revision of estimates. 5) Continued instability in tribal regions, where outbreaks may occur at any time, with corresponding adverse effects upon harvesting and collection. 6) Possible failure of internal transport to handle the necessary movement of grain from surplus to deficit areas. As the Department knows, this has been one of the most serious obstacles to the 1943-44 harvest collection program, and the problem was solved only with substantial help from the British and American Armies, UKCC, Iranian Army and other agencies.

Estimates of 1323 (1944/45) Harvest (Tons)

Region	Target	Expected	Consumption	Difference
South	209,000	159,000	178,200	- 19,200
North	178,000	138,000	114,000	+ 24,000
Other	5,000	4,500	13,000	- 8,500
Total	392,000	301,500	305,200	- 3,700

Source: A.G. Black's letter to A.C. Millspaugh, May 16, 1944.

Fortunately, the Russians had resumed cooperation. Ebling on May 31, 1944 (Dispatch 65, 891.00/3077):

> Mr. T.A. Allen who has recently been in Tabriz as a representative of the Director General of Cereals and Bread reports satisfactory collections in Azerbaijan of grain (wheat and barley) for local consumption and transport to Tehran. At the present time 24,600 tons of grain (wheat and barley) have been bought and are awaiting scaling and transportation. . . . Of the collections as indicated above 6,500 tons are due on the Azerbaijan quota for Tehran, while local consumption of available stocks will amount to about 8,000 tons. Azerbaijan will thus be in a position to furnish Tehran with 10,000 tons of grains over the original quota. Mr. Allen reports favorable reaction of the landlords and proprietors in disposing of their stocks of grain. Commendation has also been made of the cooperation afforded by the Soviet officials in arranging for the transport of the collected grains at reasonable rates. Soviet transport facilities are adequate to take care of all collected grains. Although local officers of the United Kingdom Commercial Corporation also expressed an interest in facilitating the transport of grains from Azerbaijan, no definite arrangements have been completed with them up to the present time. With the 10,000 tons of grains which Azerbaijan is able to furnish in excess of the original quota requested by Tehran, it will appear that the Government will experience little difficulty in meeting all demands up to the time the new harvest becomes available in August.

Ford on June 21, 1944 (Telegram 447, 891.5018/47):

> Second tripartite economic meeting held today was devoted principally to discussion of grain supply problem. (Reference my 395, June 3). Maximov having studied Black's estimates for coming crop collection as enclosed my despatch 968, May 31, expressed opinion that they were reasonable and as accurate as could be expected. He agreed that quantities indicated should be made available from northern areas for other sections. He also said Soviets were already cooperating in movement of certain newly discovered surpluses from last crop recently brought under Iranian Government control in Azerbaijan. . . . General atmosphere cordial.

Despite large government grain purchases in Azerbaijan, prices were falling, an indication of improving conditions. Ebling on August 21, 1944 (Dispatch 95, 891.00/8-2144):

> Landowners in the vicinity of Tabriz have recently been agitating for an increase in the price of wheat to 3000 rials (US $93.75) per ton, claiming that the price now offered by the Government is insufficient owing to present agricultural costs. Meetings have recently been held by landlords to consider means of effecting an increase in price of wheat. Upon request the Prime Minister has given assurance that some action would be taken in the matter by the Government. Local residents are apprehensive that an increase in the price of wheat will result in a higher price for bread, this adding to the present high living costs.

Continued Transport Difficulty

After a new War Department directive to General Connolly authorized him to assist in Iranian civilian needs, in February 1944 US army transport had begun hauling grain and by March 1944, US army trucks had taken over from the British army. This assistance, however, was short-lived; it was reduced in June and was terminated at the end of August 1944. Iran again faced the prospects of a transport crisis at harvest time. Ford on May 31, 1944 (Dispatch 968 and enclosures, 891.5018/41):

> Dr. Black informs the Legation that he considers this transport difficulty as potentially the most dangerous threat to the success of his operations. Renewed help from the Allied armies cannot safely be anticipated, nor is it desirable to have recourse to such expedients except in the case of dire necessity. This leaves the bulk of the road hauling to be done by the creaking Iranian Road Transport Administration, whose truck fleet is older than it was during the last harvest and which cannot be said to be out of the woods in dealing with its numerous organizational and operational problems. Furthermore, during the new crop year the transport needs may be greater than previously, since the expected uneven distribution of the harvest may make long hauls necessary not only to supply Tehran but also to feed other districts which normally draw grain supplies from their own immediate vicinity. Dr. Black also emphasizes the handicap under which his organization labors through lack of transport for its field personnel. He points out, and anyone familiar with Iran will agree, that the only way to ensure satisfactory deliveries of grain from the producers is to go personally to the villages where the grain is grown. In at least 90% of the cases this can only be done efficiently by automobile. Dr. Black says that what he really needs are jeeps or command cars or similar vehicles, since ordinary cars are not suitable for the rough roads which are the rule once one leaves the main highways between the cities. As

> evidence of the shortage of passenger vehicles (which is general throughout the Iranian Government) it may be mentioned that a recent survey made by Dr. Millspaugh showed only 39 Iranian Government cars assigned to the Cereals and Bread Section in the entire country, and it may be assumed that many of these are constantly out of service for mechanical reasons. . . . I am told by the local American military authorities that they could not release any of their vehicles and that they understand jeeps and the like are in world short supply, relative to the demand. However, if some change in the situation should make it possible to provide vehicles of this type, it might have an important effect in assuring Iranian self-sufficiency in grain.

Ford on July 8, 1944 (Telegram 485, 891.154A/7-844):

> From Hoskins. Millspaugh, Black and Shields seriously disturbed over impending withdrawal of American military personnel from Iranian Road Transport Administration. (Reference Legation's 429, June 15). Although General Connolly has acquiesced to token releases for June and July, balance of men must be released by August 26 unless orders are changed. How soon can we expect word from Landis as to results of his efforts with War Department for continued service of these men in this vital work? They are needed until January 1 if firm operating foundation is to be laid and at least until November 15 when critical harvest collection period will be past. Repeated to Cairo for Short.

The appeal was unsuccessful, and transport remained precarious. Ford on September 26, 1944 (Dispatch 45 and enclosure, 891.154A/9-2644):

> I have the honor to transmit herewith a copy of a report on the Iranian civil road transport situation made, following a recent visit to this country, by Mr. Walter A. Junge who has been temporarily attached to the American Economic Mission, Middle East to make a survey of transport conditions in the area. The report is, I think, self-explanatory. I should like, however, to emphasize three points made by Mr. Junge in conversation with officers of this Embassy: 1. Mr. Junge feels that the American heads of the Iranian Road Transport Administration have been called upon by the Middle East Supply Center and the supply agencies in Washington and London to do the impossible, i.e., to maintain a fleet of trucks under adverse operating conditions with virtually no spare parts or maintenance machinery. In his opinion, as a practical truck operator, a truck without spare parts is virtually no truck at all. Therefore, he regards it as shortsighted and ultimately highly wasteful

> from everyone's point of view to limit parts supplies to the extent that has been the practice with regard to Iran. He also considers it most important that the maintenance machinery ordered by the Road Transport Administration from the United States should come forward at once. 2. He believes that the Road Transport Administration is in great need of additional executives with wide practical experience in maintenance and direct operation of trucks on the road. . . . 3. Mr. Junge said that a great deal more attention should be paid to road maintenance, as the bad state of the roads in this country is one of the principal reasons for the rapid breakdown of trucks.

The severe shortage of spare parts had persisted. Ford on October 3, 1944 (Dispatch 63 and enclosure, 891.154A/10-344):

> I have the honor to refer to the Embassy's despatch No. 45 of September 26, 1944 forwarding a copy of a report on the Iranian civil road transport situation by Mr. Walter A. Junge. There is transmitted herewith a copy of a letter, with enclosure, from Mr. Floyd F. Shields, director of the Road Transport Administration, to the FEA (Foreign Economic Administration) representative in Tehran which will, I believe, indicate some of the difficulties being experienced by the Administration in obtaining urgently-needed maintenance equipment for its truck fleet.

Shields' letter of September 30, 1944, describes his disappointment at the failure of the MESC to deliver on its promise to supply the spare parts, and the refusal of the Allied armies to provide workshop tools and equipment for truck repair.

The approaching end of the war and the reduced haulage to Russia had relieved the transport problem. Ford in a report entitled "Present Road Transport Situation in Iran," dated November 8, 1944 (Dispatch 98 and enclosure, 891.154A/11-844):

> I have the honor to refer to the Embassy's telegram No. 820 of November 6, 1944 regarding the desire of the present American executives of the Iranian Road Transport Administration to relinquish their positions within the near future. Although it is believed that their decision has been taken primarily for personal reasons, it is also true that the general organizational and operational picture has improved greatly during the past year as a result of the measures taken by the American group and the generally improved transport position resulting from

better economic conditions and the reduction of Allied military supply operations in Iran. . . . There is enclosed herewith a copy of a memorandum prepared by Mr. Shields, setting forth his estimate of the situation and the immediate objectives he hopes to achieve, wholly or in part, during the three months he has tentatively set as the period he will remain in charge. (He indicates that he would be willing to stay a little longer if proper replacements do not reach Iran in time.) It will be noted that the memorandum contemplates substantial relaxation of government control over commercial trucks, and there is transmitted herewith a copy of Transport Regulation No. 189/17, dated October 29, 1944 (7 Aban, 1323) which initiates this relaxation. Other measures contemplated include the sale to private operators of a part of the government-owned fleet of Lend-Lease trucks and the turning over to private merchants, under government supervision, of responsibility for the distribution of tires and spare parts. These measures are made possible largely by the fall in prices in Iran which, together with the release of trucks by UKCC and Iransovtrans, has restored the element of competition to Iranian trucking and reduced the attraction of illicit hauling. It is apparent that the task of the Road Transport Administration should be less exacting in the future than in the past, as its responsibilities will progressively decrease. Present thinking of those concerned seems to envisage the eventual abolition of the organization altogether or, at least, reduction of its function to that of operator of a small government-owned fleet for special tasks, such as the movement of essential supplies in remote and unprofitable areas. However, there is still a long distance to go before that stage is reached, and opinion is unanimous that competent American directors are needed in the interim. According to Mr. Shields, much progress has been made in finding and training good Iranian subordinates, but the Iranian members of the organization are not yet capable of taking over the positions of major responsibility. Copy to Mr. Landis, Cairo.

Chapter 28

The Anglo-American Notes and Evasion of Commitments to Iran

The American and British governments had soon found an excuse to avoid their obligation to assist Iran, the Tehran Declaration notwithstanding. Ford on August 5, 1944 (Dispatch 1060, 891.6131/8-544):

> I have the honor to refer to my despatch No. 968 of May 31, 1944 regarding prospects for grain collection in Iran during 1944-45 harvest year and to report that the program prepared by the Cereals and Bread Section of the Ministry of Finance has had to be modified by the abandonment of plans to bring under government control a portion of the peasants' share of the crop. As the Department will recall, in past years the Government's collection program has envisaged compulsory sale to the Cereals and Bread Section of the greater part of the landowners' share in the crop but has not called for collections from peasants except on a voluntary basis. This year, however, faced with an uncertain harvest, the Government proposed to collect 20% of his share from each peasant who received four-fifth or more of the produce of the land cultivated by him. (In practice, this would affect only those peasants cultivating unirrigated land; where irrigation is necessary the water is supplied by the landlord and he, therefore, receives more than one-fifth of the crop as his share.) Opposition to this extension of the compulsory sale system developed as soon as the regulations were published and quickly found expression in the Majlis. So far as the Legation can determine, landowners and their associates were the principal opponents. They argued that the measure would discourage agriculture because: (a) the peasant would be left without sufficient grain for his own consumption, or (b) the peasant's economic position would

be adversely affected because he would have to sell grain at the comparatively, low official price while, at the same time, he would have to buy essential goods, such as cloth, sugar, tea, at high black market prices. It is unlikely that these arguments were either well-founded or sincere. In all probability the landlords opposed the measure because it would reduce their own opportunities for purchase of grain from the peasants and its resale at black market prices. Most peasants are unable to transport their grain to the cities, where prices are high, and are forced to sell to landlords and dealers who have transport facilities. A bill was introduced into the Majlis several weeks ago which would have prohibited the collection of grain from peasants except against payment in monopoly goods: cloth, sugar and tea. Dr. Millspaugh regarded this as administratively impracticable, since it would upset the whole program of distribution of monopoly goods and at the same time greatly increase the difficulties of grain collection. After endeavoring to persuade the deputies to drop the bill, he called the matter to the attention of the American Legation and British Embassy. Both Mr. Lascelles, British Chargé d'Affaires, and I spoke to the Prime Minister about it, pointing out that he would regret any action which could make grain collection more difficult. We emphasized that the Allies could not be expected to provide imports of grain in order to make up a deficit resulting from mismanagement on the part of the Iranian Government, especially since that Government now had an efficient organization which had demonstrated its ability to handle the grain problem if allowed to carry out its program without interference. Our representations seem to have been ineffective, however, and it became obvious a few days ago that the bill was on the verge of passage. Dr. Millspaugh therefore decided to make a virtue of necessity and himself took the step of eliminating from the regulations the provision for collection from peasants. He felt that it was better to handle the matter in this way rather than let the Majlis establish a precedent of overriding his regulations by legislative action.

Apart from the fact that Millspaugh has suffered a minor, though significant, defeat on this issue, opinions differ regarding the ultimate effect of the change on the grain situation. No one knows how much grain could have been obtained from the peasants, optimistic estimates ranging around 50,000 tons. With only the landlords to draw upon, Dr. Black thinks collections are not likely to exceed 300,000 tons, slightly under estimated urban consumption. It now appears, however, that the carry-over into the new crop year may be between 50,000 and 60,000 tons, which would seem to give a fairly safe margin, at least with comparison with previous years. On the favorable side, too, is the possibility of an early end to the war in Europe, which would bring about a general drop in prices and make producers anxious to sell grain to the Government at the official price. On the other side, Dr. Black had hoped to build up and maintain a permanent grain reserve of at least 50,000 tons, preferably substantially larger, which he now feels will be impossible. He also feels that the elimination of the peasants as a source of supply removes a safety factor which he was relying upon to offset any unfavorable developments which might prevent attainment of the targets for collections from landlords.

Leland Morris on September 7, 1944 (Dispatch 18 and enclosure, 891.6131/9-744):

I have the honor to refer to the Embassy's despatch No. 1060 of August 5, 1944, reporting the abandonment of plans to bring under Iranian Government control a portion of the peasant's share of the new grain crop. As stated in that despatch, Dr. Millspaugh, Administrator General of Finances, gave way on this point under heavy pressure from the Majlis. It was his understanding that by making this concession he would thereby save the remainder of his grain collection program from interference by the Majlis or the cabinet. This has proven not to be the case however, since strong groups of the Majlis are now pressing for the exemption of landlords having less than 1½ tons of surplus grain from any obligation to deliver cereals to the Government collecting organization. In addition pressure has been brought for the removal of all restrictions on the movement of grain by private persons from the country districts to the cities. Dr. Millspaugh has been holding discussions regarding the grain collection regulations with a specially designated committee of twelve members of the Majlis. He at first refused to make any further changes in the collection regulations, but, two or three weeks ago he proposed a compromise whereby he would remove the restrictions on private transport of grain if the Majlis would enact a law authorizing the summary arrest and imprisonment of land owners who failed to fulfill their contracts for the delivery of grain. This was agreed to and a corresponding project of law was introduced. However, on the floor of the Majlis, an amendment was tacked on to the bill providing for exemption of landlords with less than 1½ tons surplus from delivery obligations, as mentioned above. A further amendment, of less concern to Dr. Millspaugh but possibly having some importance for the Allied nations, provided that Government could not sell grain to any of the Allied Governments (meaning the United States, Great Britain and the USSR) except at a price at least double that paid by the Government to the grower. Dr. Millspaugh and Dr. Black, head of the Cereals and Bread Section of the Ministry of Finance, recently called these developments to the attention of the British and American Embassies. They expressed themselves as perturbed not only by the potential loss in grain stocks available to the Government but also by the continued disposition of the Majlis to whittle away the administrative powers granted Dr. Millspaugh. Both Embassies agreed that this was disturbing, and I think both the British Chargé d'Affaires and I regret that Millspaugh was willing to make even the partial concessions which he did offer to the Majlis in the case of the peasants' share of grain and the free movement of grain. After a considerable discussion, it was agreed that the Embassies should emphasize to the Iranian Government the importance of utilizing every possible means of collecting domestic Iranian grain crop and our alarm at the measures which had been taken or were proposed to reduce the means open to the Cereals and Bread Section to bring grain under its control. I enclose herewith a copy of a note along these lines which I have sent to the Prime Minister. A copy of the similar note presented by the British Chargé d'Affaires will be forwarded within a few days.

The note to Saed is dated September 8, 1944:

Excellency: Through the office of the Middle East Supply Center in Tehran, I have received a copy of Your Excellency's letter of August 27, 1944, to Dr. A.C. Millspaugh, Administrator General of Finances, regarding Iran's 1945 import quotas for certain commodities, among them wheat and barley. I note that in section 3 of the letter, Your Excellency says that the Iranian Government reserves the right to call upon the Middle East Supply Center for imports of grain in case Iran should find itself short of cereals at a later period in the season. This statement appears to indicate that the Iranian Government relies upon the American and British Governments to make available supplies of imported grain to cover any deficit which may develop. I think it desirable, therefore, to say that the Department of State has informed this Embassy that the American Government counts upon Iran to be self-sufficient in cereals during the present harvest year and can undertake no commitment regarding the provision of imported grain for Iranian consumption. According to the Embassy's information, the 1323 (1944/45) grain crop, although not so good as that of 1322 (1943/44), should nevertheless be sufficient to meet Iran's requirements if it is properly collected and distributed. The American Government, con-

> sequently, feels that it must give precedence to other countries, whose domestic resources are clearly inadequate to cover their needs. My attention has been called to press reports of certain measures taken or contemplated by the Iranian Government to collect the full amount of domestic grain available: 1) I understand that, on the insistence of the Majlis, the plan to collect a portion of the peasants' share of the crop has been abandoned, with the resultant possible loss to the Government of as much as 50,000 tons. 2) It is reported that a measure has been introduced in the Majlis to exempt landowners having a surplus of less than one and one-half tons from any obligation to deliver grain to the Government, an exemption which maybe expected to reduce still further the Government's collection. 3) It is also stated that certain groups in the Majlis are pressing strongly for repeal of regulations forbidding free transport of grain by private persons from producing districts to the cities. If this should be done, there seems reason to fear that it would handicap the Government's collection program by making it easier for the growers and dealers to sell grain improperly at high prices on the so-called "free market."
>
> Your Excellency will understand, of course, that I do not pretend to pass upon the circumstances which may have led the Government to consider these measures. They are obviously, internal matters for the decision of the Iranian Government alone. But I would be remiss if I did not point out that the world shipping and supply situation, coupled with the tremendous needs of the liberated countries of Europe, make it absolutely essential that Iran should exert every effort to be self-sufficient in cereals, and that the American Government cannot hold itself responsible for the supply of grain to cover a deficit attributable to failure of the Iranian Government to use every means at its disposal for the collection of a maximum share of its domestic harvest. Accept, Excellency, the renewed assurances of my highest consideration. Leland Morris.

The parallel British note of September 4, 1944, true to style, was calculated to offend (Dispatch 29 and enclosure, 891.6131/9-1144, September 11, 1944):

> Your Excellency, I have the honour to inform you that my attention has been drawn by the Middle East Supply Centre to Your Excellency's letter No. 9886 of the 27th August to the Administrator-General of the Finances, concerning the arrangements required for the supply of certain essential commodities. I have taken particular note of the fact that

in paragraph 3 (ii) of that letter Your Excellency reserves the right to call upon the Middle East Supply Centre to provide a quota of cereals if, after the collection of all engagements taken in respect to this year's crops, it is found that the quantity of cereals available in the country is insufficient to meet the needs of the population. In the same paragraph of the letter Your Excellency expressed the opinion that this year's crop, together with the surplus left over from last year's harvest, might possibly prove insufficient to meet the country's needs. All the information at my disposal confirms that this year's crop will in fact prove adequate provided that proper measures are taken to collect it. In other words, the country's own resources will suffice unless the authorities fail in their task of ensuring that these resources are made available to the population as a whole. In these circumstances I have learned with great misgiving, from reports of recent proceedings in the Majlis, of certain measures, some already implemented, others still under consideration—the effect of which can only be to curtail seriously the amount of grain available for public consumption. I refer in particular to the proposals recently tabled for the exemption of the peasants' share from compulsory collection. While these proposals were still under discussion, i.e. on June 17th last, I ventured to draw Your Excellency's especial attention to the danger which, in my view, they presented; and to warn you that the Allied supply authorities were unlikely to feel called upon to make good a deficiency which could have been avoided by exercising sufficient forethought. Nevertheless, it seems that the backing of a majority of the Majlis was subsequently secured for these proposals, and that, in consequence, the Administrator-General of the Finances was obliged—with the object, as I can only assume, of preserving the semblance of his authority—to render their passage unnecessary by the issue of an emending regulation to the same effect. The result, I am given to understand, is likely to be a decrease of some 50,000 tons in the quantity of wheat collected. I now learn that, in addition, certain important Majlis groups are pressing for the exemption from compulsory collection of any surplus of less than 1½ tons accruing to the landlords, and for the removal of the ban on the free transport of cereals within the country. These two further measures, if put into effect, can only increase further the already serious danger of a shortage during the period immediately preceding the collection of the next harvest.

In these circumstances, I feel it to be my duty to warn Your Excellency in the most friendly spirit of the bearing of these measures on the attitude likely to be adopted by the Allied supply authorities towards

> an eventual demand for a quota of imported cereals for Iran. The liberation of Europe is proceeding apace, and the liberated populations are everywhere in dire need of food supplies. Their need is the result of the German despoliation, and not of improvident economic legislation by their own authorities. It will be the clear and bounden duty of the Allied Governments to give priority to the alleviation of this unmerited distress. Vast quantities of cereals will be needed for that purpose, and Allied shipping will also be required on an unprecedented scale. I can hold out no hope—still less furnish a guarantee—that in these difficult circumstances of post-war rehabilitation the Allied Governments will feel able to deflect supplies to countries such as Iran, where the natural cereal resources are adequate and any shortage may therefore be attributed to the improvidence of the legislative or executive authorities concerned. I avail myself of this opportunity to renew to Your Excellency the assurance of my highest consideration. (Sgd.) D.W. Lascelles.

It turned out that these offensive notes were unnecessary, and with improving conditions due to the approaching end of the war, grain imports were not needed. Ebling on October 17, 1944 (Dispatch 111, 891.00/10-1744):

> During the past seven months Mr. Thomas B. Allen, representing the Administration of Cereal and Bread Section, Ministry of Finance, has been actively engaged in the collection of grains in Azerbaijan. The statement in Dr. Millspaugh's letter of October 6, 1944, to the Prime Minister that "The Government possesses the largest supply of grains in the history of Iran" illustrates the success which has been achieved in the collection of grains in Azerbaijan. It is anticipated that the final figures of the 1944 crops will show total collections of 80,000 tons, permitting the export to Tehran of about 26,000 tons. . . . Contrary to the early days of grain collection in Azerbaijan, the landed proprietors now find it advantageous to dispose of their grain on Government contract owing to the lower price of grain in the free market. . . . The operations of the Edarei Barbari (Transport Office) in Azerbaijan is another feature of the American adviser program. The transport office is actively engaged in the hauling of wheat and cereals to distributing centers, as well as controlling the transport of all products throughout the area. As previously reported, the United Kingdom Commercial Corporation has ceased operations in this district. The Iransovtrans continues its activities. . . . Local residents who have witnessed the formidable amount of war supplies transported overland via Tabriz to

> the USSR often express apprehension that with the close of hostilities, the famous war-time highways will again fall into disrepair thus restoring the former isolation of Azerbaijan with the rest of Iran. . . . The American adviser program since its inauguration in January, 1943, has met much opposition in Azerbaijan. . . . The recent decline in the prices of many staple products, such as wheat, sugar, and firewood has afforded an opportunity for the American adviser program to win friends. Since the lower price levels, many favorable comments have been registered in support of the American advisers. The merchants and traders have been on the alert to counteract any such development by circulating rumors that lower prices are due to the approaching end of the war. Nevertheless there is a growing sympathy among the people for Dr. Millspaugh's efforts and an increasing hatred toward the merchants who have been accumulating profits during the past five years due to the international situation.

Conditions had continued to improve. Morris on November 7, 1944, on "Changes in Iranian Grain Situation" (Dispatch 95 and enclosure, 891.6131/11-744):

> I have the honor to enclose herewith a copy of a memorandum prepared by Dr. Albert G. Black, chief administrator of the Cereals and Bread Section of the Iranian Ministry of Finance, in which he outlines recent favorable changes in the Iranian grain supply situation. It will be noted that Dr. Black believes all requirements for the current harvest year (ending September 1, 1945) can be met from domestic sources and that a safe reserve stock will be carried over into the following year. This memorandum was prepared just before the recent Irano-Soviet crisis brought on by refusal of the Iranian Government to act on a Soviet request for an oil concession in northern Iran. Coincidental with the development of that dispute, the Soviet authorities suspended the transport of grain by railroad from northern Iran to Tehran, a suspension which remained in force from October 16 to November 4. Had such movement been permanently cut off, the situation described by Dr. Black would have been very much less hopeful, although he believes that the Government would have been able to scrape through the year, feeding the southern areas of the country out of their own production and the fairly substantial stocks in hand from the preceding harvest year. As it is, assuming that reasonable quantities of grain will be brought down from the northern provinces to feed the southern cities, the general picture appears to be more favorable than it has been at any previous time in the past three years. Dr. Black drew up

his memorandum following an inquiry by the Embassy regarding certain regulations issued by Dr. A.C. Millspaugh, Administrator General of Finances, which increased the exemptions of landlords from obligations to deliver surplus grain to the Government. The Department will recall that, as reported in my despatch No. 18 of September 7, 1944, Dr. Millspaugh had been disturbed by the pressure brought upon him to relax restrictions on the sale and transport of grain and had appealed to the American and British Embassies for support. Consequently, the British Chargé d'Affaires and I addressed similar notes to the Prime Minister to warn him against measures which might reduce the quantity of grain brought under Iranian Government control. (I have never received a reply to that note.)

The Department will observe that Dr. Black now feels that relaxation of the restrictions, which has already been done, will not have a harmful effect, and I assume his opinion is as authoritative as any we can get. Certainly, I am entirely in accord with any steps that can safely be taken to reduce the innumerable controls burdening the Iranian economy and complicating the task of American advisers. I would like to point out, however, that this is one of the many instances in which Dr. Millspaugh has been greatly alarmed by some projected move of the Iranian Government, has appealed to this Embassy for help, and has later reversed his position, usually without notice to the Embassy. Both he and Dr. Black were definitely opposed to changes in the grain regulations when they raised the question with us in late August, yet in a few weeks they had made nearly all the suggested changes and left the Embassy to discover it by reading the new regulations after they were issued.

Black's informative memorandum follows:

Some important changes have lately been made in the Cereals and Bread Regulations. Briefly their effect is to a) give somewhat higher exemptions to the smaller landlords; b) exempt the peasants completely, and c) remove all restrictions on transport of grain. Considerable political pressure had been exerted during the last 18 months to get these very changes. The new regulations have been agreed to, however, not as a compromise or as a matter of political expediency, but because certain recent trends have so altered the situation that it has become possible to relax control without jeopardizing our essential objectives. These objectives are: a) To ensure regular supply of bread at a reasonable price in adequate amounts throughout the country; b) To maintain sufficient reserve stocks against a future failure of crops; c) To foster confidence and a sense of security in the public mind.

During the last two years it was not possible to attain these objectives without collection of the total surplus crop and the issue in towns of their full daily requirements. Now however, in view of a) the disappearing tendency to hoarding due to favorable war news, b) the recent consistent and in some cases substantial drop in the prices of grain, the removal of restrictions is expected to be a help rather than a hindrance. The grain not sold to Government is expected to move directly from the villages to the bakers or the consuming households, and to that extent Government will be relieved of collection and distribution work, and will thus avoid a waste of administrative effort and connected transport and overhead expenses. It is important from now on not to give exclusive importance to figures of total collections, as in the previous two years. We should concern ourselves instead with seeing that: a) the price of free bread is kept down by competing issues from our own stocks at controlled prices, and b) that our stock situation is maintained so that we carry over into the next harvest year at least as big and if possible a bigger reserve than last year.

Looking at this overall picture it can be stated that, although collections, due to the smaller harvest, the higher exemptions of the regulations, and relaxation on transport restrictions, etc., may be smaller than last year's, the grain left in private hands will not be hoarded, but will steadily come onto the market and will reduce our commitments. Thus the average all-Iran issues of grain which during the last harvest year were 25,000 tons per month, have recently been running at less than 20,000 tons per month. If present trends continue, our stocks at the end of the harvest year should approximate 150,000 tons. There are, however, two important considerations which may affect this matter. Firstly, if prospects for the 1324 (1945/46) harvest look bad due to inadequate precipitation this winter, a tendency to hoarding on a small scale may develop in 2 or 3 months from now, with resulting increased demands for Government bread. Secondly, if any large amount of Iranian labor now employed by the Allies is discharged, much of it might come to towns and stay there until next harvesting season, and become our responsibility in the meantime for its bread supply. Considering all factors it seems therefore reasonable to conclude that we can this year meet all our requirements and carryover stocks, at least as big and probably bigger than our carry-over of last year. The real problem now, in fact, is not that of collecting enough grain to meet requirements, but one of proper distribution and in particular that of transportation from Azerbaijan and adequate and proper storage to prevent losses from wastage and infestation. (signed) A.G. Black, Chief Administrator, Cereals & Bread Section

Chapter 29

A Malthusian Catastrophe: The Toll from Famine and Disease

An analysis of population statistics indicates that 3-4 million Iranians died of famine and disease during World War II. Iran's 1920 population was reported at 10 million and that of 1940 was reported at 15 million in the American diplomatic archives, an indication that it had grown by 2% per annum during 1920-40. Continuing to grow at the same rate, Iran's population in 1944 should have been 16 million. The population in 1944 when the famine had ended is reported at 12 million by Millspaugh in his correspondence with the Middle East Supply Center concerning Iran's import quotas, while the population figure used by the Middle East Supply Center to set Iran's import quotas was 10 million. Assuming that Iran's population at the end of the famine in 1944 was 12 million, it follows that 4 million had died of starvation and disease.

Subsequent census figures also confirm that at least 3 million Iranians died in World War II. Iran's first nation-wide population census was taken in 1956, and the population was stated at 18.95 million. In the second population census taken in 1966, the population was reported to be 25.79 million, an indication that it grew at 3.07% during the 1956-66 decade.[1] Using this growth rate and extrapolating backward, the 1945 population is found to be 13.5 million. Based on the 1940 figure and a growth rate of 2%, it should have been 16.5 million, an indication that *at least* 3 million had perished during the war. The post-war years experienced rapid population growth worldwide (baby boom years), and the growth rate declined as the war years receded. Consequently, it is more than likely that the actual population growth during 1945-55 exceeded the growth rate of 3.07% used in the latter computation and that Iran's 1945 population was *at most* 13.5 million. These results enable one to state with confidence that 3-4 million Iranians, 20-25% of the 1940 population, perished to starvation and disease during the Allied occupation of the country in World War II.

Given that 8-10 million Iranians had also died of famine and disease in World War I, one concludes that 12-14 million Iranians died in the two world wars.[2] Moreover, given that the population of Iran in 1944 (12 million) was the same as 1900, it is clear that nearly half a century of population growth had been wiped out by the famines of World War I and World War II, a very effective means of "population control," and a perfect case of Malthusian Catastrophe. With the memory of the 1917-19 famine fresh in the mind of the people, the onset of the famine in 1942 had terrified Iran, prompting unrest and rioting.

There are several obvious reasons why the toll in World War II was so much lower than in World War I. First and foremost, while Iran was a battlefield between belligerent armies resulting in heavy carnage and destruction in World War I, in contrast, Iran in World War II was not a scene of hostilities between opposing armies. While British military operations on Iranian soil had continued until 1919, foreign military operations in World War II had ceased on August 28, 1941. Another apparent reason was Allied assistance with grain collection and transport given in the fall of 1943 which had prevented the extension of the famine into a third year, as it had happened in World War I. Finally, the other obvious reason for lower casualties was the fact that Iran's pre-World War II population (15 million) was less than that of pre-World War I (18-20 million).

Until now, little was known about the Iran famine of 1942-43, and even less has been written. As noted in chapter 1, a highly praised book on the strategic role of food in World War II published nearly 70 years after World War II contained nothing on Iran, and there is reason to believe that the omission was deliberate.[3] The absence of coverage and the failure to discuss Iran's World War II famine has also been observed in the case of the 1917-1919 famine. In fact, the reaction of the academic establishment to the 2003 study of the Great Famine of 1917-1919 and the findings contained therein is most revealing, and, as the same can be expected with the present study, I take this opportunity to give a brief outline. After the initial shock and disbelief, as expected, attempts were made to discredit the work and its author. In the absence of documentary evidence to the contrary and the inability to fault the analytical reasoning used to arrive at the casualty figures, the attempts to discredit the study were notable failures and in fact tended to strengthen the findings. Willem Floor's review of the book provides an example of the attempt to disparage the work.[4] In contrast, the book struck a sympathetic and familiar chord with some Irish historians who noted the parallels between the Irish and Persian famines.[5] After the book's translation into Persian, several Iranian historians also tried to throw doubt on the findings.[6] Lacking solid documentary support, they also failed in their objective. With the publication of the second edition of the work in 2013 containing additional documentation and demographic data, it appears that attempts to discredit the work have ceased for the present, but instead some have tried to misrepresent its contents. In a 2014 study of World War I in the Middle East, Ulrichsen claims that in my 2003 book on the Great Famine it was stated that (only) one-quarter of the population of *northern* Iran was lost to famine and disease, thus implying there was no famine in southern Iran.[7] Nowhere did I make such a statement. It was shown that at least 40% of the population of Iran was lost to famine and disease.

Apart from refraining to review the study, the mainstream scholarly journals in the field of Middle East studies have declined to consider, let alone publish, an article on the Great Famine and demographic developments in early 20th century Iran.[8] Not surprisingly, in the 2014 special World War I edition of the same journal commemorating the centennial of the outbreak of the war, there is nothing on Iran nor the Great Famine.[9] From the absence of any articles on Iran in this volume the impression is conveyed that Iran was not touched by World War I and apparently was not even part of the Middle East. The continued silence on the Great Famine is amply illustrated by a 2014 book on the human toll and suffering in the Middle East in World War I.[10] In describing the military campaigns conducted on Iranian soil by the various belligerents, the book draws heavily on a work of mine.[11] But oddly, it does not even mention the Iran famine of 1917-1919, one of the greatest calamities of the Great War. Professor Fawaz's omission is the more remarkable because the Iran famine was covered in her course at the Fletcher School of Law and Diplomacy, Tufts University, with extensive assigned readings from the original 2003 edition of the book, *The Great Famine and Genocide in Persia, 1917-1919.*[12] Meanwhile, other scholars are also beginning to draw attention to some of the glaring omissions in the historiography of modern Iran.[13]

Notes

1. Iran Statistical Center. *Yearbook of Statistics, 1360 (1981/82)*. Tehran: Plan and Budget Organization, 1361 (1982/83, in Persian). 69.

2. Majd, Mohammad Gholi. *The Great Famine & Genocide in Iran: 1917-1919, 2nd Edition*. Lanham, MD: University Press of America, 2013.

3. Collingham, Lizzie. *The Taste of War: World War II and the Battle for Food*. New York: The Penguin Press, 2012.

4. Floor, Willem. "Review of The Great Famine and Genocide in Persia, 1917-1919." *Iranian Studies*, Volume 38, No. 1, March 2005, 192-196. Without providing any documentary support, Floor calls the book "sensational" and "wrong." The review is also notable for its sarcasm.

5. Walsh, Patrick. "Who Remembers the Persians . . . ?" *Irish Foreign Affairs*, Volume 3, No. 3, August 2010. 4-7.

6. Malekzadeh, Elham. "Review of The Great Famine." *Goftogoo: A Cultural and Social Quarterly*, No. 65, October 2014.143-148. For the record, my reply to the review was not even acknowledged let alone published. Similar to Malekzadeh, another historian, Majid Tafreshi, has repeatedly claimed that my results were "exaggerated." However, they do not provide any solid facts or figures to back up their claim.

7. Ulrichsen, Kristian C. *The First World War in the Middle East*. London: Hurst, 2014. 179.

8. For instance, the *International Journal of Middle East Studies* (IJMES) declined to even consider a submitted article on the WWI Iran famine. The editor, Judith E. Tucker, an expert on women and gender studies in 19th century Egypt, determined that the article was "insufficiently analytical" to be considered by IJMES. The *Middle East Journal* (MEJ) declined to consider the article on the grounds that MEJ deals only with post 1945, despite the fact the previous issue of MEJ contained an article with extensive discussion of British policy in Iraq after World War I.

9. *International Journal of Middle East Studies*, Volume 46, Special Issue No. 4 (World War I), November 2014. Guest Editor, Mustafa Aksakal; Editor, Beth Baron.

10. Fawaz, Leila Tarazi. *A Land of Aching Hearts: The Middle East in the Great War*. Cambridge, MA: Harvard University Press, 2014.

11. Majd, Mohammad Gholi. *Persia in World War I and Its Conquest by Great Britain*. Lanham: University Press of America, 2003.

12. The course was "War & Society in Historical Perspective," DHP H 261/Hist 234, Fall 2010. In a note of October 21, 2010, Professor Fawaz called the book a "valuable study."

13. Jackson, Ashley. "The Empire's War in History." *The Round Table: The Commonwealth Journal of International Affairs*, Vol. 103, No. 2, 2014, 141-144.

Index

About the Author

Mohammad Gholi Majd is the author of *The Great Famine & Genocide in Iran: 1917-1919*, 2nd Edition. University Press of America, 2013, and several other works on twentieth century Iranian history. He holds a PhD in Agricultural Economics from Cornell University.